Cancer
Survivorship

Cancer Survivorship

Today and Tomorrow

Patricia A. Ganz, M.D.
Editor

American Cancer Society Clinical Research Professor
Division of Cancer Prevention and Control Research
Jonsson Comprehensive Cancer Center
UCLA Schools of Public Health and Medicine
Los Angeles, California, USA

Foreword by Sandra J. Horning, M.D.

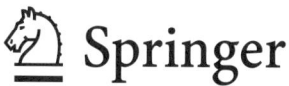 Springer

Patricia A. Ganz, M.D.
American Cancer Society Research Professor
Division of Cancer Prevention and Control Research
Jonsson Comprehensive Cancer Center
UCLA Schools of Public Health and Medicine
Los Angeles, CA 90095-6900
USA

Library of Congress Control Number: 2006925526

ISBN-10: 0-387-34349-0   e-ISBN-10: 0-387-68265-1
ISBN-13: 978-0-387-34349-5   e-ISBN-13: 978-0-387-68265-5

Printed on acid-free paper.

9 8 7 6 5 4 3 2 1

springer.com

*I would like to dedicate this book to the founding members of
the National Coalition for Cancer Survivorship (NCCS),
as well as to the many cancer patients and survivors who have taught us so much.
We have learned a lot about cancer survivorship, but there is much more to discover.*

Foreword

Cancer survivors have increased in number more than threefold over the last 30 years to the current level of 10 million and growing. Among patients diagnosed today, nearly two-thirds are expected to survive 5 or more years. This success may be attributed to the expertise of physicians and nurses from multiple disciplines, who precisely execute a complex plan based in clinical research. Yet, after a period of orchestrated and frequent interaction with healthcare professionals, bolstered by the attention and encouragement of family and friends, the cancer patient may view the end of treatment with anxiety and concern. And, what exactly is the plan? Just as healthcare providers are expected to keep up-to-date with the latest in treatment and prevention, they must now coordinate and provide comprehensive survivor care. This significant text, organized and edited by Patricia A. Ganz and involving the contributions of over 40 distinguished authors, provides a greatly needed resource for survivor care—today and tomorrow.

The current attention on cancer survivorship represents a confluence of burgeoning survivor numbers, a corpus of data on late treatment effects in children and adults, and increased public and professional awareness. Dr. Ganz and many of the contributors to this comprehensive text pioneered cancer survivorship, and they must justifiably be proud that their advocacy and commitment to survivor care and research have resulted in in-depth reports by the President's Cancer Panel, several Institute of Medicine studies, and this timely text. *Cancer Survivorship: Today and Tomorrow* is a natural evolution of these efforts, inclusive of the major areas of survivor care: surveillance for recurrence and second cancers, management of late effects, coordination of ongoing health maintenance and prevention, and the important psychosocial elements integral to the healing process after cancer treatment. Care of an entire generation of cancer survivors is needed and will be facilitated by the organization of this volume according to specific diseases, patient groups, and crosscutting topics. Yet, as valuable and current as this text is, it makes patently clear that survivorship is ever changing as diagnosis and treatment evolve, and that much more research is needed to predict and preempt undesirable late effects.

As a survivor, I appreciate the fog of a new cancer diagnosis, when the world is upended and the future uncertain. It is at this time that cancer patients need expert guidance for a personalized approach to the least-complicated as well as the most-effective therapy. The inclusion of survivorship issues in training curricula and ongoing education of healthcare professionals, consideration of age and comorbidity in treatment planning, and prospective assembly of a multidisciplinary team to deliver both cancer and survivor care are necessary to accomplish this goal. As an oncologist and a cancer survivor, I recognize the need to coordinate care for the generations at risk for second cancers and other late complications and to make their health and social outcomes the subject of ongoing scientific inquiry.

The current era of molecular medicine brings hope that effective cancer treatments will be accompanied by fewer complications and greater success. It also presents the opportunity to incorporate survivorship research from the onset in clinical investigation, as we are now better able to understand the molecular basis of treatment complications as well as efficacy. All of these tools need to be brought to bear for the current generation of cancer survivors. This comprehensive volume brings us up-to-date with cancer survivorship for the moment and sets the stage for future developments. Congratulations go to the editor and the 42 contributing colleagues for this valued text.

Sandra J. Horning, M.D.
Professor of Medicine
Department of Medicine/Oncology
Stanford University Medical Center
Stanford, California, USA

Preface

It was almost 30 years ago that I began my training in hematology/oncology. I had a special interest in the emerging field of medical oncology. While hematology had a long and distinguished history as a subspecialty focus in medicine, oncology care had been primarily the domain of surgeons and radiotherapists, with a limited role for internists. Having spent my undergraduate years working in various cardiology research laboratories, my sudden interest in cancer medicine must have surprised those around me. Myocardial infarction was a common killer of men in their early fifties, and it was not unusual to have patients admitted to the hospital with irreversible brain damage after a full cardiac arrest in the field. I was discouraged that my patients with advanced cardiovascular disease had little therapy that could control their pain and symptoms, and that it was difficult to talk with them openly about the seriousness of their diagnosis and prognosis. Little did I know that major developments in understanding the mechanisms of atherosclerosis, along with important advances in preventive treatments, would lead to the dramatic decline in cardiovascular disease we see today.

In contrast, the patients whom I met on the oncology ward seemed more able to confront their diagnoses and to discuss the options for treatment that occasionally held the possibility of cure, sometimes disease control, and, at the minimum, palliation. Only about 35% of patients could expect to live for 5 years or more, but there was enormous excitement about new drug discoveries, the development of combination chemotherapy, and the emerging cures in patients with Hodgkin's disease and childhood leukemia. Somehow, I thought that in my lifetime cancer would have a greater prospect for cure than cardiovascular disease. Well, I guess I might have made the wrong bet, not appreciating the complexity of the enemy called *cancer*, which represents more than 100 specific diseases with different etiologies and risk factors. Nevertheless, we have made great progress in the prevention, detection, and treatment of cancer during these past 3 decades. With these advances, we have seen the expansion of the number of cancer survivors and the recognition of the unique medical and psychosocial needs of this patient population.

During the past few years, there has been an increasing focus on the needs of the cancer-survivor population, with three Institute of Medicine reports providing detailed reviews of topics relevant to childhood and adult cancer survivors, as well as to the psychosocial needs of breast cancer survivors. Other recent reports by the President's Cancer Panel and the Centers for Disease Control and Prevention highlight the plight of cancer survivors and how their needs are not being adequately met by the current healthcare system. Thus, a major goal of this volume is to provide a concise and focused resource for healthcare professionals. We describe the current state of knowledge regarding the medical and psychosocial issues related to cancer survivorship, which range from general (e.g., surveillance after primary therapy) to disease specific (e.g., testicular, gynecological, prostate, breast, colorectal cancers). We also focus on topics that range from the late effects of cancer treatments to insurance, employment, and job discrimination. As the title of this book implies, this is the state of our knowledge today, as well as our hope for greater knowledge tomorrow, as further systematic research is conducted on the health outcomes of long-term cancer survivors.

Producing this volume has provided an opportunity for me to call upon many long-term friends and colleagues in the survivorship community, including Susan Leigh, who I first met in 1986 at the founding of the National Coalition for Cancer Survivorship (NCCS), and Pat Fobair, an early pioneer in the survivorship movement as the social worker in the radiation oncology department at Stanford University Medical Center. Barbara Hoffman, a young lawyer, who took up legal advocacy for cancer survivors, was another NCCS founder. I also met Ellen Stovall in the early 1990s when she took over the helm of the NCCS, which she is now leading into its twenty-first year. Others, such as Julia Rowland and Becky Silliman, have been my research colleagues in recent years, while the remaining authors are all individuals with whom I have worked or collaborated with in various ways. This volume comes from the shared experience of having seen cancer-survivorship research and care emerge as a legitimate focus in medicine today.

I would like to thank several people for their role in making this work possible: to my parents for their constant support of me throughout my childhood and as my professional career developed; to my husband and best friend, Tom, who, in spite of being a physician and laboratory scientist, seems to understand what I have been doing all of these years; and to my children, David and Rebecca, for their patience in listening to me talk about the challenges I faced in my work, as I tried to measure quality of life in cancer patients and gain acceptance for something that nobody seemed to appreciate at the time. Finally, I want to extend my thanks to Paula Callaghan, my editor at Springer, who recognized the importance of cancer survivorship as a twenty-first-century issue and made production of this volume a reality.

Patricia A. Ganz, M.D.

Contents

Contributors

Noreen M. Aziz, M.D., Ph.D., M.P.H.
Senior Program Director, Office of Cancer Survivorship, Division of Cancer Control and Population Science, National Cancer Institute, Rockville, Maryland, USA

Karen Basen-Engquist, Ph.D., M.P.H.
Associate Professor, Department of Behavioral Science, The University of Texas at M.D. Anderson Cancer Center, Houston, Texas, USA

Smita Bhatia, M.D., M.P.H.
Director, Epidemiology and Outcomes Research, Department of Pediatric Oncology, City of Hope Cancer Center, Duarte, California, USA

Diane C. Bodurka, M.D.
Associate Professor, Department of Gynecological Oncology, The University of Texas at M.D. Anderson Cancer Center, Houston, Texas, USA

Michael Boeckh, M.D.
Assistant Member, Program in Infectious Diseases, Fred Hutchinson Cancer Research Center; and Assistant Professor of Medicine, University of Washington School of Medicine, Seattle, Washington, USA

Louise J. Bordeleau, M.D., F.R.C.P.(C.), M.Sc.
Attending, Department of Medical Oncology, Mount Sinai Hospital, Toronto, Ontario, Canada

Jacqueline Casillas, M.D., M.S.H.S.
Assistant Professor, Department of Pediatrics, Division of Hematology/Oncology, David Geffen School of Medicine at UCLA, Los Angeles, California, USA

Anne Coscarelli, Ph.D.
Research Psychologist, Department of Public Health; and Director, Ted Mann Family Resource Center, University of California–David Geffen School of Medicine, Los Angeles, California, USA

Alvin A. Dahl, M.D., Ph.D.
Professor, Department of Clinical Cancer Research, National Hospital–Radium Hospital, Oslo, Norway

Suzanne C. Danhauer, Ph.D.
Assistant Professor and Associate Director, Psychosocial Oncology and Cancer Patient Support Programs, Department of Internal Medicine, Wake Forest University Baptist Medical Center, Winston-Salem, North Carolina, USA

Joachim Deeg, M.D.
Member, Clinical Research Division, Fred Hutchinson Cancer Research Center; and Professor of Medicine, University of Washington School of Medicine, Seattle, Washington, USA

Craig C. Earle, M.D., M.Sc., F.R.C.P.C.
Associate Professor of Medicine, Department of Medical Oncology, Dana–Farber Cancer Institute, Harvard Medical School, Boston, Massachusetts, USA

Patricia Fobair, L.C.S.W.
Clinical Social Worker and Group Therapist, Supportive Program, Cancer Center, Stanford University Hospital, Stanford, California, USA

Sophie D. Fosså, Ph.D.
Professor, Department of Long-Term Studies, National Hospital–Radium Hospital, University of Oslo, Oslo, Norway

Patricia A. Ganz, M.D.
Director, Division of Cancer Prevention and Control Research, Jonsson Comprehensive Cancer Center at UCLA; and Professor, Schools of Public Health and Medicine, University of California, Los Angeles, California, USA

Pamela J. Goodwin, M.D., M.Sc., F.B.P.C.
Professor, Department of Medicine, University of Toronto; and Senior Scientist, Samuel Lunenfeld Research Institute, Mount Sinai Hospital, Toronto, Ontario, Canada

Frederic W. Grannis, Jr., M.D.
Assistant Professor, Department of Thoracic Surgery, City of Hope National Medical Center, Duarte, California, USA

Barbara Hoffman, J.D.
Founding Chair, National Coalition for Cancer Survivorship, Rutgers University School of Law, Newark, New Jersey, USA

Stein Kaasa, M.D., Ph.D.
Professor, Department of Cancer Research and Molecular Medicine, Faculty of Medicine, The Norwegian University of Science and Technology and the Palliative Care Unit, St. Olavs Hospital, Trondheim, Norway

Clifford Y. Ko, M.D.
Associate Professor, Department of Surgery, UCLA School of Medicine–West Los Angeles VA Medical Center, Los Angeles, California, USA

Tracey L. Krupski, M.D.
Assistant Professor, Department of Urology, Dale University Medical School, Durham, North Carolina, USA

Wendy Landier, R.N., M.S.N., C.P.N.P.
Pediatric Nurse Practitioner, Division of Pediatrics, City of Hope Comprehensive Cancer Center, Duarte, California, USA

Susan Leigh, B.S.N., R.N.
Cancer Survivorship Consultant, Tucson, Arizona, USA

Julie Lemieux, M.D.
Attending, Department of Medicine, Mount Sinai Hospital, Toronto, Ontario, Canada

Mark S. Litwin, M.D., M.P.H.
Professor, Department of Urology and Health Services, David Geffen School of Medicine, School of Public Health, Jonsson Comprehensive Cancer Center, University of California, Los Angeles, California, USA

Jon Håvard Loge, M.D., Ph.D.
Professor, Department of Behavioral Sciences in Medicine, University of Oslo and the Centre for Palliative Medicine, Ulleval University Hospital, Oslo, Norway

Karim S. Malek, M.D.
Assistant Professor, Department of Medicine, Section of Hematology and Oncology, Boston University School of Medicine, Boston, Massachusetts, USA

Paul Martin, M.D.
Member, Clinical Research Division, Fred Hutchinson Cancer Research Center; and Professor, Department of Medicine, University of Washington School of Medicine, Seattle, Washington, USA

Matthew J. Matasar, M.D.
Instructor, Department of Medicine, Columbia University Medical Center, New York, New York, USA

Richard P. McQuellon, Ph.D.
Associate Professor and Director, Psychosocial Oncology and Cancer Patient Support Programs, Wake Forest University Health Sciences, Winston-Salem, North Carolina, USA

Alfred I. Neugut, M.D., Ph.D.
Professor, Department of Epidemiology, Mailman School of Public Health; and Department of Medicine, Herbert Irving Comprehensive Cancer Center, College of Physicians and Surgeons, Columbia University Medical Center, New York, New York, USA

Julia H. Rowland, Ph.D.
Director, Office of Cancer Survivorship, Division of Cancer Control and Population Science, National Cancer Institute, Bethesda, Maryland, USA

Linda Sarna, R.N., D.N.Sc., F.A.A.N.
Professor, School of Nursing, University of California, Los Angeles, Los Angeles, California, USA

Leslie R. Schover, Ph.D.
Professor, Department of Behavioral Science, University of Texas, M.D. Anderson Cancer Center, Houston, Texas, USA

Deborah Schrag, M.D.
Memorial Sloan-Kettering Cancer Center, New York, New York, USA

Rebecca A. Silliman, M.D., Ph.D.
Professor, Department of Medicine and Public Health; and Chief, Section of Geriatrics, Boston University School of Medicine, Boston Medical Center, Boston, Massachusetts, USA

Ellen L. Stovall
President and CEO, National Coalition for Cancer Survivorship, Silver Spring, Maryland, USA

Karen L. Syrjala, Ph.D.
Associate Member, Clinical Research Division, Fred Hutchinson Cancer Research Center, Associate Professor of Psychiatry and Behavioral Sciences, University of Washington School of Medicine, Seattle, Washington, USA

L.B. Travis
Senior Investigator, National Institutes of Health, Department of Health and Human Services, Division of Cancer Epidemiology and Genetics, National Cancer Institute, Bethesda, Maryland, USA

Steven H. Woolf, M.D., M.P.H.
Departments of Family Medicine, Epidemiology, and Community Health, Virginia Commonwealth University, Richmond, Virginia, USA

Lydia B. Zablotska, M.D., Ph.D.
Assistant Professor, Department of Epidemiology, Mailman School of Public Health, Columbia University, New York, New York, USA

Lonnie Zeltzer, M.D.
Professor, Departments of Pediatrics, Anesthesiology, Psychiatry and Biobehavioral Sciences; Director, Pediatric Pain Program, David Geffen School of Medicine at UCLA; Associate Director, Patients and Survivors Program, Division of Cancer Prevention and Control Research; and UCLA Jonsson Comprehensive Cancer Center, Los Angeles, California, USA

1

Cancer Survivors:
A Physician's Perspective

Patricia A. Ganz

During the past three decades since the declaration of a war on cancer with the National Cancer Act of 1971, we have been exposed to a very public display of both the challenges and triumphs in this war. As a young medical oncologist, I anxiously awaited each annual meeting of the American Society of Clinical Oncology (ASCO), expecting to hear the latest small advances in the treatment of leukemia, lymphoma, Hodgkin's disease, and then breast cancer (the first solid tumor that seemed to respond to multiagent chemotherapy), gradually seeing plateaus in the survival curves suggesting cure. With the phase II trials of cisplatinum, there were rumors of young men with advanced testicular cancer rising from their deathbeds after a single course of treatment. Soon thereafter, the Einhorn regimen[1] of vinblastine, bleomycin and cisplatin, brought about high cure rates in this rare but devastating cancer of young men. And of course, three decades later we all know the story of Lance Armstrong, one of the world's most famous testicular cancer survivors. However, as the breast cancer activists reminded us in the early 1990s, there were still more American women dying each year from breast cancer than U.S. deaths during the entire Vietnam War.[2]* Fortunately, in 2006, with new targeted therapies, we may now be modifying the course of disease for many other solid tumors.

So without revealing my specific age, I have told you about how I have personally observed advances that have led to the growth in the absolute numbers and relative proportion of cancer survivors, who now in the U.S. are more than 10 million strong and growing.[3] In the past two decades, the 5-year survival rate for the top 15 cancers (as identified in SEER data from 1975 to 1979 and then from 1995 to 2000) has increased from 42.7% for men and 56.6% for women, to 64% for men and to 64.3% for women.[4] Figures 1.1 to 1.4 provide the most recent statistics available on cancer survivors from the National Cancer Institute (NCI) Office of Cancer Survivorship (OCS),[5] and set the stage for why this book has been written, and the rationale for the specific chapters that are included. In this volume we focus on disease sites or patient groups who have most benefited from treatments during the past three decades.

However, the purpose of this chapter is to provide a physician's perspective on issues related to cancer survivorship, and the chapters that immediately follow present the perspectives of my colleagues in nursing and social work. In this way, we hope to make this topic relevant to various health care providers involved in the ongoing and follow-up care of cancer survivors.

In this chapter, I will discuss the following:

- the role of the physician in the care of the cancer survivor;
- strategies to address the positive and negative consequences of cancer treatments;
- how to help patients and families heal;
- managing long-term relationships and caring for multiple generations; and
- addressing the critical role of prevention among survivors.

The reader must understand that this reflects only one physician's perspective and that the content is strongly influenced by the author's most recent clinical work and research focused on breast cancer patients and survivors. However, it is clear that these observations can be generalized to other cancer sites and settings.

How Did We Get Here and What Is the Role of the Physician?

In parallel with the expansion of research associated with the National Cancer Act of 1971, there was an enormous investment of federal funds in cancer centers and training programs, fostering the expanded development of a large number of specialists to diagnose, treat, and rehabilitate cancer patients. We now have mature oncology subspecialty training programs in general surgery, thoracic oncology, urologic oncology, gynecological oncology, otolaryngology and so forth, in addition to pediatrics, internal medicine, and radiology. Subsequently, there was growing interest in early detection, screening and prevention, which were also fostered through central programs at the NCI as well as funding of the extramural research program. The NCI Cooperative Group Program, first established in the 1950s to evaluate new anticancer agents from NCI's drug development program, gradually shifted to studies of combined modality therapy approaches in cancer treatment characterized by the large phase III clinical trials that are in place today, many of which are supported by the pharmaceutical industry.

The NCI designated cancer centers and their affiliated hospitals are the setting in which most clinical oncologists

---

*Forty-four thousand women were dying each year from breast cancer. While subsequent estimates of death in Vietnam were 759,000, breast cancer activists often used this for a point (Patricia A. Ganz, personal recollection).

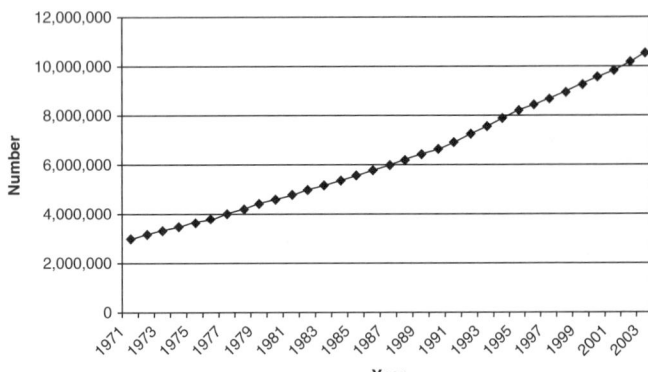

FIGURE 1.1. Estimated number of cancer survivors in the United States from 1971 to 2003. U.S. estimated prevalence counts were estimated by applying U.S. populations to SEER 9 and to historical Connecticut Limited Duration Prevalence proportions, and adjusted to represent complete prevalence. Populations from January 2003 were based on the average of the July 2002 and July 2003 population estimates from the U.S. Bureau of Census. (*Source*: 2005 submission.)

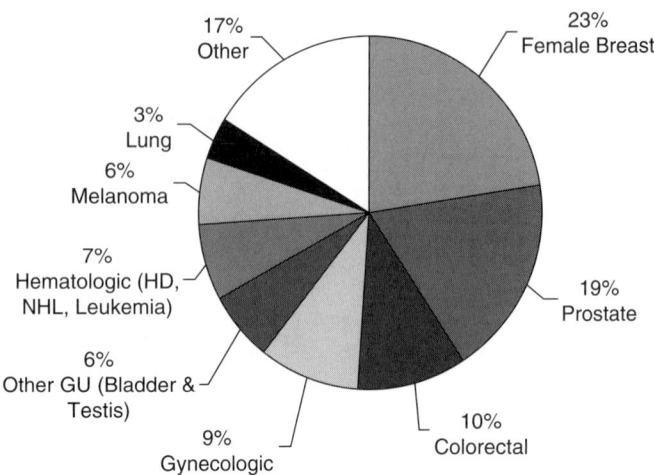

FIGURE 1.3. Estimated number of persons alive in the United States diagnosed with cancer by site (*n* = 10.5 million survivors). U.S. estimated prevalence counts were estimated by applying U.S. populations to SEER 9 and to historical Connecticut Limited Duration Prevalence proportions, and adjusted to represent complete prevalence. Populations from January 2003 were based on the average of the July 2002 and July 2003 population estimates from the U.S. Bureau of Census. (*Source*: 2005 submission.)

in practice today have been trained. This is especially true for medical oncologists, but also includes specialists trained in surgery and radiation oncology. Most trainees were introduced to clinical research through participation in cooperative group trials, investigator initiated studies, and pharmaceutical industry studies. The systematic development of cancer treatments through clinical investigation has contributed to an extensive published literature which is often summarized in evidence based reviews or guidelines that can facilitate best practices and treatment decision making. Cancer care is viewed today as multidisciplinary, requiring the input of several clinicians, including nurses, social workers and others. The gains in survival described earlier reflect the systematic approach to treatment, which benefits from the advances in clinical research as well as the diffusion of well-trained oncology specialists into the community away from specialized NCI designated cancer centers.

Unfortunately, in spite of excellent training in the curative approach to cancer treatment, most oncology specialists have had little formal training in the follow-up care of cancer survivors. However, during the past 10 to 15 years, the number of articles on the late effects of cancer treatment has grown substantially, spearheaded first by those interested in childhood cancer survivors,[6–10] and more recently by those investigating adult cancer survivors.[11–19] A recent IOM report focused on the needs of childhood cancer survivors[20] with a parallel report on adult cancer survivors in 2005.[21] For children, the price of cure is detailed extensively in Chapter 7 in this volume. It is important to note that most children with cancer in the United States are treated in specialized centers and are enrolled in cooperative group trials. This has facilitated the linkage of specific treatments to untoward late effects (e.g., second malignancies, neuropsychological impair-

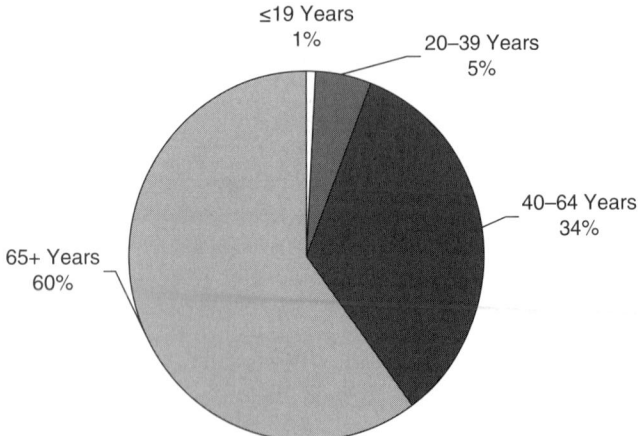

FIGURE 1.2. Estimated number of persons alive in the United States diagnosed with cancer by current age (invasive/first primary cases only, *n* = 10.5 million survivors). U.S. estimated prevalence counts were estimated by applying U.S. populations to SEER 9 and to historical Connecticut Limited Duration Prevalence proportions, and adjusted to represent complete prevalence. Populations from January 2003 were based on the average of the July 2002 and July 2003 population estimates from the U.S. Bureau of Census. (*Source*: 2005 submission.)

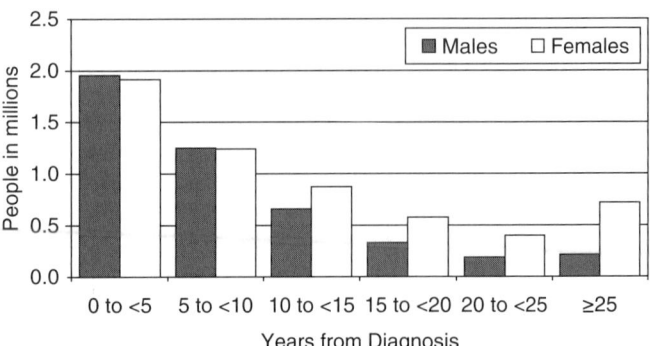

FIGURE 1.4. Estimated number of persons alive in the United States diagnosed with cancer on January 1, 2003, by time from diagnosis and gender (invasive/first primary cases only, *n* = 10.5 million survivors). U.S. estimated prevalence counts were estimated by applying U.S. populations to SEER 9 and to historical Connecticut Limited Duration Prevalence proportions, and adjusted to represent complete prevalence. Populations from January 2003 were based on the average of the July 2002 and July 2003 population estimates from the U.S. Bureau of Census. (*Source*: 2005 submission.)

ment, cardiac complications). These observations have influenced the conduct of subsequent clinical trials.

In adult oncology, where participation in clinical trials is more limited, there is less precision in understanding the incidence of late effects, whether serious or minimal. Nevertheless, there is a growing body of information, especially for survivors of breast cancer, prostate cancer, leukemia, lymphoma, Hodgkin's disease, and testes cancers, as described later in this volume. More important, as delineated in the IOM report on adult cancer survivors,[21] there is growing awareness of a distinct phase in the cancer trajectory where acute treatment is completed and the patient/survivor transitions into a period of less intensive medical follow-up that necessitates a new model for care. There is a need for coordinated care between cancer specialists and primary care physicians at this juncture, with a focus on paying attention to the short-term and late effects of cancer treatment, prevention of late sequelae (e.g., osteoporosis) and/or recurrence, surveillance for new cancers, and monitoring of adjuvant therapy (e.g., extended hormonal or maintenance treatments). In addition, someone must make sure that routine preventive health care (e.g., smoking cessation, obesity prevention, cardiovascular disease prevention) is addressed. To this end, the recent IOM report suggests that an *end-of-treatment summary and survivorship care plan* be completed, which is forward looking and anticipates these aspects of care.[21] Such a summary is currently lacking, but if used it can be the means of providing explicit communication of this information by the treating oncologist to the patient/survivor, as well as to the primary care physician and other health care professionals. It is expected that this process will influence better coordination of care during the posttreatment phase of cancer survivorship. In addition, such documentation in the medical record can be a source of information for evaluation of quality of care, as well as systematic evaluation of the linkage between treatment exposures and outcomes.

Currently, care during this phase of treatment is often shared in a nonexplicit way between oncology specialists and primary care physicians.[22,23] This leads to both under and overutilization of surveillance testing for cancer recurrence,[24,25] and lack of attention to prevention and rehabilitation services (see more detailed discussion in Chapter 5 in this volume). It is hoped that this proposed IOM recommendation will serve to better coordinate the care for survivors by defining the role(s) of each of these groups of physicians in the long-term follow-up of cancer survivors. In addition, there is likely an important potential role for other allied healthcare providers (nurse practitioners, physician assistants) in providing the ongoing care for cancer survivors within the oncology care setting. Oncology specialists and primary care physicians each have their role, and just as we recommend shared decision making in cancer treatment planning, there is also a critical role for shared care in the follow-up of cancer survivors. This proposed strategy is designed to facilitate a dialogue among all of these stakeholders so that the care and follow-up of the cancer survivors can be optimized.

Another group of medical specialists who have largely been left out of this dialogue are physical medicine and rehabilitation specialists. While rehabilitation medicine demonstration projects were a key component of the early years of the National Cancer Act,[26–28] in recent years there has been much less involvement of this group of physicians in cancer care. Possible exceptions to this have been in lymphedema management, neurological rehabilitation (e.g., brain tumor patients), postlaryngectomy patients, and for patients with stomas. However, an active and preventive role for rehabilitative medicine services across a wide variety of cancer sites needs to be considered early in the cancer treatment process, and is largely neglected in current practice.[29] The IOM adult cancer survivor report calls attention to this issue[21] and perhaps we will see more involvement of this physician community working with survivors in the future.

Facing the Positive and Negative Consequences of Therapy

Oncology physicians clearly appreciate seeing long-term survivors for return office visits, as this reminds them of the value of their efforts in managing the complexities of initial treatment. However, these physicians are often ill-equipped to identify and manage some of the lingering effects of cancer therapy. Furthermore, they may experience guilt as well as distress, at seeing patients they have treated develop serious health problems that are a result of cancer treatments (e.g., second malignancies, infertility, cognitive changes, congestive heart failure). The oncology specialist whose practice is focused on one particular cancer site (e.g., breast, prostate, lymphoma, or colorectal) can become quite expert in managing some of the common problems in these survivors. For example, most urologists are able to address the problems of erectile dysfunction and urinary incontinence in prostate cancer survivors, and they may have access to support groups for these patients and their partners. However, for the busy oncologist who sees patients with a wider variety of diagnoses and cares for only a limited number of survivors, these types of problems might be quite vexing. Oncologists might never ask questions about sexual functioning nor offer specific treatments. As a result, cancer survivors are often disappointed that no one is paying attention to the late effects they experience as a result of their cancer treatment, and that no one has a systematic approach to monitoring them after initial treatment.

How can we address this challenge? Among the best things we can do is to try to prepare our patients for the possibility of some common late effects of treatment from the outset. That means addressing the likelihood of infertility, early menopause, cardiac dysfunction, chronic side effects from treatment, and even second malignancies. This is sometimes challenging to do, given the rapidity with which cancer treatment decisions are made and the complexity of preventive interventions (e.g., sperm banking).[30,31] Nevertheless, survivors appreciate that they were at least told about the possibilities of these difficulties, even though we may not be able to predict who will develop specific side effects or long-term sequelae from treatment. (This is where more research is absolutely needed.) How much individual patients recall from these early discussions is unclear, but as part of informed consent for treatment, known risks for late effects should be disclosed.

Even though no formalized system of care exists for cancer survivors, it appears that a substantial number of oncologists are regularly caring for them. As part of a recent survey performed by ASCO's Cancer Prevention Committee,[32] a random sample of ASCO members (surgeons, medical oncologists, radiation oncologists) were asked three questions related to the care of cancer survivors. The survey respondents were asked "To what extent do you provide ongoing general medical care, including health maintenance, screening, and preventive services, to the cancer survivors in your practice?" Thirty-one percent reported "always," 48% "sometimes," 15% "rarely," and 5% "not at all or do not care for survivors." When asked whether or not it was the role of the oncology specialist to provide this type of continuing care to cancer survivors, the overwhelming majority (74%) responded "yes." Finally, they were asked whether or not they were comfortable providing ongoing general medical care to cancer survivors and 66% responded "yes."[32] So although it appears that many of ASCO's members are providing some form of care to cancer survivors, we do not know how focused that care is on surveillance for cancer recurrence *versus* health promotion, disease prevention, and monitoring/ prevention of late effects.

A major focus, however, is likely to be surveillance for recurrence and/or detection of new cancers that may be independent of the original primary or related to the original cancer (e.g., new breast or colorectal cancers in patients with a first primary). New cancers may also occur because of a past exposure history (tobacco, sunlight, infection) or as a secondary effect of past cancer treatments. The oncologist is probably the best physician member of the team to follow survivors who may have these risks, and often second cancers are detected earlier in cancer survivors. In my own practice, I have had three breast cancer survivors in whom stage I lung cancers were detected early (chest x-rays taken for minimal pulmonary symptoms). All three of these women had remote and limited histories of tobacco exposure, and had quit smoking many years earlier. There are also some cancer survivors who are just unlucky, and they may be prone to multiple primary cancers, either related to their age, past treatments, or rarely, hereditary predisposition genes. Increasingly, oncologists have taken on the responsibility for providing genetic counseling to their patients and their families.[33,34] Being proactive in addressing the risk for future cancers is often reassuring to cancer survivors, and physicians play an important role in this activity.

Helping Patients and Families Heal

Just as physicians play a critical role at the time of cancer diagnosis, describing the etiology of the specific cancer and why the patient may have developed the disease, as well as explaining the rationale for staging, diagnostic procedures, and the treatment plan, so must the physician guide the patient and family making the transition from the acute phase of survivorship to the phase that Mullan calls "extended survival."[35] This is often a difficult time psychologically, as all of life's activities that might have been put on hold during treatment (e.g., work, school, marriage, childbearing) must now be addressed and often the patient/survivor is a changed person as a result of the cancer treatment experience. This may include the enhancement of some personal relationships and the abandonment of others; a decision to change jobs; a reinvigoration of life goals and plans; separation or divorce related to longstanding marital difficulties; adoption of a healthier lifestyle; increased spirituality and focus on existential issues. The changes invoked by the

cancer experience affect patients and their families, and this is often a time when patients are most interested in obtaining psychosocial support. Patients may find that their family members and co-workers think that everything is over when the treatment ends, but in fact, the patient must continue dealing with the uncertainties of survival and the necessity of maintaining their health through regular check-ups and ongoing maintenance therapies. In the case of childhood cancer, the patient's family may require special attention, with strong evidence of posttraumatic stress in parents and aftereffects on siblings.[36,37]

Couples and families may find it useful to seek counseling or join support groups if relationship issues become apparent. Physicians can provide expert guidance at this time, being available to address the specific concerns about important life plans (e.g., pregnancy, life insurance, job discrimination). They also can provide assistance with rehabilitative issues such as diet, lifestyle, sexuality and body image concerns. For the patient entering this phase of the survivorship trajectory, there is much greater uncertainty, and reassurance and structured psychosocial and educational intervention may facilitate the patient's recovery and return of energy.

Also at this time family members may become much more concerned about their own vulnerability with regard to a cancer diagnosis. Especially concerning diseases such as breast and colorectal cancer, where hereditary predisposition genes have been identified, or in which familial risk of cancer may be heightened. Physicians are often called upon to counsel these individuals about their risk for cancer and what might be done to prevent it. Having just seen a close relative experience cancer treatment can be a catalyst for these family members to come forward and seek help and advice. Being prepared to care for the extended family of a survivor in this way is an important part of the physician's role. Increasingly, I have found myself serving as a family physician in this setting, albeit cancer focused. Helping these family members obtain an accurate estimate of their cancer risk, as well as educating them about preventive interventions, often allows them to provide better ongoing emotional support to their loved one.

As wisely stated two decades ago by physician and cancer survivor, Fitzhugh Mullan,

Since this phase is not predominantly a medical one, doctors and nurses tend to have a diminishing role in providing support and counseling. The result is a void that leaves many cancer patients and their families fending awkwardly for themselves in the "healthy world.". . . . Treatment plans for patients in this postacute phase rarely address the psychosocial problems of reentering the active world. Systematic referrals by oncologists, primary care physicians, and nurses to support services for patients at this point in their recovery would do a tremendous amount to aid adjustment, relieve suffering, and stimulate the further development of these scarce resources.[35]

Long-Term Relationships and Caring for Multiple Generations

There is a unique bond that is established between cancer patients and the physicians who treat them. The close calls of cancer treatment (e.g., febrile neutropenia) and the ups and downs of surgery, radiation or toxic therapies delivered and received for the benefit of the patient/long-term survivor, engenders the development of a strong dyadic relationship. Many years later, cancer survivors will often reminisce with fondness and/or gallows humor about their treatment experience, and they frequently maintain contact with these physicians for many years thereafter, even with relocation to another community. The cancer treatment physician is often seen as a trusted source of information, for issues related to late effects of treatment, as well as for referrals to other physicians. The intensity of the relationship may vary, but under most circumstances, that physician is a key authority figure for the cancer survivor.

As long-term survival has increased, especially with common diseases such as breast, colorectal and prostate cancers, it is not uncommon for the cancer specialist to become professionally involved with family members of the cancer patient. These new medical relationships may focus on prevention and genetic testing in close family members (e.g., daughters, sisters, brothers, children),[33] or actual treatment of cancer in close family members. In my practice, I have cared for mothers and daughters, sisters, as well as husbands and wives. Sometimes it is easier on everyone concerned to have the same familiar oncologist take on the new cancer patient in the family due to the levels of trust and personal relationship, although it may be challenging for the physician to have to go through cancer treatment once again with another member of the family. As our knowledge of risk factors (exposure and genetics) for cancer increases, physicians will need to consider the extended family as well as the patient/survivor.

Critical Role of Prevention

A cancer diagnosis can teach something to both patients and their physicians.[38,39] Faced with a life-threatening illness, survivors often want to do the best they can to reduce their risk of having another cancer episode. This may take the form of smoking cessation, dietary modifications, weight loss, exercise, use of mind-body techniques (meditation, relaxation), and exploration of various complementary and alternative medicine strategies.[19] To the extent possible, physicians must be prepared to support these survivors in making lifestyle changes, which means we need to be prepared to offer smoking cessation treatment and counseling, diet and exercise counseling, as well as access to mind-body treatments to help manage stress and enhance psychological well-being. These types of services may be part of routine care within primary care practices, but may need to be adapted to the special needs of cancer survivors. Frequently, these types of services are available at community and comprehensive cancer centers. They might also be available through some community organizations such as the American Cancer Society and American Lung Association (e.g., smoking cessation).

At the same time, physicians may be called upon by their patients to weigh in on the latest media reports of cancer cures or prevention strategies, including diet and lifestyle products that are heavily marketed to the public. We live in a health and youth oriented culture, and it is impossible to escape having to deal with these issues in medical practice. The big challenge occurs when scientific reports conflict (e.g., vitamin E prevents cancer in one study, but increases heart disease in another). Under these circumstances, it is essential to communicate to patients and survivors the incremental nature of scientific discovery, and the need for patience in sorting out conflicting results. Ultimately, it is usually large randomized clinical trials that settle many of these questions. A good example was the issue of whether or not it was safe to give hormone therapy to women after a breast cancer diagnosis. Breast cancer survivors who were either very symptomatic with vasomotor symptoms or were concerned about prevention of heart disease and dementia felt deprived of the potentially disease preventing effects of postmenopausal hormone therapy. This question for breast cancer survivors was largely resolved with the negative results from the Women's Health Initiative trial in healthy women,[40–43] and then in breast cancer patients in the HABITS trial.[44] Having randomized controlled trial data provide the strongest arguments for or against a health promoting strategy, and we may need to reinforce that with our patients and survivors.

There also has been an expanding role for chemoprevention in this target population, with many large phase III clinical trials demonstrating cancer risk reduction benefit in high risk patient groups that include cancer survivors.[45,46] Increasingly, those who care for cancer survivors will need to address the potential use of chemopreventive agents in survivors. This is now a standard of care in the management of breast cancer survivors with estrogen receptor positive tumors, where long-term endocrine therapies are used for reduction in the risk of second primaries.[47–49] Trials of chemoprevention also have been conducted in survivors of early stage colorectal cancer,[50] however, standardized approaches to chemoprevention in this setting have not taken hold. Rather surveillance with colonoscopy is the primary strategy in use for prevention.

Childhood cancer survivors are probably the group in greatest need of preventive interventions, as the risks for second cancers are so much greater in this population (see Chapters 6, 7, 15, and 17). Research suggests that these high-risk individuals do not undergo cancer screening at a frequency generally recommended in the population, and certainly not at the rate expected given their high-risk status.[51] Some work has already been done to target childhood cancer survivors who use tobacco, as they are at a substantially higher risk of developing smoking related neoplasms.[52,53] Other important interventions in this target group are sun protection, dietary and physical activity interventions. These interventions are necessary due to the high rates of basal cell carcinoma, as well as the metabolic syndrome.[38] Finally, adolescent and young adult women who receive chest irradiation as part of their cancer treatments are at high risk for breast cancer[54] and should receive high-risk screening and potentially endocrine directed chemopreventive treatments. Other detailed recommendations regarding cancer screening for childhood cancer survivors can be found in the "Children's Oncology Group Long Term Follow-up Guidelines" that are briefly reviewed in the *Journal of Clinical Oncology*[55] and can be found online at *www.survivorshipguidelines.org*.

Conclusions

During the past 4 decades, cancer has been transformed from a highly stigmatized condition that was often acutely fatal, to one in which the vast majority of individuals can expect cure. Today, few public figures can hide that they have been diagnosed with cancer and the concept of cancer survivorship has been widely popularized. We are on the brink of the widespread use of more personalized and targeted forms of cancer therapies that are likely to enhance the likelihood of cure and lead to avoidance of unnecessary toxicities in many patients. Nevertheless, there is an entire generation of cancer survivors who are living with the sequelae of our more traditional treatments (see Chapters 7, 9, 15, and 17). Just as physicians must keep abreast of the latest developments in detection and treatment, now they will be expected to be able to provide comprehensive and coordinated care for the growing number of cancer survivors. The challenge for us will be to develop systems of long-term follow-up and care for these survivors, and most importantly, expand our knowledge base regarding the most frequent late effects they might experience. In parallel, we must develop preventive interventions and comprehensive rehabilitation programs to maximize recovery and quality of life after cancer treatment ends.[54,55] This all must be done in collaboration with our patients and other members of the healthcare team.

References

1. Einhorn LH, Donohue J. Cis-diamminedichloroplatinum, vinblastine, and bleomycin combination chemotherapy in disseminated testicular cancer. Ann Intern Med 1977;87:293–298.
2. Stabiner K. To Dance with the Devil: The New War on Breast Cancer; Politics, Power, People. Delacorte Press, New York, 1997.
3. Cancer survivorship–United States, 1971–2001. MMWR Morb Mortal Wkly Rep 2004;53:526–529.
4. Jemal A, Clegg LX, Ward E, et al. Annual report to the nation on the status of cancer, 1975–2001, with a special feature regarding survival. Cancer 2004;101:3–27.
5. http://cancercontrol.cancer.gov/ocs/prevalence/prevalence.html, accessed September 26, 2006.
6. Balsom WR, Bleyer WA, Robison LL, et al. Intellectual function in long-term survivors of childhood acute lymphoblastic leukemia: protective effect of pre-irradiation methotrexate? A Children's Cancer Study Group study. Med Pediatr Oncol 1991;19:486–492.
7. Bhatia S, Meadows AT, Robison LL. Second cancers after pediatric Hodgkin's disease. J Clin Oncol 1998;16:2570–2572.
8. Haupt R, Fears TR, Robison LL, et al. Educational attainment in long-term survivors of childhood acute lymphoblastic leukemia. JAMA 1994;272:1427–1432.
9. Meadows AT, Hobbie WL. The medical consequences of cure. Cancer 1986;58:524–528.
10. Sklar CA, Mertens AC, Walter A, et al. Changes in body mass index and prevalence of overweight in survivors of childhood acute lymphoblastic leukemia: role of cranial irradiation. Med Pediatr Oncol 2000;35:91–95.
11. Gotay CC, Muraoka MY. Quality of life in long-term survivors of adult-onset cancers. J Natl Cancer Inst 1998;90:656–667.
12. Bower JE, Ganz PA, Desmond KA, et al. Fatigue in breast cancer survivors: occurrence, correlates, and impact on quality of life. J Clin Oncol 2000;18:743–753.
13. Ganz PA, Rowland JH, Desmond K, et al. Life after breast cancer: understanding women's health-related quality of life and sexual functioning. J Clin Oncol 1998;16:501–514.
14. Litwin MS, Hays RD, Fink A, et al. Quality-of-life outcomes in men treated for localized prostate cancer. JAMA 1995;273:129–135.
15. Schag CA, Ganz PA, Wing DS, et al. Quality of life in adult survivors of lung, colon and prostate cancer. Qual Life Res 1994;3:127–141.
16. Schover LR, von Eschenbach AC, Smith DB, et al. Sexual rehabilitation of urologic cancer patients: a practical approach. CA Cancer J Clin 1984;34:66–74.
17. Bloom JR, Fobair P, Gritz E, et al. Psychosocial outcomes of cancer: a comparative analysis of Hodgkin's disease and testicular cancer. J Clin Oncol 1993;11:979–988.
18. Fobair P, Hoppe RT, Bloom J, et al. Psychosocial problems among survivors of Hodgkin's disease. J Clin Oncol 1986;4:805–814.
19. Ganz PA, Desmond KA, Leedham B, et al. Quality of life in long-term, disease-free survivors of breast cancer: a follow-up study. J Natl Cancer Inst 2002;94:39–49.
20. Hewitt M, Weiner SL, Simone JV (eds). Childhood Cancer Survivorship: Improving Care and Quality of Life. Washington, DC: National Academies Press, 2003.
21. Hewitt M, Greenfield S, Stovall E (eds). From Cancer Patient to Cancer Survivor: Lost in Transition. Washington, DC: National Academies Press, 2006.
22. Earle CC, Burstein HJ, Winer EP, et al. Quality of non-breast cancer health maintenance among elderly breast cancer survivors. J Clin Oncol 2003;21:1447–1451.
23. Earle CC, Neville BA. Under use of necessary care among cancer survivors. Cancer 2004;101:1712–1719.
24. Lafata JE, Simpkins J, Schultz L, et al. Routine surveillance care after cancer treatment with curative intent. Med Care 2005;43:592–599.
25. Lash TL, Silliman RA. Medical surveillance after breast cancer diagnosis. Med Care 2001;39:945–955.
26. Lehmann JF, DeLisa JA, Warren CG, et al. Cancer rehabilitation: assessment of need, development, and evaluation of a model of care. Arch Phys Med Rehabil 1978;59:410–419.
27. DeLisa JA. A history of cancer rehabilitation. Cancer 2001;92:970–974.
28. Harvey RF, Jellinek HM, Habeck RV. Cancer rehabilitation. An analysis of 36 program approaches. JAMA 1982;247:2127–2131.
29. Gerber LH. Cancer rehabilitation into the future. Cancer 2001;92:975–979.
30. Schover LR, Brey K, Lichtin A, et al. Oncologists' attitudes and practices regarding banking sperm before cancer treatment. J Clin Oncol 2002;20:1890–1897.
31. Schover LR, Brey K, Lichtin A, et al. Knowledge and experience regarding cancer, infertility, and sperm banking in younger male survivors. J Clin Oncol 2002;20:1880–1889.
32. Ganz PA. ASCO Cancer Prevention Survey. 2005.
33. Garber JE, Offit K. Hereditary cancer predisposition syndromes. J Clin Oncol 2005;23:276–292.
34. Narod SA, Offit K. Prevention and management of hereditary breast cancer. J Clin Oncol 2005;23:1656–1663.
35. Mullan F. Seasons of survival: reflections of a physician with cancer. N Engl J Med 1985;313:270–273.
36. Kazak AE, Barakat LP, Meeske K, et al. Posttraumatic stress, family functioning, and social support in survivors of childhood leukemia and their mothers and fathers. J Consult Clin Psychol 1997;65:120–129.
37. Kazak AE, Stuber ML, Barakat LP, et al. Predicting posttraumatic stress symptoms in mothers and fathers of survivors of childhood cancers. J Am Acad Child Adolesc Psychiatry 1998;37:823–831.
38. Demark-Wahnefried W, Aziz N, Rowland JH, et al. Riding the crest of the teachable moment: promoting long-term health after the diagnosis of cancer. J Clin Oncol 2005;23:5814–5830.
39. Ganz PA. A teachable moment for oncologists: cancer survivors, 10 million strong and growing! J Clin Oncol 2005;23:5458–5460.
40. Rapp SR, Espeland MA, Shumaker SA, et al. Effect of estrogen plus progestin on global cognitive function in postmenopausal women: The Women's Health Initiative Memory Study: a randomized controlled trial. JAMA 2003;289:2663.

41. Shumaker SA, Legault C, Rapp SR, et al. Estrogen plus progestin and the incidence of dementia and mild cognitive impairment in postmenopausal women: The Women's Health Initiative Memory Study: a randomized controlled trial. JAMA 2003;289:2651.

42. Risks and benefits of estrogen plus progestin in healthy post-menopausal women: principal results from the Women's Health Initiative randomized controlled trial. JAMA 2002;288:321–333.

43. Hays J, Ockene JK, Brunner RL, et al. Effects of estrogen plus progestin on health-related quality of life. N Engl J Med 2003; 10.1056/NEJMoa030311.

44. Holmberg PL, Anderson H. HABITS (hormonal replacement therapy after breast cancer—is it safe?), a randomised comparison: trial stopped. The Lancet 2004;363:453–455.

45. Lippman SM, Levin B. Cancer prevention: strong science and real medicine. J Clin Oncol 2005;23:249–253.

46. Hong WK, Spitz MR, Lippman SM. Cancer chemoprevention in the 21st century: genetics, risk modeling, and molecular targets. J Clin Oncol 2000;18:9s–18.

47. Lippman SM, Brown PH. Tamoxifen prevention of breast cancer: an instance of the fingerpost. JNCI Cancer Spectrum 1999;91: 1809–1819.

48. Cuzick J. Aromatase inhibitors for breast cancer prevention. J Clin Oncol 2005;23:1636–1643.

49. Fabian CJ, Kimler BF. Selective estrogen-receptor modulators for primary prevention of breast cancer. J Clin Oncol 2005;23: 1644–1655.

50. Sandler RS, Halabi S, Baron JA, et al. A randomized trial of aspirin to prevent colorectal adenomas in patients with previous colorectal cancer. N Engl J Med 2003;348:883–890.

51. Yeazel MW, Oeffinger KC, Gurney JG, et al. The cancer screening practices of adult survivors of childhood cancer: a report from the Childhood Cancer Survivor Study. Cancer 2004;100:631–640.

52. Emmons K, Li FP, Whitton J, et al. Predictors of smoking initiation and cessation among childhood cancer survivors: A report from the Childhood Cancer Survivor Study. J Clin Oncol 2002; 20:1608–1616.

53. Emmons KM, Butterfield RM, Puleo E, et al. Smoking among participants in the childhood cancer survivors cohort: the partnership for health study. J Clin Oncol 2003;21:189–196.

54. Kenney LB, Yasui Y, Inskip PD, et al. Breast cancer after childhood cancer: a report from the Childhood Cancer Survivor Study. Ann Intern Med 2004;141:590–597.

55. Landier W, Bhatia S, Eshelman DA, et al. Development of risk-based guidelines for pediatric cancer survivors: the Children's Oncology Group Long-Term Follow-Up Guidelines from the Children's Oncology Group Late Effects Committee and Nursing Discipline. J Clin Oncol 2004;JCO.

56. Ganz PA. Current issues in cancer rehabilitation. Cancer 1990; 65:742–751.

57. Ganz PA. The status of cancer rehabilitation in the late 1990s. Mayo Clin Proc 1999;74:939–940.

Cancer Survivorship: A Nursing Perspective

Susan Leigh

When asked to write about cancer survivors from a nursing perspective, I realized how daunting this task could be. Could I be objective in representing my profession and colleagues? Should I share my personal perspective and why I became an oncology nurse? Would I look at the role of oncology nursing in relation to survivors, or would I focus on other areas of nursing that care for survivors in nononcology settings? From whose perspective would cancer *survivor* be defined? And where does *survivorship* fit into the continuum of care? Since there is little agreement as to the definitions of these terms and where responsibilities for survivorship care lie, I must be right upfront with my biases and explain how and why I am interested in this timely topic.

I am both a cancer survivor and an oncology nurse. It was my own personal experience surviving Hodgkin's disease in 1972 that later propelled me to specialize in the newly developing field of oncology nursing. As my years of survival added up, I became more and more concerned about what would happen to cancer survivors in the long run. For years, I took hormonal therapy for ovarian failure. I continue to take daily synthroid for hypothyroidism. My lungs are fibrotic from radiation therapy and make it difficult for me to breathe in certain situations. My neck and upper chest muscles are atrophied and cause severe weakness. But all of these conditions are essentially manageable and a seemingly fair trade-off for my extra years of life.

Then I was diagnosed with breast cancer in December of 1990. I abruptly discontinued estrogen replacement therapy and had bilateral mastectomies with reconstruction. It took over two months for my damaged tissue to heal. A few years later my pelvis was fractured in a taxicab accident, leading to pelvic pain and urinary urgency, which continued for months and now years. I received an unexpected diagnosis of carcinoma in situ of the bladder. I then went on to receive 3 years of BCG immunotherapy (1995–1998), and was also started on medication to slow the progression of osteoporosis. Even though I have experienced some late effects of treatment over 3 decades of survival, I still consider myself one of the lucky ones. I have not only done well thus far with the aftereffects of cancer treatment, but I also have access to medical care through the Veteran's Administration Medical Centers (VA), and I have an insider's advantage in navigating the healthcare system. Obviously, not all survivors are so fortunate.

So, I have seen and experienced cancer care over multiple decades and from more than one perspective. This experience of surviving a life-threatening disease has not only impacted my physical health, it has also impacted my views of life and nursing, both personally and professionally. Thus, I share this encapsulated narrative as an example of a never-ending story. We simply don't know what will happen next, and what our future will look like. Survival becomes a series of occurrences—remission, rehabilitation, rediagnosis, and more treatment—and seems more cyclic than linear. We ask questions, such as, how will we know if the cancer comes back, or how do we learn to monitor our health? How do we live with the fear and uncertainty? Who will oversee our follow-up care? When will guidelines be developed so that nononcology practitioners will know what to look for when our care is returned to them? And who will pay for this type of continued follow-up? While the questions are many, the answers, unfortunately, are few.

Obviously, this chapter already has a personal bias as it is written from both sides of the bedpan! In this chapter, I hope to:

- look at the relationship between nursing and cancer care,
- discuss the emergence of the survivorship movement and its new semantics,
- examine nursing as it is today and how it relates to survivorship, and
- explore the future of nursing in relation to long-term follow-up.

Nursing and Cancer Care

The term *survivorship* was not in the lexicon of cancer nursing when I was first diagnosed and treated for Hodgkin's disease in the early 1970s. As a matter of fact, nurses who specialized in cancer care were few in number at that time. While nurses had always cared for patients with cancer, it was historically surgical and palliative care nursing. A few of the earliest examples of hospitals specializing in cancer care were Memorial Sloan Kettering, New York (1884), Roswell Park, Buffalo, New York (1911), and MD Anderson, Houston, Texas (1941), and surgery was, of course, the primary form of treatment.[1] Physicians were advisors and mentors to nursing staff who had the responsibility to make patients as comfortable as possible as this was typically all that could be done. Meanwhile, Renilda Hilkemeyer, a pioneer in oncology nursing, describes the early days when a handful of administrators and educators started developing inservice programs, policies and procedures, nursing care manuals, and lectures specifically targeting this type of nursing.[1] In the 1950s, the handful of colleagues who worked with cancer patients, yet were isolated geographically, began an informal phone network. Finally, the American Cancer Society (ACS) organized a national nursing advisory committee that brought all of them together for face-to-face meetings.

Around this time, radiotherapy was added to the cancer treatment menu, and it was initially delivered by radiologists in general radiology departments and from low voltage machines.[1] The treatments were crude and toxic, and nurses were once again challenged to treat the side effects when patients returned to the wards. They attempted to prevent infections, manage pain, and help the patient feel more comfortable. Meanwhile, myths about cancer were abundant, such as being contagious or being a punishment for some sin or transgression, which led to fear and shunning.[2,3] Many patients were never told their diagnosis. Family members felt obligated to continue the charade of deception, and had to try and act cheerful and upbeat in arduous circumstances. Few could even utter the word *cancer* as the disease was considered a death sentence. And many nurses themselves deliberately avoided working with this population of patients as it was perceived as being depressing.

With the advent of medical oncology in the 1960s, we saw the germination of a new sense of optimism and hope. Single drug therapy evolved into multiple drug combinations, and some cancers, like Hodgkin's disease, became treatable. Cancer care began its evolution into the specialized field called oncology, and was available in a select number of hospitals and academic institutions, including the ones mentioned before. So, while I was learning about oncology as a patient, a small number of nurses around the country were learning about oncology as a new subspecialty.

Physicians involved in clinical trials and the development of new therapies often selected nurses to work with them as part of cancer care teams. With these new therapies came new jobs, positions, and on-the-job training. Many nurses found themselves working under medical rather than nursing supervisors. Cancer nurses developed and taught ostomy care, mixed drugs and gave chemotherapy, counseled patients and families, created patient education materials, collected data and specimens for medical research, and managed clinical trials. They also learned how to talk about and deal with death and dying as the majority of patients with cancer still died of their disease. And if cancer programs were really visionary and had the funds available, they may have added a social worker to the oncology team. Yet, while there was a new glimmer of hope for some people with cancer, nurses working in this new field often felt isolated from their own profession. There were few, if any, nursing colleagues to share experiences, solve problems, help with decision-making, or just be around for support. Even though some patients were now successfully treated, cancer care still took a huge toll on the professionals who worked in this area.

ACS again recognized this void for nurses, and invited anyone who was interested to attend a joint meeting with the National Cancer Institute on advances in cancer management. This was 1974. Nurses from oncology settings around the country met for the first time and discussed how they might establish some sort of formal networking and communication system for those who had been working in relative isolation.[1] The enthusiasm about this get-together was palpable, and the group decided to meet soon afterwards at the next meeting of the American Society of Clinical Oncology (ASCO) and the American Association of Cancer Research (AACR). In 1975, the informal group with an interest in cancer nursing decided to create their own formal specialty organization, and the Oncology Nursing Society (ONS) was founded. There was no way that Lisa Begg Marino, Cindy Mantz Cantril, Connie Henke Yarbro, and Daryl Maass Mathers could have envisioned what lay ahead of them in this endeavor. These were the first four officers of the fledgling ONS which has now grown to more than 35,000 members worldwide.

I attended my first national ONS meeting in 1976 as a neophyte oncology nurse. Cancer survivors were not even on the radar screen at that time. We were simply trying to find ways to deliver chemotherapy safely, treat debilitating side effects, and better support both patients and family members through the grueling cancer treatment experience. These were now nursing responsibilities, and all attention was focused on helping patients survive the traumatic therapies. As a former patient who had received chemotherapy from a variety of physicians just a few short years before, I was elated to see this expertise transferred to nurses.

It would be a number of years, though, before ONS discovered survivorship and incorporated it thematically into programs and projects. Conceptually, though, oncology nurses have always been involved in supporting survivorship without necessarily knowing it.

Survivorship and Semantics

Shortly before ONS was organized, the term cancer *survivor* was used by the insurance industry to describe the loved ones left behind after the patient died. By the time oncology nurses became official members of cancer care teams, physicians were already seeing progress in disease-free survival, especially in pediatrics. Survivors then came to be defined as those who lived beyond 5 years with no evidence of disease, and parameters were quantitative and strictly-defined within medical boundaries.[4] As pediatric oncology was the first to develop survivor clinics, their young patients were promoted or transitioned to this next step of follow-up care only after they survived for 5 years with no recurrence of the original disease.

While these parameters are needed in order to answer research questions and attempt to define and care for a very specific population, they can be limiting in that they don't necessarily reflect individual survivor experiences. As more people who had been treated for cancer lived longer, questions arose as to the quality of their lives both during and after therapy. In 1986 a network of oncology professionals, cancer survivors, family members, and cancer organizations were invited to Albuquerque, NM by Catherine Logan Carrillo, the founder of (People) Living Through Cancer, a community based resource and support center.[4] Catherine's vision was to address these issues of survival from a consumer perspective, and to develop a network of national and community organizations. At this ground-breaking meeting, the National Coalition for Cancer Survivorship (NCCS) was founded. Many in this founding group were professionals, including nurses and physicians, who also had personal histories of cancer. All had a common interest in raising awareness about the complexities of surviving cancer, about the unmet needs of those living beyond their treatments, and about the need to improve quality of life throughout the continuum of survival. Fitzhugh Mullan (NCCS co-founder, physician, and cancer survivor) had written: "When could I say simply that I was cured? Actuarial and population-based figures give us survival estimates for various cancers, but those figures do not speak to the individual patient whose experience is unique and not determined or described by aggregate data."[5]

The group decided that they needed to define their constituency, and a discussion about who is and is not a cancer survivor ensued. It must be noted that the initial defining exercise was to establish an *organizational* constituency. Little did we know at that first meeting how this exercise would eventually lead to heated debates and arguments about who is or is not a survivor, and to the plethora of other labels that would eventually define this burgeoning population. NCCS founders agreed to define *survivor* within the context of a continuum: "from the time of its discovery and for the balance of life, an individual diagnosed with cancer is a survivor."[6] No one would be excluded as everyone's survival issues would fall somewhere under one of the continuum stages. We would not be an elitist organization that would require members to be free of disease. And we would address the concerns and distress felt by family members and caregivers across the continuum of survival.

Besides defining *survivor (the individual)*, NCCS also coined the term *survivorship (the experience)*. While the term *survivor* was already used by the pediatric community as a stage of survival after treatment, the concept of survivorship was first used within the context of cancer by NCCS. Over the years it has collected almost as many meanings as has the term survivor. Even the oncology community has defined "survivorship" in different ways. From a biomedical perspective, it has been characterized as

- a time frame (after 2, 5, or 10 years, depending upon the disease);
- as a stage or phase of survival (after initial treatment ends, complete remission); or
- as an outcome of treatment (no evidence of disease/NED or cured).

While these quantitative measurements help to categorize a new population of patients who have responded favorably to treatments, they fail to account for survivors who

- indefinitely require maintenance therapy;
- live with cancer that is controlled and considered a chronic illness;
- need periodic changes in treatment modalities;
- have a recurrence of the original disease;
- develop a second primary due to past therapy or genetic predisposition; or
- experience other late effects of treatment, such as premature cardiac disease.

These inconsistencies clearly show how intricate the semantics become when the definers come from different perspectives (i.e., from scientists, clinicians, caregivers, or those surviving the disease).

In order to illustrate the qualitative components of survival, Mullan introduced his article, "Seasons of Survival" in the *New England Journal of Medicine* in 1985.[5] Mullan's early model of survival follows a linear format, and is seen as a progression of events rather than formal, clinical stages:

- Acute Stage—Patient receiving treatment
- Extended Stage—Immediately posttreatment, remission
- Permanent Stage—Long-term survival

Carter soon after described her survival model as "going through." This suggests that survival is a dynamic process rather than a static stage:[7]

Interpreting the diagnosis...Confronting mortality... Reprioritizing...Coming to terms...Moving on...Flashing back...

These two descriptions are the basis for the NCCS definition of cancer survivorship as "living with, through and beyond cancer."[3] Yet, these are not the only authors that have attempted to illustrate the survivorship experience as a continuum. A few other early examples include the following:

Fiore, 1979[8]—Diagnosis...Preoperative care...Postoperative care recovery and adjustment...Postoperative therapy ...Termination of active therapy or rehabilitation...and Post five-year survival

Mages & Mendelsohn,1980[9]—Discovery and diagnosis... Primary treatment...Remission, recurrence, dissemination ...Terminal illness

Anduri, 1997[10]—Revelation (diagnosis)...Repture (surgery, therapy)...Reentry (therapy completed)...Regeneration (recovery)

The models above all depict a sense of movement or transitioning through phases or stages, and come from medicine, nursing, psychology, sociology, and theology. While only Mages and Mendelsohn[9] have included death in their continuum, the lack of attention to this important phase of the life cycle warrants attention. Death is surely the end point for any and all models that illustrate life after cancer.

Nursing and Survivorship

How nurses relate to survivorship depends upon how they define the term and if they even have knowledge of this term. If they see survivorship as the stage of survival that begins once initial treatment ends, then oncology nurses will have decreasing contact with cancer survivors. For a limited period of time, usually up to 5 years and often regulated by insurance plans, survivors will return to the clinic where they received care and have brief check-ups and diagnostic tests essentially to see if they continue to be in remission. Nurses may or may not see the returning survivor, and if they do, their encounter usually consists of a quick hello and pat on the back. Busy clinics, time constraints, and a focus on the acutely ill all require the full attention of most oncology nurses. The one exception is the oncology nurse practitioner (NP) who has become a specialist in long-term follow-up, and helps the physician with the survivor's transition to posttreatment care.

Meanwhile, if survivorship is viewed as a process that begins at the time of diagnosis, then oncology nurses are attentive to survivorship issues along the extended continuum of care. A survival plan is often laid out shortly after diagnosis, and realistic strategies and hopes are modified over time. Survivors and their families are supported medically and emotionally throughout treatment, and, hopefully, a survivorship care plan is developed toward the end of therapy. This would ideally include detailed summaries of all diagnostic tests, surgeries, and cancer therapies, and the survivor begins the transition to life beyond cancer. Survivorship is not just about *IF* or *HOW LONG* patients live, but also about *HOW WELL* they survive and, hopefully, thrive.

The many roles of oncology nurses include caregivers, clinicians, educators and counselors. They also serve as authors, editors and lecturers. In addition they are researchers, rehabilitators, and nurse practitioners. These diverse roles illustrate how oncology nurses are changing the way care is delivered, treatments are tolerated, and palliation is presented. They also are altering the way survivors recover.

From Then to Now

Examples of changes in oncology nursing over the past 3 decades are sometimes dramatic:

- When I first gave chemotherapy in 1976, emesis basins were stacked high right next to the patient's chair. Today, patients eat lunch while receiving "chemo"!
- Thirty years ago, radiation "techs" offered day to day consistency and answered questions as well as they could. Today, radiation therapy nurses are specialized, organized, and working together to advance nursing practice in this intricate area of technology and subspecialization.
- Toward the end of my chemotherapy and radiation therapy for Hodgkin's disease in 1972, my schedule was often disrupted and finally discontinued due to bone marrow suppression. Today, colony stimulating factors keep schedules on time and with patients receiving optimal dosing.
- During the early days of oncology, a friend and colleague proposed looking at cancer survivors for her master's thesis. She was told it was an unscholarly topic for nursing, and was asked to choose another area to study. Today, Ph.D.'s in nursing are awarded to scholars researching survivorship.
- When oncology nursing began, "research" nurses assisted physicians with their medical research, including specimen and data collection. Today, we have educated, professional, oncology nurses dedicated to related nursing research. Examples of their research include fatigue, pain, cognitive dysfunction, quality of life, family issues, sexuality, spirituality, psychosocial distress, reproductive problems, hormonal changes, and long-term survival.
- And, 30 years ago, survivors dreamed of reaching that magic 5-year mark, while today we dream about dying of old age.

But these dreams do not come without a price. As lives are extended, so too are the risks of developing late or delayed effects of treatment. Since there has been no systematic follow-up of the majority of adult long-term cancer survivors, we still have much to learn about the positive and negative aspects of treatments and survival. And major questions today include who will take responsibility to monitor the health of survivors, assist in their recovery, make appropriate referrals to subspecialists, and then *pay* for this type of continued care. It is one thing to pay for research and treatment.

There must also be a commitment to pay for the continued care, rehabilitation, and psychosocial fallout after treatment ends.

Nursing and Long-Term Follow-Up

Since I attended that first NCCS gathering in 1986, I have had a dream. This dream is that survivors have continued access to systematic follow-up care by providers who understand our individual situations, have knowledge of potential risks, and can help us learn to be well again. This may be within oncology, with primary care, or with a combination of both. Close monitoring by the cancer care team is usually guaranteed for the first few years posttreatment, but the difficulty often begins once the survivor is no longer followed in the oncology clinic. Oncologists simply cannot continue to see all their long-term survivors while seeing new patients and managing those on active treatment. Yet, primary care and nononcology physicians don't really know what to do with us. The need for guidelines for long-term care is vital, yet it will be years before they can truly become evidence-based. Hopefully, consensus-based guidelines will help us fill this gap.

Meanwhile, nurses may be the most qualified oncology professionals to oversee specialized follow-up care, since many of them build on knowledge gained through delivering and monitoring treatments and managing side effects. They also develop relationships with family members and loved ones, assess for psychosocial problems, refer to appropriate specialists, and generally work within a model of wellness promotion rather than disease management. This model has worked beautifully in pediatric oncology. It has a much shorter history in the adult arena. But there is hope on the horizon. In the near future, oncology nurse practitioners will most likely play as active a role in adult follow-up care as they do in pediatrics.

Issues of long-term survival became a more noticeable priority after the introduction of the NCCS's *Imperatives for Quality Cancer Care: Access, Advocacy, Action, and Accountability.*[11] NCCS published this report in 1995. Soon afterward, the Office of Cancer Survivorship (OCS) was established at the National Cancer Institute (NCI) with the directive to focus on the needs of cancer survivors, and especially those with long-term and late effects of treatment. "Imperatives" also identified nurse practitioners and oncology clinical nurse specialists as major players on a multidisciplinary team of healthcare specialists. It stressed health promotion and wellness in survivor clinics. It identified the continued need for access to supportive care services especially for minority populations. And it called for education and rehabilitation for symptoms, such as fatigue, chronic pain, weight changes, and decreased stamina. These are all areas in which oncology nurses were already working and doing research. Yet, while this report raised awareness about the continuing needs of long-term survivors, there was no plan to implement the recommendations. It would take another 8 years before the next report was published about issues of survivorship.

More recent governmental reports include the following:

- 2003—Childhood Cancer Survivorship: Improving Care and Quality of Life. A report by the Institute of Medicine (IOM), National Research Council of the National

Academies.[12] This extensive report, solicited by the National Cancer Advisory Board (NCAB), recommends developing guidelines for follow-up care of childhood cancer survivors; developing standards for comprehensive systems to deliver survivorship care; raising awareness of late effects; improving professional education and training in the area of long-term survival; and increasing research in this area. Nurses were represented on the review board, and the National Institute of Nursing Research was included as a source for increased support. Pediatric nurse practitioners are part of the report as they have always played a major role in developing and staffing survivor clinics.

- 2004—Living Beyond Cancer: Finding a New Balance.[13] This report from the President's Cancer Panel (PCP) at NCI differentiates survivor issues across the lifespan. Over the course of a year, 5 panels were convened to look at age-specific issues, and many oncology nurses participated. This report includes long-term health issues and follow-up care, legal and regulatory protections, problems with privacy and insurance portability provisions, access to education and information, availability of psychosocial and supportive care needs, health insurance, and surveillance and research.
- 2004—A National Action Plan for Cancer Survivorship: Advancing Public Health Strategies.[14] This report is jointly sponsored by the Centers for Disease Control (CDC) and the Lance Armstrong Foundation (LAF). Prevention and control of long-term and late effects of treatment present a new challenge to public health, another area with nursing implications. This proposed National Action Plan hopefully will be used as a guide to help decrease the burden of cancer, improve the quality of life of all Americans affected by this disease, and increase funding for survivorship research and delivery of culturally appropriate care.[14] Nurses were again represented throughout the entire process of meeting and developing the plan.
- 2005—For release in November 2006 is the much anticipated report from the IOM entitled Cancer Survivorship: Charting the Course to Improve Care and Quality of Life.[15] This report will focus on adult survivors just as the 2003 IOM report focused on pediatrics. This report, more than any of the above, emphasizes the role of nursing in long-term follow-up care.

Another example illustrating the relationship between nursing and survivorship was a State of the Science Symposium on Adult Survivorship convened by the American Journal of Nursing, July 15–17, 2005, in Philadelphia. Topics from nursing and related research covered much of the holistic spectrum of survival that encompasses physiological, psychological, social, and existential categories. While the main focus was on posttreatment survivorship issues, many of the papers covered symptoms that either began during treatment, lingered after therapy was completed, or surfaced months to years later. The proceedings and papers from this meeting were published as a supplement to the American Journal of Nursing,[16] and implementation of projected projects will be encouraged.

Yet another report specific to nursing is a white paper on Nursing-Sensitive Patient Outcomes (NSPO's).[17,18] In this paper, ONS challenges oncology nurses to get involved with both research and implementation of NSPO's as this is where nursing makes a difference in oncology care. While medical outcomes describe mortality, morbidity, and disease-free survival, nursing outcomes represent changes in symptom management, functional status, safety, psychological status, or costs.[17,18] Nurses invest heavily in patient/survivor care, and attention to the results of that care is increasingly important. According to the authors of this white paper, "Outcomes matter to decision makers—patients, providers, private payors, government agencies, regulators, standards-setting organizations, and professional organizations—and society at large."[18] The continuum of care associated with these NSPO's include:

Prevention . . . Early detection and diagnosis . . . Initial treatment . . . Continuing care . . . Maintenance . . . Follow-up . . . Recurrence/progressive disease . . . and palliative/end-of-life care

There is no mention of survivorship as a stage. Rather, survivorship could be seen as the overall umbrella that unites these phases of the survival continuum.

Conclusions

After all these years with minimal attention given to survivorship issues, the topic is finally gaining momentum. Pediatric oncology identified this area as needing continuing attention well over 20 years ago. The advocacy community followed suit shortly thereafter, and a proliferation of organizations have incorporated survivorship in their missions. ONS offered its first session on survivorship at the 1987 Congress, and currently includes a Nurse Survivors Focus Group (NSFG), a Survivorship Special Interest Group (SIG), and a plethora of nursing researchers studying issues around this topic. While a mere handful of adult oncologists have been dedicated to researching and writing about long-term and late effects, cancer survivorship is now on ASCO's agenda. And LAF is now helping to fund the establishment of survivor clinics. The tide is finally turning. My question remains, "Why has it taken so long?" Some believe we have reached a critical mass and the population and issues can no longer be ignored.

The Office of Cancer Survivorship has estimated that 14% of the overall population of cancer survivors has survived for over 20 years, and this number most likely represents a growing number of survivors who were diagnosed at younger ages. The longer we survive, the greater our chances are of developing delayed or late effects from therapies. While many of us have been diagnosed with second malignancies and have had our current treatments adapted due to prior therapies, we continue to live on with varying degrees of difficulty. Others are struggling to find providers who understand the challenges of assessing the symptoms of someone treated years ago for cancer. Frustration levels run high when survivors concerns and fears are minimized, or the costs of diagnostic tests or follow-up care are denied, or someone dies unnecessarily because an appropriate diagnosis was delayed.

But hope is on the horizon. The book, The Tipping Point, is about a theory of social epidemics. It discusses the moment of critical mass, the boiling point when an idea or trend finally explodes and spreads to the masses.[19] While we have witnessed a geometric progression of interest within the survivorship movement, we have yet to identify a singular dramatic event that changed the course of awareness surrounding survivorship. So, maybe it is a critical mass of multiple exposures that have been building over the past 3 decades. Advocates, activists, physicians, researchers, social workers, mental health specialists, public policy makers, payors—and, of course, nurses—are all working together to help us survive survival. I applaud everyone who has been in the trenches fighting to get survivorship on the radar screen. But our work has just begun. Hopefully, the wisdom within these pages will help to shed light on the magnitude of the situation, and impel others to join us in this significant campaign.

References

1. Nevidjon B. Building A Legacy: Voices of Oncology Nurses. Boston, MA: Jones and Bartlett Publishers, 1995.
2. Sontag S. Illness as Metaphor and AIDS and its Metaphors. New York: Anchor, 1988.
3. Leigh S. Myths, monsters, and magic: personal perspectives and professional challenges of survival. Oncol Nurs Forum 1992; 19:1475.
4. Leigh S. Defining our destiny. In: Hoffman B, ed. A cancer survivor's almanac: charting your journey. Hoboken, NJ: John Wiley & Sons; 2004.
5. Mullan F. Seasons of survival: reflections of a physician with cancer. N Engl J Med 1985;313:270–273.
6. NCCS Charter. National Coalition for Cancer Survivorship, 1986.
7. Carter B. Going through: a critical theme in surviving breast cancer. Innov Oncol Nurs 1989;5:2.
8. Fiore NA. Fighting Cancer—one person's perspective. N Engl J Med 1979;300:284–289.
9. Mages NL, Mendelsohn GA. Effects of cancer on patient's lives: A personological approach. In: Stone GC, Cohen R, Adler NE, eds. Health psychology—a handbook. San Francisco: Jossey-Bass; 1980.
10. Anduri J. Surviving cancer: a sacred journey for the nineties. Paper presented at: A Family Journey Through Breast Cancer, Columbia Memorial Hospital; 1997; Jacksonville, FL.
11. National Coalition for Cancer Survivorship. Imperatives for Quality Cancer Care: Access, Advocacy, Action, and Accountability. Silver Spring, MD: 1996.
12. Institute of Medicine. Childhood Cancer Survivorship: Improving Care and Quality of Life. Washington, DC: National Academies Press; 2003.
13. National Cancer Institute. Living Beyond Cancer: Finding a New Balance. Available at http://pcp.cancer.gov.
14. Centers for Disease Control and Prevention and the Lance Armstrong Foundation (LAF). 2004. A National Action Plan for Cancer Survivorship: Advancing Public Health Strategies. Available at http://www.cdc.gov/cancer/survivorship/what_cdc_is_doing/symposium.htm, accessed September 24, 2006.
15. Hewitt M, Greenfield S, Stovall E (eds). From Cancer Patient to Cancer Survivor: Lost in Transition. Washington, DC: National Academies Press, 2006.
16. AJN. State of the science: Nursing and cancer survivorship. Am J Nursing. March 2006;106.
17. Given BA, Sherwood PR. Nursing-sensitive patient outcomes—A white paper. Oncol Nurs Forum 2005;32:773–784.
18. Rutledge D. ONS leads the way in oncology nursing-sensitive outcomes research. ONS News. July 2005:20.
19. Gladwell M. The Tipping Point: How Little Things Can Make a Big Difference. New York: Little, Brown & Company, 2002.

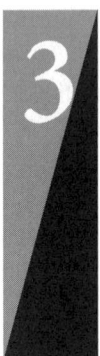

Oncology Social Work for Survivorship

Patricia Fobair

The cancer survivorship movement became part of the American scene in the 1980s with cancer patients and a physician survivor leading the way.[1–5] Cancer survivorship became a force as a result of medicine's focus on finding solutions to the problems of cancer following World War II. These solutions included the success of chemotherapy treatment in the 1960s, research into late effects and psychosocial research following cancer treatment (1970s), and the patient activist movement beginning in the 1980s. Oncology social workers have played a major role, being on the scene since the early days, delivering supportive services to cancer survivors, participating as team members in psychosocial research, and serving as members and leaders in survivorship organizations.[6] This chapter examines survivorship from the perspective of a cancer survivor and oncology social worker, one who enjoys both clinical work and research.

What Is Oncology Social Work?

Oncology social work is an important humanizing influence felt throughout the hospital or cancer center. The role was first described in 1974 with Ruth Abrams's book, *Not Alone with Cancer: A Guide for Those Who Care.*[7] This is a profession "designed to promote the patient's best utilization of the health care system, the optimal development of coping strategies and mobilization of community resources to support maximum functioning."[8] As a clinical practitioner, the oncology social worker draws upon knowledge from medical and psychosocial oncology, and, when possible, participates in research. Oncology social workers provide advocacy and clinical services to patients and families. They work as team members with other health professionals, and provide education and mentoring for younger social work professionals. Some oncology social workers become administrators and/or educators influencing the institutions in which they work and providing services to their community and profession.[8] A central role of the oncology social worker is to assess patient and family care needs and provide interventions that help patients work towards solutions that address physical, intrapsychic, interpersonal and environmental problems.[9]

Oncology social work has retained the values and practices from the early days of the nineteenth century. A few examples are "The importance of being an advocate for the survivor's point of view both within the medical system and in the community, understanding the cancer disease process, and participating as a team-member with physicians and other health professionals." Each value described by Ida Cannon[10] can be found today in the Standards of Practice in Oncology Social Work.[8]

Survivorship

The term *cancer survivor* was coined in 1985 by Fitzhugh Mullan, physician and cancer survivor, in his article, "The Seasons of Survival: Reflections of a Physician with Cancer."[5] He defined cancer survivor as "someone who has received the diagnosis of a potentially fatal form of cancer and is therefore forced to face his or her own mortality." The article resonated with survivors and physicians. A cancer survivor is "living with and beyond cancer." In 1986, Mullan joined with other cancer survivors and health professionals to form a new organization, the National Coalition of Cancer Survivorship,[11] which is on the Web at http://www.canceradvocacy.org/. Elsewhere, new magazines were created to support cancer survivors. The "Surviving!" Magazine,[12] was created in 1983 to publish stories by cancer survivors. It continued doing so until 2003. Coping Magazine, "America's consumer magazine for people whose lives have been touched by cancer," began in 1985 and continues today.[13] These events created an environment that welcomed patient participation in an era of cancer survivorship.

Mullan's definition of a survivor as one "living with and beyond cancer" continues to be used today. Web sites for the public, such as the Office of Cancer Survivorship at the National Cancer Institute[14] and the Lance Armstrong Foundation,[15] use a similar definition. Although calling oneself a "survivor" often feels more comfortable after treatment is completed, "an individual is considered a cancer survivor from the time of diagnosis, through the balance of his or her life."[16] Family members, friends, and caregivers are also affected by the survivorship experience and are included in this definition.[14]

Surviving Treatment

The aura of well-being within a person can be destroyed. One's inner attitude towards life is perhaps more fragile than we tend to recognize.

—Bruno Bettelheim

The shock of hearing that they have a cancer diagnosis leaves many patients feeling "wounded" and "out of control."[17] "A glass wall surrounded me for a few days. I felt isolated by the news."[18] The patient may experience waves of panic and thoughts of a life threat. Though physicians reassure patients of their "good chance for survival," patients' worries continue. The "glass wall" melts as decisions about treatment move forward, but negative feelings may flood one's being for some time. The first adaptive task after the discovery of cancer is to initiate appropriate treatment, yet each form of treatment holds its special terrors.[19] Newly diagnosed cancer patients are faced with the challenge of regulating their emotions while dealing with the reality of the situation and integrating the experience into the rest of their life.

Facing the reality of the illness can be tough during the first weeks after diagnosis. An interruption in a busy life, patients may feel that they "don't have time for this." The stress of coping with a cancer diagnosis can be mild to severe, often depending on the severity of the diagnosis and treatment. For some newly diagnosed patients, the degree of stress meets the criteria for "acute traumatic stress syndrome." Patients reexperience the possibility of the "life threat," and have chills of momentary panic, physical arousal, or a numbing of responsiveness. In one study, distress among patients diagnosed with cancer was 25% at the beginning of treatment and 40% four months later.[19,20] In this study, the prevalence of psychological distress among cancer patients was 35%.[20,21] Other studies have found similar figures.[23] Recognizing distress, health professionals have an opportunity to form a bond with survivors, talk with them about their fears and offer interventions which give them greater inner control.

Setting priorities for oneself and actively making one's own medical decisions helps most patients return to feeling in control. Choosing the physician they want to work with activates survivors as teammates in their treatment plan. Deciding whether to continue working or to take time off during treatment is an issue patients can control. Working is a source of normalcy and comfort for some patients, while others benefit from having extra time to recover. Choosing to stay physically active during and after treatment reduces the effects of chemotherapy and lowers symptoms of distress.[24] Avoiding isolation by finding others to talk with about issues and feelings is a step towards maintaining mental health during a stressful time. Support groups, offered by many community hospitals and agencies, are helpful in reducing emotional distress.[25] Facing cancer provided me with a pivotal moment to take stock of life. Finding meaning in the situation, reorganizing priorities, and continuing to plan for the future provides arcas of personal control that also help survivors get through treatment.

Issues in Recovery

Although there are many chapters in this book that will touch on disease-specific aspects of survivorship (e.g., issues for breast, prostate, lung, colorectal cancer survivors), in this section, we review crosscutting themes in survivorship perceived from an oncology social workers' vantage point. While cancer treatment improves survival and postpones recurrence, it often is followed by damage to the body or changes in levels of distress.[26] Research indicates that the greater the treatment needed to control the disease, the greater the possibility of body impairment, and subsequently, the greater the threat to the person's self-esteem and increased likelihood of distress.[27–30] In a large study comparing 4,878 cancer survivors with those without a history of cancer, the survivors were more likely to report being in "fair or poor health," to experience limitations of activity, functional limitations, psychological disability, and to suffer a lesser ability to work because of a health condition.[26]

Physical Functioning

From the work of Mages and Mendelsohn,[19] we learn that the adaptive task is to mourn the physical or psychological loss of health, and where possible replace or compensate for the lost body parts or functions. Maximizing other physical and psychological potential helps one maintain a sense of self-esteem and intactness.[19]

Regaining lost energy following treatment is the first pressing issue for many patients. Greene et al found that 82% of breast cancer patients reported fatigue after their first chemotherapy and 77% after their second cycle.[31] The incidence of fatigue as a result of treatment varied from over 35% to 80% in several studies.[27,32] Surveys in the United States and Ireland indicate that 53% of cancer patients experience significant fatigue daily, and 80% at least monthly.[33,34]

Reported fatigue can linger months or years after treatment for many, 37% in one study, 40% in another.[35] Reductions or losses of normal physical activity may affect as many as 43% of patients.[27] When Ganz et al compared the fatigue survivors experienced before treatment and 1 and 2 years after treatment for Hodgkin's disease, they found that both the chemotherapy and radiation therapy patients had more fatigue before treatment than the healthy reference group, and that survivor's fatigue did not improve after treatment.[36] In another study, Ganz et al found that physical functioning among breast cancer survivors treated 6.3 years earlier was excellent, but that women who received no adjuvant therapy had significantly better physical functioning (p = 0.003) when compared with those receiving chemotherapy, tamoxifen, or both.[37]

Several studies compared fatigue among survivors of Hodgkin's disease, testicular cancer and/or with healthy norms. They provided examples of how physical functioning after cancer treatment correlates with the extent of disease or treatment given. For instance, Bloom et al found that energy loss was greater among patients treated for Hodgkin's disease when compared with testicular cancer survivors.[38] Fossa et al found that patients treated for Hodgkin's disease reported more chronic fatigue than testicular survivors, and both had greater problems with fatigue than the general population.[39] Ruffer et al found that patients treated for Hodgkin's disease had greater problems with fatigue than those in the control group.[40] In addition, Van Tulder et al found that when compared with healthy controls,[41] survivors of Hodgkin's disease had greater problems with physical functioning at strenuous levels of activity, and greater problems in role functioning at work and daily activities. They also had lower perceived overall health and less satisfaction with their sex lives.

Cancer patients treated with bone marrow transplantation (BMT) have problems with fatigue and physical functioning soon after treatment[42,43] and at 3 years[44] or 5 years following a BMT.[45] McQuellon et al found that while distress improved over the first year after transplant, overall quality of life worsened at discharge but improved over time. However, concerns worsened during the first year.[43] Ten years after the transplant, Bush et al found a moderate incidence of lingering complications, including fatigue and emotional and sexual dysfunction, but the degree of distress attributed to these complications was mostly low.[46]

Progress in addressing the problem of fatigue has been made through the definition and search for underlying mechanisms. Recognizing the importance of reaching agreement on how to define posttreatment fatigue, the National Comprehensive Cancer Network (NCCN) created an algorithm to help in assessment.[47] The guideline is available at www.nccn.org. Research designed to examine the mechanisms underlying the occurrence and persistence of fatigue was initiated by Bower et al.[20,49] Bower found that fatigued breast cancer survivors had higher serum levels of several markers associated with proinflammatory cytokine activity than nonfatigued survivors, which suggested mechanisms through which immune activation might occur. The fatigued survivors also had an increased number of circulating T lymphocytes, suggesting that persistent fatigue in breast cancer survivors might be associated with a chronic inflammatory process involving the T cell compartment. The pilot work is promising. Further studies are indicated.[48,49]

Physical activity and exercise are recommended for the problem of fatigue. Research shows benefits of exercise in reducing fatigue among cancer patients[24,50] compared with control patients. When additional quality-of-life measures were examined, exercise groups exhibited less psychological distress,[51] decreased weight[52] and showed improvements in aerobic capacity.[50] Body esteem and mood were higher among physically active breast cancer survivors than among the sedentary breast cancer survivors.[53] Women whose physical activity increased following a breast cancer diagnosis scored higher on a physical health scale.[54] Physical activity may have survival benefits after a breast cancer diagnosis according to one study.[55] The collective evidence is that increasing physical activity may improve quality of life and it reduces survivor fatigue following cancer treatment.

Body Image and Sexuality

Changes in a person's functional body from cancer, surgery, or other treatment adds to the problems that patients experience. Functional impairment produces distress and can lead to loss of self-esteem, reclusive behavior, or a distortion of intimate relationships.[19] Mages et al found that 19% of an initial sample and 21% of a follow-up sample experienced high distress and impairment following treatment.[56] These patients had feelings of anger and fearfulness and were living constricted lives.[56] Broers et al found that 25% of survivors treated three years earlier with BMT experienced serious functional limitations and somatic symptoms.[44] The patients' psychological distress was related to the degree of functional distress as well as to baseline psychological functioning.[44]

Problems with body image and sexuality following treatment are reported in studies of women with breast cancer.[66] The percentage of early stage breast cancer patients concerned

with their body image following treatment varied by study from 31% to 70%[67,41] and 44% in two studies by Bukovic et al[68,69] 50%[70] Avis et al found 70% of the women in their study reporting problems with body image.[66]

Breast cancer patients who had problems with body image also had problems with self-esteem, mental health, and had partners who had difficulty in understanding them.[70] Ganz et al found that sexual functioning was worse for women who received chemotherapy than for those who did not, regardless of the type of surgery.[62] Other factors associated with problems in sexual functioning are vaginal dryness, emotional well-being, body image, and the quality of the partnered relationship.[60,70] Ganz et al found that sexual activity declined from 65% of patients at baseline to 55% an average of 6.3 years later.[37] While exploring sexual dysfunction in breast cancer survivors, Bukovic et al found 70% or more patients rated their sex lives as satisfying before cancer, but satisfaction dropped to 56% among patients with advanced disease and to 50% among early stage breast cancer patients after treatment.[69] Sexual functioning was a greater problem than lack of sexual interest in a study by Avis et al.[71] Carter et al found 67% of 20 gynecology cancer patients reporting dissatisfaction with their sex lives, and 56% reporting low levels of sexual desire.[23] Some improvement in problems of poor body image and sexuality may come with the benefits of physical activity. Regular exercisers reported higher body esteem and more positive attitudes towards their sexual attractiveness than sedentary breast cancer survivors.[53] Ganz et al found that a comprehensive menopausal assessment, education, and counseling intervention helped breast cancer survivors improve symptoms and sexual functioning.[72]

Sexual function among men may decline following primary treatment for localized prostate cancer.[73] Erectile dysfunction before treatment was reported by 31% of prostatectomy patients and by 40% of radiotherapy patients. At the 5-year follow-up these percentages were 88% dysfunction among the prostatectomy patients and 64% among the radiotherapy patients.[73] Physical activity was positively correlated with sexual functioning for men treated with external beam radiotherapy for prostate cancer.[74] In this cross-sectional study, the relationships among physical activity, sexual functioning, and treatment type were evaluated among 111 men who had undergone radiotherapy for localized prostate cancer. After statistically controlling for age, medical comorbidity, fatigue, and urinary and bowel functioning, more physical activity was significantly associated with better sexual functioning.[74] Overall, 35% of the variance in sexual functioning was accounted for by the model. The effect of physical activity on sexual function after brachytherapy and combination therapy was nonsignificant. The men who underwent external beam radiotherapy in this study had significantly greater sexual functioning scores as their physical activity increased.[74]

Problems with body image and sexuality following BMT have been tracked for survivors of multiple myeloma, breast cancer, leukemia, and other diagnoses. In three studies, about 33% of patients were found to have problems with sexual activity. Among patients treated for multiple myeloma, 34% reported disrupted sexual functioning and difficulty with body image.[30] McQuellon et al found 33% of the breast cancer patients followed pre and post treatment had problems with appearance and intimate relations, with 30% having problems with sexuality.[75] Hayden et al found 33% of leukemia survivors indicating decreased sexual functioning.[76] Sexual dissatisfaction was less of a problem in two other studies. Wingard et al[77] found 22% and Chao et al[78] found 14% sexual dissatisfaction reported, respectively, among survivors of bone marrow transplant. Addressing issues around sexual dysfunction remains a continuing challenge.

Psychosocial Issues

Mourning the loss from cancer treatment, compensating for lost function, and maximizing other potentials is the adaptive task described by Mages and Mendelsohn for maintaining a sense of self-esteem and intactness.[19] These are personal tasks, which can seem overwhelming for isolated patients or those needing professional guidance and social support.

Cognitive changes after cancer treatment are troubling for patients. In follow-up visits patients mention problems with "forgetfulness." Meyers writes that cognitive problems are underreported by patients and under diagnosed by healthcare professionals.[79] The incidence of cognitive problems after standard dose chemotherapy has been estimated as 17 to 20%, but this figure may be low.[79] In a review of 28 studies (1000 patients) showing cognitive deficits from chemotherapy, Welzel et al found that 44% treated with either chemotherapy or radiation therapy had cognitive problems after treatment, while 65% of patients treated with both radiation and chemotherapy reported cognitive problems.[80] Comparing survivors with noncancer controls, Tchen et al found that cognitive impairment was greater in the patient group.[81]

Current research promises to specify which parts of memory or cognitive processes are most at risk. In a study by Castellon et al breast cancer patients who completed chemotherapy had greater problems in verbal learning, vision-spatial functioning, and visual memory than those receiving surgery only.[82] Rausch found that breast cancer patients receiving hormone treatment showed four areas of problems with memory (4/18), while patients receiving chemotherapy experienced more areas of difficulty (14/18).[83] New studies in progress use MRI scanning techniques along with cognitive testing.[83] Results will specify the patterns of memory complaints that patients experience. Determining patterns may direct us to more effective interventions. Current interventions for the treatment of cognitive deficits include pharmacological management, behavioral strategies, lifestyle alterations, formal rehabilitation, and counseling. Pharmacological treatment, such as stimulants, can alleviate problems with concentration, psychomotor slowing, fatigue, and improve mood.[79] Cognitive therapy, education and support groups have also been helpful in providing resources that instruct and reassure patients that their experiences are not unusual.

Maintaining emotional equilibrium is a challenge for many patients recovering from treatment. Patients report symptoms of distress, depression and mood swings following diagnosis and at many points along the disease continuum. A third or more of patients report psychological distress during the early months of treatment.[84-86] Clinical depression affects around 18% to 20% of Hodgkin's survivors at various points in time.[27] Bodurka et al found that 21% of their patients met the criteria for depression, similar to results found by others.[85] Researchers have also found that some survivors have a tougher time when their diagnosis is debilitat-

ing.[85,86] Carter et al[23] found 40% of the gynecologic cancer patients suffered from depression. Pelletier et al[89] found 38% of the brain tumor patients depressed. Bukberg et al[90] and Lynch[91] found 45% depressed patients among those with advanced disease.

Psychological interventions have helped to improve mood. Depressive symptoms resulting from cancer often improve with time.[92,93,37] Yet, subgroups of survivors remain vulnerable to distress and/or depression. Patients with many types of cancer have found psychological benefit in participating in support groups.[94-97] Metastatic breast cancer patients who participated in the supportive-expressive group therapy reduced anxiety and depression, improved coping and reduced pain compared with those in the control group.[96] Classen et al found that supportive-expressive group therapy, with its emphasis on providing support and helping patients face and deal with their disease-related stress, reduced distress in patients.[98] Patients find help for depressive thoughts when they express their negative feelings, and enjoy the acknowledgment of problems and social support within a group.[99] Cordova et al found that expression of negative feelings and an attitude of realistic optimism reduced distress among survivors.[100] Levine et al found that group support was more helpful in reducing posttraumatic distress than complementary alternative interventions.[101]

In studies with cancer patients,[102-104] active coping was associated with fewer problems and less distress. Behavioral therapy has been found helpful as an intervention for patients with cancer.[105] Uitterhoeve et al conducted a review of randomized intervention studies from 1990 to 2002.[103] A total of 12 out of 13 trials evaluating behavioral therapy found positive results on one or more indicators of quality of life, such as depression.[104] In a study that compared the use of imagery with group support, Richardson et al found that imagery reduced stress and improved quality of life, while imagery and group support together improved coping, attitudes, and perception of support.[106] In a study of support-group attendance, Cameron et al found that 49% of the 110 invited women joined and participated, particularly those with stronger beliefs that the cancer was caused by altered immunity. Younger women especially had higher cancer-related distress, and lower avoidance tendencies.[107] Other sources of help for persistent mood problems include journal writing, physical activity, tai chi, chi-gong, nutrition, and prescription medications.

Complementary and alternative therapy (CAM) programs provide a sense of inner control to survivors throughout the world. Recent surveys have described survivor preferences for CAM. In the United States, the percent of survivors interested in CAM ranged from 48% to 91%.[108-112] Internationally, survivor interest was highest in China (98%),[113] but in most other countries it was generally lower, 17% to 50%.[114-120] A variety of CAM programs have been developed in community settings. A survey in Florida found that exercise, vitamins, prayer/spiritual practice, support groups, humor, self-help books, and relaxation were frequently mentioned.[121] In a California hospital massage, yoga, and qigong classes had the highest number of participants.[122] These program choices are reflected in the other studies mentioned above.

When survivors are asked why they use CAM, participants frequently say they want, "to feel more in control" and "to enhance their immune system."[110,112] Women use CAM more often than men, for example 81.5% versus 59% in

Seattle, and chose different categories of alternative providers that reflected their psychological needs.[110] Is CAM cost-effective? There is recent evidence that a self-administered stress management technique for chemotherapy patients was cost-effective when compared with usual care.[123] While not exactly CAM, many CAM therapies reflect self-management strategies and are low cost.

Relationships

Interpersonal relationships, a challenge for people throughout life, are often more vulnerable following a cancer diagnosis. The subtle task of communicating feelings and the changes in life that result from cancer, presents new challenges for everyone- patients, family and friends. Mages et al write about this issue in terms of the patient's need to maintain continuity in life following acute phases of the illness.[56] In their study, patients reported that they had been changed by the experience of cancer and had developed new attitudes towards time, mortality, work, personal relationships, and priorities in life. "The adaptive task is to understand and communicate one's changed attitudes, needs, and limitations in a way that permits formation of a new balance with the environment."[19] Several scenarios threaten to change the communication patterns among family and friends. The patient may feel isolated by the news of the diagnosis. While the spouse or family member remains helpful and attentive, the patient may feel that "they just don't get it!" Patients feel "wounded," separated from others after hearing they have a malignant disease. They recognize that their life will never be quite the same again. Some partners pull away or distance themselves from the patient leading to new problems in the relationship. In a study of 763 disease-free breast cancer survivors Ganz et al found that follow-up interviews showed a decline in sexual functioning between the two assessments, from 65% to 55% ($p = 0.001$), as well as a decline in the quality of the partnered relationship.[37] Though the decline may be age related rather than cancer related change, survivors and partners might find the loss troubling.

The more severe and visible the disability from cancer, the greater the challenge for communication between partners. In a study of 110 head and neck patients, deBoer et al found that a higher percentage of laryngectomy patients still experienced severe psychosocial distress 2 to 6 years after their last treatment.[124] The patients indicated that ineffective communication with others was a problem. Family support was the most important resource among laryngectomy patients after surgical treatment.[125] Open discussion with families was a predictor of positive outcome. Wimberly et al found that, "partner initiation of sex predicted greater marital satisfaction" among breast cancer survivors.[126] Partner adverse reaction to the scar predicted less marital satisfaction. In studies of recently treated breast cancer patients Ganz et al and Fobair et al found that the partner's difficulty in understanding the patient was associated with patients reporting sexual problems after treatment.[60,70] We can better understand communication challenges for cancer survivors and their partners when we consider that spouses experience mood changes following their partner's diagnosis. Northouse et al found that there is a high degree of correspondence between the levels of adjustment reported by women with breast cancer and their husbands.[127–130]

Depression can overtake the whole family. Spouses and family members experience distress and depression as a result of the patient's cancer, sometimes at higher levels than the patient. Cliff and MacDonagh studied 135 patients with prostate cancer and their partners[131] and found some degree of general cancer distress in 47% of patients and 76% of partners. However, severe distress was detected in only 11% of patients and 30% of partners. In their study, general cancer distress was highly prevalent and more severe in partners than in patients.[131]

When compared to couples adjusting to benign breast disease,[128] couples facing breast cancer reported greater decreases in their marital and family functioning, more uncertain appraisals of their situation, and more adjustment problems associated with the illness. Northouse et al found that spouses tended to regard a colon cancer diagnosis more negatively than did the patients.[129] Tuninstra et al found that women patients expressed more distress than men did prior to colon cancer surgery.[132] Three and six months later the women continued to express more distress than the men, regardless of being the patient or the spouse.[132] Women, whether patients or partners may have greater distress within a couple.

Some couples become closer after breast cancer. Dorval et al found that 42% of 282 couples said breast cancer brought them closer.[133] When the spouse found the patient confident, received advice from her in the first two weeks about coping with breast cancer, accompanied her to surgery, and provided more affection at three months since her diagnosis, both partners agreed that the disease brought them closer.[133] Spouses affect each other's adjustment over time, Northouse et al found.[130] Husbands' and wives' levels of adjustment at 1 year had a significant direct effect on each other's adjustment.[130] In order to test whether a psychoeducational support group for partners would be effective in improving mood, Bultz et al had 36 partners participate in a randomized controlled trial of a brief psychoeducational group program for partners only.[134] Three months after the intervention, partners had less mood disturbance than did controls. Patients whose partners received the intervention reported less mood disturbance, greater confidant support, and greater marital satisfaction.[134]

Social support takes on new meaning after cancer. Neuling and Winefield found that satisfaction with the quality of the patient's social support was matched with measures of adjustment.[135] Those patients who were satisfied with support from family members were significantly less anxious and depressed in the hospital than those who were not satisfied. The importance of social support cannot be overstated. Bloom et al found that patients' psychological well-being was related to the size and the integration of their social network.[137] Having a large integrated network of social ties has direct effects on the patient's mood and outlook in life.[137] Each result suggests that an intervention offering couples support and education provides further opportunities for them to communicate their changed attitudes, needs and limitations.

This intervention has been helpful to couples when additional education is not sufficient to improve a domestic situation. Johnson and Talitman offer emotionally focused marital therapy to help couples dealing with posttraumatic stress.[138] This is a fresh approach to couples with cancer in the family. Emotionally focused marital therapy concentrates on the creation of secure attachment.[139] An attachment injury occurs when one partner violates the expectation that the other will offer comfort and caring in times of danger or distress. Stories from men and women with cancer detail disappointments with spouses who fail to communicate their concern or withdraw from the patient following diagnosis or treatment. The injurious incident defines the relationship as insecure and maintains relationship distress because it is continually used as a standard for the dependability of the offending partner.[140] Johnson and Talitman found that among the couples dealing with trauma, the female partner's trust, her faith in her husband predicted the couples' satisfaction at follow-up.[138] A female's faith in her husband also significantly predicted the males' level of intimacy at follow-up. When wives showed trust and faith in their husbands, husbands were more comfortable with physical intimacy in the relationship. Interventions that encourage emotional self-disclosure and interpersonal trust may be specifically helpful for cancer patients following treatment.

Work Roles and Employment

Work and career are an important part of the adult life in western culture. Continuity in work roles is frequently challenged by cancer treatment. Research covering employment issues finds anywhere from 30% to 90% of patients returning to work.[141–147] Survivors who returned to full-time work were more likely to report a positive view of their body image, better energy and mood and more ambition.[147] Nevertheless, employment problems also emerge as some patients have less capacity for strenuous activity. They experience greater fatigue and are less able to enjoy leisure time activities.[148] Problems also include having difficulty in getting promotions or communicating comfortably with one's employer.[27] Comparing healthy individuals with patients treated for Hodgkin's disease, van Tulder et al found that Hodgkin's patients reported more restrictions in their role functioning in work and daily activities than the norms.[41] Hays et al found few differences between childhood survivors of cancer and matched controls in patterns of employment, but entry into the uniformed services was barred for patients, and there was difficulty in getting life insurance in the first years following treatment.[150]

Some survivors have trouble returning to work. Gruber et al reported that 31% of their patients were not able to return to work.[142] Nordstron et al found that among the 47% patients working less than full-time, some survivors returned to work only to find that their working conditions had changed.[146] Weis et al had a similar result. They found that 33% of the patients returned to work but reduced their working time or changed their job.[145] Examining patients "not employed" Fobair et al found that women outnumbered men (76 women, 41 men) and that more than a third of the women were housewives.[148,29]

Predictors of returning to employment in the Stanford study of Hodgkin's survivors were having positive co-worker support, gender (men), feeling less depressed, and a positive sense of one's body image.[147] Employment problems were more likely among those with more advanced disease at diag-nosis, more current fatigue, poor body image, less physical activity, and more severe emotional distress. Further discussion on employment issues appears in Chapter 20.

Existential Issues

Reexamining one's life choices and the meaning in one's life are important tasks for survivors of cancer. Following treatment many survivors reexamine their values and meaning in life.[152,153] In reordering personal values and priorities, some reaffirm their current life; others decide to make changes in areas of life involving stress. Many survivors find spirituality a source of comfort.

Spirituality and personal growth are quality of life issues in the psychosocial literature. Brady et al examined a large ethnically diverse sample and found a significant association between spirituality and quality of life.[153] Finding positive meaning (i.e. life purpose and coherence) in one's life has been correlated with better mood and less distress, which are both mental health aspects of quality of life.[154] A negative meaning in illness is correlated to higher levels of depression and poorer quality of life.[155] Sarna et al found that depressed mood, negative views of the meaning of life, and younger age all correlated with poorer physical, psychological, and social dimensions of quality of life in women with lung cancer.[88] Spiritual correlates of functional well-being have been found in women with breast cancer.[156] Study results confirmed the importance of spirituality and spiritual well-being with physical and functional well-being.

Severe physical challenges can lead to personal growth. When stem cell patients were compared with healthy controls they may have had poorer physical functioning, but the survivors showed greater psychological and interpersonal growth.[157] In a study of after cancer survivorship Dow et al found nine important themes: the struggle between independence and dependence, balance, wholeness, life purpose, reclaiming life, coping with multiple losses, having control, altered meaning of health, and surviving cancer from a family perspective.[158]

A spiritual disequalibrium may result when survivors are overwhelmed by fear of dying and a sense of isolation from the struggle to maintain one's self-identity after cancer.[159] In a small qualitative study of newly diagnosed breast cancer patients, Coward and Kahn found that solving spiritual disequilibria meant restoring a sense of connection to self, others, and/or a higher power, as well as regaining a positive self-identity.[159]

Coping with Advanced Disease

When primary treatment fails and metastatic disease is discovered, the survivors' landscape changes dramatically. The issues become: coping with new physical symptoms, treatment, pain, and progressive infirmity. While there can be hope for an extended remission, and periods of comfortable and productive life, the imminent life threat changes the survivor's world.[19] The challenge of maintaining self-sufficiency and control over one's life is a persistent problem. The sense of failure of one's effort and the efforts of physicians to thwart progressive disease threatens survivors with hopeless/help-less feelings. The challenge will be not to succumb to fear, despair, and passivity. The desire to control the impact of cancer on career, intimate relationships, and bodily functions poses additional problems. The adaptive task is to exercise choice where possible and to accept one's helplessness and dependence when necessary without excessive regression or turning to a magical solution in lieu of appropriate treatment.[19]

Mages et al interviewed two samples of patients: one soon after treatment and a second group three to five years after treatment.[56] In the first group, those bearing up with advanced disease were found to have fatigue, pain and physical symptoms. They were somewhat fearful, depressed and pessimistic. They sought to maintain their sense of self-sufficiency, and were undemanding. They enjoyed their family and friends, and some gained support from their religion and from the hospital services. In the second group, the patients bearing up with advanced disease had come to terms with the illness. They talked about having some pain and physical disability, but they remained independent and active, and maintained their family and social contacts.[56] When Oh et al studied breast cancer survivors following a recurrence and compared their responses with a matched sample of women free of disease, they found the women with recurrence reported a good mood, low stress, and good quality of interpersonal relationships. But they also reported higher cancer-specific stress.[160] The women with a recurrence also reported experiencing both more meaning in their lives and vulnerability as a result of breast cancer.[160] In 1999, Houck et al found that patients with advanced disease reported fatigue (100%) and anorexia (55%).[161] Patients with advanced cancer may experience weight loss, reduced appetite, fatigue and weakness. Chronic nausea and early satiety may also occur along with pain.[162] Recognizing the importance of helping patients with advanced cancer, Uitterhoeve et al reviewed the literature to determine which psychosocial interventions could be effective in improving quality of life, especially in emotional functioning.[104] They found that behavioral therapy had positive effects on one or more indicators of quality of life, such as depression.[104]

Confronting Issues and Feelings About Death

Survivors' fear of recurrence and progressive disease is most prominent in the early months and years after cancer. Though in the majority of cases, primary treatment succeeds in elim-inating detectable disease, the fear of recurrence can be acti-vated before follow-up visits or when new symptoms appear. In order to live with this fear, it is helpful to be able to put it out of mind most of the time, to continue with medical follow-ups and to take one's reality into consideration when making long range plans.[19] The challenges of coping with per-sistent or recurrent disease include maintaining one's self-suf-ficiency and control over choices in life and actively coping with feelings of hopeless or helplessness. A sense of power-lessness threatens to intrude when patients think that they have failed or that their physicians have failed them. It is important to help survivors facing persistent disease to main-tain control over their own choices and decisions as they cope with the medical, career, and family issues in front of them.

Terminal illness confronts the patient and his family with the challenge of accepting the reality to come. It is helpful when patients can work with medical assistance to find the inter-nal resources to minimize pain. Patients are challenged to retain as much self-sufficiency and personal dignity as possi-ble in facing the need to prepare to leave one's family and friends. Ideally, the terminally ill survivor faces the prospect of death without excessive denial so that the remainder of life can be lived as well as possible.[19] In a qualitative study of 12 terminally ill women on home hospice care Grumann and Spiegel found that all subjects reported thinking about their death.[163] Half of them were comfortable with their thoughts and half were troubled with thoughts of unresolved issues. The second group had higher anxiety, pain and fatigue. A majority of the 12 women wanted to talk about their impend-ing death. This finding suggests a need to offer opportunities for patients to discuss these unresolved concerns.

How Does Oncology Social Work Help?

The oncology social worker's primary goal is to help people in need and to address social problems. What do oncology social workers do to provide these services? Some of the means that oncology social workers use to provide services to survivors are summarized here: Being available, case finding with staff, locating patients "in distress" through dis-cussion with professional team members, offering support group interventions and educational forums, staying tuned to professional staff as they see "new" and "follow-up" patients, and participating in tumor board discussions.

Being There

Social workers help by "being available" when cancer patients want to talk. Being available when survivors need to talk lowers their distress. Many survivors need to talk about the stunning news of having a cancer diagnosis. It feels like a "death sentence." They feel out of control. They feel com-forted when there is someone to talk with about treatment decisions and the changes in their lives. Feeling less alone with fear, anger, and other negative feelings, survivors find more energy to work on other problems. Oncology social workers look for opportunities to share with survivors their knowledge of the emotional impact of cancer, to introduce them to other survivors who have been through the process, and to reassure them that they (the oncology social workers) will be there for the patients as they move through the treat-ment plan. Survivors benefit from interactions with oncology social workers when they recognize that their problems have been treated with dignity and their worth as a person has been reinforced.

Being the Point Person

Oncology social workers help by being the "point person" assigned by the survivor and healthcare team to assist them in managing the crises of the cancer experience.[164] Crises come up at the beginning with "news of the diagnosis," when healthcare professionals tell the patient sensitive information over the telephone rather than in person; when there is confusion over the medical decision making; when family members take too active a role on behalf of the patient; and when assistance is needed for housing or transportation to the medical facility. Sometimes recent survivors need someone outside the family to talk with about the social and emotional impact of cancer in their lives, and the rapid-fire events, "two weeks ago, I noticed a lump," that brought them to treatment. Being in treatment offers moments of crises for patients, communication problems with staff, grief in acknowledging the "life threatening" aspects of the diagnosis, problems with family insensitivity, additional needs for tangible assistance. One needs support after treatment too. "What will I do now without the support of the healthcare team?" the patient may ask. Referrals to support groups can be of particular assistance as patients finish therapy and require new sources of continuity.

Advocating for Patient

Social workers often advocate for cancer survivors and families in order to assist them in securing their rights under existing laws, and help them get the public funds and other benefits they may have been denied.[164] By supporting their cause, speaking in their favor, or pleading their case with agencies, oncology social workers become the patient's ally. This empowers patients to also act on their own behalf whenever possible. Teaching the patient or family member how to advocate for themselves in the healthcare system and in the community empowers patients and family members to cope with problems that threaten their sense of being in control.

Providing Tangible Resources

The need for cancer treatment often triggers a chain of unwished for problems, such as a sudden need for additional funds, transportation to a hospital, or securing housing for the out-of-town patient. The oncology social worker finds the resources to assist with particular needs, and contacts the hospital or community agencies that offer support for patient care. In one study, 35% of the patients came from outside the local area and required short-term housing.[165] Out-of-town patients often required help with other pressing issues such as the anxiety triggered by the diagnosis, the need to talk with others like them, the need for group support and leisure activities. Some oncology social workers excel in finding financial resources to assist survivors with particular needs. One colleague raised funds to send an international patient's family home to Sri Lanka.[165]

Helping the Survivor Cope with Employment Problems

Disruptions at work and getting worker's benefits during medical leave are common problems. Legal regulations that support working cancer patients have improved since the 1970s. Many employers are supportive of their cancer patient employees, and provide benefits and time off. Yet, some employers are less helpful to their working cancer survivors. Smaller companies, and those struggling to stay financially afloat have a harder time accommodating the survivor. Social workers can be effective in obtaining benefits and services for survivors by personally calling the company or insurance carrier involved, or going to the Social Security appeals board

with the survivor. If the survivor has an advocate the employer may become more helpful. If making a telephone contact is insufficient to stimulate an employer to provide legal benefits, showing up in behalf of the survivor or finding a public agency lawyer who will take your client's case can succeed.

Teaching Survivors to Be Assertive when Necessary

Many patients have difficulty describing their complaints to physicians or other health professionals. Oncology social workers can be helpful by coaching overwhelmed patients to be assertive. When patients are effective in speaking up and getting the assistance they need, they regain a feeling of control. Sometimes patients are effective in obtaining entitlements when they refuse to leave the office until their right to the benefit has been acknowledged. Telling survivors stories of prior experiences with others can be helpful.

Providing a Safe Place to Talk About Emotional Issues

The social worker's office is a refuge where patients can express their emotions and distress about having cancer. Very often patients need to talk about the shock and disruption cancer causes in their lives with someone other than family, as the cancer has disrupted their role in the family. With the social worker patients can plan or role-play what they wish to say to family members or to their physician.

Discussing Interpersonal Issues

Recognizing the central importance of human relationships, oncology social workers respond positively to requests from survivors to talk about interpersonal conflicts. Such discussions may involve the disclosure of intimate communication problems within the family or work force. Recognizing that cancer can challenge one's interpersonal skills, oncology social workers are not surprised when distress from cancer stimulates the need to talk about former or current family experiences, values, priorities or conflicts. Changes in sexual functioning and partner misunderstanding are topics that frequently emerge in individual and group support meetings and within the couples' groups.

Helping Patients Cope with the Issues of "Life After Treatment"

Survivors frequently drop into the oncology social worker's office on follow-up visits with their physician. Recovery issues—energy loss, fatigue, body image and sexual changes, cognitive changes, emotional mood swings, employee concerns, communication shifts in personal relationships, and changes in one's view of life—are of concern to patients who visit the oncology social worker. While emotional support is always helpful in response to a survivor's discussion of problems, providing new information offers something hopeful for the survivor as well. Social workers can stay abreast of the latest research updates with the use of the Internet and offer the latest information to patients during their visit. Referring patients to support groups offers them an opportunity to learn from each other.

Offering Group Support

Moments of clarity, identification, and connection that come with storytelling are part of the emotional healing that group therapies offer cancer survivors. Groups offer a safe place to talk about emotional issues and provide a process that helps return survivors to a sense of inner control. Survivors learn from each other. They soak up the positive energy group members offers each other. Groups can be educational or counseling focused. Groups offer survivors a place to talk with others facing similar challenges in life. Topics in group discussion include coping with negative feelings, feelings of being out of control, exploring one's desire to minimize or escape from overwhelming feelings, and solving problems through facing and coping with difficult issues. Survivors often need to talk about changes in their lives with others going through similar experiences.[95,166,100,167,168,169] They share with each other their altered sense of life and mortality, and talk about new ways of caring for themselves.[170]

Group participation is an intervention that contributes to better mood and active coping in decisions.[95,97,100,171,172] Survivors come into a group feeling distressed about having cancer and the need for treatment. When treatment is an issue, the group encourages members to seek more information. Survivors find satisfaction in assuming greater responsibility for their choices. Group members move from feeling "out of control" to choosing how they are going to handle the issues in front of them. They move from "right/wrong, all or nothing" reasoning, and seek a broader perspective with several alternatives. Group members become more self-confident, comfortable in sharing themselves, and enjoy the group process. Participating in a group has the positive effect of moving participants toward self-actualization.[173]

Reconnect Patients with Their Community

Oncology social workers encourage patients be their own advocates in the healthcare system and in other community agencies. They encourage patients to get transportation assistance through the American Cancer Society or the Red Cross and to join survivorship organizations, such as the National Coalition for Cancer Survivorship, or the Lance Armstrong Foundation. After treatment, some survivors will "want to give back" by becoming drivers for the American Cancer Society or the Red Cross, or as fund raisers for cancer research or for agencies that bring attention to the needs of survivors.

Helping Survivors and Their Families with the Issues of Recurrent Disease

Oncology social workers help patients cope with recurrent disease by encouraging them to have a hopeful attitude, by working closely with their healthcare team, and by supporting them as they choose helpful treatment. Patients with recurrent disease may want to talk about reprioritizing what is most important in their lives, or how to maintain an acceptable quality of life at home during treatment. When survivors discuss their difficulties with depression, weight loss, pain or anorexia, the oncology social worker's task becomes supporting the survivor in accepting home-based supportive services.

Helping Survivors Cope with the Issues in Terminal Illness and End-of-Life Care

Oncology social workers help terminally ill patients and their families to arrange the end-of-life care that they desire, and to offer family members support during the early months of their bereavement. There may be further choices to be made about medical care, or about additional care in the home. Sometimes family communication problems arise creating a need for the patient's or family member's acceptance and forgiveness, a need made more pressing by the pending death of the patient. Saying "goodbye" is difficult and bittersweet task, and oncology social workers can often be helpful here.

When the Oncology Social Worker Is the Survivor

Hester Hill Schnipper and I are going to tell you what it was like for us, how we coped, what we learned, and how we relate to our fellow survivors and colleagues.

What it was like for me? A social worker for 20 years in the San Francisco Bay Area, I was diagnosed with breast cancer at age 53 in 1987. Emotionally unprepared for what it felt like to have a "life threat," I was flooded with feelings of anxiety and moments of panic. I felt as if I was floating in a surrealistic space. My empathy for other survivors hadn't prepared me for the personal experience of being the patient. There was a Grand Canyon between the difference in clinical empathy and the new feelings of being emotionally "out of control" as a patient. Perhaps the chasm between roles can't be avoided. As a clinical worker I hadn't yet faced the possibility of my own death. Now, directly facing "survival," negative feelings hit me with the power of a fire hose turned on full blast.

On the surface, I coped with being a patient by organizing my home life and returning to work. I became aware of an internal "life force" that gave me a determination to live, if possible. I knew that treatment might not overwhelm the disease, but I was going to do everything I could to help that happen. My biggest challenge was coping with my emotional world. Unable to remain objective, I had troubling personal thoughts. Cancer felt like a negative judgment. There were moments of clarity, but I often felt exposed in interpersonal situations. I had trouble handling the awkward remarks of well wishers.

My physical energy and emotional health could no longer be taken for granted. I had to limit my scope of outside activities; say "no" to certain events. I had to intentionally learn to look after my emotional health. When, I felt moments of panic or feelings of being "out of control," I taught myself to discover, "the problem" that had tipped the balance. By acknowledging that I had a problem, then noticing the feeling that went with it such as, "grief" "sadness" "anxiety," I wasn't as apt to feel out of control. Sometimes, I resorted to negative coping like feelings of being "helpless." Eventually, I taught myself to counter-argue, "Only children are helpless." Finding solutions to the daily problems of being a survivor helped me feel "okay," again.

What lessons did I learn? Gratitude and forgiveness are more important to mental health than I realized. I was grateful for the help that came my way, often from unexpected places. I had a need to forgive others and myself after troubling interactions. I felt a new appreciation for the physician's capacity to comfort, and a fresh appreciation for the field of medicine. Hester's husband, Lowell E Schnipper, MD, a medical oncology specialist at Harvard, wrote some pertinent comments, which are included in the foreword to her book, *After Breast Cancer: A Common Sense Guide to Life After Treatment.*[174] He understood this reciprocal role of doctor and patient when he wrote,

The moment a woman hears a diagnosis of breast cancer, her world is forever different. Initially stunned to the point of numbness, she gradually finds an equilibrium that enables her to wind her way through a complex process. . . . While that process is all-consuming, the help of a surgical and medical oncologist offers most women a structure of relationships that conveys a sense of security, if not well-being.

As I saw my internal process with fresh insight, a new camaraderie with other survivors became a part of my world. It came from the personal knowledge of the tougher issues we had been through in facing mortality. As one of Lowell Schnipper's patients said,

To dance with death, to weep over it, to rage at it, even to laugh at it, brings a kind of resolution, an encounter with mortality that is truly a life-changing event.[174]

When it came time to retire in 2003, I found a way to retain the best part of my working week, the group support activities. The happiest part of my former work schedule is now the best part of my week.

Hester Hill Schnipper is the Chief Oncology Social Worker at Beth Israel Deaconess Medical Center in Boston. In her book, *After Breast Cancer: A Common Sense Guide to Life After Treatment*, she writes about how she coped, what she learned, and addresses her fellow patients and colleagues:

The diagnosis of breast cancer brought me to my knees. The first, the very first lesson for me was that I knew nothing about what it was really like to have breast cancer. . . . Mainly, there was no way to prepare for the feelings. I was overwhelmed with terror and grief and anger. I literally did not know where to put those emotions.

She went back to work while still in treatment, and worried that her fear and sadness might get in the way at work. Would she be as comforting or as helpful as patients needed, "when my own heart was pounding my own soul was trembling"? She found her answer in watching the patients and their relatives and "realized that I was surrounded by lessons in how to live with fear and sadness."

When Hester finished treatment she learned a second lesson, that "the crisis of diagnosis and the difficult months of physical treatment are almost the easy part. The real challenge comes with living with breast cancer. It is clear that the goal must be to live as though the cancer will never return. . . . The issues of survivorship must be appreciated for what they are: the fruits of pain and the rewards of living." Her book is intended to offer support in coping with the physical and psychological difficulties of living with cancer.

Hester writes this about her relationships with colleagues and survivors:

My style with my patients had always been one of relatively few rigid boundaries and of shared human relationships, but my own diagnosis of cancer shattered any lingering wall between us and set up a new paradigm of truly working together. . . . My own vision gradually expanded to include a life lived in parallel: therapist and patient, caregiver and care recipient. My strongest alliances shifted to stand with my patients rather than with my professional colleagues. I live a double life.

The power of symbols and of the shared connection between survivors with each other can be glimpsed in Hester's description of a basket of rocks and shells in her office. Survivors contribute stones as they return from trips around the world. Hester offers the women beginning their journey to select something from the basket to keep with them as special totem and shared good wishes. The ideas in her book represent the rocks of experiences learned from women and passed along to others.[175]

Closing Thoughts

The world of cancer survivorship has been articulated in ever expanding waves of experience and research since the 1970s. The field of psychosocial oncology was created in response to our need to know more about the quality of life of cancer survivors. Oncology social workers team up with other healthcare providers to help survivors through the acute experiences of discovery, treatment, advanced disease and, if needed, through the end of life. The oncology social worker's task remains "being there" for patients in his/her domain in order to prevent as much as can be the negative effects of being "alone" or "unsupported."

As survivors, we may not be able to avoid a cancer diagnosis, but we do have the ability to learn about treatment and its consequences, and to benefit by making choices to minimize our losses.

References

1. Morra ME. Patients as citizen advocates. Cancer Pract. 1997; 5(1):55–57.
2. O'Shea JS. The power of social change: the Women's Movement and breast cancer. Breast J. 2003;9(5):347–349.
3. Sharf BF. Out of the closet and into the legislature: breast cancer stories. Health Aff (Millwood). 2001;20(1):213–218.
4. Trillin AS. Of dragons and garden peas: a cancer patient talks to doctors. N Engl J Med. 1981;304(12):699–701.
5. Mullan F. Seasons of survival: reflections of a physician with cancer. N Engl J Med. 1985;313(4):270–273.
6. Holland JC. History of psycho-oncology: overcoming attitudinal and conceptual barriers. Psychosom Med. 2002;64(2):206–221.
7. Abrams RD. Not Alone with Cancer: A Guide for Those Who Care, What to Expect, What to Do. Springfield, Ill: Charles C. Thomas, 1974.
8. Association of Oncology Social Workers. Standards of Practice in Oncology Social Work. web site: Auailable at www.aosw.org/mission/standards.html. Accessed July 15, 2005.
9. Hermann JF, Carter J. The dimensions of oncology social work: intrapsychic, interpersonal, and environmental interventions. Semin Oncol. 1994;21(6):712–717.
10. Cannon IM. Social Work in Hospitals: Contribution to Progressive Medicine. 2nd ed. New York: Russell Sage Foundation; 1923.
11. Mullan F. National Coalition of Cancer Survivorship. Albuequerque, New Mexico, 1986 (http://www.canceradvocacy.org).
12. Fobair P. "Surviving!" Magazine. 1–20; 1983–2003:1–16.
13. Coping Magazine. 1–20; 1985–2005.
14. Office of Cancer Survivorship CCPS, Cancer Control & Population Sciences. National Cancer Institute; 2005.
15. Armstrong L. Lance Armstrong Foundation. Austin, Texas; 2005.
16. Aziz NM, Rowland JH. Trends and advances in cancer survivorship research: challenge and opportunity. Semin Radiat Oncol. 2003;13(3):248–266.
17. Bettelheim B. San Francisco Chronicle; 1981.

18. Fobair, P. Turning the switch. Surviving Magazine. 1988; (Winter):3.

19. Mages NL, Mendelsohn GA. Effects of cancer on patients' lives: a personological approach. GC Stone, F Cohen, NE Adler et al. Health Psychology—A Handbook. San Francisco: Jossey-Bass, Inc.; 1979:255–284.

20. Flatten G, Junger S, Gunkel S, Singh J, Petzold E. Traumatic and psychosocial distress in patients with acute tumors. Psychother Psychosom Med Psychol. 2003;53(3–4):191–201.

21. Zabora J, Brintzenhofe Szoc K, Curbow B, Hooker C, Piantadosi S. The prevalence of psychological distress by cancer site. Psychooncology. 2001;10(1):19–28.

22. Faller H, Olshausen B, Flentje M. Emotional distress and needs for psychosocial support among breast cancer patients at start of radiotherapy. Psychother Psychosom Med Psychol. 2003; 53(5):229–235.

23. Carter J, Rowland K, Chi D, et al. Gynecologic cancer treatment and the impact of cancer related infertility. Gynecol Oncol. 2005;97(1):90–95.

24. Courneya KS, Friedenreich CM, Quinney HA, et al. A longitudinal study of exercise barriers in colorectal cancer survivors participating in a randomized controlled trial. Ann Behav Med. 2005;29(2):147–153.

25. Goodwin PJ, Leszcz M, Ennis M, et al. The effect of group psychosocial support on survival in metastatic breast cancer. N Engl J Med. 2001;345(24):1719–1726.

26. Hewitt M, Rowland JH, Yancik R. Cancer survivors in the United States: age, health, and disability. J Gerontol A Biol Sci Med Sci. 2003;58(1):82–91.

27. Fobair P, Hoppe RT, Bloom J, Cox R, Varghese A, Spiegel D. Psychosocial problems among survivors of Hodgkin's disease. J Clin Oncol. 1986;4(5):805–814.

28. Lutgendorf SK, Anderson B, Rothrock N, Buller RE, Sood AK, Sorosky JI. Quality of life and mood in women receiving extensive chemotherapy for gynecologic cancer. Cancer. 2000;89(6): 1402–1411.

29. Sherman AC, Coleman EA, Griffith K, et al. Use of a supportive care team for screening and preemptive intervention among multiple myeloma patients receiving stem cell transplantation. Support Care Cancer. 2003;11(9):568–574.

30. Sherman AC, Simonton S, Latif U, Spohn R, Tricot G. Psychosocial adjustment and quality of life among multiple myeloma patients undergoing evaluation for autologous stem cell transplantation. Bone Marrow Transplant. 2004;33(9):955–962.

31. Greene D, Nail LM, Fieler VK, Dudgeon D, Jones LS. A comparison of patient-reported side effects among three chemotherapy regimens for breast cancer. Cancer Pract. 1994;2(1):57–62.

32. Servaes P, Verhagen S, Bleijenberg G. Determinants of chronic fatigue in disease-free breast cancer patients: a cross-sectional study. Ann Oncol. 2002;13(4):589–598.

33. Curt GA, Breitbart W, Cella D, et al. Impact of cancer-related fatigue on the lives of patients: new findings from the Fatigue Coalition. Oncologist. 2000;5(5):353–360.

34. Curt G, Johnston PG. Cancer fatigue: the way forward. Oncologist. 2003;8(suppl 1):27–30.

35. Broeckel JA, Jacobsen PB, Horton J, Balducci L, Lyman GH. Characteristics and correlates of fatigue after adjuvant chemotherapy for breast cancer. J Clin Oncol. 1998;16(5):1689–1696.

36. Ganz PA, Moinpour CM, Pauler DK, et al. Health status and quality of life in patients with early-stage Hodgkin's disease treated in Southwest Oncology Group Study 9133. J Clin Oncol. 2003;21(18):3512–3519.

37. Ganz PA, Desmond KA, Leedham B, Rowland JH, Meyerowitz BE, Belin TR. Quality of life in long-term, disease-free survivors of breast cancer: a follow-up study. J Natl Cancer Inst. 2002; 94(1):39–49.

38. Bloom JR, Fobair P, Gritz E, et al. Psychosocial outcomes of cancer: a comparative analysis of Hodgkin's disease and testicular cancer. J Clin Oncol. 1993;11(5):979–988.

39. Fossa SD, Dahl AA, Loge JH. Fatigue, anxiety, and depression in long-term survivors of testicular cancer. J Clin Oncol. 2003; 21(7):1249–1254.

40. Ruffer JU, Flechtner H, Tralls P, et al. Fatigue in long-term survivors of Hodgkin's lymphoma; a report from the German Hodgkin Lymphoma Study Group (GHSG) Eur J Cancer. 2003;39(15):2179–2186.

41. van Tulder MW, Aaronson NK, Bruning PF. The quality of life of long-term survivors of Hodgkin's disease. Ann Oncol. 1994;5(2):153–158.

42. Winer EP, Lindley C, Hardee M, et al. Quality of life in patients surviving at least 12 months following high dose chemotherapy with autologous bone marrow support. Psychooncology. 1999;8(2):167–176.

43. McQuellon RP, Russell GB, Rambo TD, Cravem BL, Radford, J, Perry JJ, et al. Quality of life and psychological distress of bone marrow transplant recipients: the "time trajectory" to recovery over the first year. Bone Marrow Transplant. 1998;21(5):477–486.

44. Broers S, Kaptein AA, Le Cessie S, Fibbe W, Hengeveld MW. Psychological functioning and quality of life following bone marrow transplantation: a 3-year follow-up study. J Psychosom Res. 2000;48(1):11–21.

45. Byar KL, Eilers JE, Nuss SL. Quality of life 5 or more years post-autologous hematopoietic stem cell transplant. Cancer Nurs. 2005;28(2):148–157.

46. Bush NE, Haberman M, Donaldson G, Sullivan KM. Quality of life of 125 adults surviving 6–18 years after bone marrow transplantation. Soc Sci Med. 1995;40(4):479–490.

47. Mock V, Atkinson A, Barsevick A, et al. NCCN Practice Guidelines for Cancer-Related Fatigue. Oncology (Williston Park). 2000;14(11A):151–161.

48. Bower JE, Ganz PA, Aziz N, Fahey JL, Cole SW. T-cell homeostasis in breast cancer survivors with persistent fatigue. J Natl Cancer Inst. 2003;95(15):1165–1168.

49. Bower JE, Ganz PA, Aziz N, Fahey JL. Fatigue and proinflammatory cytokine activity in breast cancer survivors. Psychosom Med. 2002;64(4):604–611.

50. Segal R, Evans W, Johnson D, et al. Structured exercise improves physical functioning in women with stages I and II breast cancer: results of a randomized controlled trial. J Clin Oncol. 2001; 19(3):657–665.

51. Dimeo F, Schwartz S, Fietz T, Wanjura T, Boning D, Thiel E. Effects of endurance training on the physical performance of patients with hematological malignancies during chemotherapy. Support Care Cancer. 2003;11(10):623–628.

52. Schwartz AL. Fatigue mediates the effects of exercise on quality of life. Qual Life Res. 1999;8(6):529–538.

53. Pinto BM, Trunzo JJ. Body esteem and mood among sedentary and active breast cancer survivors. Mayo Clin Proc. 2004; 79(2):181–186.

54. Kendall AR, Mahue-Giangreco M, Carpenter CL, Ganz PA, Bernstein L. Influence of exercise activity on quality of life in long-term breast cancer survivors. Qual Life Res. 2005; 14(2):361–371.

55. Holmes MD, Chen WY, Feskanich D, Kroenke CH, Colditz GA. Physical activity and survival after breast cancer diagnosis. JAMA. 2005;293(20):2479–2486.

56. Mages NL, Castro JR, Fobair P, et al. Patterns of psychosocial response to cancer: can effective adaptation be predicted? Int J Radiat Oncol Biol Phys. 1981;7(3):385–392.

57. Schover LR. The impact of breast cancer on sexuality, body image, and intimate relationships. CA Cancer J Clin. 1991;41(2): 112–120.

58. Ganz PA, Lee JJ, Sim MS, Polinsky ML, Schag CA. Exploring the influence of multiple variables on the relationship of age to quality of life in women with breast cancer. J Clin Epidemiol. 1992;45(5):473–485.

59. Ganz PA, Coscarelli A, Fred C, Kahn B, Polinsky ML, Petersen L. Breast cancer survivors: psychosocial concerns and quality of life. Breast Cancer Res Treat. 1996;38(2):183–199.

60. Ganz PA, Desmond KA, Belin TR, Meyerowitz BE, Rowland JH. Predictors of sexual health in women after a breast cancer diagnosis. J Clin Oncol. 1999;17(8):2371–2380.

61. Ganz PA, Greendale GA, Petersen L, Kahn B, Bower JE. Breast cancer in younger women: reproductive and late health effects of treatment. J Clin Oncol. 2003;21(22):4184–4193.

62. Ganz PA, Kwan L, Stanton AL, et al. Quality of life at the end of primary treatment of breast cancer: first results from the moving beyond cancer randomized trial. J Natl Cancer Inst. 2004;96(5):376–387.

63. Pozo C, Carver CS, Noriega V, et al. Effects of mastectomy versus lumpectomy on emotional adjustment to breast cancer: a prospective study of the first year postsurgery. J Clin Oncol. 1992;10(8):1292–1298.

64. Yurek D, Farrar W, Andersen BL. Breast cancer surgery: comparing surgical groups and determining individual differences in postoperative sexuality and body change stress. J Consult Clin Psychol. 2000;68(4):697–709.

65. Arora NK, Gustafson DH, Hawkins RP, et al. Impact of surgery and chemotherapy on the quality of life of younger women with breast carcinoma: a prospective study. Cancer. Sep 1 2001;92(5):1288–1298.

66. Avis NE, Crawford S, Manuel J. Quality of life among younger women with breast cancer. J Clin Oncol. 2005;23(15):3322–3330.

67. Figueiredo MI, Cullen J, Hwang YT, Rowland JH, Mandelblatt JS. Breast cancer treatment in older women: does getting what you want improve your long-term body image and mental health? J Clin Oncol. 2004;22(19):4002–4009.

68. Bukovic D, Fajdic J, Strinic T, Habek M, Hojsak I, Radakovic N. Differences in sexual functioning between patients with benign and malignant breast tumors. Coll Antropol. 2004;28(suppl 2):191–201.

69. Bukovic D, Fajdic J, Hrgovic Z, Kaufmann M, Hojsak I, Stanceric T. Sexual dysfunction in breast cancer survivors. Onkologie. 2005;28(1):29–34.

70. Fobair P, Stewart SL, Chang S, et al. Body Image and sexual problems in young women with breast cancer. Psychooncology. 2006;15:1513–1524.

71. Avis NE, Crawford S, Manuel J. Psychosocial problems among younger women with breast cancer. Psychooncology. 2004;13(5):295–308.

72. Ganz PA. Quality of life across the continuum of breast cancer care. Breast J. 2000;6(5):324–330.

73. Korfage IJ, Essink-Bot ML, Borsboom GJ, et al. Five-year follow-up of health-related quality of life after primary treatment of localized prostate cancer. Int J Cancer. 2005;116(2):291–296.

74. Dahn JR, Penedo FJ, Molton I, Lopez L, Schneiderman N, Antoni MH. Physical activity and sexual functioning after radiotherapy for prostate cancer: beneficial effects for patients undergoing external beam radiotherapy. Urology. 2005;65(5):953–958.

75. McQuellon RP, Craven B, Russell GB, et al. Quality of life in breast cancer patients before and after autologous bone marrow transplantation. Bone Marrow Transplant. 1996;18(3):579–584.

76. Hayden PJ, Keogh F, Ni Conghaile M, et al. A single-centre assessment of long-term quality-of-life status after sibling allogeneic stem cell transplantation for chronic myeloid leukaemia in first chronic phase. Bone Marrow Transplant. 2004;34(6):545–556.

77. Wingard JR, Curbow B, Baker F, Zabora J, Piantadosi S. Sexual satisfaction in survivors of bone marrow transplantation. Bone Marrow Transplant. 1992;9(3):185–190.

78. Chao NJ, Tierney DK, Bloom JR, et al. Dynamic assessment of quality of life after autologous bone marrow transplantation. Blood. 1992;80(3):825–830.

79. Meyers CA. Neurocognitive dysfunction in cancer patients. Oncology (Williston Park). 2000;14(1):75–79; 81–85.

80. Welzel G, Steinvorth S WF. Cognitive Effects of Chemotherapy and/or Cranial Irradiation. Strahlenther Onkol. 2005;181(3):141–156.

81. Tchen N, Juffs HG, Downie FP, et al. Cognitive function, fatigue, and menopausal symptoms in women receiving adjuvant chemotherapy for breast cancer. J Clin Oncol. 2003;21(22):4175–4183.

82. Castellon SA, Ganz PA, Bower JE. et al. Neurocognitive performance in breast cancer survivors exposed to adjuvant chemotherapy and tamoxifen. J Clin Exp Neuropsychol. 2004;26(7):955–969.

83. Rausch RC, Park D, Pegram C, Northfelt MD, and Pietras R. A prospective study of memory changes associated with adjuvant chemotherapy in patients with breast cancer. Breast Cancer Res Treat. 2004;88(suppl 1):138.

84. Bodurka-Bevers D, Basen-Engquist K, Carmack CL, et al. Depression, anxiety, and quality of life in patients with epithelial ovarian cancer. Gynecol Oncol. 2000;78(3):302–308.

85. Trask PC, Paterson A, Riba M, et al. Assessment of psychological distress in prospective bone marrow transplant patients. Bone Marrow Transplant. 2002;29(1):917–925.

86. Carlson LE, Angen M, Cullum J, et al. High levels of untreated distress and fatigue in cancer patients. Br J Cancer. 2004;90(12):2297–2304.

87. D'Antonio LL, Long SA, Zimmerman GJ, Peterman AH, Petti GH, Chonkich GD. Relationship between quality of life and depression in patients with head and neck cancer. Laryngoscope. 1998;108(6):806–811.

88. Sarna L, Padilla G, Holmes C, Tashkin D, Brecht ML, Evangelista L. Quality of life of long-term survivors of non-small-cell lung cancer. J Clin Oncol. 2002;20(13):2920–2929.

89. Pelletier G, Verhoef MJ, Khatri N, Hagen N. Quality of life in brain tumor patients: the relative contributions of depression, fatigue, emotional distress, and existential issues. J Neurooncol. 2002;57(1):41–49.

90. Bukberg J, Penman D, Holland JC. Depression in hospitalized cancer patients. Psychosom Med. 1984;46(3):199–212.

91. Lynch ME. The assessment and prevalence of affective disorders in advanced cancer. J Palliat Care. 1995;11(1):10–18.

92. Penman DT, Bloom JR, Fotopoulos S, et al. The impact of mastectomy on self-concept and social function: a combined cross-sectional and longitudinal study with comparison groups. Women Health. 1986;11(3–4):101–130.

93. Psychological response to mastectomy. A prospective comparison study. Psychological aspects of Breast Cancer Study Group. Cancer. 1987;59(1):189–196.

94. Linn MW, Linn BS, Harris R. Effects of counseling for late stage cancer patients. Cancer. 1982;49(5):1048–1055.

95. Spiegel D, Bloom JR, Yalom I. Group support for patients with metastatic cancer. A randomized outcome study. Arch Gen Psychiatry. 1981;38(5):527–533.

96. Spiegel D, Bloom JR, Kraemer HC, Gottheil E. Effect of psychosocial treatment on survival of patients with metastatic breast cancer. Lancet. 1989;2(8668):888–891.

97. Fawzy FI, Fawzy NW, Hyun CS, et al. Malignant melanoma. Effects of an early structured psychiatric intervention, coping, and affective state on recurrence and survival 6 years later. Arch Gen Psychiatry. 1993;50(9):681–689.

98. Classen C, Butler LD, Koopman C, et al. Supportive-expressive group therapy and distress in patients with metastatic breast cancer: a randomized clinical intervention trial. Arch Gen Psychiatry. 2001;58(5):494–501.

99. Fobair P. Cancer support groups and group therapies: part I, historical and theoretical background and research on effectiveness. Journal of Psychosocial Oncology. 1997;15(1):63–81.

100. Cordova MJ, Giese-Davis J, Golant M, et al. Mood disturbance in community cancer support groups. The role of emotional suppression and fighting spirit. J Psychosom Res. 2003;55(5):461–467.

101. Levine EG, Eckhardt J, Targ E. Change in post-traumatic stress symptoms following psychosocial treatment for breast cancer. Psychooncology. 2005;14(8):618–635.

102. Bishop SR, Warr D. Coping, catastrophizing and chronic pain in breast cancer. J Behav Med. 2003;26(3):265–281.

103. Trask PC, Paterson AG, Griffith KA, Riba MB, Schwartz JL. Cognitive-behavioral intervention for distress in patients with melanoma: comparison with standard medical care and impact on quality of life. Cancer. 2003;98(4):854–864.

104. Uitterhoeve RJ, Vernooy M, Litjens M, et al. Psychosocial interventions for patients with advanced cancer—a systematic review of the literature. Br J Cancer. 2004;91(6):1050–1062.

105. Trask PC, Paterson AG, Fardig J, Smith DC. Course of distress and quality of life in testicular cancer patients before, during, and after chemotherapy: results of a pilot study. Psychooncology. 2003;12(8):814–820.

106. Richardson MA, Post-White J, Grimm EA, Moye LA, Singletary SE, Justice B. Coping, life attitudes, and immune responses to imagery and group support after breast cancer treatment. Altern Ther Health Med. 1997;3(5):62–70.

107. Cameron LD, Booth RJ, Schlatter M, Ziginskas D, Harman JE, Benson SR. Cognitive and affective determinants of decisions to attend a group psychosocial support program for women with breast cancer. Psychosom Med. 2005;67(4):584–589.

108. Yates JS, Mustian KM, Morrow GR, et al. Prevalence of complementary and alternative medicine use in cancer patients during treatment. Support Care Cancer. 2005;13:806–811.

109. Dy GK, Bekele L, Hanson LJ, et al. Complementary and alternative medicine use by patients enrolled onto phase I clinical trials. J Clin Oncol. 2004;22(23):4810–4815.

110. Hedderson MM, Patterson RE, Neuhouser ML, et al. Sex differences in motive for use of complementary and alternative medicine among cancer patients. Altern Ther Health Med. 2004;10(5):58–64.

111. Henderson JW, Donatelle RJ. Complementary and alternative medicine use by women after completion of allopathic treatment for breast cancer. Altern Ther Health Med. 2004;10(1):52–57.

112. Navo MA, Phan J, Vaughan C, et al. An assessment of the utilization of complementary and alternative medication in women with gynecologic or breast malignancies. J Clin Oncol. 2004;22(4):671–677.

113. Cui Y, Shu XO, Gao Y, et al. Use of complementary and alternative medicine by Chinese women with breast cancer. Breast Cancer Res Treat. 2004;85(3):263–270.

114. Harris P, Finlay IG, Cook A, Thomas KJ, Hood K. Complementary and alternative medicine use by patients with cancer in Wales: a cross sectional survey. Complement Ther Med. 2003;11(4):249–253.

115. Hyodo I, Amano N, Eguchi K, et al. Nationwide survey on complementary and alternative medicine in cancer patients in Japan. J Clin Oncol. 2005;23(12):2645–2654.

116. Rakovitch E, Pignol JP, Chartier C, et al. Complementary and alternative medicine use is associated with an increased perception of breast cancer risk and death. Breast Cancer Res Treat. 2005;90(2):139–148.

117. Nagel G, Hoyer H, Katenkamp D. Use of complementary and alternative medicine by patients with breast cancer: observations from a health-care survey. Support Care Cancer. 2004;12(11):789–796.

118. Pud D, Kaner E, Morag A, Ben-Ami S, Yaffe A. Use of complementary and alternative medicine among cancer patients in Israel. Eur J Oncol Nurs. 2005;9(2):124–130.

119. Molassiotis A, Marguiles A, Fernandez-Ortega P, et al. Complementary and alternative medicine use in patients with haematological malignancies in Europe. Complement Ther Clin Pract. 2005;11(2):105–110.

120. Hana G, Bar-Sela G, Zhana D, Mashiach T, Robinson E. The use of complementary and alternative therapies by cancer patients in northern Israel. Isr Med Assoc J. 2005;7(4):243–247.

121. Hann D, Baker F, Denniston M, Entrekin N. Long-term breast cancer survivors' use of complementary therapies: perceived impact on recovery and prevention of recurrence. Integr Cancer Ther. 2005;4(1):14–20.

122. Rosenbaum E, Gautier H, Fobair P, et al. Cancer supportive care, improving the quality of life for cancer patients. A program evaluation report. Support Care Cancer. 2004;12(5):293–301.

123. Herman PM, Craig BM, Caspi O. Is complementary and alternative medicine (CAM) cost-effective? A systematic review. BMC Complement Altern Med. 2005;5:11.

124. de Boer MF, Pruyn JF, van den Borne B, Knegt PP, Ryckman RM, Verwoerd CD. Rehabilitation outcomes of long-term survivors treated for head and neck cancer. Head Neck. 1995;17(6):503–515.

125. Relic A, Mazemda P, Arens C, Koller M, Glanz H. Investigating quality of life and coping resources after laryngectomy. Eur Arch Otorhinolaryngol. 2001;258(10):514–517.

126. Wimberly SR, Carver CS, Laurenceau JP, Harris SD, Antoni MH. Perceived partner reactions to diagnosis and treatment of breast cancer: impact on psychosocial and psychosexual adjustment. J Consult Clin Psychol. 2005;73(2):300–311.

127. Northouse LL, Swain MA. Adjustment of patients and husbands to the initial impact of breast cancer. Nurs Res. 1987;36(4):221–225.

128. Northouse LL, Templin T, Mood D, Oberst M. Couples' adjustment to breast cancer and benign breast disease: a longitudinal analysis. Psychooncology. 1998;7(1):37–48.

129. Northouse LL, Schafer JA, Tipton J, Metivier L. The concerns of patients and spouses after the diagnosis of colon cancer: a qualitative analysis. J Wound Ostomy Continence Nurs. 1999;26(1):8–17.

130. Northouse LL, Templin T, Mood D. Couples' adjustment to breast disease during the first year following diagnosis. J Behav Med. 2001;24(2):115–136.

131. Cliff AM, MacDonagh RP. Psychosocial morbidity in prostate cancer: II. a comparison of patients and partners. BJU Int. 2000;86(7):834–839.

132. Tuinstra J, Hagedoorn M, Van Sonderen E, et al. Psychological distress in couples dealing with colorectal cancer: gender and role differences and intracouple correspondence. Br J Health Psychol. 2004;9:465–478.

133. Dorval M, Guay S, Mondor M, et al. Couples who get closer after breast cancer: frequency and predictors in a prospective investigation. J Clin Oncol. 2005;23(15):3588–3596.

134. Bultz BD, Speca M, Brasher PM, Geggie PH, Page SA. A randomized controlled trial of a brief psychoeducational support group for partners of early stage breast cancer patients. Psychooncology. 2000;9(4):303–313.

135. Neuling SJ, Winefield HR. Social support and recovery after surgery for breast cancer: frequency and correlates of supportive behaviours by family, friends and surgeon. Soc Sci Med. 1988;27(4):385–392.

136. Bloom J, Fobair P, Spiegel D, Cox RS, Varghese A, Hoppe R. Social supports and the social well-being of cancer survivors. Advances Med-Soc. 1991;2:95–114.

137. Bloom JR, Stewart SL, Johnston M, Banks P, Fobair P. Sources of support and the physical and mental well-being of young women with breast cancer. Soc Sci Med. 2001;53(11):1513–1524.

138. Johnson SM, Talitman E. Predictors of success in emotionally focused marital therapy. J Marital Fam Ther. 1997;23(2):135–152.

139. Johnson SM, Williams-Keeler L. Creating healing relationships for couples dealing with trauma: the use of emotionally focused marital therapy. J Marital Fam Ther. 1998;24(1):25–40.

140. Johnson SM, Makinen JA, Millikin JW. Attachment injuries in couple relationships: a new perspective on impasses in couples therapy. J Marital Fam Ther. 2001;27(2):145–155.

141. Gruber U, Fegg M, Buchmann M, Kolb HJ, Hiddemann W. The long-term psychosocial effects of haematopoetic stem cell transplantation. Eur J Cancer Care (Engl). 2003;12(3):249–256.

142. Edman L, Larsen J, Hagglund H, Gardulf A. Health-related quality of life, symptom distress and sense of coherence in adult survivors of allogeneic stem-cell transplantation. Eur J Cancer Care (Engl). 2001;10(2):124–130.

143. Duell T, van Lint MT, Ljungman P, et al. Health and functional status of long-term survivors of bone marrow transplantation. EBMT Working Party on Late Effects and EULEP Study Group on Late Effects. European Group for Blood and Marrow Transplantation. Ann Intern Med. 1997;126(3):184–192.

144. Weis J, Koch U, Geldsetzer M. Changes in occupational status following cancer. An empirical study on occupational rehabilitation. Soz Praventivmed. 1992;37(2):85–95.

145. Nordstron G, Myman CR, Theorell T. The impact on work ability of ileal conduit urinary diversion. Scand J Soc Med. 1990;18(2):115–124.

146. Demin E. The Problems of the work rehabilitation of breast cancer patients after radical treatment. Vopr Onkol. 1989;35(11):1365–1370.

147. Fobair P, Bloom J, Hoppe R, Varghese A, Cox R, Speigel D. Work Patterns Among Long-term Survivors of Hodgkin's Disease. New York: Praeger; 1989.

148. Bloom JGR, Fobair P, Hoppe R, Cox R, Varghese A, Spiegel D. Physical performance at work and at leisure: validation of a measure of biological energy in survivors of Hodgkin's disease. J Psychosocial Oncol. 1990;8(1):49–63.

149. Maunsell E, Brisson C, Dubois L, Lauzier S, Fraser A. Work problems after breast cancer: an exploratory qualitative study. Psychooncology. 1999;8(6):467–473.

150. Hays DM, Landsverk J, Sallan SE, et al. Educational, occupational, and insurance status of childhood cancer survivors in their fourth and fifth decades of life. J Clin Oncol. 1992;10(9):1397–1406.

151. Fobair P. Quality of Life in People with Hodgkin's Disease. Oncology. 1993;7(8):50–52.

152. Fobair P. Cancer Support Groups and Group Therapies. Washington, DC: NASW Press; 1998.

153. Brady MJ, Peterman AH, Fitchett G, Mo M, Cella D. A case for including spirituality in quality of life measurement in oncology. Psychooncology. 1999;8(5):417–428.

154. Degner LF, Hack T, O'Neil J, Kristjanson LJ. A new approach to eliciting meaning in the context of breast cancer. Cancer Nurs. 2003;26(3):169–178.

155. Johnson Vickberg SM, Duhamel KN, Smith MY, et al. Global meaning and psychological adjustment among survivors of bone marrow transplant. Psychooncology. 2001;10(1):29–39.

156. Levine & Targ, 2002.

157. Andrykowski MA, Bishop MM, Hahn EA, et al. Long-term health-related quality of life, growth, and spiritual well-being after hematopoietic stem-cell transplantation. J Clin Oncol. 2005;23(3):599–608.

158. Dow KF, Ferrell BR, Haberman MR, Eaton L. The meaning of quality of life in cancer survivorship. Oncology Nursing Forum. 1999;26(3):519–528.

159. Coward DD, Kahn DL. Resolution of spiritual disequilibrium by women newly diagnosed with breast cancer. Oncol Nurs Forum. 2004;31(2):E24–31.

160. Oh S, Heflin L, Meyerowitz BE, Desmond KA, Rowland JH, Ganz PA. Quality of life of breast cancer survivors after a recurrence: a follow-up study. Breast Cancer Res Treat. 2004;87(1):45–57.

161. Houck K, Avis NE, Gallant JM, Fuller AF Jr., Goodman A. Quality of life in advanced ovarian cancer: identifying specific concerns. J Palliat Med. 1999;2(4):397–402.

162. McClement S. Cancer anorexia-cachexia syndrome: psychological effect on the patient and family. J Wound Ostomy Continence Nurs. 2005;32(4):264–268.

163. Grumann MM, Spiegel D. Living in the face of death: Interviews with 12 terminally ill women on home hospice care. Palliative and Supportive Care. 2003;1(1):23–32.

164. AOSW AoOSW. Oncology Social Work Tool Box. Washington DC: AOSW; 2001.

165. Fobair P. Program planning for cancer patients. Paper presented at: The American Cancer Society Third National Conference on Human Values & Cancer; 1981, Washington, DC.

166. Spiegel D, Classen C. Group Therapy for Cancer Patients: A Research-based Handbook of Psychosocial Care. New York: Basic Books; 2000.

167. Fobair P. Cancer support groups and group therapies. Part II: Process, organizational, leadership, and patient Issues. Journal of Psychosocial Oncology. 1997;15(3/4):123–147.

168. van Wegberg B, Lienhard A, Andrey M. Does a psychosocial group intervention program alter the quality of life of cancer patients? Schweiz Med Wochenschr. 2000;130(6):177–185.

169. Miller DK, Chibnall JT, Videen SD, Duckro PN. Supportive-affective group experience for persons with life-threatening illness: reducing spiritual, psychological, and death-related distress in dying patients. J Palliat Med. 2005;8(2):333–343.

170. Begoun A. Ten Questions for Reclaiming Your Life After Breast Cancer. Palo Alto: Community Breast Health Project; 2004.

171. Giese-Davis J, Koopman C, Butler LD, et al. Change in emotion-regulation strategy for women with metastatic breast cancer following supportive-expressive group therapy. J Consult Clin Psychol. 2002;70(4):916–925.

172. Fobair P, Koopman C, DiMiceli S, et al. Psychosocial intervention for lesbians with primary breast cancer. Psychooncology. 2002;11(5):427–438.

173. Mestenhauser JA. Traveling the Unpaved Road to Democracy from Communism: A cross-cultural perspective on change. Minneapolis/St. Paul: College of Education and Human Development, Department of Educational Policy and Administration, University of Minnesota; 1996.

174. Schnipper HH. Life after breast cancer. J Clin Oncol. 2003; 21(suppl 9):104–107.

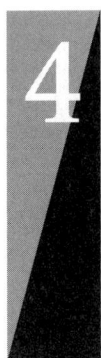

Survivorship Research: Past, Present, and Future

Julia H. Rowland

Origins of Cancer Survivorship Research

In 1884, an official ceremony was held and the cornerstone laid for an ornate and turreted building in New York City that would for many years house the first cancer treatment center in the country. The site, located on the upper west side of Central Park, then a virtual wilderness area on the larger island of Manhattan, was selected because the belief at the time was that cancer was contagious. The rounded design of the towers, where patient beds were to be located, was intended to discourage the risk of germs, which were thought to lurk in corners. Named The New York Cancer Hospital, this institution would later be moved in 1948 to its current east side location where it was, until 1960, called the Memorial Hospital for Cancer and Allied Diseases. The history of this leading center for cancer care and research, known today as the Memorial Sloan-Kettering Cancer Center, a sprawling multisite enterprise, is illustrative of where we have come in viewing cancer.[1]

At the turn of the 20th century, cancer was largely incurable, poorly understood, and associated with treatments that were often as dire as the disease itself. By midcentury, with the advent of anesthesia, antibiotics, and the introduction of multimodal cancer therapies, the number of individuals living longer (beyond 5 years) with cancer had slowly increased. However, it was not until the latter part of the 1900s that the nationally estimated 5-year cancer prevalence figures (prevalence being defined as the number of people alive at a given point in time with a history of cancer) reached 50%. From an evidence perspective, this event, which occurred between 1974 and 1976,[2] might in hindsight be considered a turning point in what would soon become the field of cancer survivorship. Arguably, without substantial numbers of survivors, issues of "survivorship" would never have become of interest; the focus of research would have remained, as it had in the past, largely on trying simply to enable an individual to become a survivor, not what the future of that person's life might be like.

The first glimpse at this new world came from pediatric oncology where, seemingly overnight, a death sentence was being converted into long-term cure. This point is well illustrated in the steady upward curve in pediatric cancer survival rates from 1950 to 1998 depicted in Figure 4.1. Introduction in the late 1960s of therapies to prevent central nervous system relapse in survivors of childhood lymphoblastic leukemia (ALL) was among several key treatment changes that would lead to a revised perspective on this disease (Figure 4.2). Because ALL is the most common form of childhood cancer, accounting today for approximately 30% of cancer cases diagnosed in children before the age of 14,[3] the impact of this breakthrough produced a dramatic shift in 5-year survival rates for pediatric cancer as a whole. It also spawned the first generation of articles calling for attention by the medical community to issues that went beyond merely curing a child to those affecting his or her quality of life after treatment.[4–6] This same process was slower to evolve in the adult cancer arena.

Development of Survivorship Researcher and Assessment Tools

Others, and most notably Jimmie Holland,[7,8] have written in detail about the confluence of both medical and societal factors that led to the recognition of the field of psychosocial oncology. Three elements essential to the growth of the field were the change within the medical community toward disclosing a cancer diagnosis, training of a cadre of researchers to address posttreatment issues related to quality of life (QOL), and development of assessment tools to measure and describe the survivorship experience. Of these, the movement toward disclosing a cancer diagnosis was the most critical.

Throughout most of the 1960s, the practice in the United States was not to tell patients their diagnosis, "never tellers" constituting an estimated 90% of physicians surveyed in a report by Oken.[9] A report published by Novack and colleagues revealed that this policy reversed in the course of a brief 10 years. By 1977, 97% of physicians stated that they told patients they had cancer at the time of diagnosis.[10] This change in practice was important because it opened the door for researchers to approach and ask patients directly about their understanding of their illness and its impact on their lives. The shift in candor about a cancer diagnosis was consequent to growing attention in the United States to patients' rights, particularly in the health arena. However, physicians' willingness to adopt this practice was also a reflection of the greater optimism about survival prospects for those diagnosed with cancer. It should be noted that sharing the diagnosis is not a universal practice. In many countries around the world, including several industrialized nations, physicians still hide this information, sometimes at the request of family members.[11–13] In Third World countries, where access to curative therapies is more limited and hence prognosis is grim,

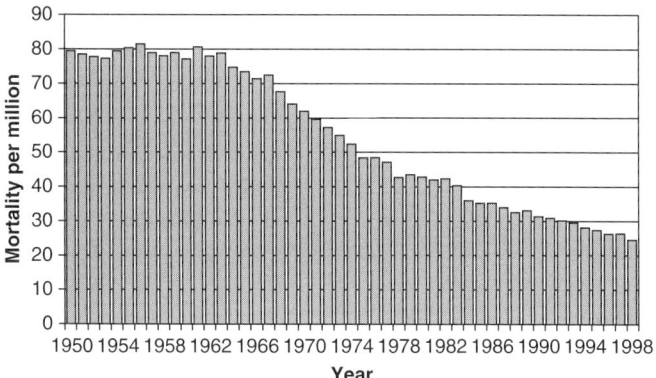

FIGURE 4.1. Remarkable past progress: childhood cancer mortality, 1950–1998.

however, had formal training in psycho-oncology, as dedicated educational programs in this field did not appear until the late 1970s and early 1980s.[7,16] Today, a number of the National Cancer Institute (NCI)-designated clinical and comprehensive cancer centers offer 2- to 3-year training programs for MDs and PhDs who wish to specialize in this area of research or care. Many also provide access to courses in psychosocial aspects of cancer research to a diversity of healthcare professionals. It also is increasingly common to see position openings for psychosocial oncology specialists announced on association-based online listserves, such as that supported by the American Psychological Association's Division 38 Health Psychology forum.

Paralleling the expertise of the early researchers, the tools used for QOL assessment of survivors' outcomes were drawn initially from the psychiatric or mental health field. Examples of frequently used instruments included the Hopkin's Symptom Checklist (better known to many as the SCL-90),[17] the Profile of Mood States,[18] and the Center for Epidemiologic Studies Depression Scale (CES-D).[19] It quickly became apparent that these measures were not well suited to the cancer survivor population, which, although experiencing distress, generally did not report symptoms at psychiatric or pathologic levels. At the same time, teasing apart symptoms that might be caused by the effects of treatment (e.g., fatigue/lack of energy, sleep disruption, problems concentrating) from signs of emotional distress created a challenge to score interpretation.[20-22] Further, many of the experiences of those treated were poorly captured by the questions asked in these tools. Frustration with the limits of these more-generic tools resulted in the birth of cancer-specific measurements, an enterprise that, although starting slowly, burgeoned in the 1980s to produce many of the QOL measures, or at least their sophisticated variants, most commonly used today.[23-26]

protecting patients from learning their diagnosis is considered more humane.[14] Even in many European countries, cancer still carries a significant social stigma. As part of its year-long study of cancer survivorship in the United States, the President's Cancer Panel held a meeting in Lisbon, Portugal, in May 2003. The purpose of this meeting was "to learn about the health services and survivorship activities in diverse European nations and health systems that might benefit survivors in this country".[15] The Panel found that the term survivor was rarely used, and in some countries no linguistic equivalent existed. It was common for European survivors, the testimony from many of whom is included in transcripts and the final report from this meeting,[15] to feel they could not publicly reveal their cancer history, or discuss their illness experience, even with family. In contrast to the situation in the United States, few prominent Europeans have disclosed their status as cancer survivors.

Early pioneers in the field of psychosocial oncology often came from mental health or nursing backgrounds. Few,

Role of Advocacy in the Growth of the Field

DEFINING THE DOMAIN

The shift in focus and language to recognition of people with a history of cancer as "survivors" and their health and social outcomes as constituting "survivorship research" has its own history. In 1985, a young pediatrician working for the Public Health Service, Fitzhugh Mullan, wrote about his experience of living with cancer in a short piece for the *New England Journal of Medicine*. He referred to his journey as the "Seasons of Survival" and in his text first gave name to issues of survivorship.[27] In October 1986, he and an intrepid group of about two dozen fellow survivors, cancer healthcare providers and advocates, met in Albuquerque, New Mexico, and established the National Coalition for Cancer Survivorship (NCCS).[28] The standard medical definition of a survivor at the time of that gathering, and the only definition commonly applied, held that only those individuals who remained disease free for a minimum of 5 years could be labeled as survivors. At the founding NCCS meeting, the group declared that a person should be viewed as, and was entitled to call himself or herself, a survivor, "from the moment of diagnosis and for the balance of his or her life, regardless of the ultimate cause of death."

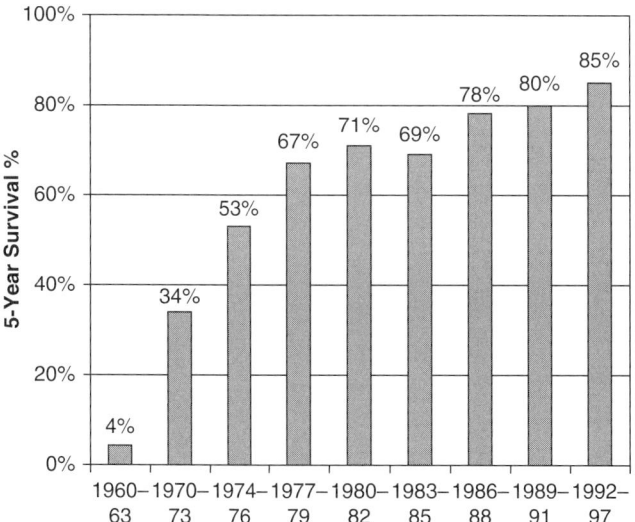

FIGURE 4.2. Remarkable past progress: childhood acute lymphoblastic anemia (ALL) survival rates, 1960–1997.

The group's argument for advancing this new definition was that it was only by endorsing such thinking that survivors would be able to significantly alter the prevailing medical culture. Specifically, they sought to encourage the cancer practitioner community to move away from its more narrow focus on starting treatment as quickly as possible to one that recognized that a person's unique needs, desires, and ultimate health and life outcomes must be acknowledged in this process. Ideally this would start on day 1, after diagnosis. Although controversial at the time, and certainly not uniformly embraced even today, this broader definition of a cancer survivor has taken hold, at least in the United States. In a search of *Pub Med* from 1981 to 1985, the 5-year period before the founding of the NCCS, 28 research articles (among humans, published in English), were identified using the terms cancer survivorship. Using the same approach to examine the "hits" in 5-year increments since then yielded the following: 1986–1990, 1,700 citations; 1991–1995, 8,417; 1996–2000, 10,574; 2001 to current (with 16 months still remaining to come during this 5-year period), 7,673. Although many of the citations identified would not be classified by many as addressing issues related to living with or beyond cancer (i.e., many still focus on survival, not survivorship), the numbers speak for themselves. On the public side, since 1987 the first Sunday in June has been celebrated as National Cancer Survivors' Day. Many of the large cancer centers in major cities now hold their own "Cancer Survivors Day" celebrations, often in association with special presentations by survivors, scientists, and advocates. The most significant evidence that the field of cancer survivorship had finally come into its own was the creation of an Office of Cancer Survivorship within the world's premier cancer research center, the U.S. National Cancer Institute.

A BRIEF HISTORY OF THE OFFICE OF CANCER SURVIVORSHIP

Had NCCS members decided to stop at endorsing a new definition of survivor, it is not clear how rapidly the broader field of survivorship research might have progressed. Fortunately, they were not content to merely draw attention to the needs of those living with a history of cancer. NCCS members began to advocate for specific resources to further identify and address these needs. In anticipation of what would become the first NCCS Congress, held in Washington, D.C., in November 1995, the Coalition sought the input of scores of researchers, clinicians, and survivors on what questions remained unanswered, who should be charged with addressing these, and how best were we going to achieve optimal cancer care for all. Response to this inquiry was combined in a white paper entitled Imperatives for Quality Cancer Care: Access, Advocacy, Action & Accountability. In spring 1996, Ellen Stovall, Executive Director for NCCS, gave a copy of this document to the director of the NCI, Dr. Richard Klausner. After reading this paper, Dr. Klausner called for the creation of the Office of Cancer Survivorship (OCS).

Formally inaugurated at a ceremony held in the Rose Garden of the White House in October 1996, the OCS was established in recognition of the growing population of cancer survivors and their unique and poorly understood needs.[29] The overall mission of the office is to enhance the length and quality of survival of all those diagnosed with cancer. The OCS achieves this by serving as a focus for the support and direction of research that will lead to a clearer understanding of, and the ultimate prevention of, or reduction in, the adverse psychosocial, physical, and economic outcomes of cancer and its treatment. Survivorship research is seen as encompassing the medical, functional, and health-related QOL of children and adults diagnosed with cancer, as well as that of their families. It also includes within its domain issues related to healthcare delivery, access, and follow-up care as they relate to survivors. Because considerable work had been done in elucidating the needs and care of those newly diagnosed and in active treatment, particular emphasis in creating the OCS was placed on developing and supporting research that addresses the health and well-being of individuals who are posttreatment or in remission. The OCS also has as its purview a commitment to educating healthcare providers, as well as survivors themselves, about issues and practices critical to their patients (or in the case of survivors, their own) optimal well-being. Finally, the OCS works to foster and promote the training of the next generation of survivorship researchers and clinicians.

In 2001, members of the OCS, the NCI Director's Consumer Liaison Group, and a number of community researchers and advocates independently suggested that NCI leadership consider advancing cancer survivorship as an area for special focus along with other previously identified topics such as Genes and the Environment, Cancer Imaging, Research on Tobacco and Tobacco-Related Cancers, and Cancer Communications. This recommendation met with approval and elevated Cancer Survivorship to special status in NCI's Fiscal Year 2004 and 2005 budgets[31,32] (pp 88–93 and 66–71, respectively). Successful adoption of cancer survivorship as an extraordinary opportunity for investment by the NCI was in significant measure due to the specific intercession of Dr. Andrew von Eschenbach. Dr. von Eschenbach's appointment as NCI Director by the President of the United States brought to the Institute in February 2002, for the first time, a cancer survivor as its director. Throughout his leadership, Dr. von Eschenbach has been outspoken about his own cancer experience as a three-time survivor and an unflagging champion for survivorship research.

The breadth of attention to cancer survivorship as an area of public health interest is reflected in a number of recent events at the national level. These events include the release in 2002 by the Institute of Medicine's National Cancer Policy Board of its report *Childhood Cancer Survivorship: Improving Care and Quality of Life* (and the adult companion *From Cancer Patient to Cancer Survivor: Lost in Transition*)[32]; the decision by the President's Cancer Panel to pursue cancer survivorship as a theme for its planned hearings in 2003 and 2004, the report from which activities, *Living Beyond Cancer: Finding a New Balance*, was released at the annual meetings of the American Society of Clinical Oncology held in New Orleans in June 2004[33]; and the publication in April 2004 of *A National Action Plan for Cancer Survivorship: Advancing Public Health Strategies* by the Centers for Disease Control and Prevention (CDC) and the Lance Armstrong Foundation.[34] The latter two initiatives bear the important contribution of Lance Armstrong. Lance, seven-time winner of the world's most grueling bicycle race, the Tour de France, an accomplishment achieved after his diagnosis with and treatment for metastatic testicular cancer, was nominated in 2002 by President Bush to serve as one of three members of the President's Cancer Panel. The foundation that bears his name underwrote the CDC effort to produce the *National Action Plan* document. During this same period, 2002–2004, five separate bills were introduced in Congress that included language identifying cancer survivorship as an area warranting more attention and funds from the U.S. Department of Health and Human Services (DHHS); one of these would have formally authorized the office by an act of Congress. None of these bills ultimately became law. However, the fact that they were put forward (with others of similar intent likely to follow) is strong evidence that the nation acknowledges that it is not enough for our scientists to find a cure for cancer; we must also, as a country, ensure the quality of the lives of those treated. In the Congressional appropriations document for 2003 (Senate Report 107-216; Department of Labor, Health and Human Services, and Education, and Related Agencies Appropriation Bill), members of the Senate wrote "...More must be done to improve the understanding of the growing cancer survivorship population, including determinations of the physiological and psychological late effects, prevalence of secondary cancers, as well as further development of effective survivorship interventions. The Committee supports an aggressive expansion of the NCI Office of Cancer Survivorship activities...."

Function of Survivorship Research in Cancer Control and Care

The world of cancer survivorship research has expanded far beyond that originally envisioned. In the early 1970s, the function of such research was largely limited to describing the "terrain" of survival. By the early 1980s, researchers sought not simply to elucidate the impact of cancer on the lives of individuals and their families but to use this information to develop interventions to help survivors cope better with their illness.[35,36] In the case of pediatrics, the findings from survivorship research were being used to refine cancer therapies so as to reduce their associated morbidity without diminishing the gains achieved in reduced mortality.[37] As we race into the new millennium, this vision, along with the approach to as well as application of survivorship research, has vastly expanded and come to encompass the entire cancer control continuum (Figure 4.3). Originally occupying just one part of the continuum, cancer survivorship research and care now have the potential to address and affect issues along the entire continuum. For example, with more young survivors expected to live full or lengthened lifetimes, they need to be counseled to reduce the risk of (primary prevention) and screened for (secondary prevention) other unrelated malignancies for which they would be at risk across the course of life/normal aging.[38]

Clinically, the primary function of survivorship research is fivefold. Information about survivors is critical if we are to help patients make decisions now about treatment options that will affect their future; understand the action of and tailor therapies to maximize cure while minimizing adverse treatment-related effects; develop and disseminate evidence-based interventions that reduce cancer morbidity as well as mortality and facilitate adaptation among cancer survivors; improve quality of care and control costs; and equip the next generation of physicians, nurses, and other healthcare profes-

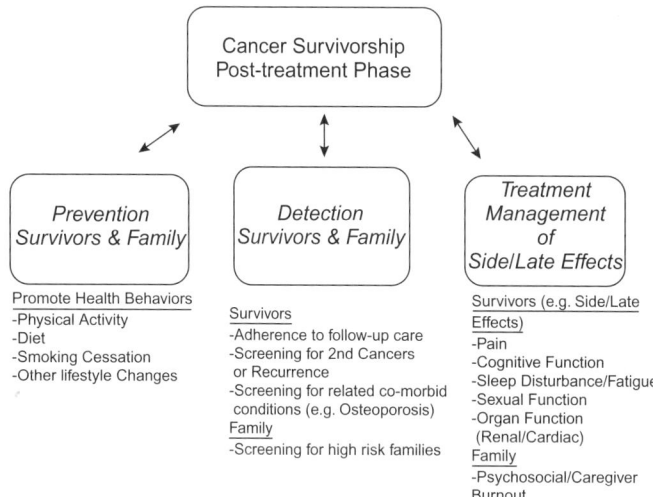

FIGURE 4.3. Aspects of cancer survivorship interventions.

sionals to provide not just the science but also the art of comprehensive cancer medicine.

The New Generation of Survivors: Who are They?

Profile of the Current Survivor Population

"The new population of survivors hanging in there can be found everywhere...in offices and factories, on bicycles and cruise ships, on tennis courts and beaches, and in bowling alleys. You see them in all ages, shapes, sizes, colors, usually unremarkable in their appearance, sometimes remarkable for the way they learn to live with disabilities." (Natalie Davis Spingarn,[39] p. 69)

In 1982, Natalie Davis Spingarn became one of a feisty vanguard of cancer survivors, and vocal patient advocates, to publish a book about their encounter with cancer. Her volume, titled *Hanging in There, Living Well on Borrowed Time*,[39] chronicled her experience of being diagnosed as a young woman (under age 50) and living long term with metastatic breast cancer. A journalist and investigative reporter by training, Natalie provided information often hard for fellow cancer travelers to find and encouraged them to become active participants in their care, a quite provocative message for those more comfortable operating in the paternalistic model of care of the times. In 1999 she published an update of this journey in a book titled *The New Cancer Survivors: Living with Grace, Fighting with Spirit*.[40] In this second volume she describes what she recognized as a new and emerging generation of survivors who come from all walks of life, seek an equal or at a minimum a partnership role in their health-related decision making and care, and expect to be treated as whole persons, not as a particular disease (cancer) or body site (breast patient).

The main driver behind interest in issues of cancer survivorship is necessarily the growing population of survivors. Cancer survival in the United States has risen steadily over the past three decades for all cancers combined. When Nixon declared "the war" on cancer in 1971, there were only

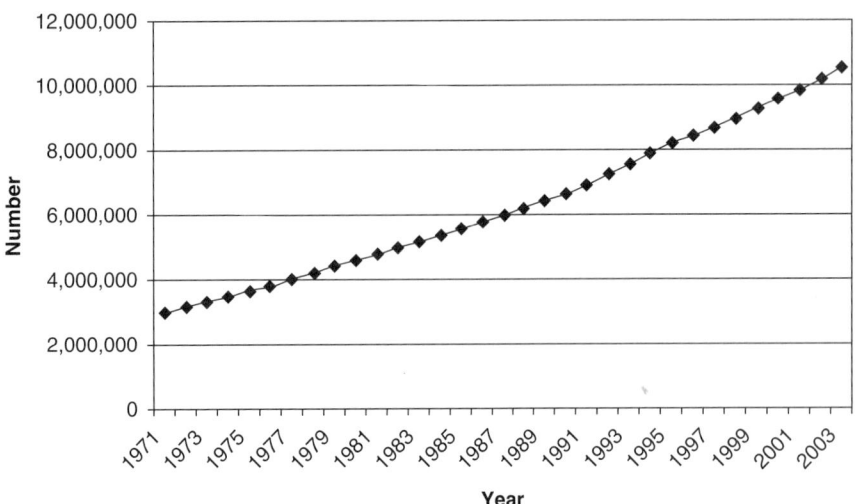

FIGURE 4.4. Estimated number of cancer survivors in the United States from 1971 to 2003. U.S. estimated prevalence counts were estimated by applying U.S. populations to Surveillance Epidemiology and End Results (SEER) 9 Limited Duration Prevalence proportions. Populations from January 2003 were based on the average of the 2002 and 2003 population estimates from the U.S. Bureau of Census. (*Source:* November 2005 submission.)

3 million survivors. Today, there are approximately 24.5 million cancer survivors worldwide; an estimated 10.5 million of these live in the United States alone, representing between 3% and 4% of the population (Figure 4.4).[41a] In the absence of other competing causes of death, current figures indicate that for adults diagnosed during 1995 to 2000, 64% could expect to be alive in 5 years; this is up from 50% estimated for those diagnosed during 1974 to 1976. The relative 5-year survival rate for those diagnosed as children (less than 19 years of age) is even higher. Of children diagnosed with cancer between 1974 and 1976, while 80% survived beyond 1 year, little more than half (56%) were still alive 5 years later. Today, 79% of childhood cancer survivors will be alive at 5 years, and the 10-year survival is approaching 75%. If these trends in survival continue, we may reasonably expect to reach the *2010 Healthy People* goal of 70% 5-year survival for all those diagnosed with cancer.

Of the 10.5 million survivors in the United States, an impressive 14% were diagnosed 20 or more years ago (Figure 4.5).[41a] More women than men are survivors. The higher proportion of men who are within 5 years of diagnosis is consistent with the larger number of males versus females

diagnosed annually with cancer. At the other end of the survivorship continuum, more women survive longer than men due to the higher proportion found to have more readily detected and treatable cancers (e.g., breast, gynecologic), the fact that fewer women (n = 80,660) than men (n = 93,110) develop lung cancer or die of it (females, 68,510 versus males, 91,930) annually,[3] and the generally lower all-cause mortality rate among women versus men in this country.

Of the prevalent cancer population, the largest constituent group comprises breast cancer survivors (23%), followed by survivors of prostate cancer (19%), colorectal cancer (10%), and gynecologic cancer (9.9%) (Figure 4.6).[41a] Consonant with the fact that cancer is a disease associated with aging [median age of cancer patients at diagnosis based on

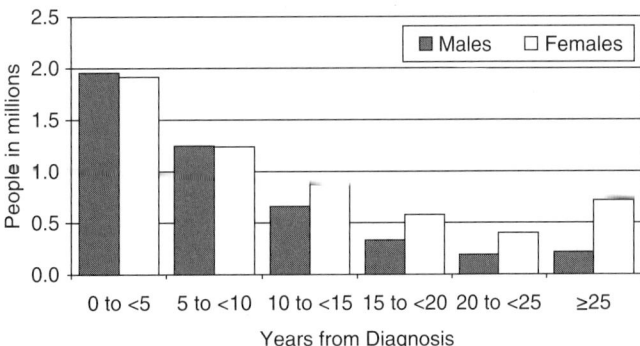

FIGURE 4.5. Estimated number of persons alive in the United States diagnosed with cancer on January 1, 2003, by time from diagnosis and gender (invasive/first primary cases only; n = 10.5 million survivors). U.S. prevalence counts were estimated by applying U.S. populations to SEER-9 Limited Duration Prevalence proportions. Populations from January 2003 were based on the average of the 2002 and 2003 population estimates from the U.S. Bureau of Census. (*Source:* 2005 submission.)

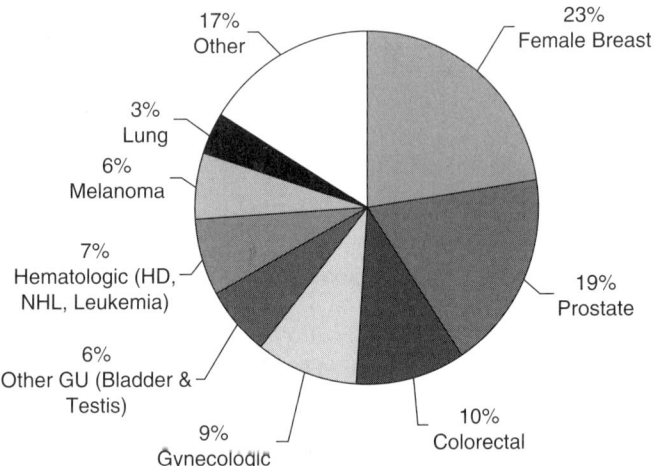

FIGURE 4.6. Estimated number of persons alive in the United States diagnosed with cancer by site. Starting *clockwise from 12:00 position:* female breast (23%), prostate (19%), colorectal (10%), gynecologic (9%), other genitourinary (GU, bladder and testis) (6%), hematologic [Hodgkin's Disease (HD), non-Hodgkin's lymphoma (NHL), leukemia] (7%), melanoma (6%), lung (3%), and other (17%). U.S. Estimated Prevalence counts were estimated by applying U.S. populations to SEER 9 for All Races, White, and Black, SEER 11 for Asian/Pacific Islander, and SEER 11 (excluding Hawaii and Detroit for Hispanic) Limited Duration Prevalence proportions. Populations from January 2003 were based on the average of the 2002 and 2003 population estimates from the U.S. Bureau of Census. (*Source:* 2005 submission.)

SEER (Surveillance, Epidemiology, and End Results) 12 data from 1997 to 2001 was 67 years; an estimated 56.8% of new cancers are diagnosed in patients 65 and older],[42] the majority (61%) of our survivors are aged 65 or older, while 33% are between ages 40 and 64, 5% are aged from 20 to 39 years, and fewer than 1% are 19 or younger. It is currently estimated that one of every six persons over the age of 65 is living with a history of cancer. Although it is unknown what impact the use of chemopreventive agents such as tamoxifen will have on the larger figures for breast cancer incidence, as past and future advances in cancer detection, treatment, and care diffuse into clinical practice, the number of survivors can be expected to increase. Fewer deaths from cardiovascular disease and the aging of the population will contribute to this trend.

Projected Population of the Future

Realization that the world's population is aging is sobering.[43] In 2011, the first members of the baby boomer generation (those born between 1946 and 1964) will turn 65. It is estimated that by the year 2030 one in five individuals will be age 65 or older and 40% will be from minority groups. At the same time, it is recognized that older cancer patients tend to be in poorer health (34% versus 10% of the general population), often have two or more chronic medical conditions (16% versus 4%), report functional limitations (nearly 70% versus less than 30%), and experience more limitations in activities of daily living (ADL) or instrumental ADL (17% versus 3%).[44] Given these figures, it is clear that planning for the care and ongoing health of our aging population, many of whom will become cancer survivors, constitutes a critical public health challenge for the future.[43]

The OCS includes family or caregivers as "secondary" survivors in its definition of survivors. This concept reflects the growing appreciation of the critical role they play in a loved one's or family member's illness. The American Cancer Society (ACS) in its *Facts and Figures* publication for 1996 estimated that three of every four families would have an affected family member. Recent data on caregiving in America suggest that 21% of those over the age of 18 provide unpaid care for an adult 18 and older. The second most common reason for a recipient to need care, after old age, is cancer.[45] Data obtained from cancer survivors identified by the National Health Interview Survey in 1992 indicated that approximately 24% of adult cancer survivors (1.3 million) had a child 18 years of age or younger living in the home.[46] To date, relatively little is known about the impact of living with someone who has cancer on other family members in general; even less is known about cancer's impact on the current or future health behaviors and well-being of younger and potentially highly vulnerable family members.

With advances in our understanding of genomics and proteomics and the application of novel delivery systems, many project that future antineoplastic therapies will be more targeted to cancer cells and less toxic to normal tissue, resulting in significant reductions in treatment-associated morbidity. This is not to say cancer therapy will be entirely benign, as few pharmacological treatments are ever entirely without side effects. Monitoring for the novel, potentially subtle, and late-appearing or unexpected effects of newer approaches to cure represents a challenge to future researchers. Of equal importance will be our ability to assess the impact of delivery of these molecularly targeted treatments. Many agents will be administered orally, shifting the responsibility for delivery and monitoring away from the medical team and to the patient. Appreciating the obstacles faced by patients and families to understand and adhere to regimens will be critical if we are to understand not just drug effectiveness but also survivors' QOL and health-related outcomes.

Domains of Survivorship Research: Multidimensionality

In the early era of research on the psychosocial and physical impact of cancer, the common practice was to use global (e.g., Karnofsky) or summary scores representing overall function across a range of activities of daily living activities (e.g., FLIC, functional living index-cancer; LASA, linear analog self assessment). Perhaps unique to cancer QOL studies (as opposed to those for other chronic illnesses) is their history of emphasis on the importance of patient-based outcomes. What was quickly apparent in instrument selection and development was the need for patient (versus physician)-based measures.[47–49] The few clinician-rated scales still commonly in use represent measures to assess patient status for clinical trials (e.g., ECOG, Eastern Collaborative Oncology Group, status) or were designed for use when a patient might be too sick to complete a self-assessment, e.g., the Spitzer Quality of Life Index.[50]

As clinicians began looking more closely at patient-focused outcomes and more behavioral scientists joined the field of inquiry, four primary areas of QOL impact emerged: physical (symptoms), functional (capacity to engage in activities of daily living), emotional (mood/affective and cognitive status), and social (role functioning and/or support, financial burden). Examples of early scales with these four domains include the Quality of Life Index[51] and the Sickness Impact Profile.[52] These four domains remain at the core of contemporary scales.

An early challenge for the field was the need to develop and test cancer-specific tools. As already noted, initial studies of mental health outcomes for survivors relied heavily on the use of instruments borrowed from the psychiatric arena, for example, the Hopkins Symptom Checklist (SCL-90) and the Profile of Mood States (POMS). Even when studies became more sophisticated and expanded to include such domains as sexual functioning, the available measures (e.g., Derogatis Sexual Functioning Inventory) were often poorly designed to assess cancer patients' functioning or unique areas or types of dysfunction. It is of note that the recent interest in examining benefit finding among survivors led clinical researchers to reflexively go back to the psychiatric literature for tools (e.g., posttraumatic stress scale, civilian version; posttraumatic growth inventory) before realizing that they would need to develop measures better suited to capturing the cancer experience.

The most recent generation of cancer-specific measures is designed to assess domains of well-being that represent newer foci of attention. These measures include, for example, items or scales to assess fatigue, cognitive dysfunction, and menopausal or hot flash symptoms, as well as bowel and urologic status in colorectal, select gynecologic, and prostate cancer survivors. (See the Cancer Outcomes Measurement Working group-generated publication for an excellent review of current measurement tools.[53]) The two newest areas of attention in measurement development are long-term survivorship scales[54-56] and measures of postcancer health behaviors.[57-60] Curiously, although fear of recurrence is probably the single most common concern of those living with a history of cancer, efforts to create instruments designed specifically to measure this domain have languished.[61-63]

There has been considerable debate as to whether current measures assess QOL or simply health-related quality of life (HRQOL).[64,65] Many argue that individual QOL is intangible and almost impossible to meaningfully measure. Although the majority of survivorship researchers today use the terms QOL and HRQOL interchangeably, when pressed most agree that our common assessment tools are most accurate in providing (and often specifically designed to generate or elicit) information on survivors' perception of their health-related quality of life than QOL per se. One of the more recently appreciated challenges to the field of QOL assessment among cancer survivors is interpreting the impact cancer has over time in individuals' lives. Cancer researchers are (re)learning what others have reported for decades,[66] that humans are incredibly adaptable and, given time and support, can adapt to considerable limitations. The manifestation of this resilience is seen in what researchers now refer to as "response shift" in subjects' report of functioning and well-being when measured over time.[67] In this paradigm, respondents, as they accommodate to a loss or disability, are less likely to report being upset by it, even though the impairment may continue to cause the same level of, and sometimes greater, disability over time. Trying to make sense of this phenomenon while teasing out what health-promoting interventions may or may not be most helpful for survivors' recovery has become a respected field of inquiry in itself.

Trends in Survivorship Research

Past

The historical research on survivorship has been well reviewed by others.[35,36] General themes have evolved over time. In the early era of survivorship research, most studies focused on the psychological impact of cancer or the delineation of specific sequelae of treatment (e.g., impact of stomas, lymphedema, amputation).[68,69] As the number of survivors grew and length of survival increased, attention expanded to include examination of the social (interpersonal, family, work, school) and sexual well-being of survivors.[6,70-72] By the mid-1980s, researchers, responding to the observation by many survivors that they continued to reexperience aspects of the events associated with their diagnosis and treatment, began to conceptualize cancer as a "traumatic event." A new wave of studies sought to determine the extent to which cancer produced symptoms of posttraumatic stress disorder (PTSD).[73,74] In pursuing this path, investigators began to hear from survivors, particularly in studies that contained

qualitative analyses or open-ended formats, that cancer also caused them to recognize the positive aspects of their lives. The consequence of this observation is that a current trend in research is to examine the role of benefit finding in promoting and/or mediating and moderating survivorship outcomes.[75-77]

Since the establishment of psychosocial oncology as a field of its own in the early 1970s, clinical researchers have actively sought to take what they learned in their surveys and apply it to interventions that would reduce cancer's toll on survivors and their families. Relatively little of this research, however, was designed exclusively to meet the needs of those posttreatment.[78,79] This picture is slowly changing.

Present

Since 2000, the NCI's Office of Cancer Survivorship has conducted annual analyses of the number and types of grants in the area of cancer survivorship funded across the National Institutes of Health. (These data are updated and posted yearly online.[80]) Included in this analysis are grants that examine the health or behavior of individuals after treatment for cancer or that of their family members. Excluded from this review are studies that consider patients solely during active treatment or early posttreatment (less than 2 months follow-up) or survivors with recurrent or advanced disease. When the OCS was originally established in 1996, only 24 National Institutes of Health (NIH) grants could be identified that met these narrower criteria. In the philosophy of "build it and they will come," the NCI's commitment to this area of science, with the creation of the OCS, appears to have been successful.

Judging by the numbers, the research community is slowly being enticed to advance its expertise to tackle issues further along the cancer control continuum. In fiscal year 2003 (encompassing October 2002 through September 2003), the period for which most complete data exist, a total of 179 grants were identified as addressing survivorship issues. Of these, 154 (86%) were funded through the NCI. The remainder were supported by the National Institute for Nursing Research ($n = 14$), National Institutes of Mental Health ($n = 5$), National Institute on Aging ($n = 4$), and the National Institute of Dental and Craniofacial Research ($n = 2$). That many grants end up at institutes other than the NCI reflects the fact that many of the issues faced by survivors (e.g., depression, aging, family challenges, pain syndromes) are not always unique to cancer. In keeping with past patterns, the majority of studies supported were descriptive or analytic in nature (54%). However, 42% of the funded research projects contained an intervention component designed to improve the psychosocial well-being, physical status, and/or health behaviors of survivors and/or their family members. This latter figure is important as it denotes the transition that is occurring in the research arena away from mere identification of problems (discovery) to the development and testing of interventions designed to reduce posttreatment morbidity and mortality (development). Most of the studies continue to be unique to or include samples of breast cancer survivors ($n = 79$, 44%), who, for a variety of reasons, have historically been the focus of the majority of the psychosocial research conducted in cancer.[81] Other leading cancer sites represented in this work include hematologic, prostate, and colorectal.

A clear testament to the success of the NCI's efforts to grow in survivorship research, and the readiness of the research community to pursue questions in this area, is reflected in the response to its request for applications (RFA) for studies addressing long-term cancer survivorship (defined as studies among cancer survivors diagnosed 5 or more years ago). In 1997 the OCS presented its first such RFA (CA 97-018), which attracted 79 applications. In 2003, the RFA was reissued (CA 04-003). A total of 125 applications were received in response to this second call. Of the 125 grants received, 50 (40%) were from investigators new to the field of cancer survivorship research.

One of the reasons that the NCI reissued the Long-Term Survivors RFA was that without this impetus few investigators appeared willing to take on the additional challenges of studying individuals years posttreatment. A review of the research portfolio conducted before the RFA reissuance revealed that only 27 of 126 grants analyzed were studying survivors 5 or more years postdiagnosis; 21 of these were developed in response to the initial RFA. Critical barriers to long-term survivorship research include finding this population, obtaining access to them, including negotiating the many hurdles consequent to the recently implemented Health Insurance Portability and Accountability Act (HIPAA) regulations, developing tools that measure outcomes of relevance to the long-term survivorship experience, identifying appropriate control or comparison groups, and coordinating a team invested in addressing these issues.

Future

Staff at the American Cancer Society took advantage of the opportunity to poll investigators engaged in behavioral, psychosocial, and policy research in cancer about their current interests and expectations for future research foci when compiling a directory of these individuals in 1997 and again when they updated the directory for release in 2002.[82] Addressing psychosocial issues and treatment and outcomes remained key interest areas over time, a finding not altogether surprising given the target survey participants. However, two important areas for future research emerged in this report: the need to address special populations, a future direction voiced by members of all five of the disciplines represented (behavioral scientist, epidemiologist, nurse, physician, psychologist), and growing attention to health education and communication. Interesting in this study was the low endorsement of interest in survivorship research. Less than 10% said they were engaged in this type of research in 1997 (7.3%), and only 1.5% in 2002. However, in 2002, 11.7% thought it was going to be an important area of research in the future.

Ongoing analysis of the NIH-wide survivorship portfolio highlights a number of areas where our knowledge is lacking. Two of these areas echo themes identified for future targeting by Nehl and colleagues[82]: (1) the exploration of outcomes for our diverse population of survivors, specifically those from ethnoculturally diverse backgrounds, those from low-income or low educational backgrounds, rural survivors, elderly survivors, and survivors from common cancer sites under-

represented in the literature (lung, colorectal, gynecologic, hematologic)[83]; and (2) effective communication about survivorship-related issues. To these, four more areas are added, including (3) research on the impact of cancer on the family or caregiver; (4) studies addressing the economic impact of cancer on survivors and survivorship; (5) assessment of the nature, delivery, and outcomes of follow-up care to survivors; and (6) measurement tool development, including that which would enable us to compare survivors with those without a cancer history while also controlling for other comorbid illness states.

As the field of survivorship research has matured, change has occurred not only in the focus of the research being conducted but also in how and by whom this research is being carried out. The typical published cancer survivorship study has evolved from a largely descriptive outcome report based on a small single institution sample[84,85] to one involving multidisciplinary teams accruing large cohorts and applying complex outcome and intervention assessments.[86,87] A concrete measure of the growing sophistication of this body of research is the expectation by standing members of study sections (peer review groups) to see power analyses, detailed rationales for measurement choices, adequate representation by appropriate diverse scientific experts, and demonstrated sensitivity to the unique needs and experience of the target survivor group in grants submitted for review, with general impatience with studies that appear to "rediscover" what is already documented. Table 4.1 provides an overview of some of these trends over time.

Looking to the future, it is expected that a healthy balance needs to be maintained between the identification of problematic long-term and late effects of cancer and our ability to address these. The roughly 60%/40% split in current NIH-funded research between studies aimed at identifying problem areas and those designed to develop and test interventions that reduce the negative effects of cancer is probably a reasonable balance. With respect to the intervention arena, two new trends are of note. It is increasingly apparent that to be successful this research must (a) attempt to explain the biopsychosocial interaction between what is being delivered and its impact on health outcomes[88,89] and (b) control or account for the costs associated with its delivery.[90] Although psychoneuroimmunology (PNI) research in cancer is by no means new,[91–93] attention to mind–body links is expanding as researchers seek to explain what is going on inside the proverbial "black box," in particular, in the context of psychosocial interventions that might mediate or moderate the impact of these trials on cancer recurrence or survival. Further, although drug interventions are relatively low cost, most psychosocial or behavioral interventions are labor intensive and hence more expensive to deliver. Despite this, there is good evidence to suggest they can reduce medical costs.[94] In recognition of this, investigators are working hard to design interventions that can be either self-administered,[90,95] delivered readily by available healthcare staff with minimal training,[96] and/or, the newest piece in these models, made available online.[97,98] This last point is critical if we are to have any hope of taking into the broader community interventions that hold the promise of significantly reducing the burden of cancer on individuals and society.

TABLE 4.1. Trends in cancer survivorship research design.

	Past	Present	Future
Target samples	Generally small convenience samples, often single institution based and mainly white, middle class, and middle age; largely breast cancer, or mixed, some colorectal, gynecologic; also pediatric, but largely leukemia	Moderate to large samples; often multiinstitutional; some clinical trials and population- or registry-based; increasing diversity of survivor groups by age and site (especially prostate, Hodgkin's disease, other gynecologic); still limited ethnocultural, income, and geographic diversity; more focus on family/caregivers	Mix of large (e.g., cohort, population-based) and moderate size; largely multiinstitutional; greater representation of more diverse cancer sites and previously neglected populations (e.g., by ethnic/income/geographic/age groups); more use of clinical trials samples
Team	Physicians, nurses, and some mental health professionals	Multidisciplinary teams; behavioral scientists leading in many areas; nurses with strong role as well; increasing role of advocates/survivors in research design	Truly multidisciplinary teams; attention to addition of basic scientists and psychoneuroimmunology (PNI) researchers to understand mind–body implications and impact of research findings for recurrence/survival, risk, and treatments; customary role for advocates/survivors in research
Basic design	Descriptive; limited interventions; often atheoretical and exploratory in nature; almost exclusively cross-sectional designs	Increase in hypothesis- and model-driven designs; complex multicomponent interventions growing; replication studies appearing; longitudinal studies increasing	Sophisticated model building and hypothesis testing; emphasis on building on prior studies, including research to take interventions to different audiences, settings, deliverers; intervention designs incorporating biologic markers and/or economic and health services endpoints or outcomes; longitudinal/cohort research
Topic	Focus almost exclusively on documenting dysfunction: distress, disability, impairment; a few coping studies; limited risk modeling	HRQOL instrument development; shift to evaluate both benefits and deficits of illness; modeling of risk for poor outcomes; examining role of caregivers in survivor outcomes and vice versa; growing attention to treatment effects and focused attention to specific problems, e.g., sexual dysfunction, fatigue, cognitive impairment; beginning attention to health after treatment	HRQOL development for long-term survivors (including comparison to other chronic illness groups and controlling for comorbid conditions); identifying/describing late, as yet unknown effects of cancer and novel problems associated with newer treatments and risk for these; targeting and tailoring interventions to survivors; identifying who may need what delivered by whom and when in the course of care; establishing the unique human and economic burden of cancer (versus other chronic illnesses); health promotion, follow-up care studies

HRQOL, health-related quality of life.

Challenges for the Future

Looking to the future, investigators face a number of challenges in advancing cancer survivorship research.[99] These challenges can be seen as falling into three broad categories: (1) identifying the most salient topics for study, (2) creating or enhancing the resources necessary to conduct the research, and (3) developing ways to make use of what is discovered.

Discovery

One of the greatest challenges to engaging in survivorship research is keeping up with the rapid pace of change in cancer treatments and care, as is particularly well illustrated in the context of breast cancer. In the past 10 years we have seen the uptake into standard practice of the use of sentinel node biopsies (replacing axillary node dissections), neoadjuvant (presurgical administration of) chemotherapy for large tumors, dose-intense and dense regimens of adjuvant chemotherapy with their greater attendant exposure to growth factors, testing for Her2 and consideration of herceptin, autologous tissue implants (over saline or silicone implants) for breast reconstruction, and aromatase inhibitors

in the adjuvant setting, as well as a shift away from use of stem cell transplant as a treatment option. Each of these alterations in practice has implications for QOL outcomes for women treated. For example, elimination for many women of the need for axillary node dissection may result in far fewer women developing lymphedema as a consequence of their breast cancer therapy.[100,101] Nevertheless, greater exposure to more-intense chemotherapy regimens will likely increase the number of women at risk for persistent problems with pain (related to the accompanying use of growth factors)[102] and memory problems (or chemo brain).[103] Meanwhile, continued changes in the healthcare delivery system are transforming significantly the availability of and access to resources that have been shown to buffer the adverse effects of care (e.g., access to social support, information and education, and rehabilitation services). In an effort to control rising medical costs and respond to diminished insurance reimbursements, many hospitals and medical centers have sought to decrease the number of patient hospitalizations and length of stay, eliminate or downsize the types of support services as well as the number of social workers in their systems, and shift the delivery of oncology care largely to the outpatient setting.[104,105] Third-party payers in turn have placed constraints on patients' ability to use specialized providers and/or services. Combined, these changes in the delivery of cancer care have put enormous pressure on cancer survivors and their family members or caregivers to be more self-sufficient or in some cases to do without the support or services they might wish to have in facilitating optimal recovery.[106] This burden is borne disproportionately by minority and underserved members of our society.[107] Curiously, while research consistently shows that providing education and support is important for survivors' capacity to cope with cancer, access to this help is diminishing.

The implication of these changes for researchers is that what may have been critically important for one cohort of survivors may be less relevant to the next generation of individuals treated. For example, body image was a major focus of research in early studies of breast cancer outcomes when mastectomy was the treatment of choice.[68] Today, most women have a choice (often involving several options) in how to treat the breast and deal with the cosmetic impact of breast cancer. As a consequence, body image disruption is less salient as either an outcome or research issue. Of more concern is how breast cancer treatment may alter sexual function and/or menopausal symptoms, given that more than 50% of women diagnosed now receive some form of adjuvant chemotherapy or hormonal therapy.[108] Increasingly, researchers are finding themselves caught between the need to identify emerging chronic or late effects of newer therapies and chronicling and addressing the long-term effects of older ones. This dilemma can become problematic if, at review, scientific peers around the table cannot see the relevance of long-term outcomes studies (given this picture), or when forced to make a choice about limited funding dollars, opt to support studies about current therapies only.

Some of the more recently identified "hot" areas of symptom research include a focus on memory problems, fatigue, weight gain, long-term cardiac health, osteoporosis, and persistent pain syndromes (associated with exposure to taxanes and/or use of growth factors). Interest in all these concerns has occurred in direct response to survivors' accounts of specific problems with these conditions (e.g., memory problems, fatigue, weight gain, pain), or clinicians' concerns about known potential toxicities of treatment (e.g., second malignancies, cardiac dysfunction, osteoporosis). As already observed, the recent advances in modern computer and laboratory technology and the associated explosion of discovery in the molecular sciences lend hope that future therapies can be designed to have fewer adverse effects on healthy tissue. Nevertheless, listening carefully to patients' experience of these new approaches is critical if we are to identify and evaluate in future generations of survivors the impact of cancer on health.

On a larger scale, with so many individuals living longer following a diagnosis of cancer, growing attention is being given to researching the efficacy of more generic interventions in improving the future health of survivors, not merely in diminishing their current symptoms. There is a growing movement in particular to develop interventions that include elements with the potential to be generalized to other noncancer conditions. Two good examples of this are the work being done by Antoni and colleagues in the area of stress management[109,110] and that of Courneya and colleagues on delivery of physical activity interventions.[111,112] With the baby boomers fast entering the years of greatest cancer risk, under-

standing the role of comorbidities on cancer outcomes and care is critical to both evaluating and reducing the burden of cancer.[43,44,113,114] At the same time, a pressing need continues for us to understand the enormous and growing divide between survival—and necessarily the survivorship experience—of our communities of color, low income, low education, and rural status, versus the Caucasian and Asian survivor populations about whom we have the most data.[83,115]

Development

To accomplish any of this work will take some very specific resources and infrastructure or capacity building. First is access to relevant study samples. A continuing challenge for many researchers is identifying and reaching long-term survivors, in particular those diagnosed more than 5 years earlier.[116] Tumor registries can help,[117] but loss to follow-up is common. Clinical trials groups, an obvious place to partner to obtain long-term follow-up data, also often lose track of their participants over time.[118] The introduction of new federal privacy laws (Health Insurance Portability and Accountability Act, or HIPAA), by requiring individual consent for the conduct of specific studies and data sharing, has made access to survivors and their medical records even more cumbersome. This problem is not unique to the United States.[119] Establishment of the NCI-supported Childhood Cancer Survivor Study cohort currently provides a rich resource for survivorship information generated from its ascertained sample of roughly 14,000 survivors of childhood cancer diagnosed between 1978 and 1986 and the companion sample of more than 3,800 siblings.[120] To date, no such repository exists for survivors of adult cancer.

A second critical need is a steady flow of researchers. Despite the fact that the field of psycho-oncology (or psychosocial oncology), and the more-specific area of posttreatment survivorship research, has grown steadily in the past two decades, the number of researchers devoted to this science is still very limited. Further, there continue to be only a handful of training centers across the country devoted to the education and support of the next generation of researchers invested in survivorship research. With the recent creation of the American Society of Psychosocial Oncology (APOS), now independent from the older International Psycho-Oncology Society, there is hope that this picture may change. Further, the advances in computer technology, use of self-training programs for credit, and online access to a world of expertise may help close this gap in investigator resources. In this regard, APOS and the American Society of Clinical Oncology are pioneering efforts to promote the pursuit of continuing education by members in this and related symptom management and assessment domains.[121,122] Further, colleagues around the world are beginning to develop programs that promise to ensure a future cadre of talented clinicians and researchers.[123,124]

A third area of necessary development is on the provider side. Some in the pediatric oncology community have been heard to lament that fewer physicians are choosing to pursue careers in this specialty, assuming (incorrectly) that with survival figures already so high, few challenges or opportunities remain to make breakthroughs in this field. Adult oncology, by contrast, continues to offer diverse challenges; one of these being to better understand the long-term and late consequences of treatment as a way to improve cancer diagnosis, treatment, and care. Inadequate support for young physicians to engage in research remains a barrier to ensuring more oncologists will seek to expand their expertise in the survivorship arena. In a 2002 review of professional education and training in cancer survivorship commissioned by the National Cancer Policy Board (NCPB), Roger Winn found that although oncology textbooks were beginning to incorporate pieces about this aspect of care (in particular, the incidence and pathophysiology of chronic or late effects), often the material was fragmented and provided few guidelines for evaluation and care. There were, however, notable exceptions to this, including the Harris et al. volume *Diseases of the Breast*, and the monograph produced for the benefit of its members by the American Association of Family Practitioners on *Cancer Survivors*.

The picture in nursing appears to be quite different. Nurses were among the leaders in pioneering psychosocial research and QOL instrument development in cancer.[51,54-56] In a review also commissioned in 2002 by the NCPB, Betty Ferrell and Rose Virani found that all the major nursing textbooks of oncology nursing had sections or information on cancer survivorship and addressing late and long-term effects of disease. The Oncology Nursing Society has had a Special Interest Group in this area for several years.

Engaging the entire medical community (including nurses, primary care physicians, mental health professionals, and rehabilitation specialists) is necessary to ensure that we ask the right questions in survivorship research and use the best approaches to conduct this science. All this activity will require fiscal resources. Already there has been a rapid growth in the number of federal dollars being expended on survivorship research. This amount of money remains small, nevertheless, when compared to that being invested in cancer biology, detection, and treatment. In 2003, the OCS supported $17 million in grant-related research; NCI-wide investment in survivorship research, broadly defined to include studies among individuals across the survivorship continuum from diagnosis to end of life, was estimated at $160 million, less than 4% of the NCI budget for that year. Further, the end of the doubling of the NIH budget with FY 2004 and expected spending limits projected for the near future threaten to make competition for this still-nascent area of research a critical source of challenge.

On the positive side, a number of additional funders committed to supporting research on survivors' outcomes have appeared on the scene; these include the Lance Armstrong Foundation, the Avon Foundation, the Susan G. Komen Foundation, and the California Breast Cancer Research Program. Recently reframed as constituting a public health issue,[34] cancer survivorship is also beginning to appear on the agenda of the Center for Disease Control and Prevention. In addition, as noted earlier, Congress has put forward a number of bills in the past 2 years indicating their intention that the NIH in general and NCI in particular continue to invest in this science. The creation of the Office of Cancer Survivorship at the NCI provided a critical infrastructure and platform from which to oversee, track, and direct cancer survivorship research at the Federal level. Its existence within the NCI serves as a reminder of the importance of this aspect of the cancer control continuum both across NCI and nationally. Staff from the CDC, National Association of American Cancer Registries, ACS, NCI, and American College of Surgeons recently put forward recommendations for elements of the framework necessary to move cancer control forward in the next 20 years.[125] Similarly, members of NCI's Division of Cancer Control and Population Sciences have outlined where we need to go in the future to advance quality of cancer care across the continuum.[126]

Delivery

The final challenge faced is how best to disseminate and use the information gleaned from the growing body of cancer survivorship research. To date, this process has been painstakingly slow, in particular in the adult oncology arena. Delivering on what we already know represents, both historically[127] and at the present time, the least developed area of cancer survivorship research and constitutes one of the most significant challenges for the future.[128-130] This problem is well illustrated in a recent publication of the Institute of Medicine (IOM) entitled *Meeting the Psychosocial Needs of Women with Breast Cancer*.[131] In this volume, the multiple authors provide a wealth of evidence indicating that we already understand the kinds of problems faced by women treated for this disease, the handful of risk factors that increase risk for poor QOL, and the types of interventions that may help improve women's outcomes. Translating this into practice remains the biggest hurdle. This need includes educating healthcare providers about the psychosocial and behavioral effects of cancer and training them to incorporate psychosocial concerns into standard treatment planning and posttreatment monitoring, as well as designing and funding healthcare delivery systems that support this activity.[128] It is of note that, even in the nation's comprehensive cancer centers, programs for survivors who have completed their cancer therapy remain limited.[132] In addition, in many of these centers, researchers engaged in survivorship research are not routinely connected with the clinics or care centers.

These same kinds of struggles play out differently in the area of childhood cancer. In pediatrics, attention to the "total child" and his or her family is simply part of standard care.[133] Further, most pediatric care, whether in the cancer or non-cancer setting, is designed around promoting normal development and preventing or minimizing risk of disease. Pediatric oncologists, perhaps because of the dramatic advances made in curing childhood cancers, have been at the forefront of efforts to tailor therapies to reduce morbidity without compromising cure. For example, once trials began to show that use of central nervous system prophylaxis dramatically altered the survival for children with ALL in the late 1960s and early 1970s, clinicians quickly turned their attention to finding less-toxic ways to provide this coverage that would eliminate the need for or reduce the dose of cranial radiation to which children would be exposed.[37] Equivalent evidence for this approach in adult oncology is harder to identify. The movement away from more-radical excisions to greater tissue-sparing approaches to surgery, as seen in breast and colorectal cancer, are good examples of efforts to modify treatment to improve QOL without adversely affecting cure. These surgical oncology examples notwithstanding, the general trend in adult oncology remains heavily focused on delivering more, not less, treatment, even if the length of time over which these therapies are administered is shrinking.

More recently, both the pediatric and adult oncology communities have engaged in efforts to decide how best to follow themselves, or engage the larger adult healthcare delivery system to care for, the growing population of young and maturing adults previously treated as children.[134,135] The Children's Oncology Group (COG) has taken a leadership role in shaping this effort. In spring 2004 COG publicly released the first set of comprehensive, long-term follow-up guidelines.[136] Unique to this document is its attention to the long-term and late sequelae of curative therapies. Unlike currently available guidelines for adult survivors who are posttreatment (e.g., as developed by ASCO, American Society of Clinical Oncology, and NCCN, National Comprehensive Cancer Network) that focus exclusively on cancer surveillance, the childhood cancer follow-up guidelines are constructed around identification and management of risk-based, exposure-related problems that may be screened for and potentially addressed after treatment. Largely unknown is how nononcology professionals view and care for the survivors in their patient population.[137] What evidence we have suggests that many survivors are not receiving care that might be expected for peers without a cancer history.[38,59,138,139] In this regard, data from two NCI-led SEER-based research studies on hematologic (non-Hodgkin's lymphoma, NHL) and selected solid tumor (breast, colorectal, prostate, gynecologic) survivors' experience of posttreatment care that will be available starting in 2005 should be informative.

A final criterion for the success of what one might call the cancer survivorship research enterprise is whether it is having an impact on the outcomes of present and future survivors and/or their families and caregivers. This aspect of survivorship research is as yet the least developed of all. Benchmarks for success exist in other realms of cancer control. For example, one can track the reduction in smoking rates to assess prevention efforts, the uptake of screening modalities (e.g., mammography, colonoscopy) by the appropriate populations to monitor inroads in promoting early detection, and survival curves to determine global cancer control. However, it is not clear what the markers of success are for improved survivorship (not to be confused with survival) outcomes.[140] Should this be return to school for children? Return to work for younger adults? Self-reported QOL compared to the general population for cohorts of survivors? Decrease in medical care use among survivors receiving a supportive intervention? If we have learned anything from survivors it is that being disease free does not mean being free of your disease. It is not enough to cure or enable individuals to live long term with a chronic illness without attending to what they are being returned. Because so many cancer survivors are older and present with a history of other comorbid conditions and experience, determining and alleviating what may be the unique burden of cancer is an area that remains to be fully addressed.[44,113,114,141] At a minimum, we need to be able to provide more than an estimate of the number of individuals who are living beyond a diagnosis of cancer. Finding ways to quantify how those individuals are faring in the main, and where they are on the cancer trajectory (i.e., recently diagnosed, in active treatment, posttreatment, living with or dying of progressive disease) is critical, particularly if we are to establish benchmarks against which to measure our progress. Efforts to do this are under way in Europe[142] and here in the United States.[143,144]

In summary, the evidence is clear that cancer survivorship, once merely a nascent field, is fast entering its adolescence, its pace of maturation driven by the progress made in controlling the many diseases we call cancer. Although still modest for most cancers, the body of research identifying the long-term and late effects of illness, as detailed in Chapter 101 by Aziz in this volume, is growing rapidly. At the same time, investment in the study of interventions to eliminate or reduce adverse cancer- or treatment-related outcomes is increasing. The cancer advocacy community has matured and provides an invaluable resource for ensuring continued attention to survivorship issues.[145-147] However, it is becoming apparent daily that improvements in cancer survivors' outcomes will likely be affected most by what happens to our healthcare delivery system in the years to come. We already know a great deal about what harms or helps those diagnosed and treated for cancer; delivering on the promise of care that conforms to that knowledge should be our most significant overarching goal for the foreseeable future.

References

1. A History of Commitment: 1884–Today. New York: Memorial Sloan-Kettering Cancer Center, Public Affairs Department booklet, 1994.
2. Jemal A, Clegg LX, Ward E, et al. Annual report to the nation on the status of cancer, 1975–2001, with a special feature regarding survival. Cancer (Phila) 2004;101:3–27.
3. Cancer Facts and Figures 2004. Atlanta, GA: American Cancer Society, 2004.
4. D'Angio GJ. Pediatric cancer in perspective: cure is not enough. Cancer (Phila) 1975;35:866–870.
5. Meadows AT, D'Angio GJ, Evans AE, et al. Oncogenesis and other late effects of cancer treatment in children. Radiology 1975;114:175–180.
6. Koocher G, O'Malley J. The Damocles Syndrome. New York: McGraw-Hill, 1981.
7. Holland JC. Historical overview. In: Holland JC, Rowland JH (eds). Handbook of Psychooncology: Psychological Care of the Patient with Cancer. Oxford: Oxford University Press, 1989:3–12.
8. Dolbeault S, Szporn A, Holland JC. Psycho-oncology: where have we been? Where are we going? Eur J Cancer 1999;35:1554–1558.
9. Oken D. What to tell cancer patients: a study of medical attitudes. JAMA 1961;175:1120–1128.
10. Novack DH, Plumer R, Smith RL, et al. Changes in physicians' attitudes toward telling the cancer patient. JAMA 1979;241:897–900.
11. Mystakidou K, Parpa E, Tsilila E, et al. Cancer information disclosure in different cultural contexts. Support Care Cancer 2004;12(3):147–154.
12. Surbone A. Persisting differences in truth telling throughout the world. Support Care Cancer 2004;12(3):143–146.
13. Wang S-Y, Chen C-H, Chen Y-S, Huang H-L. The attitude toward truth telling of cancer in Taiwan. J Psychosom Res 2004;57:53–58.
14. Holland JC. IPOS Sutherland Memorial Lecture: An international perspective on the development of psychosocial oncology: overcoming cultural and attitudinal barriers to improve psychosocial care. Psycho-Oncology 2004;13(7):445–459.
15. Reuben SH (ed). Living Beyond Cancer: A European Dialogue. President's Cancer Panel 2003–2004 Annual Report Supplement. Bethesda, MD: U.S. Department of Health and Human Services, NIH, NCI, May 2004.
16. Die-Trill M, Holland JC. A model curriculum for training in psycho-oncology. Psycho-Oncology 1995;4:169–182.

17. Derogatis LR, Lipman RS, Covi L. SCL-90: an outpatient psychiatric rating scale: preliminary report. Psychopharmacol Bull 1973;9:13–28.

18. NcNair DM, Lorr M, Droppleman R. EITS Manual for the Profile of Mood States. San Diego, CA: Educational and Industrial Testing Service, 1971.

19. Radloff LS. The CES-D scale: a self-report depression scale for research in the general population. Appl Psychol Meas 1977; 1:385–401.

20. Endicott J. Measurement of depression in patients with cancer. Cancer (Phila) 1984;53:2243–2249.

21. Kathol RG, Noyes R, Williams J, et al. Diagnosing depression in patients with medical illness. Psychosomatics 1990;31(4): 434–440.

22. Cohen-Cole SA, Brown FW, McDainel JS. Assessment of depression and grief reactions in the medically ill. In: Stoudemire A, Fogel BS (eds). Psychiatric Care of the Medical Patient. New York: Oxford University Press, 1993:53–69.

23. Schipper H, Clinch J, McMurray A, Levitt M. Measuring the quality of life of cancer patients: The Functional Living Index—Cancer: development and validation. J Clin Oncol 1984;2(5):475–483.

24. Schag CAC, Heinrich RL. Development of a comprehensive quality of life measurement tool: CARES. Oncology 1990;4(5): 135–138.

25. Aaronson NK, Ahmedzai S, Bergman B, et al. The European Organization for Research and Treatment of Cancer QLQ-C30: a quality of life instrument for use in international clinical trials in oncology. J Natl Cancer Inst 1993;85(5):365–376.

26. Cella DF, Tulsky DS, Gray G, et al. The Functional Assessment of Cancer Therapy Scale: development and validation of the general measure. J Clin Oncol 1993;11(3):570–579.

27. Mullan F. Seasons of survival: reflections of a physician with cancer. N Engl J Med 1985;313:270–273.

28. Hoffman B (ed) National Coalition for Cancer Survivorship. A cancer survivor's almanac. Charting your journey. Minneapolis: Chronimed Publishing, 1996:XII–XIII. http://www.canceradvocacy.org

29. http://www.survivorship.cancer.gov

30. The Nation's Investment in Cancer Research: A plan and budget proposal for fiscal year 2004. NIH Publication No. 03-4373. Prepared by the Director, National Cancer Institute. Bethesda, MD: National Institutes of Health, USDHHS, October 2002; Hewitt M, Greenfield S, Stovall E (eds). From Cancer Patient to Cancer Survivor: Lost in Transition. Washington, DC: National Academies Press, 2006.

31. The Nation's Investment in Cancer Research: A plan and budget proposal for fiscal year 2005. NIH Publication No. 03-5446. Prepared by the Director, National Cancer Institute. Bethesda: National Institutes of Health, USDHHS, October 2003.

32. Hewitt M, Weiner SL, Simone JV (eds). Childhood Cancer Survivorship. Improving Care and Quality of Life. Washington, DC: National Academies Press, 2003.

33. Living Beyond Cancer: Finding a New Balance. President's Cancer Panel 2003 Annual Report. Bethesda, MD: U.S. Department of Health and Human Services, NIH, NCI, May 2004.

34. CDC, Lance Armstrong Foundation. A national action plan for cancer survivorship: advancing public health strategies. Atlanta, GA: U.S. Department of Health and Human Services, CDC, 2004.

35. Tross S, Holland JC. Psychological sequelae in cancer survivors. In: Holland JC, Rowland JH (eds). Handbook of Psychooncology: Psychological Care of the Patient with Cancer. Oxford: Oxford University Press, 1989:101–116.

36. Kornblith AB. Psychosocial adaptation of cancer survivors. In: Holland JC (ed). Psycho-Oncology. New York: Oxford University Press, 1998:223–241.

37. Meadows AT. Pediatric cancer survivors: past history and future challenges. Curr Probl Cancer 2003;27:112–126.

38. Yeazel MW, Oeffinger KC, Gurney JG, et al. The cancer screening practices of adult survivors of childhood cancer: a report from the Childhood Cancer Survivors Study. Cancer (Phila) 2004; 100:631–640.

39. Spingarn ND. Hanging in There: Living Well on Borrowed Time. New York: Stein & Day, 1982.

40. Spingarn ND. The New Cancer Survivors: Living With Grace, Fighting with Spirit. Baltimore: Johns Hopkins University Press, 1999.

41. Cancer survivorship–United States, 1971–2001. MMWR 2004; 53(24):526–529; and 41a. http://cancercontrol.cancer.gov/ocs/prevalence/prevalence.html, accessed September 16, 2006.

42. http://www.seer.cancer.gov/seerstat

43. Yancik R, Ries LA. Cancer in older persons: an international issue in an aging world. Semin Oncol 2004;31:128–136.

44. Hewitt M, Rowland JH, Yancik R. Cancer survivors in the United States: age, health, and disability. J Gerontol A Biol Sci Med Sci 2003;58(1):82–91.

45. Caregiving in the U.S. A report by the National Alliance for Caregiving and AARP, 2004, http://www.caregiving.org/pubs/data.htm

46. Hewitt M, Breen N, Devesa S. Cancer prevalence and survivorship issues: analyses of the 1992 National Health Interview Survey. J Natl Cancer Inst 1999;91:1480–1486.

47. Cella DF, Tulsky DS. Quality of life in cancer: definition, purpose and method of measurement. Cancer Invest 1993;11:327–336.

48. Sprangers MAG, Aaronson NK. The role of health care providers and others in evaluating the quality of life of patients with chronic disease: a review. J Clin Epidemiol 1992;45:743–760.

49. Fromme EK, Eilers KM, Mori M, et al. How accurate is clinician reporting of chemotherapy adverse effects? A comparison with patient-reported symptoms from the Quality-of-Life Questionnaire C30. J Clin Oncol 2004;22:3485–3490.

50. Sptizer QO, Dobson AJ, Hall J, et al. Measuring the quality of life of cancer patients: a concise QL-Index for use by physicians. J Chron Dis 1981;34:585–597.

51. Padilla GV, Presant C, Grant MM, et al. Quality of Life Index for patients with cancer. Res Nurs Health 1983;6:117–126.

52. Bergner M, Bobbitt RA, Careter WB, Gilson BS. The Sickness Impact Profile: development and final revision of a health status measure. Med Care 1981;19:787–806.

53. Lipscomb J, Gotay CC, Snyder CF. Outcomes Assessment in Cancer: Measures, Methods, and Applications. Cambridge, England: Cambridge University Press, 2005.

54. Ferrell BR, Dow KH, Grant M. Measurement of quality of life in cancer survivors. Qual Life Res 1995;4:523–531.

55. Wyatt GK, Friedman LL. Development and testing of a quality of life model for long-term female cancer survivors. Qual Life Res 1996;5:387–394.

56. Ferrans CE, Power MJ. Quality of life index: development and psychometric properties. Ann Nurs Sci 1995;8:15–24.

57. Pinto B, Eakin E, Maruyama N. Health behavior changes after a cancer diagnosis: what do we know and where do we go from here? Ann Behav Med 2000;22:38–52.

58. Blanchard CM, Denniston M, Baker F, et al. Do adults change their lifestyle behaviors after a cancer diagnosis? Am J Health Behav 2003;27:246–256.

59. Oeffinger KC, Mertens AC, Hudson MM, et al. Health care of young adult survivors of childhood cancer; a report from the Childhood Cancer Survivor Study. Ann Fam Med 2004;2:61–70.

60. Holmes MD, Kroenke CH. Beyond treatment: lifestyle choices after breast cancer to enhance quality of life and survival. Womens Health Issues 2004;14:11–13.

61. Northouse LL. Mastectomy patients and the fear of cancer recurrence. Cancer Nurs 1981;4:213–220.

62. Lee-Jones C, Humphris G, Dixon R, Hatcher M. Fear of cancer recurrence: a literature review and proposed cognitive formulation to explain exacerbation of recurrence fears. Psycho-Oncology 1997;6:95–105.

63. Vickberg SM. The Concerns About Recurrence Scale (CARS): a systematic measure of women's fears about the possibility of breast cancer recurrence. Ann Behav Med 2003;25(1):16–24.

64. Doward LC, McKennssa SP. Evolution of quality of life assessment. In: Rajagopalan R, Sheretz EF, Anderson RT (eds). Care Management of Skin Disease: Life Quality and Economic Impact. New York: Dekker, 1997:9–33.

65. Guyatt GH, Feeny DH, Patrick DL. Measuring health-related quality of life. Ann Intern Med 1993;118:622–629.

66. Bonanno GA. Loss, trauma and human resilience. Have we underestimated the human capacity to thrive after extremely aversive events? Am Psychol 2004;59:20–28.

67. Sprangers MA. Quality-of-life assessment in oncology. Achievements and challenges. Acta Oncol 2002;41:229–237.

68. Bard M, Sutherland AM. The psychological impact of cancer and its treatment: IV. Adaptation to radical mastectomy. Cancer (Phila) 1955;8:656–672.

69. Holmes HA, Holmes FF. After ten years, what are the handicaps and life styles of children treated for cancer? Clin Pediatr 1975;14:819–823.

70. Rieker P, Edbril SD, Garnick MB. Curative testis cancer therapy: psychosocial sequelae. J Clin Oncol 1985;3:1117–1126.

71. Cella DF, Tross S. Psychological adjustment to survival from Hodgkin's disease. J Consult Clin Psychol 1986;54:616–622.

72. Rapoport Y, Keritler S, Chaitchik S, et al. Psychosocial problems in head-and-neck cancer patients and their change with time since diagnosis. Ann Oncol 1993;4:69–73.

73. Green BL, Krupnick JL, Rowland JH, et al. Trauma history as a predictor of psychologic symptoms in women with breast cancer. J Clin Oncol 2000;18:1084–1093.

74. Cordova MJ, Andrykowski MA. Responses to cancer diagnosis and treatment: posttraumatic stress and posttraumatic growth. Semin Clin Neuropsychiatry 2003;8:286–296.

75. Lechner SC, Zakowski SG, Antoni MH, et al. Do sociodemographic and disease-related variables influence benefit-finding in cancer patients? Psycho-Oncology 2003;12:491–499.

76. Sears SR, Stanton AL, Danoff-Burg S. The yellow brick road and the emerald city: benefit finding, positive reappraisal coping and post-traumatic growth in women with early-stage breast cancer. Health Psychol 2003;22:487–497.

77. Tomich PL, Helgeson VS. Is finding something good in the bad always good? Benefit finding among women with breast cancer. Health Psychol 2004;23:16–23.

78. Meyer TJ, Mark MM. Effects of psychosocial interventions with adult cancer patients. A meta-analysis of randomized experiments. Health Psychol 1995;14:101–108.

79. Devine EC, Westlake SK. The effects of psychoeducational care provided to adults with cancer: metaanalysis of 116 studies. Oncol Nurs Forum 1995;22:1369–1381.

80. http://dccps.nci.nih.gov/ocs/portfolio.asp

81. Rowland JH. Psycho-oncology and breast cancer: a paradigm for research and intervention. Breast Cancer Res Treat 1994;31(2–3):315–324.

82. Nehl EJ, Blanchard CM, Stafford JS, et al. Research interests in the field of behavioral, psychosocial, and policy cancer research. Psycho-Oncology 2003;12:385–392.

83. Aziz NM, Rowland JH. Cancer survivorship research among ethnic minority and medically underserved groups. Oncol Nurs Forum 2002;29(5):789–801.

84. Schottenfeld D, Robbins GF. Quality of survival among patients who have had radical mastectomy. Cancer (Phila) 1970;26:650–654.

85. Li FP, Stone R. Survivors of cancer in childhood. Ann Intern Med 1976;84:551–553.

86. Ganz PA, Kwan L, Stanton AL, et al. Quality of life at the end of primary treatment of breast cancer: first results from the moving beyond cancer randomized trial. J Natl Cancer Inst 2004;96:376–387.

87. Kroenke CH, Rosner B, Chen WY, et al. Functional impact of breast cancer by age at diagnosis. J Clin Oncol 2004;22:1849–1856.

88. Andersen BL, Farrar WB, Golden-Kreutz DM, et al. Psychological, behavioral, and immune changes after a psychological intervention: a clinical trial. J Clin Oncol 2004;22:3570–3580.

89. Abercrombie HC, Giese-Davis J, Sephton S, et al. Flattened cortisol rhythms in metastatic breast cancer patients. Psychoneuroendocrinology 2004;29:1082–1092.

90. Jacobsen PB, Meade CD, Stein KD, et al. Efficacy and costs of two forms of stress management training for cancer patients undergoing chemotherapy. J Clin Oncol 2002;20:2851–2862.

91. Bovbjerg D. Psychoneuroimmunology and cancer. In: Holland JC, Rowland JH (eds). Handbook of Psychooncology. Psychological Care of the Patient with Cancer. New York: Oxford University Press, 1989:727–734.

92. Bauer-Wu SM. Psychoneuroimmunology. Part II: Mind-body interventions. Clin J Oncol Nurs 2002;6:243–246.

93. Antoni MH. Psychoneuroendocrinology and psychoneuroimmunology of cancer: plausible mechanisms worth pursuing? Brain Behav Immun 2003(suppl 1):S84–S91.

94. Sobel DS. The cost-effectiveness of mind-body medicine interventions. Prog Brain Res 2000;122:393–412.

95. Angell KL, Kreshka MA, McCoy R, et al. Psychosocial intervention for rural women with breast cancer: the Sierra–Stanford Partnership. J Gen Intern Med 2003;18:499–507.

96. Fawzy NW. A psychoeducational nursing intervention to enhance coping and affective state in newly diagnosed malignant melanoma patients. Cancer Nurs 1995;18:427–438.

97. Gustafson DH, Hawkins RP, Boberg EW, et al. CHESS: 10 years of research and development in consumer health informatics for broad populations, including the underserved. Int J Med Inform 2002;65:169–177.

98. Lierberman MA, Golant M, Giese-Davis J, et al. Electronic support groups for breast carcinoma: a clinical trial of effectiveness. Cancer (Phila) 2003;97:920–925.

99. Aziz NM, Rowland JH. Trends and advances in cancer survivorship research: challenge and opportunity. Semin Radiat Oncol 2003;13:248–266.

100. Schijven MP, Vingerhoets AJ, Rutten HJ, et al. Comparison of morbidity between axillary lymph node dissection and sentinel node biopsy. Eur J Surg Oncol 2003;29(4):341–350.

101. Blanchard DK, Donohue JH, Reynolds C, Grant CS. Relapse and morbidity in patients undergoing sentinel lymph node biopsy alone or with axillary dissection for breast cancer. Arch Surg 2003;138(5):482–487.

102. Ingham J, Seidman A, Yao TJ, et al. An exploratory study of frequent pain measurement in a cancer clinical trial. Qual Life Res 1996;5:503–507.

103. Tannock IF, Ahles TA, Ganz PA, van Dam FS. Cognitive impairment associated with chemotherapy for cancer: report of a workshop. J Clin Oncol 2004;22:2233–2239.

104. Hewitt M, Simone JV (eds) Ensuring Quality Cancer Care. Washington, DC: National Academy Press, 1999.

105. Chassin MR, Galvin RW. The urgent need to improve health care quality. Institute of Medicine National Roundtable on Health Care Quality. JAMA 1998;280:1000–1005.

106. Hewitt M, Rowland JH. Mental health service use among adult cancer survivors: analyses of the National Health Interview Survey. J Clin Oncol 2002;20(23):4581–4590.

107. Freeman HP, Reuben SH (eds) Voices of a Broken System: Real People, Real Problems. President's Cancer Panel Report of the Chairman, 2000–2001. NIH Publication No. 03-5301. Bethesda, MD: National Institutes of Health, National Cancer Institute, December 2002.

108. Rowland JH, Desmond KA, Meyerowitz BE, et al. Role of breast reconstructive surgery in physical and emotional outcomes among breast cancer survivors. J Natl Cancer Inst 2000;92(17):1422–1429.

109. McGregor BA, Antoni MH, Boyers A, et al. Cognitive-behavioral stress management increases benefit finding and immune function among women with early-stage breast cancer. J Psychosom Res 2004;56:1–8.

110. Antoni MH. Stress Management Intervention for Women with Breast Cancer (accompanied by Therapist's Manual and Participant's Workbook). Washington, DC: American Psychological Association Press, 2003.

111. Courneya KS, Mackey JR, Bell GJ, et al. Randomized controlled trial of exercise training in postmenopausal breast cancer survivors: cardiopulmonary and quality of life outcomes. J Clin Oncol 2003;21(9):1660–1668.

112. Courneya KS. Exercise in cancer survivors: an overview of research. Med Sci Sports Exerc 2003;35(11):1846–1852.

113. Piccirillo JF, Tierney RM, Costas I, et al. Prognostic importance of comorbidity in a hospital-based cancer registry. JAMA 2004;291:2441–2447.

114. Yabroff KR, Lawrence WF, Clauser S, et al. Burden of illness in cancer survivors; findings from a population-based national sample. J Natl Cancer Inst 2004;96:1322–1330.

115. Meyerowitz BE, Richardson J, Hudson S, Leedham B. Ethnicity and cancer outcomes: behavioral and psychosocial considerations. Psychol Bull 1998;123:47–70.

116. Ganz PA. Why and how to study the fate of cancer survivors: observations from the clinic and the research laboratory. Eur J Cancer 2003;39(15):2136–2141.

117. Pakilit AT, Kahn BA, Petersen L, et al. Making effective use of tumor registries for cancer survivorship research. Cancer (Phila) 2001;92:1305–1314.

118. Robison L. Research involving long-term survivors of childhood and adolescent cancer: methodologic considerations. Curr Probl Cancer 2003;27:212–224.

119. Ward HJT, Cousens SN, Smith-Bathgate B, et al. Obstacles to conducting epidemiological research in the UK general population. BMJ 2004;329:277–279.

120. http://www.cancer.umn.edu/ltfu

121. http://www.apos-society.org/webcasts.asp

122. http://www.asco.org/ac/1,1003,_12-002303-00_18-0012404,00.asp

123. Loiselle CG, Bottorff JL, Butler L Degner LF. PORT: Psychosocial oncology research training: a newly funded strategic initiative in health research. Can J Nurs Res, 2004;36:159–164.

124. Fallowfield L, Jenkins V, Farewell V, Solis-Trapala I. Enduring impact of communication skills training: results of a 12-month follow-up. Br J Cancer 2003;20:1445–1449.

125. Wingo PA, Howe HL, Thun MJ, et al. A national framework for cancer surveillance in the United States. Cancer Causes Control 2005;16:151–170.

126. Lipscomb J, Donaldson MS, Arora NK, et al. Cancer outcomes Research. Natl Cancer Inst Momogr 2004;33:178–192.

127. Greer S. Psycho-oncology: its aims, achievements and future tasks. Psycho-Oncology 1994;3:87–101.

128. Holland JC. Psychological care of patients: psycho-oncology's contribution. J Clin Oncol 2003;21:253s–265s.

129. Greer S. Psychological intervention. The gap between research and practice. Acta Oncol 2002;41:238–243.

130. Nicassio PM, Meyerowitz BE, Kerns RD. The future of health psychology interventions. Health Psychol 2004;23:132–137.

131. Hewitt M, Herdman R, Holland J (eds). Meeting the Psychosocial Needs of Women with Breast Cancer. Washington, DC: National Academies Press, 2004.

132. Tesauro GM, Rowland JH, Lustig C. Survivorship resources for post-treatment cancer survivors. Cancer Pract 2002;10:277–283.

133. Rowland JH. Looking beyond cure: pediatric cancer as a model. J Pediatr Psychol 2005;30:1–3.

134. Mertens AC, Cotter LK, Foster BM, et al. Improving health care for adult survivors of childhood cancer: recommendations from a Delphi panel of health policy experts. Health Policy 2004;69:169–178.

135. Kattlove H, Winn RJ. Ongoing care of patients after primary treatment for their cancer. CA Cancer J Clin 2003;54:172–196.

136. http://www.survivorshipguidelines.org

137. McMurchie M. Life after cancer. Aust Fam Physician 1991;20:1444–1451.

138. Earle CC, Burstein JH, Winer EP, Weeks JC. Quality of non-breast cancer health maintenance among elderly breast cancer survivors. J Clin Oncol 2003;21:1447–1451.

139. Earle CC, Neville BA. Under use of necessary care among cancer survivors. Cancer (Phila) 2004;101:1712–1719; 2004; epub.

140. Ganz PA. What outcomes matter to patients: a physician-researcher point of view. Med Care 2002;40(6 suppl):III-1–III-9.

141. Yancik R, Ganz PA, Varricchio CG, Conley B. Perspectives on comorbidity and cancer in older patients; approaches to expand the knowledge base. J Clin Oncol 2001;19:1147–1151.

142. Gatta G, Capocaccia R, Berrino F, et al., and EUROPREVAL Working Group. Colon cancer prevalence and estimation of differing care needs of colon cancer patients. Ann Oncol 2004;15:1136–1142.

143. Earle CC, Nattinger AB, Potosky AL, et al. Identifying cancer relapse using SEER-Medicare data. Med Care 2002;40:5–81.

144. Mariotto A. Surveillance Research Program, Division of Cancer Control and Population Sciences. National Cancer Institute, NIH/DHHS, Bethesda, MD. Personal communication.

145. Leigh S. The culture of survivorship. Semin Oncol Nurs 2001;17:234–235.

146. Zebrack B. An advocate's perspective on cancer survivorship. Semin Oncol Nurs 2001;17:284–287.

147. Stovall E, Gesme D. Coming together to conquer cancer. J Clin Oncol 1999;17:730.

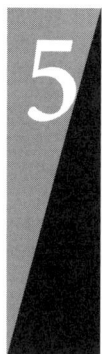

5

Surveillance after Primary Therapy

Craig C. Earle

Primary treatment for cancer is often a very regimented experience, with schedules and protocols. These provide comfort to patients because of their certainty. Constant contact with the medical staff helps patients feel that everything must be under control for now, and that if anything develops, someone will notice it. Yet as the end of treatment approaches, it is not uncommon for anxiety levels of patients to rise.

When patients treated with curative intent finish their primary therapy, they often request a detailed plan for surveillance. In part, this is to preserve confidence that someone knows exactly what should happen now. Physicians also yearn for guidance in the selection, timing, and sequence of diagnostic tests following primary cancer therapy. However, there is wide variation in recommendations for surveillance among experts.[1] In recent years, an increasing focus on evidence-based medicine that has coincided with increased concern about costs and efficiencies in medicine has caused a reevaluation of surveillance practices. Unfortunately, there is currently little in the way of evidence-based guidelines for cancer patient follow-up.

Rationales offered for surveillance after cancer include: detecting local or distant recurrence at a time in which treatment can be more effective or even curative; detecting metachronous cancers, whether due to a genetic predisposition or common environmental exposures, in the same or another organ; detecting long-term or late effects of treatment, including iatrogenic second malignancies; auditing the results of therapy; and providing general primary care, such as routine health maintenance, screening, counseling about modifiable risk factors, and the incidental detection of unrelated comorbid disease. The questions one must ask when considering whether a surveillance strategy is justified are (1) Whether it will detect recurrence of the cancer earlier than it would otherwise become apparent; (2) If so, whether earlier intervention will improve patient outcomes; and (3) If so, whether this is achieved in a cost-effective manner? In this chapter, we will discuss the conceptual underpinnings of surveillance and examine some if its evidence base.

Screening Tests

Although we have an expanding armamentarium of diagnostic tests that can be performed on patients after curative treatment, it is unclear whether we should actually use them, how often they should be applied, and for how long. All tests have the potential for false positive results due to biologic or circadian fluctuations and analytic variation, the latter including everything from instrument calibration to interpretation of images on a scan. The more often a test is done, generally the more likely it is that there will be a false positive result. The psychological impact and mental anguish from receiving a positive test can be immense. Positive tests usually lead to further tests, possibly invasive ones like biopsy, that can lead to other complications and add expense. If it turns out to be a false positive, all of this will have been done for no benefit. Tests also have false negative rates, and in fact, for a patient destined to recur, any test that does not detect that recurrence was, in retrospect, a false negative.

Surveillance after cancer is essentially a type of screening in high-risk individuals. As a result, many of the epidemiological issues around screening studies also apply to surveillance. Advances in diagnostic imaging can lead to a lowering of the threshold of tumor detection, which lead in turn to earlier diagnosis of relapse. Unless treatment in this newly expanded detectable pre-clinical phase leads to improved outcomes, however, the patient has not benefited.

Nonrandomized studies of screening or surveillance tests are prone to several biases, in particular lead-time and length-time biases. Lead time bias occurs if a cancer recurrence is detected early because of a test, and even though the day the patient dies is the same as it would have been if the recurrence had not been detected early, the test appears to have improved survival by making the patient live longer with the diagnosis of terminal cancer. Length time bias occurs when a test picks up more indolent cases of cancer. Aggressive cancers will become clinically apparent quickly, yet the indolent ones are more likely to remain undetected until a test is applied. As a result, test-detected recurrences will appear to have a better prognosis than those picked up clinically because the detected cases are associated with longer survival even if they have not been detected early.

Overdiagnosis, the detection of small, clinically insignificant cancers that would never cause overt illness, is another concern related to screening. Many Prostate-Specific Antigen (PSA)-detected prostate cancers are thought to be overdiagnosed. However, overdiagnosis is probably less of a concern with cancer surveillance than it is with cancer screening. Recurrence of a previous invasive cancer is likely to have clinical consequences eventually.

The only way to really control for lead-time and length-time biases is to do a randomized trial. If there truly is a detectable preclinical phase in which early detection can improve outcome, then screened patients will have superior overall outcomes than the unscreened. Any other trial design is prone to bias. The obvious prerequisite, then, is that there must be an effective intervention, i.e., one that can result in cure or at least in prolonging life, in order for surveillance to make sense. As a result, it makes sense to try to find a local recurrence of breast cancer after breast conserving surgery, but does not make sense to look for asymptomatic local recurrence of pancreatic cancer after a Whipple procedure.

Components of Surveillance

There is wide variation in recommendations for surveillance among experts. One textbook that solicited surveillance strategies from international cancer leaders found that "it was . . . uncommon for any two authors . . . to agree on one follow-up strategy for a given cancer."[1,2] There are those who argue that after primary therapy for cancer, most patients would be just as well off if they were discharged from the clinic and instructed to call if they experienced a problem.[3,4] Indeed, anxiety and cost may decrease as a result.[5] When patient expectations are different from physician intent, however, it can lead to controversy and confusion. One can spend a lot of time with patients and explain the evidence and rationale behind a less aggressive surveillance regime, but when relapse is eventually discovered, these same patients still often confront their doctors with "Shouldn't we have been getting tests to find this earlier?"[6]

The components of surveillance strategies generally are

- office visits to take history and give a physical examination;
- blood work, particularly tumor markers;
- imaging studies; and
- visualization—endoscopy, second-look surgery, or other examination of the primary organ.

Because of the diverse nature of cancer, each of these components has different characteristics with different cancer types.

It usually makes sense to take the patient's history and give him or her a physical examination. These are inexpensive procedures, and anything picked up represents, by definition, clinically apparent disease that merits further investigation and treatment. Evaluation generally focuses on the signs and symptoms of local and distant recurrence. A carefully taken expert history can sometimes correctly identify misattributed recurrence (e.g., the "sciatica" caused by a rectal cancer recurrence) that could benefit from intervention. Similarly, clinically apparent disease on the exam, such as a pleural effusion, is likely to become symptomatic soon if not attended to. Physical examination is more likely to be useful for diseases in which the primary tumor and regional lymph nodes are accessible (e.g., head and neck, breast, melanoma, or anal cancers). Of note, studies have shown that a significant proportion of patients do not seek care for relevant symptoms. This makes regularly scheduled follow-up visits, as opposed to patient-initiated contacts, potentially important,[7,8] as long as they do not prompt patients to delay seeking care until their next scheduled follow-up visit.[9]

Tumor markers exist for breast, colorectal, pancreatic, liver, ovarian, prostate, and testicular cancers.[10] These are often the first indication of recurrence, and they can prompt further investigation and intervention if appropriate. For example, in prostate cancer, PSA monitoring can guide the timing of postsurgical radiotherapy, initiation of hormonal treatment, and postradiotherapy salvage prostatectomy. However, tumor markers also give false positive results. For example, Carcino-Embryonic Antigen (CEA), a cell adhesion glycoprotein that can be detected in the serum and is overexpressed by adenocarcinomas, can be elevated in smokers, patients with pulmonary or gastrointestinal infections, inflammatory bowel disease, cirrhosis, hepatitis, pancreatitis, and renal failure. In fact, adjuvant chemotherapy can increase the CEA.[11] Tumor markers may also be too sensitive at times, which indicate that the cancer has likely recurred before imaging studies can determine the location and extent of metastases. As a result, patients and clinicians are left in the uncomfortable situation of knowing that something is happening, but having to wait perhaps months for the disease to declare itself before a treatment plan can be made. Nontumor marker blood work is usually not helpful and so it is not recommended in guidelines,[12] yet it is commonly done.

The use of imaging studies is one of the main areas of controversy in surveillance because studies are relatively expensive and are usually aimed at finding distant, often incurable, recurrence. In some diseases, however, such as Hodgkin's disease and potentially curable forms of non-Hodgkin's lymphoma, there is evidence that salvage (in this case, bone marrow transplantation) is more effective if performed earlier after relapse in patients with minimal disease.[13] In these situations, intensive surveillance at least has a rationale. Even in this example, though, the majority of relapses are detected because of symptoms, and many others are apparent on physical examination. Simple blood work (e.g. LDH in lymphoma) can usually detect the rest.[14] Directed imaging studies and nuclear medicine imaging are more likely to confirm an otherwise apparent recurrence, rather than be the only indication of relapse. Consequently, their routine use is controversial. In contrast, there is no expectation of benefit from anything more than clinical follow-up of patients with low-grade, incurable, non-Hodgkin's lymphoma. Monoclonal antibody scans, such as a radiolabelled CEA scan, are available. However, they have not yet been demonstrated to improve outcomes and require more clinical evaluation.

Visual inspection of the primary site can detect local recurrences of some cancers when they can still be cured. Examples include endoscopic surveillance of rectal cancer and head and neck malignancies. However, if local recurrence is not curable, visualization is not useful. For example, second-look surgeries for ovarian and pancreatic cancers have not been associated with improved outcomes.[15] Without curative second-line treatments, it is difficult to justify these procedures. As a result they are disappearing from practice.

Detection of Recurrence

Recurrences can generally be divided into two categories: local-regional and distant. Local recurrence generally means that the initial cancer-directed therapy failed to eradicate the tumor. Distant recurrence means that seeding, whether by hematogenous, lymphatic, or serosal routes, already occurred before primary therapy. It just wasn't evident at the time. Regional recurrence can occur for any of these reasons.

Local Recurrence

Local recurrence of cancer can often be salvaged in sites of cancer. The patient managed initially with surgery might be cured with a secondary surgical procedure or radiation after local recurrence (e.g., breast cancer). Resection of recurrences in a surgical incision site can also effect cure. Similarly, patients treated with primary radiation may be salvaged with surgery (e.g., anal cancer). Local recurrences at other sites, however, do not have effective salvage and are generally incurable (e.g., esophageal, lung, and pancreatic cancers).

Detection of Distant Metastases

This rationale for surveillance is an extrapolation of the notion that if a cancer is found "early" it can be treated more successfully. Distant recurrence however, after primary therapy is not early disease, and as such is rarely curable. In most cases in which a recurrence can be cured, it is not clear whether early detection influences the likelihood of cure. There are a few examples where either surgery (e.g., for colorectal [described below] or renal cell carcinoma metastases) or chemotherapy for distant disease (e.g., testicular cancer, lymphoma, or bladder cancer) can result in long-term disease-free survival. If a cure is not possible, however, the goal sometimes becomes to institute palliative therapy at a time when it *may* be more effective, and maintain functioning. Unfortunately, there is little clear evidence in most cases that early institution of palliative chemotherapy in asymptomatic patients provides benefit.[16]

Another reason put forward for surveillance to find incurable disease early is to detect potentially catastrophic complications (e.g., by intervening before spinal cord compression or pathological fracture occurs). However, such events are usually preceded by clinical symptoms or signs such as pain. In a randomized trial of oncologist versus primary care physician (PCP) surveillance by Grunfeld et al, specialist surveillance did not prevent these occurrences.[17] Last, some say that finding incurable recurrences early yields patients better able to participate in clinical trials by virtue of having better performance status and a longer period with metastatic disease (because of lead-time). The fact that only a few percent of cancer patients participate in clinical trials weakens this argument.[18]

Detection of Secondary Cancers

Cancer survivors are at risk for developing new cancers for a variety of reasons. Whatever caused the index cancer could still be having an effect, either on second primaries in the same organ, or on related cancers in other organs. This can be due to genetic predisposition, as is the case with breast or colorectal cancer. It also can be due to widespread genetic damage from environmental exposures that results in "field cancerization", as is the case with hepatoma, skin cancer, bladder cancer, or in the relationships between head and neck

and lung cancers in patients who have smoked. For example, patients cured of head and neck cancer remain at a 3% to 6% risk per year of developing lung cancer.[19–22]

Risk of secondary malignancies may also be due to the late effects of treatment. Breast and lung cancers, for instance, can develop at the edge of a mantle radiation field 20 years after treatment. Myelodysplasia or acute leukemia can follow adjuvant chemotherapy for breast cancer or curative chemotherapy for Hodgkin's disease. Ongoing treatment with tamoxifen after breast cancer can increase the risk of endometrial cancer. Note that in this latter example, it is generally not advisable to screen for endometrial cancer with ultrasound in an asymptomatic woman, as prospective studies have found low yield and complications.[23,24] This has prompted concerns that a false positive test may lead to discontinuation of tamoxifen, which could have a more negative effect on long-term health than even a missed, generally highly curable, endometrial cancer.[25]

Detection and Treatment of Functional Disabilities Related to Primary Treatment

Cancer treatment can leave patients with a host of chronic medical problems. For example, hypothyroidism and dental issues are common after neck irradiation. Lymphedema can be a sequela of local surgical management or radiation. Accelerated cardiovascular disease can accompany chest irradiation or certain drugs. Bone marrow transplant patients are at risk for cataracts and effects of Graft Versus Host Disease (GVHD). They also may have lost a significant amount of their immunity and require readministration of their routine vaccinations. Patients who have had either surgical or functional splenectomy require immunization against encapsulated organisms. Hormonal treatments for cancer, including steroids, can result in impaired bone health, sexual dysfunction, and menopausal symptoms. Detailed discussions of these issues appear elsewhere in this text.

Prevention

Surveillance visits present an opportunity to prevent future cancers and other illnesses. For example, physicians can counsel patients on lifestyle modifications such as smoking and alcohol cessation and decreasing sun exposure. Recently, chemoprevention has become available in some circumstances, such as tamoxifen for breast cancer[26] and aspirin for colorectal cancer.[27] There is also emerging evidence that lifestyle factors like diet and exercise may also play a role in preventing recurrence,[28] though randomized confirmation is needed. If a hereditary predisposition to cancer is suspected, genetic counseling and testing may lead to interventions that could prevent future cancers in the cancer survivor and the survivor's relatives.

Non-Cancer-Related Care

Given that 70% of cancer patients survive their disease, it is important that general medical care not be ignored. There is evidence that cancer survivors may be less likely to receive recommended care for chronic conditions across a wide range of diseases.[29] For example, 5-year colorectal cancer survivors with angina, congestive heart failure, and chronic lung disease have been observed to be less likely than matched controls to have recommended follow-up. Diabetic survivors are less likely to have preventive eye examination, and there has been a trend towards less intensive monitoring of the HbA1c. General health maintenance in women, including influenza vaccination, cholesterol screening, PAP smears, and bone densitometry are all less common among cancer survivors. It is important that cancer patients maintain a relationship with a primary care physician, as this has been a strong predictor of receiving high quality general medical care.[29,30] While some oncologists are willing and able to act as a primary care physician, surveys have shown that most are not.[31]

Psychological Effects of Surveillance

Whether surveillance provides psychological benefit is debatable[5,32] and probably patient-specific. Fear of recurrence is a dominant psychological sequela of cancer.[33] As a result, reassurance that there is no sign of the cancer at follow-up can understandably have positive effects on anxiety.[34] However, the inconvenience and often discomfort of surveillance testing, and the stress of waiting for test results and visits with clinicians can by themselves generate anxiety.[35] Moreover, if all of the tests are not completely normal, the patient will not be reassured.[6] Therefore, detection of anxiety and depression during follow-up, with appropriate referral to a mental health professional, could be construed as both a harm and a benefit of surveillance. While patients report in surveys that they prefer routine follow-up and derive reassurance from clinic visits,[36] Muss et al. found that this is often because they incorrectly assume that early detection of recurrence will improve their chance of cure, or at least prolong survival.[37] Randomized trials of surveillance after breast cancer have not found any overall positive psychological effects with more intensive surveillance strategies.[5,36]

Psychological effects can extend to physicians as well. Primary treatment for cancer is focused on cure. It may be very difficult for some doctors to tell a patient that all that can be done has been done, and that they no longer have influence on the ultimate outcome. Moreover, the message that if a recurrence occurs, there will not be an attempt to eradicate it, can seem like a breaking of the trust and aligned goals that have developed in the doctor-patient relationship.

Incorporating Risk Prediction into Surveillance Strategies

It seems logical and tempting to try to stratify patients based on their risk of recurrence and follow those at highest risk more intensively. However, it is not clear that this is either more effective or more cost-effective than following all patients similarly in most cases. High-risk patients are more likely to recur. Therefore, surveillance is more likely to find a recurrence in these patients.[6] But those at highest risk of recurrence will also likely have their clinical course dictated by the biological behavior of the tumor, and those recurrences

will tend to become clinically evident relatively quickly anyway. It may be that the patient with an overall good prognosis who simply had a tumor cell "get away" before surgery and who could be cured by early detection of oligometastatic disease is the one who could benefit the most from intensive surveillance. An example would be two patients, one with stage IIIc colon cancer and another with stage II, with 15/15 lymph nodes negative. While the patient with stage IIIc clearly has a much higher risk of recurrence, studies have shown that following metastatectomy, one of the predictors of cure is a node-negative primary.[38] It actually may make more clinical sense to follow the stage II patient more closely. The stage IIIc patient may very well be doomed if there is a recurrence. Similarly, the rationale for more intensive surveillance in the early years when there is a greater risk of relapse could be challenged. Cancers that relapse quickly are probably more aggressive and therefore less likely to be curable. It is perhaps the indolent metastases with the highest chance of cure that we should focus on. Unfortunately, surveillance trials generally have not been stratified for recurrence risk, although some have attempted to do this.[39] At this point in time, molecular genetic prognostic markers have not yet been identified for most cancers proven to refine prognosis beyond that provided by traditional anatomic staging and pathological features, in order to identify a subgroup of patients who could forgo surveillance.

However, tests establishing a genetic predisposition to cancer can alter surveillance. For example, it is known that patients with one of the mutations leading to Hereditary Non-Polyposis Colorectal Cancer (HNPCC) can have accelerated carcinogenesis and as a result are at risk for "interval" cancers between colonoscopies. Therefore, they are generally followed up yearly with endoscopy and may also undergo screening for other cancers.[40]

Another place where risk prediction can be incorporated is in the interpretation of otherwise equivocal findings. For example, the patient with high-risk colon cancer and a CEA still within the normal range but rising may prompt earlier investigation than one with a low risk for whom the CEA results may simply reflect normal fluctuation. Similarly, small lung nodules ("ditzels"), liver hypodensities, or bone scan abnormalities may be interpreted differently for patient with high or low risk of recurrence. These approaches speak to the concept of "pre-test probability," in this case, determined by the clinical risk of recurrence. After applying a test whose threshold for normal and abnormal results may have come from analysis of its "Receiver Operating Characteristics" (ROC) curves, and with certain performance characteristics that can be summarized by a likelihood ratio, there is a resultant posttest probability of disease. The pretest probability multiplied by the likelihood ratio, calculated as (the probability of disease)/(1-the probability of disease), gives the posttest probability. The higher pretest probability of high-risk patients means that there is less likely to be false positive test results in this group. Further discussion of these issues in screening and diagnostic testing is beyond the scope of this chapter and can be obtained from standard clinical epidemiology texts.

Current practice has largely evolved from consensus and tradition rather than data. Consequently, physicians should be aware of the limitations of most surveillance recommendations. Indeed, surveys have found that surveillance practices generally do not differ across stages.[41,42] This indicates that physicians don't routinely incorporate risk assessment into surveillance strategies. Until tailoring surveillance practice to risk is shown to affect outcomes, it is probably prudent not to complicate surveillance recommendations unnecessarily. Simple guidelines are more likely to be adhered to.

Frequency of Surveillance

Assuming we have established what tests are useful for surveillance of patients with a given type of cancer, the next challenge is to decide how often to conduct them. In cancer screening a one-time screen at a time of high risk is the most important and cost-effective.[43-45] The marginal cost for achieving the diminishing returns gained by increasingly frequent screening eventually becomes prohibitively expensive and not a good use of society's limited resources. The same is likely true for surveillance.

In some diseases there can be a biologic rationale to guide practice. For example, in colorectal cancer it has been observed that to go from normal appearing mucosa to invasive cancer in less than 3 to 5 years is very uncommon.[46] Therefore, physicians can be confident that a screening interval of this length after a normal colonoscopy (i.e., without polyps) is safe. If polyps are found, it may be a marker for an inherited predisposition that increases the pace of mutation, resulting in "interval" cancers between routine screenings; therefore, colonoscopy should be repeated in a year. Because it would be extremely expensive to conduct randomized trials to try to determine the optimal frequency of screening, it is most reasonable to let the frequency of screening be dictated by knowledge of the natural history of the disease.

Duration of Surveillance

Most solid tumors recur within the first few years and are much less common after 5 years. Some, however, like breast cancer or melanoma, can recur decades later. Furthermore, advances in adjuvant therapy, in addition to increasing the cure rate, appear to delay recurrence in many of those destined to ultimately relapse.[47] As a result, surveillance generally becomes less intense after the first few years and is often discontinued after 5 years. Alternatively, some argue that surveillance should continue until the survival expectation approximates that of age-matched controls.[48] Patients with a personal history of cancer are often at increased risk for new primaries, as described above. Therefore, one might argue that lifelong follow-up may be appropriate in some cases.

Specific Surveillance Examples

In this section we illustrate the considerations surrounding surveillance for three different situations: (1) a cancer for which there is emerging consensus that most surveillance is of little value (breast cancer), (2) one for which there remains heated controversy (colorectal cancer), and (3) one for which there is little debate about the usefulness of follow-up (testicular cancer).

Breast Cancer

There has been a dramatic evolution in attitudes towards surveillance of potentially cured breast cancer patients. In the 1990s, high-dose chemotherapy with stem cell support was holding out the promise of curing metastatic disease and so it seemed to make sense to try to find it in a low volume state. However, it has since become clear that metastatic disease cannot be cured and this makes the early detection of such disease of questionable value. In fact, studies have indicated that intensive surveillance offers no survival advantage or quality-of-life benefit, and as a result is not cost-effective.

SURVEILLANCE FOR LOCAL RECURRENCE

Local recurrence can still be cured over half the time,[49] with mastectomy if the original surgery was breast conserving therapy, or radiation if the patient has already had a mastectomy. Furthermore, new primaries in the contralateral breast occur at a rate approaching 1% per year,[50,51] over twice the rate in the general population. The risk is particularly high in women with lobular carcinoma in situ or a hereditary cancer syndrome. While there are no randomized trials demonstrating that surveillance for contralateral breast cancer or local recurrence in breast cancer survivors improves survival, extrapolation from screening studies and indirect evidence showing smaller recurrences at the time of detection support recommendations for surveillance.[52]

After mastectomy, clinical examination is most useful for detecting recurrences. Unfortunately, these can be cured in only a minority of patients as they are usually accompanied by distant metastases. Patients are encouraged to alert their physicians if they detect any changes at the mastectomy site, but it is not clear whether regular self-examination provides benefit. Clinical breast examination, performed by a trained healthcare provider, includes inspection and palpation of the mastectomy site, contralateral breast, and the axillary lymph nodes. Mammography of the chest wall after mastectomy is generally not helpful.[53,54]

After breast conserving surgery, on the other hand, mammography and clinical breast examination are complementary methods for detecting the 5% to 15% of ipselateral recurrences.[52] Current recommendations are for monthly self-examination, follow-up visits and examinations every 3 months for 3 years, every 6 months for 2 more years, and then annually, with annual or every other year mammography.[55-58] Magnetic resonance imaging has shown promise in high-risk screening,[59,60] though its role in surveillance after breast cancer is not yet defined.

SURVEILLANCE FOR DISTANT RECURRENCE

Surveillance for asymptomatic distant recurrence is no longer recommended. It has become clear that metastatic breast cancer cannot be cured with current treatments, and that early application of systemic therapy in asymptomatic patients does not prolong survival. While tumor markers such as CEA and CA 27–29 can be elevated in up to 50% of recurrences, they are not recommended due to lack of effective treatment.[55] The Italian Gruppo Interdisciplinare Valutazione Interventi in Oncologia (GIVIO) did a randomized trial comparing intensive surveillance to investigation guided by symptoms in 1320 women under the age of 70 with stages

I to III breast cancer followed in one of 20 hospitals in Italy.[36] Both groups had office visits every 3 months for the first 2 years, then every 6 months for 3 more years, and annual mammograms. For the 655 patients in the intensive arm, surveillance also consisted of liver function studies every 3 months, chest X-rays every 6 months, and annual abdominal ultrasounds and bone scans. The 665 in the control arm were investigated only if symptoms occurred. Despite detecting more distant disease with intensive surveillance there was no difference in survival or quality of life at 5 years.

A second multicenter trial of 1,243 women also carried out in Italy was of very similar design, except that bone scans were done every 6 months instead of annually, similarly found no survival benefit at 5 years.[61] A meta-analysis of these two trials confirmed that there was no benefit from intensive surveillance in any subgroup of patients.[62] Based on these results, a study of "on demand" follow-up of patients found this to be an acceptable strategy.[4]

As a result of these findings, the goals of follow-up in breast cancer are early detection of local recurrence and new primaries, and investigating symptoms that may portend distant relapse. Guidelines generally do not recommend intensive surveillance.[55–58,63,64]

Colorectal Cancer

The controversy surrounding surveillance in colon cancer comes from the observation that, unlike most other solid tumors, there is a small proportion of patients who recur with oligometastatic disease and can be operated on for cure.[38] This makes early detection of recurrences potentially desirable.

SURVEILLANCE FOR LOCAL RECURRENCE

Several organizations have made recommendations about colorectal cancer surveillance.[12,65–68] In colon cancer, local recurrences are uncommon. Colonoscopy, therefore, is used to find synchronous or metachronous second primaries. The colon should be completely evaluated either prior to surgery, or if the patient presents with obstruction that precludes complete evaluation, within 6 months of primary surgery. It should then be repeated at one year. If polyps are found, colonoscopy should be repeated yearly until all polyps are removed. Then it should be repeated every 3 to 5 years, as the National Polyp Study showed that a colonoscopy every 3 years after an initial colonoscopic polypectomy is equivalent to annual surveillance for patients with sporadic disease (as opposed to those with HNPCC).[46]

Rectal cancer has a much higher risk of local recurrence, and depending on the primary therapy, salvage options may remain. Therefore, endoscopy is recommended every 6 months for at least 3 years.[12]

SURVEILLANCE FOR DISTANT RECURRENCE

It is the surveillance of metastatic disease that is the most controversial. Patterns of distant spread are different for colon and rectal cancers. Colon cancer tends to spread through the portal system to the liver first. Rectal cancer spreads up the paravertebral veins and can bypass the liver, frequently showing up as isolated lung metastases. Liver and lung metastases have both been successfully resected for cure. However, because the yield is small, some investigators question whether the expense and anxiety of intense monitoring is justified.[11,69] Of patients who receive definitive treatment for stage II or III CRC, approximately 50% will eventually relapse.[70,71] A maximum of 10% to 15% will recur with potentially resectable metastases,[72] and at most about a third of those will be cured.[38] Therefore, only about 3% to 5% of CRC patients can be cured by identification and resection of isolated metastases. Because approximately 60% of patients with isolated metastases seek medical attention on their own due to symptoms, the maximum benefit surveillance could have on cure rates is only about 2%. Clinical trials have to be quite large to detect this small a difference. It has been observed, however, that patients detected asymptomatically are more likely to undergo resection for potential cure.[72,73]

There have been seven randomized trials comparing different surveillance strategies.[39,74–79] Only one had a no surveillance control arm.[75] The others compared more aggressive with less aggressive surveillance. Only two trials showed significantly improved survival for the more aggressive surveillance,[39,79] others showed at least a trend in favor of more intense surveillance.[75–78] These trials showed that with more intensive surveillance, recurrences were recognized earlier (though not more often), and patients were more likely to have surgery for recurrence with curative intent. Some of these studies had insufficient sample size to detect small differences in survival, however.[78]

Meta-analyses of these randomized trials have indicated that trials in which patients received more intensive surveillance, including the subgroup that included CEA, showed more of a survival advantage than trials with less intensive surveillance.[80,81,82] Recommendations until now have been against routine imaging studies. However, meta-analyses have demonstrated more benefit for surveillance schedules that include imaging,[81–83] indicating that surveillance can impact survival by detecting extramural recurrences. Imaging makes intuitive sense because the CEA can be normal in up to 30% of patients with detectable metastases,[42,84] especially poorly differentiated tumors.[85] If the CEA is elevated preoperatively, then one can be comfortable that it will serve as a good marker. However, it may be normal because of early-stage disease, or not measured at all prior to surgery. Consequently, guidelines are beginning to recommend that periodic follow-up is reasonable, for example with history, physical examination, and CEA determination every 3 months, combined with intermittent imaging like yearly CT scans.[65]

Such recommendations are usually limited to the subset of patients who would and could undergo potentially curative surgery.[86] This restriction could be challenged, however. Patient preferences around potentially curable surgery can change drastically after recurrence is detected. Moreover, there are increasingly less invasive options, such as ablation or stereotactic radiation, that can provide local control for a subset of the less hardy patients.

Testicular Cancer

Testicular cancer is a major success in oncology. It is one of the few tumors for which cure is the expectation no matter what the presenting stage. As a result, efforts have tried to focus on minimizing long-term toxicity. One approach to this is with less aggressive primary treatment followed by intensive surveillance and early intervention at the first sign of recurrence, thereby sparing those cured by primary therapy alone the morbidity of adjuvant treatments.

SURVEILLANCE FOR LOCAL RECURRENCE

Physical examination should include examination of the contralateral testicle, as the cumulative risk of a second primary is 3.9% over 15 years.[87]

SURVEILLANCE FOR DISTANT RECURRENCE

After inguinal orchiectomy for stage I or II seminoma, standard treatment has been radiation of the ipsilateral pelvic and paraaortic lymph nodes. A randomized trial has demonstrated that the pelvic lymph node radiation can be safely omitted in stage I disease with less toxicity.[88] For early-stage nonseminomas, retroperitoneal lymph node dissection has been standard, with chemotherapy added for poor risk stage I disease and those with stage II (disease involving the retroperitoneal nodes). These treatments can be associated with a variety of long-term effects, including adhesions, infertility and ejaculatory dysfunction, pulmonary toxicity, and secondary malignancies. However, in many of these cases, patients may be able to be spared this with a program of intense surveillance. While the specifics of the program can vary slightly among practitioners,[89] they are generally along the lines of repeated office visits with physical examination and monitoring of tumor markers every 1 to 2 months, and radiological screening with alternating chest X-rays and CT scans of the chest, abdomen, and pelvis.[90–93] Most recurrences occur in the first two years. Therefore, this is continued throughout the first 6 to 12 months, and then the frequency gradually decreases over the ensuing 5 years. For example, follow-up could decrease to bimonthly in the second year, quarterly in the third, every 4 months in the fourth, and biannually in the fifth, and then yearly. In a randomized trial comparing chemotherapy to surveillance in patients with stage II nonseminomatous germ cell tumors, of the 98 patients on surveillance, 49% relapsed, but all but 5 were cured with subsequent chemotherapy.[94] Of the 97 treated with upfront chemotherapy, 94 survived, and it was concluded that there was no detectable difference between the strategies. Although the relapse rate is higher, approaching 25%, without the adjuvant treatments, overall survival is similar because radiation and/or chemotherapy can be successfully applied when relapse is detected. More recently, the utility of chest imaging in surveillance has been questioned,[95–98] though it is still part of most surveillance recommendations.[90–93]

For more advanced stages (III) of disease, treated with chemotherapy, or those with earlier stage cancer who received definitive adjuvant radiotherapy, surveillance is similar[90] based on evidence that the extent of disease at relapse may affect the chance of salvage,[99] though some expect, but not all, recommend a less intense schedule.[87]

Who Should Do Surveillance?

In most cases it is not important which type of physician is doing surveillance, as long as there is a clearly identified coordinating physician. Randomized trials have shown that PCPs given explicit directions are as good at surveillance as specialists,[17,100–103] and that they are willing to take on this role.[104] Direction is important, however, as generalists have ordered more tests than specialists, thereby possibly increasing cost.[105] Some instances in which specialized surveillance may be required are for certain procedures such as endoscopy, and arguably, some specialized physical examinations like examining the irradiated breast. On the other hand, coordination is important following multimodality treatment. If not achieved, each specialist can review a patient every few months within weeks of each other, even ordering the same imaging studies. Patients go along with it, understandably assuming that the scan ordered by the surgeon is different from that of the medical oncologist. A randomized study of breast cancer surveillance indicated that patients might actually prefer follow-up by their primary physician, rather than a specialist.[5] This may decrease the compliance to an intensive surveillance regimen carried out by specialists, thus eroding its benefits. Therefore, whether specialists or generalists are better suited to carry out surveillance is debatable and likely depends on the inclinations of the combination of patient and physicians involved.

Economic Evaluation of Surveillance

Economic studies require clear specification of the research question and perspective from which the study is being undertaken, comparison of relevant options, identification and quantification of all important costs and benefits, the use of discounting to account for time preferences, sensitivity analyses to test the robustness of the study's results, and, finally, transparent reporting of those results. Economic analysis of surveillance after cancer treatment presents several methodological challenges.

There are four types of commonly used economic evaluations. Each involves a comparison of both the costs and consequences of alternative strategies, but they differ primarily in the methods used to measure consequences. *Cost-minimization analysis* is used when the options are equally effective and cost is the only difference between them. The costs associated with each strategy are compared, and the least costly strategy is preferred. If the strategies being assessed are not of equal effectiveness, then the life years gained, cases successfully treated, or cases averted are related to cost by calculating ratio of incremental cost per unit of incremental benefit (e.g., cost per life year gained). These *cost-effectiveness analyses* are the most common approach to economic evaluation in healthcare.[106] The cost per life year gained looks only at the survival benefits of an intervention, and not at its complications, inconvenience, or effects on quality of life. *Cost-utility analyses* are similar to cost-effectiveness analyses, but they also incorporate quality of life data into the effectiveness measure, commonly as a quality adjusted life year (QALY).[107] Quality of life is approximated by a *utility*, which is a measure of preference for a given health state rated on a scale between 0 and 1, where 0 equals death and 1 equals perfect health. *Cost-benefit analysis* takes cost-utility analysis one step further by attempting to determine whether the benefits of an intervention outweigh its cost. A dollar value is attached to the quality-adjusted life years, and an intervention is "cost-beneficial" if its benefits (measured in currency) are greater than its costs. Because these analyses always produce a monetary outcome, it is relatively easy to compare very different potential uses of society's resources, including uses outside of health care. This is important because the real cost of an intervention is the value of the alternative uses of the same resources. As a result, cost-benefit analysis is in theory the preferred form of economic evaluation. However, placing a monetary value on the outcomes of health care, in particular the value of a life, is problematic, making true cost-benefit analyses rare.

Each economic study requires a clearly defined research question involving rational comparisons. If appropriate, a "do nothing" option should be included to determine whether there should be any surveillance at all. In addition, guidelines have proposed that the least costly[108] and the most commonly used[109] alternatives should be assessed. In the case of cancer surveillance strategies, the issues are likely to center around: (1) the cost of surveillance tests for a defined population of cancer survivors; (2) the cost of subsequently treating the detected disease; (3) savings from not having to treat more advanced disease; and (4) the quality-adjusted life-years saved by surveillance. Ideally, a full economic evaluation should include the costs and benefits to all sectors of society affected by the interventions. For example, intensive surveillance of younger patients will result in a certain amount of lost productivity due to time off, work, travel, and childcare expenses.

While many studies report on cost-consequences (e.g., cost per recurrence detected or cost per operable or potentially cured patient), the only outcomes of any real importance are an increase in the quantity and/or quality of life. For surveillance this means survival benefits accrued from early detection of recurrence, and/or positive effects on quality of life and patient preferences from treating early disease as opposed to treating late disease. Of these, the most important parameter is survival. Even an expensive surveillance test that results in aggressive early treatment can provide good value if it can be shown to cure patients or, importantly, improve survival. Conversely, a surveillance strategy that is costly and simply results in patients receiving futile treatments over a longer period of time won't be cost effective.

Because the costs are spent upfront in surveillance, while the benefits are uncertain and accrue only in the future, the calculation of cost-effectiveness for surveillance strategies becomes less attractive due to discounting. In reporting economic studies, costs and benefits that occur in the future should be adjusted, or discounted, to their present value. This is because of "time preference"—we generally prefer to incur benefits sooner rather than later, and costs later rather than sooner. Thus, future costs and benefits carry less weight than current costs and benefits, and are usually accounted for by multiplying them by a constant discount rate.[110] Such adjustment has the effect of favoring therapeutic procedures that provide immediate benefit, while making preventive and screening programs, which require immediate expenditure for future benefits, less attractive. There is a lack of consensus over the appropriate discount rate, but recent American guidelines suggest 3% per year.[111] It is also debated whether benefits and costs should be discounted at the same rate since empirical studies have demonstrated that people do not have the same preferences for future health benefits as they do for future costs.[112–115]

The 5-year costs of cancer surveillance can be significant. One text[116] reported average costs across all cancers of $14,534 in 1996, which fell to $8,409 when stem cell transplant patients were not included.[116] Variations in surveillance programs recommended by experts in different countries resulted in variation in cost of over $25,000 for surveillance of esophageal cancer, and over $100,000 (approximately 50-fold) for different recommendations for surveillance of patients who had a stem cell transplant. A common proposal to reduce these costs is to shift surveillance into the primary care setting, as there is a perception that specialist care is more intense, and therefore more expensive. In support of this, physicians in one survey who were most averse to generalist surveillance did tend to propose more expensive surveillance strategies.[41] Given the cost implications, one must ask whether each increment of intensity is really likely to improve outcome. This incredible variation calls for guidelines to standardize practice, and indeed some organizations have taken this on to a limited extent. However, in most cases the lack of data impedes these efforts.

Medicolegal Considerations

Fear of a lawsuit can affect clinical practice, at least in the United States. In oncology, unfortunately, the outcomes are commonly poor, and in some of those cases patients and their families vent their anger by becoming litigious. "Failure to diagnose" is the most common cancer-related cause of a lawsuit. In the case of surveillance, these lawsuits can take the form of failing to diagnose a treatable recurrence or a new primary, whether related or not. This likely leads to increased intensity of surveillance as physicians practice defensive medicine.

Challenges of Surveillance Research

While it is apparent that randomized trials are necessary in order to definitively answer important questions regarding cancer surveillance, they are logistically difficult and expensive to carry out. It is not logical to do clinical trials of surveillance strategies in situations there is no curative treatment for recurrence. This limits the sites for which trials are conceivable to a few, such as colorectal cancer. Studies in low-risk patients with good prognoses necessitate sample sizes in the thousands, as only small improvements in outcome are possible due to surveillance. Moreover, what is tested is generally a complex strategy, so critics might argue: "if only scan X was done more frequently, the results would have been different."

Conclusion

The preponderance of evidence suggests that in most cases, surveillance serves only to shorten the disease-free interval without improving patients' overall survival, quality of life, or psychological well-being. On the other hand, it could be argued that it is paternalistic of us to purposefully not try to obtain information for our patients. Perhaps a patient would make some different life choices if s/he knew that the cancer was recurring, even if detection of recurrence did not improve his/her survival. In this time of patient autonomy, we are not charged with protecting patients from the truth. The cogent patient has a right to know the status of his or her disease. Whether the healthcare system can afford such a luxury is another question. Unfortunately, without high-level evidence to guide most recommendations, surveillance practices evolve based on a mixture of expert consensus, patient demands, medico-legal concerns, and the constraints of third-party payers.[117] Although such situations usually result in a call for more research, in the case of surveillance, the cost of obtaining comparative data on the efficacy of different strategies must be carefully weighed in each case.

References

1. Johnson FE. Overview. In: Johnson FE, Virgo KS, eds. Cancer Patient Follow-Up. St. Louis: Mosby; 1997:4.
2. Virgo KS, Johnson FE. Costs of surveillance after potentially curative treatment for cancer. In: Johnson FE, Virgo KS, eds. Cancer Patient Follow-Up. St. Louis: Mosby; 1997:44.
3. Pfister DG, Benson AB, Somerfield MR. Clinical practice. Surveillance strategies after curative treatment of colorectal cancer. N Engl J Med 2004;350:2375–2382.
4. Gulliford T, Opomu M, Wilson E, et al. Popularity of less frequent follow up for breast cancer in randomised study: initial findings from the hotline study. BMJ. 1997;314:174–177.
5. Grunfeld E, Mant D, Yudkin P, et al. Routine follow-up of breast cancer in primary care: randomised trial. BMJ. 1996;313:665–669.
6. Loprinzi CL, Hayes D, Smith T. Doc, shouldn't we be getting some tests? J Clin Oncol 2000;18:2345–2348.
7. Walsh GL, O'Connor M, Willis KM, et al. Is follow-up of lung cancer patients after resection medically indicated and cost-effective? Ann Thorac Surg 1995;60:1563–1570.
8. Briele HA, Beattie CW, Ronan SG, et al. Late recurrence of cutaneous melanoma. Arch Surg 1983;118:800–803.
9. Bruinvels DJ, Stiggelbout AM, Kievit J, et al. Follow-up of patients with colorectal cancer. A meta-analysis. Ann Surg 1994;219:174–182.
10. Bast RCJ, Ravdin P, Hayes DF, et al. 2000 update of recommendations for the use of tumor markers in breast and colorectal cancer: clinical practice guidelines of the American Society of Clinical Oncology. J Clin Oncol 2001;19:1865–1878.
11. Moertel CG, Fleming TR, Macdonald JS, et al. An evaluation of the carcinoembryonic antigen (CEA) test for monitoring patients with resected colon cancer. JAMA 1995;270:943–947.
12. Benson AB, Desch CE, Flynn PJ, et al. 2000 update of American Society of Clinical Oncology colorectal cancer surveillance guidelines. J Clin Oncol 2000;18:3586–3588.
13. Anderson JE, Litzow MR, Appelbaum FR, et al. Allogeneic, syngeneic, and autologous marrow transplantation for Hodgkin's disease: the 21-year Seattle experience. J Clin Oncol 1993;11:2342–2350.
14. Weeks JC, Yeap BY, Canellos GP, et al. Value of follow-up procedures in patients with large-cell lymphoma who achieve a complete remission. J Clin Oncol 1991;9:1196–1203.
15. NIH consensus conference. Ovarian cancer. Screening, treatment, and follow-up. NIH Consensus Development Panel on Ovarian Cancer. JAMA 1995;273:491–497.
16. Nordic Gastrointestinal Tumor Adjuvant Therapy Group. Expectancy or primary chemotherapy in patients with advanced asymptomatic colorectal cancer: a randomized trial. J Clin Oncol 1992;10:904–911.
17. Grunfeld E, Levine M, Julian JA, et al. A randomized controlled trial of routine follow-up for early stage breast cancer: a comparison of primary care versus specialist care. J Clin Oncol, 2004 Annual Meeting Proceedings (Post-Meeting Edition). 2004;22 (14S) (July 15 Suppl)(Abstract 665).
18. Cocchetto DM, Jones DR. Faster access to drugs for serious or life-threatening illnesses through use of the accelerated approval regulation in the United States. Drug Information Journal 1998; 32:27–35.
19. Wynder EL, Mushinski MH, Spivak JC. Tobacco and alcohol consumption in relation to the development of multiple primary cancers. Cancer 1977;40:1872–1878.
20. Vikram B. Changing patterns of failure in advanced head and neck cancer. Arch Otolaryngol 1984;110:564–565.
21. Vikram B, Strong EW, Shah JP, et al. Second malignant neoplasms in patients successfully treated with multimodality treatment for advanced head and neck cancer. Head Neck Surg 1984;6:734–737.
22. Vikram B, Strong EW, Shah JP, et al. Failure at distant sites following multimodality treatment for advanced head and neck cancer. Head Neck Surg 1984;6:730–733.
23. Barakat RR, Gilewski TA, Almadrones L, et al. Effect of adjuvant tamoxifen on the endometrium in women with breast cancer: a prospective study using office endometrial biopsy. J Clin Oncol 2000;18:3459–3463.
24. Gerber B, Krause A, Muller H, et al. Effects of adjuvant tamoxifen on the endometrium in postmenopausal women with breast cancer: a prospective long-term study using transvaginal ultrasound. J Clin Oncol 2000;18:3464–3470.
25. Edge SB, Levine EG, Arredondo MA, Tezcan H. Breast carcinoma. In: Johnson FE, Virgo KS, eds. Cancer Patient Follow-Up. St. Louis: Mosby; 1997:292.
26. Chlebowski RT, Collyar DE, Somerfield MR, et al. American Society of Clinical Oncology technology assessment on breast cancer risk reduction strategies: tamoxifen and raloxifene. J Clin Oncol 1999;17:1939–1955.
27. Fuchs C, Meyerhardt JA, Heseltine DL, et al. Influence of regular aspirin use on survival for patients with stage II colon cancer: findings from Intergroup trial CALGB 89803. J Clin Oncol, 2005 ASCO Annual Meeting Proceedings. 2005;23(16S, Part I of II) (June 1 Suppl):3530.
28. Meyerhardt JA, Heseltine DL, Niedzwiecki D, et al. The impact of physical activity on patients with stage III colon cancer: findings from Intergroup trial CALGB 89803. J Clin Oncol, 2005 ASCO Annual Meeting Proceedings. 2005;23(16S, Part I of II) (June 1 Suppl):3534.
29. Earle CC, Neville BA. Underuse of necessary care among elderly colorectal cancer survivors. Cancer 2004.
30. Earle CC, Burstein HJ, Winer EP, et al. Quality of non-breast cancer health maintenance among elderly breast cancer survivors. J Clin Oncol 2003;21:1447–1451.
31. American Society of Clinical Oncology. Status of the medical oncology workforce. J Clin Oncol 1996;14:2612–2621.
32. Stiggelbout AM, de Haes JC, Vree R, et al. Follow-up of colorectal cancer patients: quality of life and attitudes towards follow-up. Br J Cancer 1997;75:914–920.
33. Wolff SN, Nichols C, Ulman D, et al. Survivorship: An unmet need of the patient with cancer-implications of a survey of the Lance Armstrong Foundation (LAF). J Clin Oncol, 2005 ASCO Annual Meeting Proceedings. 2005;23(16S, Part I of II)(June 1 Suppl):6032.
34. Kjeldsen BJ, Thorsen H, Whalley D, et al. Influence of follow-up on health-related quality of life after radical surgery for colorectal cancer. Scand J Gastroenterol 1999;34:509–515.
35. Lampic C, Wennberg A, Schill JE, et al. Anxiety and cancer-related worry of cancer patients at routine follow-up visits. Acta Oncol 1994;33:119–125.
36. The GIVIO Investigators. Impact of follow-up testing on survival and health-related quality of life in breast cancer patients. A multicenter randomized controlled trial. JAMA 1994;271:1587–1592.
37. Muss HB, Tell GS, Case LD, et al. Perceptions of follow-up care in women with breast cancer. Am J Clin Oncol 1991;14:55–59.
38. Fong Y, Cohen AM, Fortner JG, et al. Liver resection for colorectal metastases. J Clin Oncol 1997;15:938–946.

39. Secco GB, Fardelli R, Gianquinto D, et al. Efficacy and cost of risk-adapted follow-up in patients after colorectal cancer surgery: a prospective, randomized and controlled trial. Eur J Surg Oncol 2002;28:418–423.

40. Stoffel EM, Garber JE, Grover S, et al. Cancer surveillance is often inadequate in people at high risk for colorectal cancer. J Med Genet 2003;40:e54-Stoffel E.

41. Earle CC, Grunfeld E, Coyle D, et al. Cancer physicians' attitudes toward colorectal cancer follow-up. Ann Oncol 2003;14:400–405.

42. Vernava AM, Longo WE, Virgo KS, et al. Current follow-up strategies after resection of colon cancer. Results of a survey of members of the American Society of Colon and Rectal Surgeons. Dis Colon Rectum 1994;37:573–583.

43. Eddy DM. Breast cancer screening in women younger than 50 years of age: what's next? Ann Intern Med 1997;127:1035–1036.

44. Eddy DM. Screening for colorectal cancer. Ann Intern Med 1990;113:373–384.

45. Eddy DM. Screening for cervical cancer. Ann Intern Med 1990;113:214–226.

46. Winawer SJ, Zauber AG, O'Brien MJ, et al. Randomized comparison of surveillance intervals after colonoscopic removal of newly diagnosed adenomatous polyps. The National Polyp Study Workgroup. N Eng J Med 1993;328:901–906.

47. Andre T, Boni C, Mounedji-Boudiaf L, et al. Oxaliplatin, fluorouracil, and leucovorin as adjuvant treatment for colon cancer. N Engl J Med 2004;350:2343–2351.

48. Meropol NJ, Smith JL. Gastric carcinoma. In: Johnson FE, Virgo KS, eds. Cancer Patient Follow-Up. St. Louis: Mosby; 1997: 94.

49. Emens LA, Davidson NE. The follow-up of breast cancer. Semin Oncol 2003;30:338–348.

50. Rosen PP, Groshen S, Kinne DW, et al. Contralateral breast carcinoma: an assessment of risk and prognosis in stage I (T1N0M0) and stage II (T1N1M0) patients with 20-year follow-up. Surgery 1989;106:904–910.

51. McCredie JA, Inch WR, Alderson M. Consecutive primary carcinomas of the breast. Cancer 1975;35:1472–1477.

52. Grunfeld E, Noorani H, McGahan L, et al. Surveillance mammography after treatment of primary breast cancer: a systematic review. The Breast 2002;11:228–235.

53. Fajardo LL, Roberts CC, Hunt KR. Mammographic surveillance of breast cancer patients: should the mastectomy site be imaged? Am J Roentgenol 1993;161:953–955.

54. Rissanen TJ, Makarainen HP, Mattila SI, et al. Breast cancer recurrence after mastectomy: diagnosis with mammography and US. Radiology 1993;188:463–467.

55. Smith TJ, Davidson NE, Schapira DV, et al. American Society of Clinical Oncology 1998 update of recommended breast cancer surveillance guidelines. J Clin Oncol 1999;17:1080–1082.

56. Pestalozzi BC, Luporsi-Gely E, Jost LM, et al. ESMO Minimum Clinical Recommendations for diagnosis, adjuvant treatment and follow-up of primary breast cancer. Ann Oncol 2005;16(suppl 1):i7–i9.

57. National Comprehensive Cancer Network (NCCN) Web site. Practice Guidelines in Oncology: Breast cancer. Available at http://www.nccn.org/professionals/physician_gls/PDF/breast.pdf. Accessed May 30, 2005.

58. Grunfeld E, Dhesy-Thind S, Levine M. Clinical practice guidelines for the care and treatment of breast cancer: follow-up after treatment for breast cancer (summary of the 2005 update). CMAJ 2005;172:1319–1320.

59. Kriege M, Brekelmans CT, Boetes C, et al. Efficacy of MRI and mammography for breast-cancer screening in women with a familial or genetic predisposition. N Eng J Med 2004;351:427–437.

60. Warner E, Plewes DB, Hill KA, et al. Surveillance of BRCA1 and BRCA2 mutation carriers with magnetic resonance imaging, ultrasound, mammography, and clinical breast examination. JAMA 2004;292:1317–1325.

61. Rosselli DT, Palli D, Cariddi A, et al. Intensive diagnostic follow-up after treatment of primary breast cancer. A randomized trial. National Research Council Project on Breast Cancer follow-up. JAMA 1994;271:1593–1597.

62. Rojas MP, Telaro E, Russo A, et al. Follow-up strategies for women treated for early breast cancer. Cochrane Database Syst Rev CD001768, 2005.

63. Tomiak E, Piccart M. Routine follow-up of patients after primary therapy for early breast cancer: changing concepts and challenges for the future. Ann Oncol 1993;4:199–204.

64. Tomiak EM, Piccart MJ. Routine follow-up of patients following primary therapy for early breast cancer: what is useful? Acta Clin Belg 1993;15(suppl):38–42.

65. Van Cutsem EJ, Kataja VV. ESMO Minimum Clinical Recommendations for diagnosis, adjuvant treatment and follow-up of colon cancer. Ann Oncol 2005;16(suppl 1):i16–i17.

66. Tveit KM, Kataja VV. ESMO Minimum Clinical Recommendations for diagnosis, treatment and follow-up of rectal cancer. Ann Oncol 2005;16(suppl 1):i20–i21.

67. National Comprehensive Cancer Network (NCCN) Web site. Practice Guidelines in Oncology: Colon cancer. Available at http://www.nccn.org/professionals/physician_gls/PDF/colon.pdf. Accessed May 30, 2005.

68. National Comprehensive Cancer Network (NCCN) Web site. Practice Guidelines in Oncology: Rectal cancer. Available at http://www.nccn.org/professionals/physician_gls/PDF/rectal.pdf. Accessed May 30, 2005.

69. Edelman MJ, Meyers FJ, Siegel D. The utility of follow-up testing after curative cancer therapy: a critical review and economic analysis. J Gen Intern Med 1997;12:318–331.

70. Moertel CG, Fleming TR, MacDonald JS, et al. Fluorouracil plus Levamisole as effective adjuvant therapy after resection of stage III colon carcinoma: a final report. Ann Intern Med 1995;122:321–326.

71. O'Connell MJ, Laurie JA, Kahn M, et al. Prospectively randomized trial of postoperative adjuvant chemotherapy in patients with high-risk colon cancer. J Clin Oncol 1998;16:295–300.

72. Goldberg RM, Fleming TR, Tangen CM, et al. Surgery for recurrent colon cancer: strategies for identifying resectable recurrence and success rates after resection. Eastern Cooperative Oncology Group, the North Central Cancer Treatment Group, and the Southwest Oncology Group. Ann Intern Med 1998;129:27–35.

73. Quentmeier A, Schlag P, Smok M, et al. Re-operation for recurrent colorectal cancer: the importance of early diagnosis for resectability and survival. Eur J Surg Oncol 1990;16:319–325.

74. Northover JM, Houghton J, Lennon T. CEA to detect recurrences of colon cancer (letter). JAMA 1994;272:31.

75. Ohlsson B, Breland U, Ekberg H, et al. Follow-up after curative surgery for colorectal carcinoma. Randomized comparison with no follow-up. Dis Colon Rectum 1995;38:619–626.

76. Makela JT, Laitinen SO, Kairaluoma MI. Five-year follow-up after radical surgery for colorectal cancer. Results of a prospective randomized trial. Arch Surg 1995;130:1062–1067.

77. Kjeldsen BJ, Kronborg O, Fenger C, et al. A prospective randomized study of follow-up after radical surgery for colorectal cancer. Br J Surg 1997;84:666–669.

78. Schoemaker D, Black R, Giles L, et al. Yearly colonoscopy, liver CT, and chest radiography do not influence 5-year survival of colorectal cancer patients. Gastroenterology 1998;114:7–14.

79. Pietra N, Sarli L, Costi R, et al. Role of follow-up in management of local recurrences of colorectal cancer: a prospective, randomized study. Diseases of the Colon & Rectum 1998;41:1127–1133.

80. Rosen M, Chan L, Beart RWJ, et al. Follow-up of colorectal cancer: a meta-analysis. Dis Colon Rectum 1998;41:1116–1126.

81. Renehan AG, Egger M, Saunders MP, et al. Impact on survival of intensive follow up after curative resection for colorectal

cancer: systematic review and meta-analysis of randomised trials. BMJ 2002;324:1–8.

82. Jeffrey GM, Hickey BE, Hider P. Follow-up strategies for patients treated for non-metastatic colorectal cancer. Cochrane Database of Systematic Reviews 2002, CD 002200. DOI: 10. 1002/14651858. CD 002200.

83. Figueredo A, Rumble RB, Maroun J, et al. Follow-up of patients with "curatively resected" colorectal cancer: A practice guideline. BMC Cancer 2003;3:26.

84. Fletcher RH. Carcinoembryonic antigen. Ann Intern Med 1986;104:66–73.

85. Goslin R, Steele G, Macintyre J. The use of preoperative plasma CEA levels for the stratification of patients after curative resection of colorectal cancers. Ann Surg 1990;182:747–751.

86. Cancer Care Ontario Program in Evidence-Based Care. Follow-up of patients with curatively resected colorectal cancer. Available at http://www.cancercare.on.ca/pdf/pebc2-9f.pdf. Accessed May 30, 2005.

87. Kondagunta GV, Sheinfeld J, Motzer RJ. Recommendations of follow-up after treatment of germ cell tumors. Semin Oncol 2003;30:382–389.

88. Fossa SD, Horwich A, Russell JM, et al. Optimal planning target volume for stage I testicular seminoma: a Medical Research Council randomized trial. Medical Research Council Testicular Tumor Working Group. J Clin Oncol 1999;17:1146.

89. Raghavan D. Testicular carcinoma. In: Johnson FE, Virgo KS, eds. Cancer Patient Follow-Up. St. Louis: Mosby; 1997: 408–1431.

90. Huddart RA, Kataja VV. ESMO Minimum Clinical Recommendations for diagnosis, treatment and follow-up of testicular seminoma. Ann Oncol 2005;16(suppl 1):i40–i42.

91. Huddart RA, Purkalne G. ESMO Minimum Clinical Recommendations for diagnosis, treatment and follow-up of mixed or non-seminomatous germ cell tumors (NSGCT). Ann Oncol 2005;16(suppl 1):i37–i39.

92. National Comprehensive Cancer Network (NCCN) Web site. Practice Guidelines in Oncology: Testicular cancer. Available at http://www.nccn.org/professionals/physician_gls/PDF/testicular.pdf. Accessed May 30, 2005.

93. Cancer Care Ontario Program in Evidence-Based Care. Surveillance programs for early stage non-seminomatous testicular cancer. Available at http://www.cancercare.on.ca/pdf/pebc3-5f.pdf. Accessed May 30, 2005.

94. Williams SD, Stablein DM, Einhorn LH, et al. Immediate adjuvant chemotherapy versus observation with treatment at relapse in pathological stage II testicular cancer. N Engl J Med 1987;317:1433–1438.

95. Harvey ML, Geldart TR, Duell R, et al. Routine computerised tomographic scans of the thorax in surveillance of stage I testicular non-seminomatous germ-cell cancer—a necessary risk? Ann Oncol 2002;13:237–242.

96. Sharir S, Jewett MA, Sturgeon JF, et al. Progression detection of stage I nonseminomatous testis cancer on surveillance: implications for the followup protocol. J Urol 1999;161:472–475.

97. Gietema JA, Meinardi MT, Sleijfer DT, et al. Routine chest X-rays have no additional value in the detection of relapse during routine follow-up of patients treated with chemotherapy for disseminated non-seminomatous testicular cancer. Ann Oncol 2002;13:1616–1620.

98. White PM, Adamson DJ, Howard GC, et al. Imaging of the thorax in the management of germ cell testicular tumours. Clin Radiol 1999;54:207–211.

99. Birch R, Williams S, Cone A, et al. Prognostic factors for favorable outcome in disseminated germ cell tumors. J Clin Oncol 1986;4:400–407.

100. Grunfeld E, Mant D, Yudkin P, et al. Routine follow up of breast cancer in primary care: randomised trial. BMJ 1996;313:665–669.

101. Grunfeld E, Yudkin P, Adewuyl-Dalton R, et al. Follow up in breast cancer. Quality of life unaffected by general practice follow up. BMJ 1995;311:54.

102. Grunfeld E, Mant D, Vessey MP, et al. Evaluating primary care follow-up of breast cancer: methods and preliminary results of three studies. Ann Oncol 1995;6(suppl 2):47–52.

103. Grunfeld E, Fitzpatrick R, Mant D, et al. Comparison of breast cancer patient satisfaction with follow-up in primary care versus specialist care: results from a randomized controlled trial. Br J Gen Pract 1999;49:705–710.

104. Grunfeld E, Mant D, Vessey MP, et al. Specialist and general practice views on routine follow-up of breast cancer patients in general practice. Fam Pract 1995;12:60–65.

105. Grunfeld E, Gray A, Mant D, et al. Follow-up of breast cancer in primary care vs specialist care: results of an economic evaluation. Br J Cancer 1999;79:1227–1233.

106. Williams C, Coyle D, Gray A, et al. European School of Oncology advisory report to the Commission of the European Communities for the "Europe Against Cancer Programme" cost-effectiveness in cancer care. Eur J Cancer 1995; 31A:1410–1424.

107. Gudex, C. and Kind, P. The QALY Toolkit. Centre for Health Economics. Discussion Paper 38. 1988. University of York. (GENERIC) Ref. Type: Pamphlet.

108. Ontario Ministry of Health. Guidelines for preparation of economic analysis in submission to drug programs branch for listing in the Ontario Benefit Formulary/Comparative Drug Index. Toronto: 1991.

109. Commonwealth of Australia. Guidelines for the pharmaceutical industry on preparation of submissions to the Pharmaceutical Benefits Advisory Committee: Including submissions involving economic analyses. Canberra: Department of Health, Housing and Community Services, 1992.

110. Drummond MF, Stoddart GL, Torrance GW. Methods for the Economic Evaluation of Health Care Programmes. Oxford: Oxford University Press; 1987.

111. Siegel JE, Weinstein MC, Russell LB, et al. Recommendations for reporting cost-effectiveness analyses. JAMA 1996; 276:1339–1341.

112. Parsonage M, Neuberger H. Discounting and health benefits. Health Econ 1992;1:71–79.

113. Coyle D, Tolley K. Discounting of health benefits in the pharmacoeconomic analysis of drug therapies: an issue for debate? Pharmacoeconomics 1992;2:153–162.

114. Cairns J. Discounting and health benefits: another perspective. Health Economics 1992;1:76–79.

115. Sheldon TA. Discounting in health-care decision-making—time for a change. J Public Health Med 1992;14:250–256.

116. Virgo KS, Johnson FE. Costs of surveillance after potentially curative treatment for cancer. In: Virgo KS, Johnson FE, eds. Cancer Patient Follow-Up. St. Louis: Mosby; 1997: 45.

117. Johnson FE. Overview. In: Johnson FE, Virgo KS, eds. Cancer Patient Follow-Up. St. Louis: Mosby; 1997: 7.

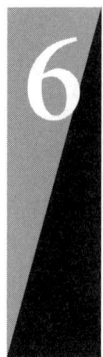

6

Late Effects of Cancer Treatments

Noreen M. Aziz

Background and Significance

With continued advances in strategies to detect cancer early and treat it effectively, along with the aging of the population, the number of individuals living years beyond a cancer diagnosis can be expected to continue to increase. Statistical trends show that, in the absence of other competing causes of death, 64% of adults diagnosed with cancer today can expect to be alive in 5 years.[1–4] Relative 5-year survival rates for those diagnosed as children (age less than 19 years) are even higher, with almost 79% of childhood cancer survivors estimated to be alive at 5 years and 75% at 10 years.[5]

Survival from cancer has seen dramatic improvements over the past three decades, mainly as a result of advances in early detection, therapeutic strategies, and the widespread use of combined modality therapy (surgery, chemotherapy, and radiotherapy).[6–10] Medical and sociocultural factors such as psychosocial and behavioral interventions, active screening behaviors, and healthier lifestyles may also play an integral role in the length and quality of that survival.[11]

Although beneficial and often lifesaving against the diagnosed malignancy, most therapeutic modalities for cancer are associated with a spectrum of late complications ranging from minor and treatable to serious or, occasionally, potentially lethal.[2,6,12–15] While living for extended periods of time beyond their initial diagnosis, many cancer survivors often face various chronic and late physical and psychosocial sequelae of their disease or its treatment. Additionally, as the number of survivors and their length of survival expand, long-term health issues specific to cancer survival are also fast emerging as a public health concern. Questions of particular importance to cancer survivors include surveillance for the adverse sequelae, or late and long-term effects, of treatment; the development of new (second) cancers; and recurrence of their original cancer. One-fourth of *late deaths* occurring among survivors of childhood cancer during the extended survivorship period, when the chances of primary disease recurrence are negligible, can be attributed to a treatment-related effect such as a second cancer or cardiac dysfunction.[16] The most *frequently observed* medical sequelae among pediatric cancer survivors include endocrine complications, growth hormone deficiency, primary hypothyroidism, and primary ovarian failure. Also included within the rubric of late effects are second cancers arising as a result of genetic predisposition (e.g., familial cancer syndromes) or the mutagenic effects of therapy. These factors may act independently or synergistically. Synergistic effects of mutagenic agents

such as cigarette smoke or toxins such as alcohol are largely unknown.[2,6,12]

Thus, there is today a greater recognition of symptoms that persist after the completion of treatment and which arise years after primary therapy. Both acute organ toxicities such as radiation pneumonitis and chronic toxicities such as congestive cardiac failure, neurocognitive deficits, infertility, and second malignancies are being described as the price of cure or prolonged survival.[2,6,12] The study of late effects, originally within the realm of pediatric cancer, is now germane to cancer survivors at all ages because concerns may continue to surface throughout the life cycle.[2,6] These concerns underscore the need to follow up and screen survivors of cancer for toxicities such as those mentioned and also to develop and provide effective interventions that carry the potential to prevent or ameliorate adverse outcomes.

The goal of survivorship research is to focus on the *health and life* of a person with a history of cancer *beyond* the acute diagnosis and treatment phase. Survivorship research seeks to examine the causes of, and to prevent and control the adverse effects associated with, cancer and its treatment and to optimize the physiologic, psychosocial, and functional outcomes for cancer survivors and their families. A hallmark of survivorship research is its emphasis on understanding the integration/interaction of multidisciplinary domains.

This chapter presents definitional issues relevant to cancer survivorship; examines late effects of cancer treatment among survivors of pediatric and adult cancer; and articulates gaps in knowledge and emerging research priorities in cancer survivorship research relevant to late effects of cancer treatment. It draws heavily from pediatric cancer survivorship research because a paucity of data continue to exist for medical late effects of treatment for survivors of cancer diagnosed as adults. Research on late effects of cancer treatment began in the realm of pediatric cancer and continues to yield important insights for the impact of cancer therapies among those diagnosed as adults.

Definitional Issues

Fitzhugh Mullan, a physician diagnosed with and treated for cancer himself, first described cancer survivorship as a concept.[17] Definitional issues for cancer survivorship encompass three related aspects:[2,6] (1) *Who is a cancer survivor?* Philosophically, anyone who has been diagnosed with cancer is a survivor, from the time of diagnosis to the end of life.[1] Caregivers and family members are also included within this definition as secondary survivors. (2) *What is cancer survivorship?* Mullan described the survivorship experience as similar to the seasons of the year. Mullan recognized three seasons or phases of survival: acute (extending from diagnosis to the completion of initial treatment, encompassing issues dominated by treatment and its side effects); extended (beginning with the completion of initial treatment for the primary disease, remission of disease, or both, dominated by watchful waiting, regular follow-up examinations, and, perhaps, intermittent therapy); and permanent survival (not a single moment; evolves from extended disease-free survival when the likelihood of recurrence is sufficiently low). An understanding of these phases of survival is important for facilitating an optimal transition into and management of survivorship. (3) *What is cancer survivorship research?* Cancer survivorship research seeks to identify, examine, prevent, and control adverse cancer diagnosis and treatment-related outcomes (such as late effects of treatment, second cancers, and quality of life); to provide a knowledge base regarding optimal follow-up care and surveillance of cancer survivors; and to optimize health after cancer treatment.[2,6]

Other important definitions include those for long-term cancer survivorship and late versus long-term effects of cancer treatment. Generally, *long-term cancer survivors* are defined as those individuals who are 5 or more years beyond the diagnosis of their primary disease and embody the concept of permanent survival described by Mullan. *Late effects* refer specifically to unrecognized toxicities that are absent or subclinical at the end of therapy and become manifest later with the unmasking of hitherto unseen injury caused by any of the following factors: developmental processes; the failure of compensatory mechanisms with the passage of time; or organ senescence. *Long-term effects* refer to any side effects or complications of treatment for which a cancer patient must compensate; also known as persistent effects, they begin during treatment and continue beyond the end of treatment. Late effects, in contrast, appear months to years after the completion of treatment. Some researchers classify cognitive problems, fatigue, lymphedema, and peripheral neuropathy as long-term effects while others classify them as late effects.[18–21]

This chapter focuses largely on the *physiologic* or *medical* long-term and late effects of cancer treatment. Physiologic sequelae of cancer treatment can also be further classified as follows:

a. System-specific (e.g., organ damage, failure, or premature aging, immunosuppression or issues related to compromised immune systems, and endocrine damage);
b. Second malignant neoplasms (such as an increased risk of recurrent malignancy, increased risk of a certain cancer associated with the primary malignancy, and/or increased risk of secondary malignancies associated with cytotoxic or radiologic cancer therapies (this topic is not covered in detail in this chapter as it is reviewed comprehensively elsewhere in this book); and
c. Functional changes such as lymphedema, incontinence, pain syndromes, neuropathies, fatigue; cosmetic changes

such as amputations, ostomies, and skin/hair alterations; and comorbidities such as osteoporosis, arthritis, and hypertension.

Late and Long-Term Effects of Cancer and Its Treatment: Overview and Generalizations

Consequent to the phenomenal success in treating cancer effectively and detecting it early, we are faced today with an increasing population of individuals who, although cancer free for many years, have issues and concerns regarding the persistent (chronic) and the late (delayed) effects of cancer therapies on their health, longevity, and quality of life. The long-term impact of cancer and its treatment can include premature mortality and long-term morbidity. The two most frequent causes of premature mortality in disease-free cancer survivors are (1) cardiac disease and (2) second malignant neoplasms.[22,23] The subject of late effects among children treated for cancer has been the topic of numerous reviews.[21,24–28] To varying degrees, it has been shown that disease- or treatment-specific subgroups of long-term survivors are at risk of developing adverse outcomes. These adverse consequences of cancer treatment include early death, second neoplasms, organ dysfunction (e.g., cardiac, pulmonary, gonadal), reduced growth and development, decreased fertility, impaired intellectual function, difficulties obtaining employment and insurance, and a decreased quality of life. This chapter summarizes selected aspects of the spectrum of outcomes relating to the late effects of therapy among individuals (adults, children, and adolescents) treated for cancer.

Generalizations About Late Effects

Several generalizations can be made.[2,6,29] It is now possible to anticipate certain types of late effects on the basis of specific therapies to which the survivor was exposed, the age of the survivor at the time of treatment, combinations of treatment modalities used, and the dosage administered. There are differences in susceptibility between pediatric and adult patients. Generally, chemotherapy results in acute toxicities that can persist whereas radiation leads to sequelae that are not apparent immediately and surface after a latent period. Combinations of chemotherapy and radiation therapy are more often associated with late effects in the survivorship period.[2,6,29]

Toxicities related to chemotherapy, especially those of an acute but possibly persistent nature, may be related to proliferation kinetics of individual cell populations as these drugs are usually cell cycle dependent. Thus, organs or tissues most susceptible are those with high cell proliferation (turnover) rates such as the skin (epidermis), bone marrow, gastrointestinal mucosa, liver, and testes. Theoretically, the least susceptible organs and tissues are those that replicate very slowly or not at all and include muscle cells, neurons, and the connective tissue.[2,6,29]

Issues Unique to Certain Cancer Sites

Late effects have been studied in greater depth for certain cancer sites. The examination of late effects for childhood cancers such as acute lymphoblastic leukemia, Hodgkin's

---

[1]From the National Coalition for Cancer Survivorship.

disease, and brain tumors have provided the foundation for this area of research. A body of knowledge on late effects of radiation and/or chemotherapy is subsequently being developed for adult sites such as breast cancer. For example, recent studies have evaluated and reported on the development of neurocognitive deficits after chemotherapy for breast cancer, a late effect that was initially observed among survivors of childhood cancer receiving cranial irradiation and/or chemotherapy. Late effects of bone marrow transplant have been studied for both adult and childhood cancer survivors, as have sequelae associated with particular chemotherapeutic regimens such as those for Hodgkin's disease or breast cancer.

Chemotherapeutic drugs for which late effects have been reported most frequently include adriamycin, bleomycin, vincristine, methotrexate, cytoxan, and many others (Table 6.1).

The side effects of radiotherapy, both alone and in conjunction with chemotherapy, have been reported fairly comprehensively for most childhood cancer sites associated with good survival rates. It is important to bear in mind that most cancer treatment regimens consist of chemotherapy in conjunction with surgery and/or radiation, and multidrug chemotherapeutic regimens are the rule rather the exception. As such, the risk of late effects must always be considered in light of all other treatment modalities to which the patient has been exposed.

Special Considerations of Primary Diagnosis and Treatment in Childhood

Cancer therapy may interfere with development in terms of physical and musculoskeletal growth, neurocognitive/intellectual growth, and pubertal development. These effects may be most *notable* during the adolescent growth spurt, even though they occur during the childhood period. These specific sequelae are covered in greater detail in the chapter by Bhatia et al. (see Chapter 7) and are not discussed here. A brief classification follows:

a. Alterations in physical growth
   i. Linear growth effects[30–32]
   ii. Impact of early puberty on growth[33,34]
   iii. Hypoplasia[35]
b. Alterations in intellectual development[36–39]
c. Altered pubertal development[40]
d. Obesity[41–43]

Special Considerations of Primary Diagnosis and Treatment During Adulthood

Some late effects of chemotherapy may assume special importance depending on the adult patient's age at the time of diagnosis and treatment. Diagnosis and treatment during the *young adult or reproductive years* may call for a special cognizance of the importance of maintaining reproductive

TABLE 6.1. Possible late effects of radiotherapy and chemotherapy.

Organ system	Late effects/sequelae of radiotherapy	Late effects/sequelae of chemotherapy	Chemotherapeutic drugs responsible
Bone and soft tissues	Short stature; atrophy, fibrosis, osteonecrosis	Avascular necrosis	Steroids
Cardiovascular	Pericardial effusion; pericarditis; CAD	Cardiomyopathy; CHF	Anthracylines Cyclophosphamide
Pulmonary	Pulmonary fibrosis; decreased lung volumes	Pulmonary fibrosis; interstitial pneumonitis	Bleomycin, BCNU Methotrexate, adriamycin
Central nervous system (CNS)	Neuropsychologic deficits, structural changes, hemorrhage	Neuropsychologic deficits, structural changes Hemiplegia; seizure	Methotrexate
Peripheral nervous system		Peripheral neuropathy; hearing loss	Cisplatin, vinca alkaloids
Hematologic	Cytopenia, myelodysplasia	Myelodyplastic syndromes	Alkylating agents
Renal	Decreased creatinine clearance	Decreased creatinine clearance	Cisplatin Methotrexate
	Hypertension	Increased creatinine Renal filtration Delayed renal filtration	Nitrosoureas
Genitourinary	Bladder fibrosis, contractures	Bladder fibrosis; hemorrhagic cystitis	Cyclophosphamide
Gastrointestinal	Malabsorption; stricture; abnormal LFT	Abnormal LFT; hepatic fibrosis; cirrhosis	Methotrexate, BCNU
Pituitary	Growth hormone deficiency; pituitary deficiency		
Thyroid	Hypothyroidism; nodules		
Gonadal	Men: risk of sterility, Leydig cell dysfunction.	Men: sterility	Alkylating agents
	Women: ovarian failure, early menopause	Women: sterility, premature menopause	Procarbazine
Dental/oral health	Poor enamel and root formation; dry mouth		
Opthalmologic	Cataracts; retinopathy	Cataracts	Steroids

CAD, coronary artery disease; CCF, congestive cardiac failure; LFT, liver function tests; BCNU, carmustine.

Source: Data from Ganz (1998, 2001)[12,13] and Aziz (2002, 2003).[2,6]

function and the prevention of second cancers. These are also key issues for children whose cancers are diagnosed during childhood.

Cancer patients diagnosed and treated during *middle age* may need specific attention to sequelae such as premature menopause, issues relating to sexuality and intimacy, pros and cons of using estrogen replacement therapy (ERT), prevention of neurocognitive, cardiac, and other sequelae of chemotherapy, and the prevention of coronary artery disease and osteoporosis. It has been reported that sexual dysfunction persists after breast cancer treatment, despite recovery in other domains, and includes vaginal discomfort, hot flashes, and alterations in bioavailable testosterone, luteinizing hormone, and sex hormone-binding globulin.[44] Menopausal symptoms such as hot flashes, vaginal dryness, and stress urinary incontinence are very common in breast cancer survivors and cannot be managed with standard estrogen replacement therapy.[45] The normal life expectancy of survivors of early-stage cancers during these years of life underscores the need to address their long-term health and quality of life issues.

Although *older patients* (65 years and over) bear a disproportionate burden of cancer, advancing age is associated with increased vulnerability to other age-related health problems and concurrent ailments such as diabetes, chronic obstructive pulmonary disease, heart disease, arthritis, and/or hypertension. Any of these could potentially affect treatment choice, prognosis, and survival. Hence, cancer treatment decisions may need to be made in the context of the older individual's preexisting health problems (comorbidities). Measures that can help evaluate the existence, nature, and severity of comorbidities among older cancer patients in a reliable manner are needed. Currently, there is little information on how comorbid age-related conditions influence treatment decisions, the subsequent course of the disease, the way that already-compromised older cancer patients tolerate the stress of cancer and its treatment, and how concomitant comorbid conditions are managed.[46]

Review of Late and Long-Term Effects by Organ System or Tissues Affected[2]

System-Specific Physiologic Sequelae[3]

CARDIAC SEQUELAE

The heart may be damaged by both therapeutic irradiation and chemotherapeutic agents commonly used in the treatment for cancer. Several types of damage have been reported, including pericardial, myocardial, and vascular. Cardiac damage is most pronounced after treatment with the anthracycline drugs doxorubicin and daunorubicin, used widely in the treatment of most childhood cancers and adjuvant chemotherapy for breast and many other adult cancers. An additive effect has also been reported when anthracyclines are

used in conjunction with cyclophosphamide and radiation therapy. Anthracyclines cause myocardial cell death, leading to a diminished number of myocytes and compensatory hypertrophy of residual myocytes.[47] Major clinical manifestations include reduced cardiac function, arrhythmia, and heart failure. Chronic cardiotoxicity usually manifests itself as cardiomyopathy, pericarditis, and congestive heart failure.

Cardiac injury that becomes clinically manifest during or shortly after completion of chemotherapy may progress, stabilize, or improve after the first year of treatment. This improvement may either be of a transient nature or last for a considerable length of time. There is also evidence of a continuum of injury that will manifest itself throughout the lives of these patients.[48] From a risk factor perspective, patients who exhibit reduced cardiac function within 6 months of completing chemotherapy are at increased risk for the development of late cardiac failure.[49] However, a significant incidence of late cardiac decompensation manifested by cardiac failure or lethal arrhythmia occurring 10 to 20 years after the administration of these drugs has also been reported.[50]

In a recent study of Hodgkin's disease (HD) survivors, investigators reported finding cardiac abnormalities in the majority of the participants.[51] This is an important finding especially because the sample consisted of individuals who did not manifest symptomatic heart disease at screening and described their health as "good." Manifestations of cardiac abnormalities included (a) restrictive cardiomyopathy (suggested by reduced average left ventricular dimension and mass without increased left ventricular wall thickness); (b) significant valvular defects; (c) conduction defects; (d) complete heart block; (e) autonomic dysfunction (suggested by a monotonous heart rate in 57%); (f) persistent tachycardia; and (g) blunted hemodynamic responses to exercise. The peak oxygen uptake (VO_{2max}) during exercise, a predictor of mortality in heart failure, was significantly reduced (less than $20\,mL/kg/m^2$) in 30% of survivors and was correlated with increasing fatigue, increasing shortness of breath, and a decreasing physical component score on the SF-36. Given the presence of these clinically significant cardiovascular abnormalities, investigators recommend serial, comprehensive cardiac screening of HD survivors who fit the profile of having received mediastinial irradiation at a young age.

Congestive cardiomyopathy is directly related to the total dose of the agent administered; the higher the dose, the greater the chance of cardiotoxicity. Subclinical abnormalities have also been noted at lower doses. The anthracyclines doxorubicin and daunorubicin are well-known causes of cardiomyopathy that can occur many years after completion of therapy. The incidence of anthracycline-induced cardiomyopathy, which is dose dependent, may exceed 30% among patients receiving cumulative doses in excess of $600\,mg/m^2$. A cumulative dose of anthracyclines greater than $300\,mg/m^2$ has been associated with an 11-fold-increased risk of clinical heart failure, compared with a cumulative dose of less than $300\,mg/m^2$, the estimated risk of clinical heart failure increasing with time from exposure and approaching 5% after 15 years.

A reduced incidence and severity of cardiac abnormalities was reported in a study of 120 long-term survivors of acute lymphoblastic leukemia (ALL) who had been treated with lower anthracycline doses ($90–270\,mg/m^2$), compared with previous reports in which subjects had received moderate

---

[2]Common to both children and adults depending on cancer site and treatment(s) received.

[3]These include organ damage, failure, or premature aging resulting from chemotherapy, hormone therapy, radiation, surgery, or any combination thereof.

anthracycline doses (300–550 mg/m²).[52,53] Twenty-three percent of the patients were found to have cardiac abnormalities, 21% had increased end-systolic stress, and only 2% had reduced contractility. The cumulative anthracycline dose within the 90 to 270 mg/m² range did not relate to cardiac abnormalities. The authors concluded that there may be no safe anthracycline dose to completely avoid late cardiotoxicity. A recent review of 30 published studies in childhood cancer survivors found that the frequency of clinically detected anthracycline cardiac heart failure ranged from 0% to 16%.[54] In an analysis of reported studies, the type of anthracycline (e.g., doxorubicin) and the maximum dose given in a 1-week period (e.g., more than 45 mg/m²) was found to explain a large portion of the variation in the reported frequency of anthracycline-induced cardiac heart failure.

Cyclophosphamide has been associated with the development of congestive cardiomyopathy, especially when administered at the high doses used in transplant regimens. Cardiac toxicity may occur at lower doses when mediastinal radiation is combined with the chemotherapeutic drugs mentioned above. Late onset of congestive heart failure has been reported during pregnancy, rapid growth, or after the initiation of vigorous exercise programs in adults previously treated for cancer during childhood or young adulthood as a result of increased afterload and the impact of the additional stress of such events on marginal cardiac reserves. Initial improvement in cardiac function after completion of therapy appears to result, at least in part, from compensatory changes. Compensation may diminish in the presence of stressors such as those mentioned earlier and myocardial depressants such as alcohol.

The incidence of subclinical anthracycline myocardial damage has been the subject of considerable interest. Steinherz et al. found 23% of 201 patients who had received a median cumulative dose of doxorubicin of 450 mg/m² had echocardiographic abnormalities at a median of 7 years after therapy.[55] In a group of survivors of childhood cancer who received a median doxorubicin dose of 334 mg/m², it was found that progressive elevation of afterload or depression of left ventricular contractility was present in approximately 75% of patients.[47] A recent review of the literature on subclinical cardiotoxicity among children treated with an anthracycline found that the reported frequency of subclinical cardiotoxicity varied considerably across the 25 studies reviewed (frequency ranging from 0% to 57%).[56] Because of marked differences in the definition of outcomes for subclinical cardiotoxicity and the heterogeneity of the patient populations investigated, it is difficult to accurately evaluate the potential long-term outcomes within anthracycline-exposed patient populations or the potential impact of the subclinical findings.

Effects of radiation on the heart may be profound, and include valvular damage, pericardial thickening, and ischemic heart disease. Patients with radiation-related cardiac damage have a markedly increased relative risk of both angina and myocardial infarction [relative risk (RR), 2.56] years after mediastinal radiation for Hodgkin's disease in adult patients, whereas the risk of cardiac death is 3.1.[57] This risk was greatest among patients receiving more than 30 Gy of mantle irradiation and those treated before 20 to 21 years of age. Blocking the heart reduced the risk of cardiac death due to causes other than myocardial infarction.[58]

In general, among anthracycline-exposed patients, the risk of cardiotoxicity can be increased by mediastinal radiation,[59] uncontrolled hypertension,[60,61] underlying cardiac abnormalities,[62] exposure to nonanthracycline chemotherapeutic agents (especially cyclophosphamide, dactinomycin, mitomycin C, dacarbazine, vincristine, bleomycin, and methotrexate),[63,64] female gender,[65] younger age,[66] and electrolyte imbalances such as hypokalaemia and hypomagnesaemia.[67] Previous reports have suggested that doxorubicin-induced cardiotoxicity can be prevented by continuous infusion of the drug.[68] However, Lipshultz et al. compared cardiac outcomes in children receiving either bolus or continuous infusion of doxorubicin, and reported that continuous doxorubicin infusion over 48 hours for childhood leukemia did not offer a cardioprotective advantage over bolus infusion.[69] Both regimens were associated with progressive subclinical cardiotoxicity, thus suggesting that there is no benefit from continuous infusion of anthracyclines.

Chronic cardiotoxicity associated with radiation alone most commonly involves pericardial effusions or constrictive pericarditis, sometimes in association with pancarditis. Although a dose of 40 Gy of total heart irradiation appears to be the usual threshold, pericarditis has been reported after as little as 15 Gy, even in the absence of radiomimetic chemotherapy.[70,71] Symptomatic pericarditis, which usually develops 10 to 30 years after irradiation, is found in 2% to 10% of patients.[72] Subclinical pericardial and myocardial damage, as well as valvular thickening, may be common in this population.[73,74] Coronary artery disease has been reported after radiation to the mediastinum, although mortality rates have not been significantly higher in patients who receive mediastinal radiation than in the general population.[58]

Given the known acute and long-term cardiac complications of therapy, prevention of cardiotoxicity is a focus of active investigation. Several attempts have been made to minimize the cardiotoxicity of anthracyclines, such as the use of liposomal-formulated anthracyclines, less-cardiotoxic analogues, and the additional administration of cardioprotective agents. The advantages of these approaches are still controversial, but there are ongoing clinical trials to evaluate the long-term effects. Certain analogues of doxorubicin and daunorubicin, with decreased cardiotoxicity but equivalent antitumour activity, are being explored. Agents such as dexrazoxane, which are able to remove iron from anthracyclines, have been investigated as cardioprotectants. Clinical trials of dexrazoxane have been conducted in children, with encouraging evidence of short-term cardioprotection[75]; however, the long-term avoidance of cardiotoxicity with the use of this agent has yet to be sufficiently determined. The most recent study by Lipshultz et al. reported that dexrazoxane prevents or reduces cardiac injury, as reflected by elevations in troponin T, that is associated with the use of doxorubicin for childhood ALL without compromising the antileukemic efficacy of doxorubicin. Longer follow-up will be necessary to determine the influence of dexrazoxane on echocardiographic findings at four years and on event-free survival.[76]

Another key emerging issue is the interaction of taxanes with doxorubicin. Epirubicin–taxane combinations are active in treating metastatic breast cancer, and ongoing research is focusing on combining anthracyclines with taxanes in an effort to continue to improve outcomes following adjuvant therapy.[77] Clinically significant drug interactions have been reported to occur when paclitaxel is administered with doxorubicin, cisplatin, or anticonvulsants (phenytoin, carbamazepine, and phenobarbital), and pharmacodynamic interactions have been reported to occur with these agents that are sequence- or schedule dependent.[78] Because the taxanes undergo hepatic oxidation via the cytochrome P-450 system, pharmacokinetic interactions from enzyme induction or inhibition can also occur. A higher than expected myelotoxicity has been reported. However, there is no enhanced doxorubicinol formation in human myocardium, a finding consistent with the cardiac safety of the regimen.[79] Investigators have suggested that doxorubicin and epirubicin should be administered 24 hours before paclitaxel and the cumulative anthracycline dose be limited to $360 \, mg/m^2$, thereby preventing the enhanced toxicities caused by sequence- and schedule-dependent interactions between anthracyclines and paclitaxel.[78] Conversely, they also suggest that paclitaxel should be administered at least 24 hours before cisplatin to avoid a decrease in clearance and increase in myelosuppression. With concurrent anticonvulsant therapy, cytochrome P-450 enzyme induction results in decreased paclitaxel plasma steady-state concentrations, possibly requiring an increased dose of paclitaxel. A number of other drug interactions have been reported in preliminary studies for which clinical significance has yet to be established.[78]

The human epidermal growth factor receptor (HER) 2 is overexpressed in approximately 20% to 25% of human breast cancers and is an independent adverse prognostic factor. Targeted therapy directed against this receptor has been developed in the form of a humanized monoclonal antibody, trastuzumab. Unexpectedly, cardiac toxicity has developed in some patients treated with trastuzumab, and this has a higher incidence in those treated in combination with an anthracycline.[80,81] Both clinical and in vitro data suggest that cardiomyocyte HER2/erbB2 is uniquely susceptible to trastuzumab.[82] Tratuzumab has shown activity as a single agent in metastatic breast cancer both before chemotherapy and in heavily pretreated patients, and its use in combination with an anthracycline or paclitaxel results in a significant improvement in survival, time to progression, and response.[80] The HER2 status of a tumor is a critical determinant of response to trastuzumab-based treatment; those expressing HER2 at the highest level on immunohistochemistry, 3+, derive more benefit from treatment with trastuzumab than those with overexpression at the 2+ level. Interactions between the estrogen receptor and HER2 pathway has stimulated interest in using trastuzumab in combination with endocrine therapy. Current clinical trials are investigating the role of this agent in the adjuvant setting.

Neurocognitive Sequelae

Long-term survivors of cancer may be at risk of neurocognitive and neuropsychologic sequelae. Among survivors of childhood leukemia, neurocognitive late effects represent one of the more intensively studied topics. Adverse outcomes are generally associated with whole-brain radiation and/or therapy with high-dose systemic or intrathecal methotrexate or cytarabine.[83–85] High-risk characteristics, including higher dose of central nervous system (CNS) radiation, younger age at treatment, and female sex, have been well documented. Results from studies of neurocognitive outcomes are directly

responsible for the marked reduction (particularly in younger children) in the use of cranial radiation, which is currently reserved for treatment of very high risk subgroups or patients with CNS involvement.[86]

A spectrum of clinical syndromes may occur, including radionecrosis, necrotizing leukoencephalopathy, mineralizing microangiopathy and dystropic calcification, cerebellar sclerosis, and spinal cord dysfunction.[87] Leukoencephalopathy has been primarily associated with methotrexate-induced injury of white matter. However, cranial radiation may play an additive role through the disruption of the blood–brain barrier, thus allowing greater exposure of the brain to systemic therapy.

Although abnormalities have been detected by diagnostic imaging studies, the abnormalities observed have not been well demonstrated to correlate with clinical findings and neurocognitive status.[88,89] Chemotherapy- or radiation-induced destruction in normal white matter partially explains intellectual and academic achievement deficits.[90] Evidence suggests that direct effects of chemotherapy and radiation on intracranial endothelial cells and brain white matter as well as immunologic mechanisms could be involved in the pathogenesis of central nervous system damage.

Neurocognitive deficits, as a general rule, usually become evident within several years following CNS radiation and tend to be progressive in nature. Leukemia survivors treated at a younger age (i.e., less than 6 years of age) may experience significant declines in intelligence quotient (IQ) scores.[91] However, reductions in IQ scores are typically not global, but rather reflect specific areas of impairment, such as attention and other nonverbal cognitive processing skills.[92] Affected children may experience information-processing deficits, resulting in academic difficulties. These children are particularly prone to problems with receptive and expressive language, attention span, and visual and perceptual motor skills, most often manifested in academic difficulties in the areas of reading, language, and mathematics. Accordingly, children treated with CNS radiation or systemic or intrathecal therapy with the potential to cause neurocognitive deficits should receive close monitoring of academic performance. Referral for neuropsychologic evaluation with appropriate intervention strategies, such as modifications in curriculum, speech and language therapy, or social skills training, implemented in a program tailored for the individual needs and deficits of the survivor should be taken into consideration.[93] Assessment of educational needs and subsequent educational attainment have found that survivors of childhood leukemia are significantly more likely to require special educational assistance, but have a high likelihood of successfully completing high school.[37,94] However, when compared with siblings, survivors of leukemia and non-Hodgkin's lymphoma (NHL) are at greater risk of not completing high school. As would be anticipated from the results of neurocognitive studies, it has been shown that survivors, particularly those under 6 years of age at treatment, who received cranial radiation and/or intrathecal chemotherapy were significantly more likely to require special education services and least likely to complete a formal education.[86,95,96]

Progressive dementia and dysfunction have been reported in some long-term cancer survivors as a result of whole-brain radiation with or without chemotherapy, and occur most often in brain tumor patients and patients with small cell lung cancer who have received prophylactic therapy. Neuropsychologic abnormalities have also been reported after CNS prophylaxis utilizing whole-brain radiation for leukemia in childhood survivors. In fact, cognitive changes in children began to be recognized as treatments for childhood cancer, especially ALL, became increasingly effective. These observations have resulted in changes in treatment protocols for childhood ALL.[97,98]

Several recent studies have reported cognitive dysfunction in women treated with adjuvant therapy for breast cancer.[99,100] In one study,[101] investigators compared the neuropsychologic performance of long-term survivors of breast cancer and lymphoma treated with standard-dose chemotherapy who carried the epsilon 4 allele of the apolipoprotein E (APOE) gene to those who carry other APOE alleles. Survivors with at least one epsilon 4 allele scored significantly lower in the visual memory (P less than 0.03) and the spatial ability (P less than 0.05) domains and tended to score lower in the psychomotor functioning (P less than 0.08) domain as compared to survivors who did not carry an epsilon 4 allele. No group differences were found on depression, anxiety, or fatigue. The results of this study provide preliminary support for the hypothesis that the epsilon 4 allele of APOE may be a potential genetic marker for increased vulnerability to chemotherapy-induced cognitive decline.

Although cranial irradiation is the most frequently identified causal factor in both adults and children, current work in adults indicates that cognitive problems may also occur with surgery, chemotherapy, and biologic response modifiers.[102–104] These findings need to be validated in prospective studies along with the interaction between treatment with chemotherapeutic agents, menopausal status, and hormonal treatments. Emotional distress also has been related to cognitive issues in studies of patients beginning cancer treatment.

Patients have attributed problems in cognition to fatigue, and others have reported problems with concentration, short-term memory, problem-solving, and concerns about "chemo-brain" or "mental pause."[105] Comparisons across studies are difficult because of different batteries of neuropsychologic tests used, and differences among patient samples by diagnosis, age, gender, or type of treatment received, and, finally, inconsistency in the timing of measures in relation to treatment landmarks. Despite these methodologic issues, studies have shown impairments in verbal information processing, complex information processing, concentration, and visual memory.[106–109]

Current studies indicate that cognitive deficits are often subtle but are observed consistently in a proportion of patients, may be durable, and can be disabling.[110] Deficits have been observed in a range of cognitive functions. Although underlying mechanisms are unknown, preliminary studies suggest a genetic predisposition. Cognitive impairment may be accompanied by changes in the brain detectable by neuroimaging. Priorities for future research include (1) large-scale clinical studies that use both a longitudinal design and concurrent evaluation of patients with cancer who do not receive chemotherapy—such studies should address the probability and magnitude of cognitive deficits, factors that predict them, and underlying mechanisms; (2) exploration of discrepancies between subjective reports of cognitive dysfunction and the objective results of cognitive testing; (3) studies of cognitive

function in patients receiving treatment for diseases other than breast cancer, and in both men and women, to address the hypothesis that underlying mechanisms relate to changes in serum levels of sex hormones and/or to chemotherapy-induced menopause; (4) development of interventions to alleviate these problems; and (5) development of animal models and the use of imaging techniques to address mechanisms that might cause cognitive impairment.

ENDOCRINOLOGIC SEQUELAE

THYROID
Radiation exposure to the head and neck is a known risk factor for subsequent abnormalities of the thyroid. Among survivors of Hodgkin's disease and, to a lesser extent, leukemia survivors, abnormalities of the thyroid gland, including hypothyroidism, hyperthyroidism, and thyroid neoplasms, have been reported to occur at rates significantly higher than found in the general population.[111–114] Hypothyroidism is the most common nonmalignant late effect involving the thyroid gland. Following radiation doses above 15 Gy, laboratory evidence of primary hypothyroidism is evident in 40% to 90% of patients with Hodgkin's disease, NHL, or head and neck malignancies.[113,115,116] In a recent analysis of 1,791 5-year survivors of pediatric Hodgkin's disease (median age at follow-up, 30 years), Sklar et al. reported the occurrence of at least one thyroid abnormality in 34% of subjects.[114] The risk of hypothyroidism was increased 17 fold compared with sibling control subjects, with increasing dose of radiation, older age at diagnosis of Hodgkin's disease, and female sex as significant independent predictors of an increased risk. The actuarial risk of hypothyroidism for subjects treated with 45 Gy or more was 50% at 20 years following diagnosis of their Hodgkin's disease. Hyperthyroidism was reported to occur in only 5%.

HORMONES AFFECTING GROWTH
Poor linear growth and short adult stature are common complications after successful treatment of childhood cancers.[117] The adverse effect of CNS radiation on adult final height among childhood leukemia patients has been well documented, with final heights below the fifth percentile occurring in 10% to 15% of survivors.[43,118,119] The effects of cranial radiation appear to be related to age and gender, with children younger than 5 years at the time of therapy and female patients being more susceptible. The precise mechanisms by which cranial radiation induces short stature are not clear. Disturbances in growth hormone production have not been found to correlate well with observed growth patterns in these patients.[31,120] The phenomenon of early onset of puberty in girls receiving cranial radiation may also play some role in the reduction of final height.[33,121] In childhood leukemia survivors not treated with cranial radiation, there are conflicting results regarding the impact of chemotherapy on final height.[122]

HORMONAL RATIONALE FOR OBESITY
An increased prevalence of obesity has been reported among survivors of childhood ALL.[123–125] Craig et al. investigated the relationship between cranial irradiation received during treatment for childhood leukemia and obesity.[126] Two hundred thirteen (86 boys and 127 girls) irradiated patients and 85 (37

boys and 48 girls) nonirradiated patients were enrolled. For cranially irradiated patients, an increase in the body mass index (BMI) Z score at the final height was associated with female sex and lower radiation dose but not with age at diagnosis. Severe obesity, defined as a BMI Z score greater than 3 at final height, was only present in girls who received 18 to 20 Gy irradiation at a prevalence of 8%. Both male and female nonirradiated patients had raised BMI Z scores at latest follow-up, and there was no association with age at diagnosis. The authors concluded that these data demonstrated a sexually dimorphic and dose-dependent effect of cranial irradiation on BMI. In a recent analysis from the Childhood Cancer Survivor Study, Oeffinger et al. compared the distribution of BMI of 1,765 adult survivors of childhood ALL with that of 2,565 adult siblings of childhood cancer survivors.[127] Survivors were significantly more likely to be overweight (BMI, 25–30) or obese (BMI, 30 or more). Risk factors for obesity were cranial radiation, female gender, and age from 0 to 4 years at diagnosis of leukemia. Girls diagnosed under the age of 4 years who received a cranial radiation dose greater than 20 Gy were found to have a 3·8-fold-increased risk of obesity.

GONADAL DYSFUNCTION

Treatment-related gonadal dysfunction has been well documented in both men and women following childhood malignancies.[128] However, survivors of leukemia and T-cell non-Hodgkin's lymphoma treated with modern conventional therapy are at a relatively low risk of infertility and delayed or impaired puberty. Treatment-related gonadal failure or dysfunction, expressed as amenorrhea or azoospermia, can lead to infertility in both male and female cancer survivors, and may have its onset during therapy.[129] Infertility can be transient, especially in men, and may recover over time after therapy. Reversibility is dependent on the dose of gonadal radiation or alkylating agents. Ovarian function is unlikely to recover long after the immediate treatment period because long-term amenorrhea commonly results from loss of ova. Cryopreservation of sperm before treatment is an option for men,[130] but limited means are available to preserve ova or protect against treatment-related ovarian failure for women.[131–133] A successful live birth after orthotopic autotransplantation of cryopreserved ovarian tissue has been recently reported.[134–137] A reasonable body of research on topics relating to the long-term gonadal effects of radiation and chemotherapy exists[138–161] and provides a basis for counseling patients and parents of the anticipated outcomes on pubertal development and fertility. For greater detail on this topic, please see Chapter 19.

Among survivors of adult cancer, the risk of premature onset of menopause in women treated with chemotherapeutic agents such as alkylating agents and procarbazine or with abdominal radiation therapy is age related, with women older than age 30 at the time of treatment having the greatest risk of treatment-induced amenorrhea and menopause, and sharply increased rates with chemotherapy around the age of 40 years. Tamoxifen has not been associated with the development of amenorrhea so far.[162] Cyclophosphamide at doses of 5 g/m² is likely to cause amenorrhea in women over 40, whereas many adolescents will continue to menstruate even after more than 20 g/m².[163] Although young women may not become amenorrheic after cytotoxic therapy, the risk of early

menopause is significant. Female disease-free survivors of cancer diagnosed at ages 13 to 19 who were menstruating at age 21 were at fourfold-higher risk of menopause compared to controls.[140]

FERTILITY AND PREGNANCY OUTCOMES

Fertility The fertility of survivors of childhood cancer, evaluated in the aggregate, is impaired. In one study, the adjusted relative fertility of survivors compared with that of their siblings was 0.85 [95% confidence interval (CI), 0.78, 0.92]. The adjusted relative fertility of male survivors (0.76; 95% CI, 0.68, 0.86) was slightly lower than that of female survivors (0.93; 95% CI, 0.83, 1.04). The most significant differences in the relative fertility rates were demonstrated in male survivors who had been treated with alkylating agents with or without infradiaphragmatic irradiation.[164]

Fertility can be impaired by factors other than the absence of sperm and ova. Conception requires delivery of sperm to the uterine cervix and patency of the fallopian tubes for fertilization to occur and appropriate conditions in the uterus for implantation. Retrograde ejaculation occurs with a significant frequency in men who undergo bilateral retroperitoneal lymph node dissection. Uterine structure may be affected by abdominal irradiation. Uterine length was significantly reduced in 10 women with ovarian failure who had been treated with whole-abdomen irradiation. Endometrial thickness did not increase in response to hormone replacement therapy in 3 women who underwent weekly ultrasound examination. No flow was detectable with Doppler ultrasound through either uterine artery of 5 women and through one uterine artery in 3 additional women.[165,166] Similarly, 4 of 8 women who received 1,440 cGy total-body irradiation had reduced uterine volume and undetectable uterine artery blood flow.[167] These data are pertinent when considering the feasibility of assisted reproduction for these survivors.

Pregnancy Most chemotherapeutic agents are mutagenic, with the potential to cause germ cell chromosomal injury. Possible results of such injury include an increase in the frequency of genetic diseases and congenital anomalies in the offspring of successfully treated childhood and adolescent cancer patients. Several early studies of the offspring of patients treated for diverse types of childhood cancer identified no effect of previous treatment on pregnancy outcome and no increase in the frequency of congenital anomalies in the offspring.[168–170] However, a study of offspring of patients treated for Wilm's tumor demonstrated that the birth weight of children born to women who had received abdominal irradiation was significantly lower than that of children born to women who had not received such irradiation,[171] a finding that was confirmed in several subsequent studies.[172–174] The abnormalities of uterine structure and blood flow reported after abdominal irradiation might explain this clinical finding.

Prior studies of offspring of childhood cancer survivors were limited by the size of the population of offspring and the number of former patients who had been exposed to mutagenic therapy. Several recent studies that attempted to address some of these limitations did not identify an increased frequency of major congenital malformations,[175–180] genetic disease, or childhood cancer[181,182] in the offspring of former pediatric cancer patients, including those conceived after bone marrow transplantation.[183] However, there are data suggesting a deficit of males in the offspring of the partners of male survivors in the Childhood Cancer Survivor Study cohort,[184] as well as an effect of prior treatment with doxorubicin or daunorubicin on the percentage of offspring with a birth weight less than 2,500 g born to female survivors in the Childhood Cancer Survivor Study who were treated with pelvic irradiation.[185]

Pulmonary Sequelae

The *acute* effects of chemotherapy on the lungs may be lethal, may subside over time, may progress insidiously to a level of clinical pulmonary dysfunction, or may be manifested by abnormal pulmonary function tests. Classically, high doses of bleomycin have been associated with pulmonary toxicity. However, drugs such as alkylating agents, methotrexate, and nitrosoureas may also lead to pulmonary fibrosis, especially when combined with radiation therapy. Radiation is thus an important contributor to pulmonary sequelae of chemotherapy.[186] Alkylating agents can injure the lung parenchyma, cause restrictive lung disease by inhibiting chest wall growth, and lead to thin anteroposterior chest diameters even 7 years after completion of therapy. Bleomycin may cause pulmonary insufficiency and interstitial pneumonitis.[187]

Pulmonary fibrosis can cause late death in the survivorship period. Among children treated for brain tumors with high doses of nitrosurea and radiotherapy, 35% died of pulmonary fibrosis, 12% within 3 years and 24% after a symptom-free period of 7 to 12 years.[188] The risk for overt decompensation continues for at least 1 year after cessation of therapy and can be precipitated by infection or exposure to intraoperative oxygen. In terms of long-term outcomes, a recent study noted that 22% of Hodgkin's disease patients with normal pulmonary function tests at the end of therapy (three cycles each of mechlorethamine (nitrogen mustard), vincristine, procarbazine, prednisone (MOPP) and adriamycin (doxovubicin), bleomycin, vinblastic, dacarbazine (ABVD) or two cycles of each plus 2,550 cGy of involved-field radiotherapy) developed abnormalities with follow-up of 1 to 7 years.

The long-term outcome of pulmonary toxicity is determined by factors such as the severity of the acute injury, the degree of tissue repair, and the level of compensation possible. Pulmonary dysfunction is usually subclinical and may be manifested by subconscious avoidance of exercise owing to symptoms. Premature respiratory insufficiency, especially with exertion, may also become evident with aging. Recent aggressive lung cancer treatment regimens consisting of surgery, radiation, and chemotherapy may well put patients at high risk for decreased pulmonary function and respiratory symptoms.

Genitourinary Tract

Several drugs such as cisplatin, methotrexate, and nitrosoureas have been associated with both acute and chronic toxicities such as glomerular and tubular injury.[189] Glomerular injury may recover over time whereas tubular injury generally persists. Hemodialysis to counteract the effects of chronic renal toxicity may be warranted for some patients. Ifosfamide may cause Fanconi's syndrome with glycosuria, phosphaturia, and aminoaciduria, and may affect glomerular

filtration. Hypophosphatemia may result in slow growth with possible bone deformity if untreated.

Radiation therapy may cause tubular damage and hypertension as a result of renal artery stenosis, especially in doses greater than 20 Gy, especially among children.[190] Radiation and chemotherapy may act synergistically, the dysfunction occurring with only 10 to 15 Gy.

The bladder is particularly susceptible to certain cytotoxic agents. Acrolein, a metabolic by-product of cyclophosphamide and ifosfamide, may cause hemorrhagic cystitis, fibrosis, and occasionally diminished bladder volume. An increased risk of developing bladder cancer also exists. Radiation may lead to bladder fibrosis, diminished capacity, and decreased contractility, the severity proportional to dose and area irradiated. The resultant scarring may diminish urethral and ureteric function.

Gastrointestinal/Hepatic

There are few studies describing long-term effects to this system, either due to underdetection or to a longer latency period than for other organs. Hepatic effects may result from the deleterious effects of many chemotherapeutic agents and radiotherapy. Transfusions may increase the risk of viral hepatitis. Hepatitis C has also been identified in increasing numbers of survivors, 119 of 2,620 tested. Of these patients, 24 of 56 who agreed to participate in a longitudinal study underwent liver biopsy. Chronic hepatitis was noted in 83%, fibrosis in 67%, and cirrhosis in 13%. Fibrosis and adhesions are known to occur after radiotherapy to the bowel.

Compromised Immune System

Hematologic and immunologic impairments can occur after either chemotherapy or radiation and are usually acute in nature. They are temporally related to the cancer treatment. Occasionally, persistent cytopenias may persist after pelvic radiation or in patients who have received extensive therapy with alkylating agents. Alkylating agents may cause myelodysplastic syndrome or leukemia as a late sequela. Immunologic impairment is seen as a long-term problem in Hodgkin's disease, relating to both the underlying disease and the treatments used. Hodgkin's disease patients are also at risk for serious bacterial infections if they have undergone splenectomy.

Peripheral Neuropathies

These effects are particularly common after taxol, vincristine, and cisplatin. However, despite the frequent use of such chemotherapeutic agents, few studies have characterized the nature and course of neuropathies associated with these drug regimens or dose levels.[191,192] Peripheral neuropathy may or may not resolve over time, and potential residual deficits are possible. Clinical manifestations include numbness and tingling in the hands and feet years after completion of cancer treatment.

Second Malignant Neoplasms and Recurrence

Second malignant neoplasms occur as result of an increased risk of second primary cancers associated with (a) the primary malignancy or (b) the iatrogenic effect of certain cancer therapies.[193–196] Examples include the development of breast cancer after Hodgkin's disease, ovarian cancer after primary breast cancer, and cancers associated with the HNPCC gene. Survivors of childhood cancer have an 8% to 10% risk of developing a second malignant neoplasm within 20 years of the primary diagnosis[197,198]; this is attributable to the mutagenic risk of both radiotherapy and chemotherapy.[199–213] This increased risk may be further potentiated in patients with genetic predispositions to malignancy.[214–220] The risk of secondary malignancy induced by cytotoxic agents is related to the cumulative dose of drug or radiotherapy (dose dependence). The risk of malignancy with normal aging results from the risk of cumulative cellular mutations. Compounding the normal aging process by exposure to mutagenic cytotoxic therapies results in an increased risk of secondary malignancy, particularly after radiotherapy, alkylating agents, and podophyllotoxins. Commonly cited secondary malignancies include (a) leukemia after alkylating agents and podophyllotoxins[221]; (b) solid tumors such as breast, bone, and thyroid cancer in the radiation fields in patients treated with radiotherapy[222]; (c) bladder cancer after cyclophosphamide; (d) a higher risk of contralateral breast cancer after primary breast cancer; and (e) ovarian cancer after breast cancer. Please refer to Chapter 17 for a detailed discussion of this significant issue.

Ancillary Sequelae

LYMPHEDEMA

Lymphedema can occur as a persistent or late effect of surgery and/or radiation treatment, and has been reported most commonly after breast cancer treatment, incidence rates ranging between 6% and 30%.[223] Lymphedema can occur in anyone with lymph node damage or obstruction to lymphatic drainage. Women undergoing axillary lymph node dissection and high-dose radiotherapy to the axilla for breast cancer are regarded as the highest risk group. Clinically, lymphedema symptoms may range from a feeling of fullness or heaviness in the affected limb to massive swelling and major functional impairment. Recommendations from the American Cancer Society conference on lymphedema in 1998 emphasize the need for additional research on prevention, monitoring, early intervention, and long-term treatment. Treatments suggested encompass multiple treatment modalities including skin care, massage, bandaging for compression, and exercise. Intermittent compression pumps were recommended only when used as an adjunct to manual approaches within a multidisciplinary treatment program, and routine use of medications such as diuretics, prophylactic antibiotics, bioflavinoids, and benzopyrones was discouraged in the absence of additional research. The impact of sentinel node biopsy in lieu of extensive axillary node dissection procedures for breast cancer on the incidence of lymphedema is not known at this time. A recent review by Erickson et al. found that arm edema was a common complication of breast cancer therapy, particularly when axillary dissection and axillary radiation therapy were used, and could result in substantial functional impairment and psychologic morbidity.[224] The authors note that although recommendations for "preventive" measures (e.g., avoidance of trauma) are anecdotally available, these measures have not been well studied. They found that nonpharmacologic treat-

ments, such as massage and exercise, have been shown to be effective therapies for lymphedema, but the effect of pharmacologic interventions remains uncertain.

FATIGUE

Fatigue has been reported as persistent side effect of treatment in many studies.[225–228] This is especially true among patients who have undergone bone marrow transplant.[229] Treatment-related fatigue may be associated with various factors such as anemia, infection, changes in hormonal levels, lack of physical activity, cytokine release, and sleep disorders.[230] The impact of exercise interventions on fatigue is a promising area of research. Fatigue is an important influence on quality of life for both the patient and the family and needs to be managed effectively.

SEXUALITY AND INTIMACY

Sexuality encompasses a spectrum of issues ranging from how one feels about one's body to the actual ability to function as a sexual being and has been reported as a persistent effect of treatment. In a recent study on breast, colon, lung, and prostate cancer survivors, issues related to sexual functioning were among the most persistent and severe problems reported. Preexisting sexual dysfunction may also be exacerbated by cancer and its treatment.[231] Please refer to Chapter 19 for further details.

Surgical and Radiation-Induced Toxicities

Surgical effects include increased risk of infections and physiologic comprise associated with nephrectomy (lifestyle changes to prevent trauma to remaining kidney), splenectomy (increased risk for sepsis resulting from encapsulated bacteria), and limb amputation.

Radiation therapy may especially exert effects on the musculoskeletal system and soft tissues among children and young adults, causing injury to the growth plates of long bones and muscle atrophy, osteonecrosis, and fractures.[2,5] Short stature can occur as a result of direct bone injury or pituitary radiation and resultant growth hormone deficiency. Chronic pain, the result of scarring and fibrosis in soft tissues surrounding the joints and large peripheral nerves, is a particularly distressing problem among patients who have received moderately high doses of radiation. Soft tissue sarcomas, skin cancers at previously irradiated sites, and pregnancy loss due to decreased uterine capacity in young girls after abdominal radiation are also possible.

Cancer Survivors, Healthcare Utilization, and Comorbid Conditions

Cancer survivors are high healthcare utilizers affecting distinct healthcare domains.[232,233] Data clearly show that cancer survivors are at greater risk for developing secondary cancers, late effects of cancer treatment, and chronic comorbid conditions. Exposures leading to these risks include cancer treatment, genetic predisposition and/or common lifestyle factors.[234–236] Although the threat of progressive or recurrent disease is at the forefront of health concerns for a cancer survivor, increased morbidity and decreased functional status and disability that result from cancer, its treatment, or health-related sequelae also are significant concerns. The impact of chronic comorbid conditions on cancer and its treatment is heightened more so among those diagnosed as adults and those who are elderly at the time of diagnosis.

Presented next is a brief overview of some factors potentiating the risk for chronic comorbid conditions among cancer survivors. A brief discussion of the major comorbid illnesses observed among survivors is also presented.

Metabolic Syndrome-Associated Diseases: Obesity, Diabetes, and Cardiovascular Disease

Obesity is a well-established risk factor for cancers of the breast (postmenopausal), colon, kidney (renal cell), esophagus (adenocarcinoma), and endometrium; thus, a large proportion of cancer patients are overweight or obese at the time of diagnosis.[237,238] Additional weight gain also can occur during or after active cancer treatment, an occurrence that has been frequently documented among individuals with breast cancer, but recently has been reported among testicular and gastrointestinal cancer patients as well.[239,240] Given data that obesity is associated with cancer recurrence in both breast and prostate cancer, and reduced quality of life among survivors, there is compelling evidence to support weight control efforts in this population.[14,15,241] Also, gradual weight loss has proven benefits in controlling hypertension, hyper-insulinemia, pain, and dyslipidemia and in improving levels of physical functioning, conditions that reportedly are significant problems in the survivor population.[14,15,21,242] Accordingly, the ACS Recommendations for Cancer Survivors list the "achievement of a healthy weight" as a primary goal.[14]

Obesity represents one of several metabolic disorders that are frequently manifest among cancer survivors, disorders that are grouped under the umbrella of "the metabolic syndrome" and include diabetes and cardiovascular disease (CVD). Insulin resistance is the underlying event associated with the metabolic syndrome, and either insulin resistance, co-occurring hyperinsulinemia, or diabetes have been reported as health concerns among cancer survivors.[243–245] As Brown and colleagues observed,[234] diabetes may play a significant role in the increased number of noncancer-related deaths among survivors; however, its role in progressive cancer is still speculative.

Although there is one study that suggests that older breast cancer patients derive a cardioprotective benefit from their diagnosis and/or associated treatments (most likely tamoxifen),[246] most reports indicate that CVD is a major health issue among survivors, evidenced by mortality data that show that half of noncancer-related deaths are attributed to CVD.[10] Risk is especially high among men with prostate cancer who receive hormone ablation therapy, as well as patients who receive adriamycin and radiation treatment to fields surrounding the heart.[247] Although more research is needed to explore the potential benefits of lifestyle interventions specifically within survivor populations, the promotion of a healthy weight via a low saturated fat diet with ample amounts of fruits and vegetables and moderate levels of physical activity is recommended.[14,15]

Osteoporosis

Osteoporosis and osteopenia are prevalent conditions in the general population, especially among women. Despite epidemiologic findings that increased bone density and low fracture risk are associated with increased risk for breast cancer,[248–256] clinical studies suggest that osteoporosis is still a prevalent health problem among survivors.[257–260] Data of Twiss et al.[258] indicate that 80% of older breast cancer patients have T-scores less than –1 and thus have clinically confirmed osteopenia at the time of their initial appointment. Other cancer populations, such as premenopausal breast and prostate cancer patients, may possess good skeletal integrity at the onset of their disease, but are at risk of developing osteopenia that may ensue with treatment-induced ovarian failure or androgen ablation.

Decreased Functional Status

Previous studies indicate that functional status is lowest immediately after treatment and tends to improve over time; however, the presence of pain and co-occurring diseases may affect this relationship.[261] In the older cancer survivor, regardless of duration following diagnosis, the presence of comorbidity, rather than the history of cancer per se, correlates with impaired functional status.[262] Cancer survivors have almost a twofold increase in having at least one functional limitation; however, in the presence of another comorbid condition, the odds ratio increases to 5.06 (95% CI, 4.47–5.72).[263] These findings have been confirmed by other studies in diverse populations of cancer survivors.[264–266] A cost analysis by Chirikos et al.[266] indicates that "the economic consequence of functional impairment exacts an enormous toll each year on cancer survivors, their families and the American economy at large."

Grading of Late Effects

The assessment and reporting of toxicity, based on the toxicity criteria system, plays a central role in oncology. Grading of late effects can provide valuable information for systematically monitoring the development and/or progression of late effects.[267] Although multiple systems have been developed for grading the adverse effects[4] of cancer treatment, there is, to date, no universally accepted grading system.[3] In contrast to the progress made in standardizing acute effects, the use of multiple late effects grading systems by different groups hinders the comparability of clinical trials, impedes the development of toxicity interventions, and encumbers the proper recognition and reporting of late effects. The wide adoption of a standardized criteria system can facilitate comparisons between institutions and across clinical trials.

---

[4]Any new finding or undesirable event that may or may not be attributed to treatment.

Some adverse events are clinical changes or health problems unrelated to the cancer diagnosis or its treatment.

A definitive assignment of attribution cannot always be rendered at the time of grading.

Multiple systems have been developed and have evolved substantially since being first introduced more than 20 years ago.[268] Garre et al. developed a set of criteria to grade late effects by degree of toxicity as follows: grade 0 (no late effect), grade 1 (asymptomatic changes not requiring any corrective measures, and not influencing general physical activity), grade 2 (moderate symptomatic changes interfering with activity), grade 3 (severe symptomatic changes that require major corrective measures and strict and prolonged surveillance), and grade 4 (life-threatening sequelae).[269] The SPOG (Swiss Pediatric Oncology Group) grading system has not been validated so far. It also ranges from 0 to 4: grade 0, no late effect; grade 1, asymptomatic patient requiring no therapy; grade 2, asymptomatic patient, requires continuous therapy, continuous medical follow-up, or symptomatic late effects resulting in reduced school, job, or psychosocial adjustment while remaining fully independent; grade 3, physical or mental sequelae not likely to be improved by therapy but able to work partially; and grade 4, severely handicapped, unable to work independently).[270]

The National Cancer Institute Common Toxicity Criteria (CTC) system was first developed in 1983. The most recent version, CTCAE v3.0 (Common Terminology Criteria for Adverse Events version 3.0) represents the first comprehensive, multimodality grading system for reporting *both* acute and late effects of cancer treatment. This new version requires changes in two areas: (1) application of adverse event criteria (e.g., new guidelines regarding late effects, surgical and pediatric effects, and issues relevant to the impact of multimodal therapies); and (2) reporting of the *duration* of an effect. This instrument carries the potential to facilitate the standardized reporting of adverse events and a comparison of outcomes between trials and institutions.

It is important to be aware that tools for grading late effects of cancer treatment are available, to validate them in larger populations, and to examine their utility in survivors of adult cancers. Oncologists, primary care physicians, and ancillary providers should be educated and trained to effectively monitor, evaluate, and optimize the health and well-being of a patient who has been treated for cancer. Additional research is needed to provide adequate knowledge about symptoms that persist following cancer treatment or those that arise as late effects, especially among survivors diagnosed as adults. Prospective studies that collect data on late effects will provide much needed information regarding the temporal sequence and timing of symptoms related to cancer treatment. It may be clinically relevant to differentiate between onset of symptoms during treatment, immediately posttreatment, or months later. Continued, systematic follow-up of survivors will result in information about the full spectrum of damage caused by cytotoxic and/or radiation therapy and possible interventions that may mitigate these adverse effects. We also need to examine the role of comorbidities on the risk for, and development of, late effects of cancer treatment among, especially, adult cancer survivors. Practice guidelines for follow-up care of cancer survivors and evaluation and management of late effects need to be developed so that effects can be mitigated when possible. Clearly, survivors can benefit from guidelines established for the primary prevention of secondary cancers as well as continued surveillance.[271,272]

Follow-Up Care for Late and Long-Term Effects

Optimal follow-up of survivors includes both ongoing monitoring and assessment of persistent and late effects of cancer treatment and the successful introduction of appropriate interventions to ameliorate these sequelae. The achievement of this goal is challenging, and inherent in that challenge is the recognition of the importance of preventing premature mortality from the disease and/or its treatment and the prevention or early detection of both the physiologic and psychologic sources of morbidity. The prevention of late effects, second cancers, and recurrences of the primary disease requires watchful follow up and optimal utilization of early detection screening techniques. Physical symptom management is as important in survivorship as it is during treatment, and effective symptom management during treatment may prevent or lessen lasting effects.

Regular monitoring of health status after cancer treatment is recommended, because this should (1) permit the timely diagnosis and treatment of long-term complications of cancer treatment; (2) provide the opportunity to institute preventive strategies such as diet modification, tobacco cessation, and other lifestyle changes; (3) facilitate screening for, and early detection of, a second cancer; (4) timely diagnosis and treatment of recurrent cancer; and (5) the detection of functional or physical or psychologic disability.

There has been no consensus on overall recommendations for routine follow-up after cancer therapy for *all* cancer survivors. A recent review by Kattlove and Winn can help guide oncologists in providing quality continuing care for their patients—care that spans a broad spectrum of medical areas ranging from surveillance to genetic susceptibility.[273] Health promotion is a key concern of patients once acute management of their disease is complete. Increasingly, cancer survivors are looking to their oncology care providers for counsel and guidance with respect to lifestyle change that will improve their prospects of a healthier life and possibly a longer one as well. Although complete data regarding lifestyle change among cancer survivors have yet to be determined, and there remains an unmet need for behavioral interventions with proven efficacy in various cancer populations,[274] the oncologist can nonetheless make use of extant data to inform practice and also should be attentive to new developments in the field.

Follow-up care and monitoring for late effects is usually done more systematically and rigorously for survivors of childhood cancer while they continue to be part of the program or clinic where they were treated. The monitoring of adult cancer sites for the development of late effects, particularly outside the oncology practice, is neither thorough nor systematic. It is important that survivors of both adult and childhood cancers be monitored for the late and long-term effects or treatment, as discussed in preceding sections, at regular intervals.

It is now recognized that cancer survivors may experience various late physical and psychologic sequelae of treatment and that many healthcare providers may be unaware of actual or potential survivor problems.[275] Until recently, there were no clearly defined, easily accessible risk-based guidelines for cancer survivor follow-up care. Such clinical practice guidelines can serve as a guide for doctors, outline appropriate methods of treatment and care, and address specific clinical situations (disease-oriented) or use of approved medical products, procedures, or tests (modality-oriented). In response to this growing mandate, the Children's Oncology Group has now developed and published its guidelines for long-term follow-up for Survivors of Childhood, Adolescent, and Young Adult Cancers.[275] These risk-based, exposure-related clinical practice guidelines are intended to promote earlier detection of and intervention for complications that may potentially arise as a result of treatment for pediatric malignancies, and are both evidence based (utilizing established associations between therapeutic exposures and late effects to identify high-risk categories) and grounded in the collective clinical experience of experts (matching the magnitude of risk with the intensity of screening recommendations). Importantly, they are intended for use beginning 2 or more years following the completion of cancer therapy and are not intended to provide guidance for follow-up of the survivor's primary disease.

Of great significance to survivors of adult cancer, using the best available evidence, the American Society of Clinical Oncology (ASCO) expert panels have also identified and developed practice recommendations for posttreatment follow-up of specific cancer sites (breast and colorectal; source: www.asco.org). In addition, ASCO has also created an expert panel tasked with the development of follow-up care guidelines geared toward the prevention or early detection of late effects among survivors diagnosed and treated as adults.

To facilitate optimal follow-up during the posttreatment phase, the patient's age at diagnosis, side effects of treatment reported or observed during treatment, calculated cumulative doses of drugs or radiation, and an overview of late effects most likely for a given patient given the treatment history should be summarized and kept on file. A copy of this summary should be provided to the patient or to the parent of a child who has undergone treatment for cancer. The importance of conveying this detailed treatment history to primary care providers should be clearly communicated, especially if follow-up will occur in the primary/family care setting. Finally, screening tests that may help detect subclinical effects that could become clinically relevant in the future should be listed.

Recommendations for regular, ongoing follow-up of cancer survivors are summarized in Table 6.2. For the prevention or early detection of second malignant neoplasms occurring as a late effect of treatment, providers should remain ever vigilant for the possibility. A detailed history and physical examination is always appropriate, in conjunction with screening at age-appropriate intervals or as outlined by consensus panel recommendations.

Physicians, caregivers, and the family must be able to hear and observe what the patient is trying to communicate, reduce fear and anxiety, counter feelings of isolation, correct misconceptions, and obtain appropriate symptom relief. Practitioners inheriting care for child or adult survivors need to understand the effects of cytotoxic therapies on the growing child or the adult at varying stages/ages of life and be knowledgeable about interventions that may mitigate the effects of these treatments.

Patient education should guide lifestyle and choices for follow-up care, promote adaptation to the disease or relevant sequelae, and help the patient reach an optimal level of wellness and functioning, both physical and psychologic, within the context of the disease and treatment effects.

Research Implications of Long-Term and Late Effects of Cancer

Cancer survivorship research continues to provide us with a growing body of evidence regarding the unique and uncharted consequences of cancer and its treatment among those diagnosed with this disease. It is becoming an acknowledged fact that most cancer treatment options available and in use today will affect the future health and life of those diagnosed with this disease. Adverse cancer treatment-related sequelae thus carry the potential to contribute to the ongoing burden of illness, health care costs, and decreased length and quality of survival.

Data and results from ongoing survivorship studies, examining outcomes among both adult and pediatric cancer survivors, are continuing to demonstrate that (a) there may be long latencies for potentially life-threatening late effects (e.g., cardiac failure secondary to the cardiotoxic effects of cancer treatment); (b) both late and chronic toxicities (e.g., fatigue, sexual dysfunction, cognitive impairment, neuropathies) are persistent, worsen over time, and carry significant potential to adversely affect the health and well being of survivors; (c) early interventions may hold the promise of reducing adverse outcomes; and (d) there may be a continued need for extended follow-up of survivors to prevent, detect early, control, or manage adverse sequelae of cancer or its treatment.

Among childhood cancer survivors, residual endocrine disorders have been shown to be as high as 40%.[276] A recent study found the cumulative frequency of congestive heart failure to be 17.4% at 20 years after diagnosis[277, (5)] and that risk factors such as female gender, higher cumulative doxorubicin doses, and lung and left abdominal irradiation increased the likelihood of heart failure in this population, variables that may affect practice in terms of initial cancer treatment, recommendations for posttreatment follow-up care, and interventions (behavioral, medical, or pharmacologic) to decrease future risk. Others have reported that there may be an increased risk of fetal malposition and premature labor among girls who received flank radiation therapy as part of their treatment for Wilm's tumor, and, among their offspring, an elevated risk for low birth weight, premature birth (less than 36 weeks gestation), and congenital malformations. These risks carry distinct implications for the obstetrical management of female survivors of Wilm's tumor.[278] Finally, data continue to show that survivors of acute lymphoblastic leukemia are at significant risk of being overweight or obese when compared to sibling controls.[125] Because premature coronary artery disease has been reported in this population, these findings underscore the importance of lifestyle and health promotion interventions.

Studies have also begun to demonstrate the deleterious impact of cancer treatment among those diagnosed with this disease as adults. Even after adjustment for age, baseline functional health status, and multiple covariates, long-term breast

---

(5)Among survivors of Wilm's tumor treated with doxorubicin.

TABLE 6.2. Follow-up care and surveillance for late effects.

Follow-up visit	Content of clinic visit	Suggested evaluative procedures and ancillary actions
Chemotherapy treatment cessation visit	1. Review complete treatment history 2. Calculate cumulative dosages of drugs 3. Document regimen(s) administered 4. Radiation ports, dosage, machine 5. Document patient age at diagnosis/treatment 6. Side effects during treatment 7. Identify likely late effects 8. Baseline "grading" of late effects (Garre or SPOG)	Develop late effect risk profile Summarize all information in previous column Provide copy to patient (or parent if minor child) Instruct that this summary should be provided to primary care or other healthcare providers Keep copy of summary in patient chart
General measures at every visit	1. Detailed history 2. Complete physical examination 3. Review systems 4. Meds, maintenance, prophylactic antibiotics 5. Education: GPA, school performance 6. Employment history 7. Menstrual status/cycle 8. Libido, sexual activity 9. Pregnancy and outcome	Evaluate symptomatology, patient reports of issues Review any intercurrent illnesses Evaluate for disease recurrence, second neoplasms Systematic evaluation of long-term (persistent) and late effects (see specific measures) Grade long-term and late effects: Garre or SPOG criteria CBC; urinalysis; other tests depending on exposure history and late effect risk profile
Specific measures to evaluate late effects Relevance differs by: 1. Age at diagnosis/treatment 2. Specific drugs, regimens 3. Combinations of treatment modalities 4. Dosages administered 5. Expected toxicities (based on mechanics of action of cytotoxic drugs (cell-cycle-dependent; proliferation kinetics) 6. Exceptions occur to the theoretical assumption that least susceptible organs/tissues are those that replicate slowly or not at all (vinca, methotrexate, adriamycin) 7. Combinations of radiation/chemotherapy more often associated with late effects	Growth: includes issues such as short stature, scoliosis, hypoplasia Cardiac Neurocognitive Neuropathy Gonadal toxicity Pulmonary Urinary Thyroid Weight history Lymphedema Fatigue Surgical toxicity Gastrointestinal/hepatic	Monitor growth (growth curve); sitting height, parental heights, nutritional status/diet, evaluate scoliosis, bone age, growth hormone assays, thyroid function, endocrinologist consult; orthopedic consult EKG, echo, afterload reduction, cardiologist consult Counsel against isometric exercises if high risk, advise ob/gyn risk of cardiac failure in pregnancy History and exam Communicate: school, family, special education Compensatory remediation techniques Neuropsychology consult; CT or MRI; CSF; basic myelin protein Written instructions, appointment cards History/exam: neurologic exam, sensory changes hands/feet, paresthesias, bladder, gait, vision, muscle strength Neurologist consult History for primary vs. secondary dysfunction, gonadal function (menstrual cycle, pubertal development/delay, libido); hormone therapy; interventions (bromocriptine) Premature menopause: hormone replacement unless contraindicated; DXA scans for osteoporosis; calcium Endocrinologist consult Reproductive technologies Chest X-ray; pulmonary function tests; pulmonologist consultation Urinalysis; BUN/creatinine; urologist if hematuria Annual TSH; thyroid hormone replacement; endocrinologist Evaluate dietary intake (food diary)/physical activity Nutritionist and/or endocrinologist consult History/exam: swelling, sensations of heaviness/fullness Rule out hypothyroidism; anemia, cardiac/pulmonary sequelae; evaluate sleep habits Evaluate physical fitness and activity levels Regular physical activity unless contraindicated Antibiotic prophylaxis (splenectomy) Liver function, hepatitis screen, gastroenterologist consult
Screening for second malignant neoplasms	Screening guidelines differ by age Oncologist consult	Follow guidelines for age-appropriate cancer screening (mammogram, Pap smear, FOBT/flexible sigmoidoscopy) Mammogram at age 30 if history of mantle radiation for Hodgkins Screen for associated cancers in HNPCC family syndrome Screen for ovarian cancer if history of breast cancer and BRCAI II.
Assess/manage comorbidities	Osteoporosis; heart disease; arthritis, etc.	History/exam; be cognizant of risk; appropriate consult

Evaluations are suggestions only. Relevance will differ by treatment history and late effect risk profile.

Source: Data from Aziz (2002, 2003).[2,6]

cancer survivors are more likely to experience persistent significant declines in *physical* health status when compared to cancer-free controls, with younger or socially isolated survivors faring worse than those middle-aged or older in both physical and psychosocial dimensions.[279] These findings have been substantiated by another recent study where breast cancer survivors were found to be at significantly higher risk of physical declines in health status compared to age-matched controls.[280]

Outcomes of cancer and its treatment may be even more complex among medically underserved or ethnoculturally diverse populations. It has been reported that African-American survivors experience poorer functional health and consistently higher levels of comorbidities, decreased physical functioning, and general health vulnerability after cancer diagnosis and treatment compared to age-matched Caucasian patients.[281] From an economic standpoint, survivors working at the time of diagnosis may experience a significant reduction in annual market earnings,[6] the adverse economic impact being worse among survivors with the greatest declines in health status.[282] Long reported as a late effect among pediatric survivors, the adverse neurocognitive impact of cancer treatment is now increasingly reported as a potentially devastating outcome among adult survivors. Breast and lymphoma survivors exposed to systemic chemotherapy are at increased risk for neurocognitive deficits affecting memory, concentration, and attention. Diffuse white and gray matter changes have been reported in magnetic resonance imaging studies, and early data indicate that APOEe4 may be a potential genetic marker for risk.[283,284] Sexual dysfunction continues to be a persistent finding among both men and women years after cancer treatment.[285,286] Finally, the extent to which women's daily living is affected by lymphedema is not recognized routinely by healthcare providers even today.[287]

There are promising findings from intervention studies among both adult and childhood cancer survivors. Daily consumption of aspirin may result in a significant reduction in relative risk of death from breast cancer.[7] Dexrazoxane (DEXRA or Zinecard) administered during active treatment may prevent or reduce acute cardiac injury associated with doxorubicin therapy.[288,289] Methylphenidate (Ritalin) may provide at least a short-term benefit in childhood cancer survivors who experience clinically significant learning problems and deficits in attention and memory.[290]

Home-based educational interventions can help to improve cancer knowledge, self-efficacy (coping), and awareness of resources among both white and African-American breast cancer survivors.[291]

Self-reported depression burden may significantly influence the severity and number of side effects experienced by breast cancer survivors, and self-help interventions may reduce fatigue, pain, and nausea burden in women with breast cancer.[292] Last but not least, cognitive-behavioral stress management interventions may successfully reduce the prevalence of moderate depression and increase generalized optimism and positive reframing, lending support to the importance of examining positive responses to traumatic events.[293]

Thus, research that examines the effects of cancer and its treatment among individuals diagnosed with the disease and their family members is critical if we are to help patients make decisions about treatment options that could affect their future. Cancer survivorship research carries the potential to enable providers of care to tailor therapies to maximize cure while minimizing adverse treatment-related effects. The development and dissemination of evidence-based interventions may help us to reduce cancer morbidity as well as mortality and facilitate adaptation among cancer survivors. Finally, knowledge gained from survivorship research could help improve quality of care, control costs, and equip the next generation of physicians, nurses, and other healthcare professionals to provide not just the science but also the art of comprehensive cancer medicine.

Conclusions

A large and growing community of cancer survivors is one of the major achievements of cancer research during the past three decades. Both length and quality of survival are important endpoints. Many cancer survivors are at risk for, and develop, physiologic late effects of cancer treatment that may lead to premature mortality and morbidity. As in the past when treatments were modified to decrease the chance of developing toxicities among survivors of childhood cancer, the goal of future research and treatment should also be to evaluate late effects systematically and further modify toxicities without diminishing cures. Interventions and treatments that can ameliorate or manage effectively both persistent and late physical effects of treatment should be developed and promoted for use in this population. Oncologists, primary care physicians, and ancillary providers should be educated and trained to effectively monitor, evaluate, and optimize the health and well-being of a patient who has been treated for cancer.

Additional research is needed to provide adequate knowledge about symptoms that persist following cancer treatment or those that arise as late effects. Prospective studies that collect data on late effects prospectively are needed as most of the literature on late effects is derived from cross-sectional studies in which it is not clear if the symptom began during treatment or immediately after treatment. Continued, systematic follow-up of survivors will provide information about the full spectrum of damage caused by cytotoxic or radiation therapy and possible interventions that may mitigate the effects. Interventions, therapeutic or lifestyle, that can treat or ameliorate these late effects need to be developed. Practice guidelines for follow-up care of cancer survivors and evaluation and management of late effects need to be developed so that effects can be mitigated when possible.

Our knowledge about the late effects of cancer treatment, in large part, comes from studies conducted among survivors of pediatric cancer. We need to explore further the impact cancer treatment on late effects in survivors diagnosed as adults. We also need to examine the role of comorbidities on the risk for, and development of, late effects of cancer treatment among these adult cancer survivors.

---

[6]Compared to age-matched cancer free controls.
[7]Holmes MA. Personal communication.

Although there has been considerable research on the late outcomes among survivors of cancer, future research must be directed toward identification of risks associated with more-recent treatment regimens, as well as the very late occurring outcomes resulting from treatment protocols utilized three or more decades ago. As treatment- and patient-related factors impact the subsequent risk of late-occurring adverse outcomes, clear delineation of those survivors who are at high risk of specific adverse outcomes is essential for the rational design of follow-up guidelines, prevention, and intervention strategies.

Each person with cancer has unique needs based on the extent of the disease, effects of treatment, prior health, functional level, coping skills, support systems, and many other influences. This complexity requires an interdisciplinary approach by all health professionals that is organized, systematic, and geared toward the provision of high-quality care. This ambience may facilitate the adaptation of cancer survivors to temporary or permanent sequelae of the disease and its treatment.

References

1. American Cancer Society. Cancer Facts and Figures, 2003. Atlanta, GA: American Cancer Society, 2004.
2. Aziz N, Rowland J. Trends and advances in cancer survivorship research: challenge and opportunity. Semin Radiat Oncol 2003; 13:248–266.
3. Jemal A, Clegg LX, Ward E, et al. Annual report to the nation on the status of cancer, 1875–2001, with a special feature regarding survival. Cancer (Phila) 2004;101:3–27.
4. Rowland J, Mariotto A, Aziz N, et al. Cancer survivorship—United States, 1971–2001. MMWR 2004;53:526–529.
5. Ries LAG, Smith MA, Gurney JG, et al. (eds). Cancer incidence and survival among children and adolescents: United States SEER program 1975–1995. NIH Publication 99–4649. Bethesda, MD: National Cancer Institute, 1996.
6. Aziz NM. Long-term survivorship: late effects. In: Berger AM, Portenoy RK, Weissman DE (eds). Principles and Practice of Palliative Care and Supportive Oncology, 2nd ed. Philadelphia: Lippincott Williams & Wilkins, 2002:1019–1033.
7. Chu KC, Tarone RE, Kessler LG. Recent trends in U.S. breast cancer incidence, survival, and mortality rates. J Natl Cancer Inst 1996;88:1571–1579.
8. McKean RC, Feigelson HS, Ross RK. Declining cancer rates in the 1990s. J Clin Oncol 2000;18:2258–2268.
9. Ries LAG, Wing PA, Miller DS. The annual report to the nation on the status of cancer, 1973–1997, with a special section on colorectal cancer. Cancer (Phila) 2000;88:2398–2424.
10. Shusterman S, Meadows AT. Long term survivors of childhood leukemia. Curr Opin Hematol 2000;7:217–220.
11. Demark-Wahnefried W, Peterson B, McBride C. Current health behaviors and readiness to pursue life-style changes among men and women diagnosed with early stage prostate and breast carcinomas. Cancer (Phila) 2000;88:674–684.
12. Ganz PA. Late effects of cancer and its treatment. Semin Oncol Nurs 2001;17(4):241–248.
13. Ganz PA. Cancer Survivors: Physiologic and Psychosocial Outcomes. Alexandria, VA: American Society of Clinical Oncology, 1998:118–123.
14. Schwartz CL. Long-term survivors of childhood cancer: the late effects of therapy. Oncologist 1999;4:45–54.
15. Brown ML, Fintor L. The economic burden of cancer. In: Greenwald P, Kramer BS, Weed DL (eds). Cancer Prevention and Control. New York: Dekker, 1995:69–81.
16. Sklar CA. Overview of the effects of cancer therapies: the nature, scale and breadth of the problem. Acta Paediatr (Suppl) 1999;88: 1–4.
17. Mullan F. Seasons of survival: reflections of a physician with cancer. N Engl J Med 1995;313:270–273.
18. Loescher LJ, Welch-McCaffrey D, Leigh SA. Surviving adult cancers. Part 1: Physiologic effects. Ann Intern Med 1989;111: 411–432.
19. Welch-McCaffrey D, Hoffman B, Leigh SA. Surviving adult cancers. Part 2: Psychosocial implications. Ann Intern Med 1989;111:517–524.
20. Herold AH, Roetzheim RG. Cancer survivors. Primary Care 1992;19:779–791.
21. Marina N. Long-term survivors of childhood cancer. The medical consequences of cure. Pediatr Clin N Am 1997;44: 1021–1041.
22. Green DM. Late effects of treatment for cancer during childhood and adolescence. Curr Probl Cancer 2003;27(3):127–142.
23. Mertens AC, Yasui Y, Neglia JP, et al. Late mortality experience in five-year survivors of childhood and adolescent cancer: The Childhood Cancer Survivor Study. J Clin Oncol 2001;19: 3163–3172.
24. Robison LL, Bhatia S. Review: Late-effects among survivors of leukaemia and lymphoma during childhood and adolescence. Br J Haematol 2003;122:345–356.
25. Boulad F, Sands S, Sklar C. Late complications after bone marrow transplantation in children and adolescents. Curr Probl Pediatr 1998;28:273–304.
26. Bhatia S, Landier W, Robison LL. Late effects of childhood cancer therapy. In: DeVita VT, Hellman S, Rosenberg SA (eds). Progress in Oncology. Sudbury: Jones and Bartlett, 2002:171–213.
27. Dreyer ZE, Blatt J, Bleyer A. Late effects of childhood cancer and its treatment. In: Pizzo PA, Poplack DG (eds). Principles and Practice of Pediatric Oncology, 4th ed. Philadelphia: Lippincott, Williams & Wilkins, 2002:1431–1461.
28. Hudson M. Late complications after leukemia therapy. In: Pui CG (ed). Childhood Leukemias. Cambridge: Cambridge University Press, 1991:463–481.
29. Blatt J, Copeland DR, Bleyer WA. Late effects of childhood cancer and its treatment. In: Pizzo PA, Poplack DG (eds). Principles and Practice of Pediatric Oncology, revised ed. Philadelphia: Lippincott, 1997:1091–1114.
30. Kirk JA, Raghupathy P, Stevens MM, et al. Growth failure and growth-hormone deficiency after treatment for acute lymphoblastic leukemia. Lancet 1987;1:190–193.
31. Blatt J, Bercu BB, Gillin JC, et al. Reduced pulsatile growth hormone secretion in children after therapy for acute lymphoblastic leukemia. J Pediatr 1984;104:182–186.
32. Silber JH, Littman PS, Meadows AT. Stature loss following skeletal irradiation for childhood cancer. J Clin Oncol 1990; 8:304–312.
33. Leiper AD, Stanhope R, Preese MA, et al. Precocious or early puberty and growth failure in girls treated for acute lymphoblastic leukemia. Horm Res 1988;30:72–76.
34. Ogilvy-Stuart AL, Clayton PE, Shalet SM. Cranial irradiation and early puberty. J Clin Endocrinol Metab 1994;78:1282–1286.
35. Furst CJ, Lundell M, Ahlback SO. Breast hypoplasia following irradiation of the female breast in infancy and early childhood. Acta Oncol 1989;28(4):519–523.
36. Meyers CA, Weitzner MA. Neurobehavioral functioning and quality of life in patients treated for cancer of the central nervous system. Curr Opin Oncol 1995;7:197–200.
37. Haupt R, Fears TR, Robeson LL, et al. Educational attainment in long-term survivors of childhood acute lymphoblastic leukemia. JAMA 1994;272:1427–1432.
38. Stehbens JA, Kaleih TA, Noll RB, et al. CNS prophylaxis of childhood leukemia: what are the long-term neurological,

neuropsychological and behavioral effects? Neuropsychol Rev 1991;2:147–176.

39. Ochs J, Mulhern RK, Faircough D et al. Comparison of neuropsychologic function and clinical indicators of neurotoxicity in long-term survivors of childhood leukemia given cranial irradiation or parenteral methotrexate: a prospective study. J Clin Oncol 1991;9:145–151.

40. Ash P. The influence of radiation on fertility in man. Br J Radiol 1990;53:155–158.

41. Didi M, Didcock E, Davies HA, et al. High incidence of obesity in young adults after treatment of acute lymphoblastic leukemia in childhood. J Pediatr 1995;127:63–67.

42. Oberfield SE, Soranno D, Nirenberg A, et al. Age at onset of puberty following high-dose central nervous system radiation therapy. Arch Pediat Adolesc Med 1996;150:589–592.

43. Sklar C, Mertens A, Walter A, et al. Final height after treatment for childhood acute lymphoblastic leukemia: comparison of no cranial irradiation with 1,800 and 2,400 centigrays of cranial irradiation. J Pediatr 1993;123:59–64.

44. Greendale GA, Petersen L, Zibecchi L, Ganz PA. Factors related to sexual function in postmenopausal women with a history of breast cancer. Menopause 2001;8:111–119.

45. Ganz PA, Greendale GA, Petersen L, Zibecchi L, Kahn B, Belin TR. Managing menopausal symptoms in breast cancer survivors: results of a randomized controlled trial. J Natl Cancer Inst 2000;5:1054–1064.

46. Yancik R, Ganz PA, Varricchio CG, Conley B. Perspectives on comorbidity and cancer in older patients: approaches to expand the knowledge base. J Clin Oncol 2001;19:1147–1151.

47. Lipshultz SE, Colan SD, Gelber RD, et al. Late cardiac effects of doxorubicin therapy for acute lymphoblastic leukemia in childhood. N Engl J Med 1991;324:808–814.

48. Bu'Lock FA, Mott MG, Oakhill A, et al. Left ventricular diastolic function after anthracycline chemotherapy in childhood: relation with systolic function, symptoms and pathophysiology. Br Heart J 1995;73:340–350.

49. Goorin AM, Borow KM, Goldman A, et al. Congestive heart failure due to adriamycin cardiotoxicity: its natural history in children. Cancer (Phila) 1981;47:2810–2816.

50. Steinherz LJ, Steinherz PG. Cardiac failure and dysrhythmias 6–19 years after anthracycline therapy: a series of 15 patients. Med Pediatr Oncol 1995;24:352–361.

51. Adams MJ, Lipsitz SR, Colan SD, et al. Cardiovascular status in long-term survivors of Hodgkin's disease treated with chest radiotherapy. J Clin Oncol 2004;22(15):3139–3148.

52. Kremer LCM, van Dalen EC, Offringa M, Otenkamp J, Voute PA. Anthracycline-induced clinical heart failure in a cohort of 607 children: long-term follow-up study. J Clin Oncol 2001;19:191–196.

53. Sorensen K, Levitt G, Chessells J, Sullivan I. Anthracycline dose in childhood acute lymphoblastic leukemia: issues of early survival versus late cardiotoxicity. J Clin Oncol 1997;15:61–68.

54. Kremer LCM, van Dalen EC, Offringa M, Voute PA. Frequency and risk factors of anthracycline-induced clinical heart failure in children: a systematic review. Ann Oncol 2002;13:503–512.

55. Steinherz LJ, Steinherz PG, Tan CT, Heller G, Murphy ML. Cardiac toxicity 4–20 years after completing anthracycline therapy. JAMA 1991;266:1672–1677.

56. Kremer LCM, van der Pal HJH, Offringa M, van Dalen EC, Voute PA. Frequency and risk factors of subclinical cardiotoxicity after anthracycline therapy in children: a systematic review. Ann Oncol 2002;13:819–829.

57. Hancock SL, Tucker MA, Hoppe RT. Factors affecting late mortality from heart disease after treatment of Hodgkin's disease. JAMA 1993;270:1949–1955.

58. Hancock SL, Donaldson SS, Hoppe RT. Cardiac disease following treatment of Hodgkin's disease in children and adolescents. J Clin Oncol 1993;11:1199–1203.

59. Fajardo L, Stewart J, Cohn K. Morphology of radiation-induced heart disease. Arch Pathol 1968;86:512–519.

60. Minow RA, Benjamin RS, Gottlieb JA. Adriamycin (NSC-123127) cardiomyopathy: an overview with determination of risk factors. Cancer Chemother Rep 1975;6:195–201.

61. Prout MN, Richards MJ, Chung KJ, Joo P, Davis HL Jr. Adriamycin cardiotoxicity in children: case reports, literature review, and risk factors. Cancer (Phila) 1977;39:62–65.

62. Von Hoff DD, Layard MW, Basa P, et al. Risk factors for doxorubicin-induced congestive heart failure. Ann Intern Med 1979;91:710–717.

63. Kushner JP, Hansen VL, Hammar SP. Cardiomyopathy after widely separated courses of adriamycin exacerbated by actinomycin-D and mithramycin. Cancer (Phila) 1975;36:1577–1584.

64. Von Hoff DD, Rozencweig M, Piccart M. The cardiotoxicity of anticancer agents. Semin Oncol 1982;9:23–33.

65. Lipshultz SE, Lipsitz SR, Mone SM, et al. Female sex and drug dose as risk factors for late cardiotoxic effects of doxorubicin therapy for childhood cancer. N Engl J Med 1995;332:1738–1743.

66. Pratt CB, Ransom JL, Evans WE. Age-related adriamycin cardiotoxicity in children. Cancer Treat Rep 1978;62:1381–1385.

67. Pai VB, Nahata MC. Cardiotoxicity of chemotherapeutic agents: incidence, treatment and prevention. Drug Saf 2000;22:263–302.

68. Legha SS, Benjamin RS, Mackay B, et al. Reduction of doxorubicin cardiotoxicity by prolonged continuous intravenous infusion. Ann Intern Med 1982;96:133–139.

69. Lipshultz SE, Giantris AL, Lipsitz SR, et al. Doxorubicin administration by continuous infusion is not cardioprotective: the Dana-Farber 91-01 Acute Lymphoblastic Leukemia Protocol. J Clin Oncol 2002;20:1677–1682.

70. Marks RD Jr, Agarwal SK, Constable WC. Radiation induced pericarditis in Hodgkin's disease. Acta Radiol Ther Phys Biol 1973;12:305–312.

71. Martin RG, Ruckdeschel JC, Chang P, Byhardt R, Bouchard RJ, Wiernik PH. Radiation-related pericarditis. Am J Cardiol 1975;35:216–220.

72. Ruckdeschel JC, Chang P, Martin RG, et al. Radiation-related pericardial effusions in patients with Hodgkin's disease. Medicine (Baltim) 1975;54:245–259.

73. Perrault DJ, Levy M, Herman JD, et al. Echocardiographic abnormalities following cardiac radiation. J Clin Oncol 1985;3:546–551.

74. Kadota RP, Burgert EO Jr, Driscoll DJ, Evans RG, Gilchrist GS. Cardiopulmonary function in long-term survivors of childhood Hodgkin's lymphoma: a pilot study. Mayo Clin Proc 1988;63:362–367.

75. Wexler LH. Ameliorating anthracycline cardiotoxicity in children with cancer: clinical trials with dexrazoxane. Semin Oncol 1998;25:86–92.

76. Lipshultz SE, Rifai N, Dalton VM, et al. The effect of dexrazoxane on myocardial injury in doxorubicin-treated children with acute lymphoblastic leukemia. N Engl J Med 2004;351(2):145–153.

77. Gluck S. The expanding role of epirubicin in the treatment of breast cancer. Cancer Control 2002;9(suppl 2):16–27.

78. Baker AF, Dorr RT. Drug interactions with the taxanes: clinical implications. Cancer Treat Rev 2001;27(4):221–233.

79. Sessa C, Perotti A, Salvatorelli E, et al. Phase IB and pharmacological study of the novel taxane BMS-184476 in combination with doxorubicin. Eur J Cancer 2004;40(4):563–570.

80. Jones RL, Smith IE. Efficacy and safety of trastuzumab. Expert Opin Drug Saf 2004;3(4):317–327.

81. Schneider JW, Chang AY, Garratt A. Trastuzumab cardiotoxicity: speculations regarding pathophysiology and targets for further study. Semin Oncol 2002;29(3 suppl 11):22–28.

82. Schneider JW, Chang AY, Rocco TP. Cardiotoxicity in signal transduction therapeutics: erbB2 antibodies and the heart. Semin Oncol 2001;28:18–26.

83. Meadows AT, Gordon J, Massari DJ, Littman P, Fergusson J, Moss K. Declines in IQ scores and cognitive dysfunctions in children with acute lymphocytic leukaemia treated with cranial irradiation. Lancet 1981;2:1015–1018.

84. Jankovic M, Brouwers P, Valsecchi MG, et al. Association of 1800 cGy cranial irradiation with intellectual function in children with acute lymphoblastic leukaemia. ISPACC. International Study Group on Psychosocial Aspects of Childhood Cancer. Lancet 1994;344:224–227.

85. Hertzberg H, Huk WJ, Ueberall MA, et al. CNS late effects after ALL therapy in childhood. Part I. Neuroradiological findings in long-term survivors of childhood ALL: an evaluation of the interferences between morphology and neuropsychological performance. The German Late Effects Working Group. Medical and Pediatric Oncology, 1997;28:387–400.

86. Green DM, Zevon MA, Rock KM, Chavez F. Fatigue after treatment for Hodgkin's disease during childhood or adolescence. Proc Am Soc Clin Oncol 2002;21:396a.

87. Price R. Therapy-related central nervous system diseases in children with acute lymphocytic leukemia. In: Mastrangelo R, Poplack DG, Riccardi R (eds). Central Nervous System Leukemia: Prevention and Treatment. Boston: Martinus-Nijhoff, 1983:71–83.

88. Peylan-Ramu N, Poplack DG, Pizzo PA, Adornato BT, Di Chiro G. Abnormal CT scans of the brain in asymptomatic children with acute lymphocytic leukemia after prophylactic treatment of the central nervous system with radiation and intrathecal chemotherapy. N Engl J Med 1978;298:815–818.

89. Riccardi R, Brouwers P, Di Chiro G, Poplack DG. Abnormal computed tomography brain scans in children with acute lymphoblastic leukemia: serial long-term follow-up. J Clin Oncol 1985;3:12–18.

90. Mulhern RK, Reddick WE, Palmer SL, et al. Neurocognitive deficits in medulloblastoma survivors and white matter loss. Ann Neurol 1999;46:834–841.

91. Packer RJ, Sutton LN, Atkins TE, et al. A prospective study of cognitive function in children receiving whole-brain radiotherapy and chemotherapy: 2-year results. J Neurosurg 1989;70:707–713.

92. Peckham VC, Meadows AT, Bartel N, Marrero O. Educational late effects in long-term survivors of childhood lymphocytic leukemia. Pediatrics 1988;81:127–133.

93. Moore IM, Packer RJ, Karl D, Bleyer WA. Adverse effects of cancer treatment on the central nervous system. In: Schwarta CL, Hobbie WL, Constine WL, Ruccione KS (eds). Survivors of Childhood Cancer: Assessment and Management. St. Louis: Mosby, 1994:81–95.

94. Mitby PA, Robison LL, Whitton JA, et al. Utilization of special education services among long-term survivors of childhood cancer: a report from the Childhood Cancer Survivor Study. Cancer (Phila) 2003;97:1115–1126.

95. Loge JH, Abrahamsen AF, Ekeberg O, Kaasa S. Hodgkin's disease survivors more fatigued than the general population. J Clin Oncol 1999;17:253–261.

96. Knobel H, Loge JH, Lund MB, Forfang K, Nome O, Kaasa S. Late medical complications and fatigue in Hodgkin's disease survivors. J Clin Oncol 2001;19:3226–3233.

97. Chessells JM. Recent advances in the management of acute leukaemia. Arch Dis Child 2000;82:438–442.

98. Pui CH. Acute lymphoblastic leukemia in children. Curr Opinion Oncol 2000;12:2–12.

99. van Dam FS, Schagen SB, Muller MJ, et al. Impairment of cognitive function in women receiving adjuvant treatment for high-risk breast cancer: high-dose versus standard-dose chemotherapy. JNCI 1998;90:210–218.

100. Brezden CB, Phillips KA, Abdolell M, et al. Cognitive function in breast cancer patients receiving adjuvant chemotherapy. J Clin Oncol 2000;18:2695–2701.

101. Ahles TA, Saykin AJ, Noll WW, et al. The relationship of APOE genotype to neuropsychological performance in long-term cancer survivors treated with standard dose chemotherapy. Psychooncology 2003;12(6):612–619.

102. Ganz PA. Cognitive dysfunction following adjuvant treatment of breast cancer: a new dose-limiting toxic effect? JNCI 1998;90:182–183.

103. Hjermstad M, Holte H, Evensen S, Fayers P, Kaasa S. Do patients who are treated with stem cell transplantation have a health-related quality of life comparable to the general population after 1 year? Bone Marrow Transplant 1999;24:911–918.

104. Walker LG, Wesnes KP, Heys SD, Walker MB, Lolley J, Eremin O. The cognitive effects of recombinant interleukin-2 therapy: a controlled clinical trial using computerised assessments. Eur J Cancer 1996;32A:2275–2283.

105. Curt GA, Breitbart W, Cella D, et al. Impact of cancer related fatigue on the lives of patients: new findings from the Fatigue Coalition. Oncologist 2000;5:353–360.

106. Ahles TA, Tope DM, Furstenberg C, Hann D, Mill L. Psychologic and neuropsychologic impact of autologous bone marrow transplantation. J Clin Oncol 1996;14:1457–1462.

107. Ahles TA, Silberfarb PM, Maurer LH, et al. Psychologic and neuropsychologic functioning of patients with limited small-cell lung cancer treated with chemotherapy and radiation therapy with or without warfarin: a study by the Cancer and Leukemia Group B. J Clin Oncol 1998;16:1954–1960.

108. Mulhern RK, Kepner JL, Thomas PR, Armstrong FD, Friedman HS, Kun LE. Neuropsychologic functioning of survivors of childhood medulloblastoma randomized to receive conventional or reduced-dose craniospinal irradiation: a Pediatric Oncology Group study. Clin Oncol 1998;16:1723–1728.

109. Raymond-Speden E, Tripp G, Lawrence B, Holdaway D. Intellectual, neuropsychological, and academic functioning in long-term survivors of leukemia. J Pediatr Psychol 2000;25:59–68.

110. Tannock IF, Ahles TA, Ganz PA, Van Dam FS. Cognitive impairment associated with chemotherapy for cancer: report of a workshop. J Clin Oncol 2004;22(11):2233–2239.

111. Shalet SM, Beardwell CG, Twomey JA, Jones PH, Pearson D. Endocrine function following the treatment of acute leukemia in childhood. J Pediatr 1977;90:920–923.

112. Robison LL, Nesbit ME Jr, Sather HN, Meadows AT, Ortega JA, Hammond GD. Height of children successfully treated for acute lymphoblastic leukemia: a report from the Late Effects Study Committee of Childrens Cancer Study Group. Med Pediatr Oncol 1985;13:14–21.

113. Hancock SL, Cox RS, McDougall IR. Thyroid diseases after treatment of Hodgkin's disease. N Engl J Med 1991;325:599–605.

114. Sklar C, Whitton J, Mertens A, et al. Abnormalities of the thyroid in survivors of Hodgkin's disease: data from the Childhood Cancer Survivor Study. J Clin Endocrinol Metab 2000;85:3227–3232.

115. Glatstein E, McHardy-Young S, Brast N, Eltringham JR, Kriss JP. Alterations in serum thyrotropin (TSH) and thyroid function following radiotherapy in patients with malignant lymphoma. J Clin Endocrinol Metab 1971;32:833–841.

116. Rosenthal MB, Goldfine ID. Primary and secondary hypothyroidism in nasopharyngeal carcinoma. JAMA 1976;236:1591–1593.

117. Sklar CA. Growth and neuroendocrine dysfunction following therapy for childhood cancer. Pediatr Clin N Am 1997;44:489–503.

118. Berry DH, Elders MJ, Crist W, et al. Growth in children with acute lymphocytic leukemia: a Pediatric Oncology Group study. Med Pediatr Oncol 1983;11:39–45.

119. Papadakis V, Tan C, Heller G, Sklar C. Growth and final height after treatment for childhood Hodgkin disease. J Pediatr Hematol/Oncol 1996;18:272–276.

120. Shalet SM, Price DA, Beardwell CG, Jones PH, Pearson D. Normal growth despite abnormalities of growth hormone secretion in children treated for acute leukemia. J Pediatr 1979;94:719–722.

121. Didcock E, Davies HA, Didi M, Ogilvy Stuart AL, Wales JK, Shalet SM. Pubertal growth in young adult survivors of childhood leukemia. J Clin Oncol 1995;13:2503–2507.

122. Katz JA, Pollock BH, Jacaruso D, Morad A. Final attained height in patients successfully treated for childhood acute lymphoblastic leukemia. J Pediatr 1993;123:546–552.

123. Odame I, Reilly JJ, Gibson BE, Donaldson MD. Patterns of obesity in boys and girls after treatment for acute lymphoblastic leukaemia. Arch Dis Child 1994;71:147–149.

124. Van Dongen-Melman JE, Hokken-Koelega AC, Hahlen K, De Groot A, Tromp CG, Egeler RM. Obesity after successful treatment of acute lymphoblastic leukemia in childhood. Pediatr Res 1995;38:86–90.

125. Sklar CA, Mertens AC, Walter A, et al. Changes in body mass index and prevalence of overweight in survivors of childhood acute lymphoblastic leukemia: role of cranial irradiation. Med Pediatr Oncol 2000;35:91–95.

126. Craig F, Leiper AD, Stanhope R, Brain C, Meller ST, Nussey SS. Sexually dimorphic and radiation dose dependent effect of cranial irradiation on body mass index. Arch Dis Child 1999;81:500–510.

127. Oeffinger KC, Mertens AC, Sklar CA, et al. Obesity in adult survivors of childhood acute lymphoblastic leukemia: a report from the Childhood Cancer Survivor Study. J Clin Oncol 2003; 21:1359–1365.

128. Thomson AB, Critchley HOD, Wallace WHB. Fertility and progeny. Eur J Cancer 2002;38:1634–1644.

129. Lamb MA. Effects of cancer on the sexuality and fertility of women. Semin Oncol Nurs 1995;11:120–127.

130. Brougham MF, Kelnar CJ, Sharpe RM, Wallace WH. Male fertility following childhood cancer: current concepts and future therapies. Asian J Androl 2003;5(4):325–337.

131. Wallace WH, Anderson R, Baird D. Preservation of fertility in young women treated for cancer. Lancet Oncol 2004;5(5): 269–270.

132. Opsahl MS, Fugger EF, Sherins RJ. Preservation of reproductive function before therapy for cancer: new options involving sperm and ovary cryopreservation. Cancer J 1997;3:189–191.

133. Oktay K, Newton H, Aubard Y, Salha O, Gosden RG. Cryopreservation of immature human oocytes and ovarian tissue: an emerging technology? Fertil Steril 1998;69:1–7.

134. Donnez J, Dolmans MM, Demylle D, et al. Livebirth after orthotic transplantation of cryopreserved ovarian tissue. Lancet 2004;364(9443):1405–1410.

135. Wallace WH, Pritchard J. Livebirth after cryopreserved ovarian tissue autotransplantation. Lancet 2004;364(9451):2093–2094.

136. Bath LE, Tydeman G, Critchley HO, Anderson RA, Baird DT, Wallace WH. Spontaneous conception in a young woman who had ovarian cortical tissue cryopreserved before chemotherapy and radiotherapy for a Ewing's sarcoma of the pelvis: case report. Hum Reprod 2004;19(11):2569–2572.

137. Wallace WH, Kelsey TW. Ovarian reserve and reproductive age may be determined from measurement of ovarian volume by transvaginal sonography. Hum Reprod 2004;19(7):1612–1617.

138. Chapman RM, Sutcliffe SB, Malpas JS. Cytotoxic-induced ovarian failure in Hodgkin's disease. II. Effects on sexual function. JAMA 1979;242:1882–1884.

139. Waxman JHX, Terry YA, Wrigley PFM, et al. Gonadal function in Hodgkin's disease: long-term follow-up of chemotherapy. Br Med J 1982;285:1612–1613.

140. Byrne J, Fears TR, Gail MH, et al. Early menopause in long-term survivors of cancer during adolescence. Am J Obstet Gynecol 1992;166:788–793.

141. Madsen BL, Giudice L, Donaldson SS. Radiation-induced premature menopause: a misconception. Int J Radiat Oncol Biol Phys 1995;32:1461–1464.

142. Li FP, Gimbreke K, Gelber RD, et al. Outcome of pregnancy in survivors of Wilms' tumor. JAMA 1987;257:216–219.

143. Constine LS, Rubin P, Woolf PD, et al. Hyperprolactinemia and hypothyroidism following cytotoxic therapy for central nervous system malignancies. J Clin Oncol 1987;5:1841–1851.

144. Lushbaugh CC, Casarett GW. The effects of gonadal irradiation in clinical radiation therapy: a review. Cancer (Phila) 1976;37:1111–1125.

145. Stillman RJ, Schinfeld JS, Schiff I, et al. Ovarian failure in long-term survivors of childhood malignancy. Am J Obstet Gynecol 1981;139:62–66.

146. Wallace WHB, Thomson AB, Kelsey TW. The radiosensitivity of the human oocyte. Hum Reprod 2003;18:117–121.

147. DaCunha MF, Meistrich ML, Fuller LM, et al. Recovery of spermatogenesis after treatment for Hodgkin's disease: limiting dose of MOPP chemotherapy. J Clin Oncol 1984;2:571–577.

148. Narayan P, Lange PH, Fraley EE. Ejaculation and fertility after extended retroperitoneal lymph node dissection for testicular cancer. J Urol 1982;127:685–688.

149. Schlegel PN, Walsh PC. Neuroanatomical approach to radical cystoprostatectomy with preservation of sexual function. J Urol 1987;138:1402–1406.

150. Rowley MJ, Leach DR, Warner GA, Heller CG. Effect of graded doses of ionizing radiation on the human testis. Radiat Res 1974;59:665–678.

151. Speiser B, Rubin P, Casarett G. Aspermia following lower truncal irradiation in Hodgkin's disease. Cancer (Phila) 1973;32:692–698.

152. Shamberger RC, Sherins RJ, Rosenberg SA. The effects of postoperative adjuvant chemotherapy and radiotherapy on testicular function in men undergoing treatment for soft tissue sarcoma. Cancer (Phila) 1981:47:2368–2374.

153. Green DM, Brecher ML, Lindsay AN, et al. Gonadal function in pediatric patients following treatment for Hodgkin disease. Med Pediatr Oncol 1981;9:235–244.

154. Sklar C. Reproductive physiology and treatment-related loss of sex hormone production. Med Pediatr Oncol 1999;33:2–8.

155. Shalet SM, Horner A, Ahmed SR, Morris-Jones PH. Leydig cell damage after testicular irradiation for lymphoblastic leukaemia. Med Pediatr Oncol 1985;13:65–68.

156. Leiper AD, Grant DB, Chessells JM. Gonadal function after testicular radiation for acute lymphoblastic leukaemia. Arch Dis Child 1986;61:53–56.

157. Sklar CA, Robison LL, Nesbit ME, et al. Effects of radiation on testicular function in long-term survivors of childhood acute lymphoblastic leukemia: a report from the Children Cancer Study Group. J Clin Oncol 1990;8:1981–1987.

158. Chapman RM, Sutcliffe SB, Malpas JS. Cytotoxic-induced ovarian failure in women with Hodgkin's disease. I. Hormone function. JAMA 1979;242:1877–1881.

159. Whitehead E, Shalet SM, Jones PH, Beardwell CG, Deakin DP. Gonadal function after combination chemotherapy for Hodgkin's disease in childhood. Arch Dis Child 1982;57:287–291.

160. Ortin TT, Shostak CA, Donaldson SS. Gonadal status and reproductive function following treatment for Hodgkin's disease in childhood: the Stanford experience. Int J Radiat Oncol Biol Phys 1990;19:873–880.

161. Mackie EJ, Radford M, Shalet SM. Gonadal function following chemotherapy for childhood Hodgkin's disease. Med Pediatr Oncol 1996;27:74–78.

162. Goodwin PJ, Ennis M, Pritchard KI, et al. Risk of menopause during the first year after breast cancer diagnosis. J Clin Oncol 1999;17:2365–2370.

163. Koyama H, Wada T, Nishzawa Y, et al. Cyclophosphamide induced ovarian failure and its therapeutic significance in patients with breast cancer. Cancer (Phila) 1977;39:1403–1409.

164. Byrne J, Mulvihill JJ, Myers MH, et al. Effects of treatment on fertility in long-term survivors of childhood or adolescent cancer. N Engl J Med 1987;317:1315–1321.

165. Critchley HOD, Wallace WHB, Shalet SM, et al. Abdominal irradiation in childhood: the potential for pregnancy. Br J Obstet Gynecol 1992;99:392–394.

166. Critchley HOD. Factors of importance for implantation and problems after treatment for childhood cancer. Med Pediatr Oncol 1999;33:9–14.

167. Bath LE, Critchley HO, Chambers SE, et al. Ovarian and uterine characteristics after total body irradiation in childhood and adolescence: response to sex steroid replacement. Br J Obstet Gynaecol 1999;106:1265–1272.

168. Li FP, Fine W, Jaffe N, et al. Offspring of patients treated for cancer in childhood. J Natl Cancer Inst 1979;62:1193–1197.

169. Hawkins MM, Smith RA, Curtice LJ. Childhood cancer survivors and their offspring studied through a postal survey of general practitioners: preliminary results. J R Coll Gen Pract 1988;38:102–105.

170. Byrne J, Rasmussen SA, Steinhorn SC, et al. Genetic disease in offspring of long-term survivors of childhood and adolescent cancer. Am J Hum Genet 1998;62:45–52.

171. Green DM, Fine WE, Li FP. Offspring of patients treated for unilateral Wilms' tumor in childhood. Cancer (Phila) 1982;49:2285–2288.

172. Byrne L, Mulvihill JJ, Connelly RR, et al. Reproductive problems and birth defects in survivors of Wilms' tumor and their relatives. Med Pediatr Oncol 1988;16:233–240.

173. Li FP, Gimbrere K, Gelber RD, et al. Outcome of pregnancy in survivors of Wilms' tumor. JAMA 1987;257:216–219.

174. Hawkins MM, Smith RA. Pregnancy outcomes in childhood cancer survivors: probable effects of abdominal irradiation. Int J Cancer 1989;43:399–402.

175. Hawkins MM. Is there evidence of a therapy-related increase in germ cell mutation among childhood cancer survivors? J Natl Cancer Inst 1991;83:1643–1650.

176. Green DM, Zevon MA, Lowrie G, et al. Pregnancy outcome following treatment with chemotherapy for cancer in childhood and adolescence. N Engl J Med 1991;325:141–146.

177. Nygaard R, Clausen N, Siimes MA, et al. Reproduction following treatment for childhood leukemia: a population-based prospective cohort study of fertility and offspring. Med Pediatr Oncol 1991;19:459–466.

178. Dodds I, Marrett LD, Tomkins DJ, et al. Case-control study of congenital anomalies in children of cancer patients. Br Med J 1993;307:164–168.

179. Kenny LB, Nicholson HS, Brasseux C, et al. Birth defects in offspring of adult survivors of childhood acute lymphoblastic leukemia. Cancer (Phila) 1996;78:169–176.

180. Green DM, Fiorello A, Zevon MA, et al. Birth defects and childhood cancer in offspring of survivors of childhood cancer. Arch Pediatr Adolesc Med 1997;151:379–383.

181. Mulvihill JJ, Myers MH, Connelly RR, et al. Cancer in offspring of long-term survivors of childhood and adolescent cancer. Lancet 1987;2:813–817.

182. Hawkins JJ, Draper GJ, Smith RA. Cancer among 1,348 offspring of survivors of childhood cancer. Int J Cancer 1989;43:975–978.

183. Sanders JE, Hawley J, Levy W, et al. Pregnancies following high-dose cyclophosphamide with or without high-dose busulfan or total-body irradiation and bone marrow transplantation. Blood 1996;87:3045–3052.

184. Green DM, Whitton JA, Stovall M, et al. Pregnancy outcome of partners of male survivors of childhood cancer. A report from the Childhood Cancer Survivor Study. J Clin Oncol 2003;21:716–721.

185. Green DM, Whitton JA, Stovall M, et al. Pregnancy outcome of female survivors of childhood cancer. A report from the Childhood Cancer Survivor Study. Am J Obstet Gynecol 2002;187:1070–1080.

186. Horning SJ, Adhikari A, Rizk N. Effect of treatment for Hodgkin's disease on pulmonary function: results of a prospective study. J Clin Oncol 1994;12:297–305.

187. Samuels ML, Douglas EJ, Holoye PV, et al. Large dose bleomycin therapy and pulmonary toxicity. JAMA 1976;235:1117–1120.

188. O'Driscoll BR, Hasleton PS, Taylor PM, et al. Active lung fibrosis up to 17 years after chemotherapy with carmustine (BCNU) in childhood. N Engl J Med 1990;323:378–382.

189. Vogelzang NJ. Nephrotoxicity from chemotherapy: prevention and management. Oncology 1991;5:97–112.

190. Dewit L, Anninga JK, Hoefnagel CA, et al. Radiation injury in the human kidney: a prospective analysis using specific scintigraphic and biochemical endpoints. Int J Radiat Oncol Biol Phys 1990;19:977–983.

191. Hilkens PHE, Verweij J, Vecht CJ, Stoter G, Bent MHvd. Clinical characteristics of severe peripheral neuropathy incuded by docetaxel, taxotere. Ann Oncol 1997;8:187–190.

192. Tuxen MK, Hansen SW. Complications of treatment: neurotoxicity secondary to antineoplastic drugs. Cancer Treat Rev 1994;20:191–214.

193. Bhatia S, Robison LL, Meadows AT, LESG Investigators. High risk of second malignant neoplasms (SMN) continues with extended follow-up of childhood Hodgkin's disease (HD) cohort: report from the Late Effects Study Group. Blood 2001;98:768a.

194. van Leeuwen FE, Klokman WJ, Stovall M, et al. Roles of radiotherapy and smoking in lung cancer following Hodgkin's disease. J Natl Cancer Inst 1995;87:1530–1537.

195. Kreiker J, Kattan J. Second colon cancer following Hodgkin's disease. A case report. J Med Libanais 1996;44:107–108.

196. Deutsch M, Wollman MR, Ramanathan R, Rubin J. Rectal cancer twenty-one years after treatment of childhood Hodgkin disease. Med Pediatr Oncol 2002;38:280–281.

197. Hawkins MM, Draper GJ, Kingston JE. Incidence of second primary tumors among childhood cancer survivors. Br J Cancer 1984;56:339–347.

198. Meadows AT, Baum E, Fossati-Bellani F, et al. Second malignant neoplasms in children: an update from the Late Effects Study Group. J Clin Oncol 1985;3:532–538.

199. Bhatia S, Robison LL, Oberlin O, et al. Breast cancer and other second neoplasms after childhood Hodgkin's disease. N Engl J Med 1996;334:745–751.

200. Malkin D, Li FP, Strong LC, et al. Germline p53 mutations in a familial syndrome of breast cancer, sarcomas, and other neoplasms. Science 1990;250:1333–1338.

201. Neglia JP, Friedman DL, Yasui Y, et al. Second malignant neoplasms in five-year survivors of childhood cancer: childhood cancer survivor study. J Natl Cancer Inst 2001;93:618–629.

202. Bhatia S, Sather HN, Pabustan OB, Trigg ME, Gaynon PS, Robison LL. Low incidence of second neoplasms among children diagnosed with acute lymphoblastic leukemia after 1983. Blood 2002;99:4257–4264.

203. Neglia JP, Meadows AT, Robison LL, et al. Second neoplasms after acute lymphoblastic leukemia in childhood. N Engl J Med 1991;325:1330–1336.

204. Relling MV, Rubnitz JE, Rivera GK, et al. High incidence of secondary brain tumours after radiotherapy and antimetabolites. Lancet 1999;354:34–39.

205. Hawkins MM, Wilson LM, Stovall MA, et al. Epipodophyllotoxins, alkylating agents, and radiation and risk of secondary leukaemia after childhood cancer. Br Med J 1992;304:951–958.

206. Tucker MA. Solid second cancers following Hodgkin's disease. Hematol-Oncol Clin N Am 1993;7:389–400.

207. Beatty O III, Hudson MM, Greenwald C, et al. Subsequent malignancies in children and adolescents after treatment for Hodgkin's disease. J Clin Oncol 1995;13:603–609.

208. Bhatia S, Robison LL, Oberlin O, et al. Breast cancer and other second neoplasms after childhood Hodgkin's disease. N Engl J Med 1996;334:745–751.

209. Jenkin D, Greenberg M, Fitzgerald A. Second malignant tumours in childhood Hodgkin's disease. Med Pediatr Oncol 1996;26:373–379.

210. Sankila R, Garwicz S, Olsen JH, et al. Risk of subsequent malignant neoplasms among 1,641 Hodgkin's disease patients diagnosed in childhood and adolescence: a population-based cohort study in the five Nordic countries. Association of the Nordic Cancer Registries and the Nordic Society of Pediatric Hematology and Oncology. J Clin Oncol 1996;14:1442–1446.

211. Wolden SL, Lamborn KR, Cleary SF, Tate DJ, Donaldson SS. Second cancers following pediatric Hodgkin's disease. J Clin Oncol 1998;16:536–544.

212. Green DM, Hyland A, Barcos MP, et al. Second malignant neoplasms after treatment for Hodgkin's disease in childhood or adolescence. J Clin Oncol 2000;18:1492–1499.

213. Metayer C, Lynch CF, Clarke EA, et al. Second cancers among long-term survivors of Hodgkin's disease diagnosed in childhood and adolescence. J Clin Oncol 2000;18:2435–2443.

214. Wrighton SA, Stevens JC. The human hepatic cytochromes P450 involved in drug metabolism. Crit Rev Toxicol 1992;22:1–21.

215. Hayes JD, Pulford DJ. The glutathione S-transferase supergene family: regulation of GST and the contribution of the isoenzymes to cancer chemoprotection and drug resistance. Crit Rev Biochem Mol Biol 1995;30:445–600.

216. Raunio H, Husgafvel-Pursiainen K, Anttila S, Hietanen E, Hirvonen A, Pelkonen O. Diagnosis of polymorphisms in carcinogen-activating and inactivating enzymes and cancer susceptibility: a review. Gene (Amst) 1995;159:113–121.

217. Smith G, Stanley LA, Sim E, Strange RC, Wolf CR. Metabolic polymorphisms and cancer susceptibility. Cancer Surv 1995;25:27–65.

218. Felix CA, Walker AH, Lange BJ, et al. Association of CYP3A4 genotype with treatment-related leukemia. Proc Natl Acad Sci U S A 1998;95:13176–13181.

219. Naoe T, Takeyama K, Yokozawa T, et al. Analysis of genetic polymorphism in NQO1, GST-M1, GST-T1, and CYP3A4 in 469 Japanese patients with therapy-related leukemia/myelodysplastic syndrome and de novo acute myeloid leukemia. Clin Cancer Res 2000;6:4091–4095.

220. Blanco JG, Edick MJ, Hancock ML, et al. Genetic polymorphisms in CYP3A5, CYP3A4 and NQO1 in children who developed therapy-related myeloid malignancies. Pharmacogenetics 2002;12:605–611.

221. Zim S, Collins JM, O'Neill D, et al. Inhibition of first-pass metabolism in cancer chemotherapy: interaction of 6-mercaptopurine and allopurinol. Clin Pharmacol Ther 1983;34:810–817.

222. Hildreth NG, Shore RE, Dvortesky PM. The risk of breast cancer after irradiation of the thymus in infancy. N Engl J Med 1989;321:1281–1284.

223. Petrek JA, Heelan MC. Incidence of breast carcinoma-related lymphedema. Cancer (Phila) 1998;83(suppl 12):2776–2781.

224. Erickson VS, Pearson ML, Ganz PA, Adams J, Kahn KL. Arm edema in breast cancer patients. JNCI 2004;93:96–111.

225. Andrykowski MA, Curran SL, Lightner R. Off-treatment fatigue in breast cancer survivors: a controlled comparison. J Behav Med 1998;21:1–18.

226. Broeckel JA, Jacobsen PB, Horton J, Balducci L, Lyman GH. Characteristics and correlates of fatigue after adjuvant chemotherapy for breast cancer. J Clin Oncol 1998;16:1689–1696.

227. Greenberg DB, Kornblith AB, Herndon JE, et al. Quality of life for adult leukemia survivors treated on clinical trials of Cancer and Leukemia Group B during the period 1971–1988. Cancer (Phila) 1997;80:1936–1944.

228. Loge JH, Abrahamsen AF, Ekeberg O, Kaasa S. Hodgkin's disease survivors more fatigued than the general population. J Clin Oncol 1999;17:253–261.

229. Bush NE, Haberman M, Donaldson G, Sullivan KM. Quality of life of 125 adults surviving 6–18 years after bone marrow transplant. Social Sci Med 1995;40:479–490.

230. Mock V, Piper B, Escalante C, Sabbatini P. National Comprehensive Cancer Network practice guidelines for the management of cancer-related fatigue. Oncologist 2000;14(11A):151–161.

231. Ganz PA, Schag CAC, Lee JJ, et al. The CARES: a generic measure of health-related quality of life for cancer patients. Qual Life Res 1992;1:19–29.

232. Demark-Wahnefried W, Aziz NM, Rowland JH, Pinto BM. Riding the Crest of the Teachable Moment: Promoting Long-Term Health after the Diagnosis of Cancer. J Clin Oncol, 2005.

233. Day RW. Future need for more cancer research. J Am Diet Assoc 1998;98:523.

234. Brown BW, Brauner C, Minnotte MC. Noncancer deaths in white adult cancer patients. JNCI 1993;85:979–997.

235. Meadows AT, Varricchio C, Crosson K, et al. Research issues in cancer survivorship. Cancer Epidemiol Biomarkers Prev 1998;7:1145–1151.

236. Travis LB. Therapy-associated solid tumors. Acta Oncol 2002;41:323–333.

237. Bergstrom A, Pisani P, Tenet V, et al. Overweight as an avoidable cause of cancer in Europe. Int J Cancer 2001;91:421–430.

238. World Health Organization. IARC Handbook of Cancer Prevention, vol 6. Geneva: World Health Organization, 2002.

239. Chlebowski RT, Aiello E, McTiernan A. Weight loss in breast cancer patient management. J Clin Oncol 2002;20:1128–1143.

240. Nuver J, Smit AJ, Postma A, et al. The metabolic syndrome in long-term cancer survivors, an important target for secondary measures. Cancer Treat Rev 2002;28:195–214.

241. Freedland SJ, Aronson WJ, Kane CJ, et al. Impact of obesity on biochemical control after radical prostatectomy for clinically localized prostate cancer: a report by the Shared Equal Access Regional Cancer Hospital database study group. J Clin Oncol 2004;22:446–453.

242. Argiles JM Lopez-Soriano FJ. Insulin and cancer. Int J Oncol 2001;18:683–687.

243. Bines J, Gradishar WJ. Primary care issues for the breast cancer survivor. Compr Ther 1997;23:605–611.

244. Yoshikawa T, Noguchi Y, Doi C, et al. Insulin resistance in patients with cancer: relationships with tumor site, tumor stage, body-weight loss, acute-phase response, and energy expenditure. Nutrition 2001;17:590–593.

245. Balkau B, Kahn HS, Courbon D, et al. Paris Prospective Study. Hyperinsulinemia predicts fatal liver cancer but is inversely associated with fatal cancer at some other sites: the Paris Prospective Study. Diabetes Care 2001;24:843–849.

246. Lamont EB, Christakis NA, Lauderdale DS. Favorable cardiac risk among elderly breast carcinoma survivors. Cancer (Phila) 2003;98:2–10.

247. Hull MC, Morris CG, Pepine CJ, et al. Valvular dysfunction and carotid, subclavian, and coronary artery disease in survivors of Hodgkin lymphoma treated with radiation therapy. JAMA 2003;290:2831–2837.

248. Buist DS, LaCroix AZ, Barlow WE, et al. Bone mineral density and endogenous hormones and risk of breast cancer in postmenopausal women (United States). Cancer Causes Control 2001;12:213–222.

249. Buist DS, LaCroix AZ, Barlow WE, et al. Bone mineral density and breast cancer risk in postmenopausal women. J Clin Epidemiol 2001;54:417–422.

250. Cauley JA, Lucas FL, Kuller LH, et al. Bone mineral density and risk of breast cancer in older women: the study of osteoporotic fractures. Study of Osteoporotic Fractures Research Group. JAMA 1996;276:1404–1408.

251. Lamont EB, Lauderdale DS. Low risk of hip fracture among elderly breast cancer survivors. Ann Epidemiol 2003;13: 698–703.

252. Lucas FL, Cauley JA, Stone RA, et al. Bone mineral density and risk of breast cancer: differences by family history of breast cancer. Study of Osteoporotic Fractures Research Group. Am J Epidemiol 1998;148:22–29.

253. Newcomb PA, Trentham-Dietz A, Egan KM, et al. Fracture history and risk of breast and endometrial cancer. Am J Epidemiol 2001;153:1071–1078.

254. van der Klift M, de Laet CE, Coebergh JW, et al. Bone mineral density and the risk of breast cancer: the Rotterdam Study. Bone (NY) 2003;32:211–216.

255. Zhang Y, Kiel DP, Kreger BE, et al. Bone mass and the risk of breast cancer among postmenopausal women. N Engl J Med 1997;336:611–617.

256. Zmuda JM, Cauley JA, Ljung BM, et al. Study of Osteoporotic Fractures Research Group. Bone mass and breast cancer risk in older women: differences by stage at diagnosis. JNCI 2001;93: 930–936.

257. Schultz PN, Beck ML, Stava C, et al. Health profiles in 5836 long-term cancer survivors. Int J Cancer 2003;104:488–495.

258. Twiss JJ, Waltman N, Ott CD, et al. Bone mineral density in postmenopausal breast cancer survivors. J Am Acad Nurse Pract 2001;13:276–284.

259. Ramaswamy B, Shapiro CL. Osteopenia and osteoporosis in women with breast cancer. Semin Oncol 2003;30:763–775.

260. Diamond TH, Higano CS, Smith MR, et al. Osteoporosis in men with prostate carcinoma receiving androgen-deprivation therapy: recommendations for diagnosis and therapies. Cancer (Phila) 2004;100:892–899.

261. Ko CY, Maggard M, Livingston EH: Evaluating health utility in patients with melanoma, breast cancer, colon cancer, and lung cancer: a nationwide, population-based assessment. J Surg Res 2003;114:1–5.

262. Garman KS, Pieper CF, Seo P, et al. Function in elderly cancer survivors depends on comorbidities. J Gerontol A Biol Sci Med Sci 2003;58:M1119–M1124.

263. Hewitt M, Rowland JH, Yancik R. Cancer survivors in the U.S.: age, health and disability. J Gerontol Biol Sci Med Sci 2003; 58:82–91.

264. Ashing-Giwa K, Ganz PA, Petersen L. Quality of life of African-American and white long term breast carcinoma survivors. Cancer (Phila) 1999;85:418–426.

265. Baker F, Haffer S, Denniston M. Health-related quality of life of cancer and noncancer patients in Medicare managed care. Cancer (Phila) 2003;97:674–681.

266. Chirikos TN, Russell-Jacobs A, Jacobsen PB. Functional impairment and the economic consequences of female breast cancer. Womens Health 2002;36:1–20.

267. Trotti A. The evolution and application of toxicity criteria. Semin Radiat Oncol 2002;12(1 suppl 1):1–3.

268. Hoeller U, Tribius S, Kuhlmey A, Grader K, Fehlauer F, Alberti W. Increasing the rate of late toxicity by changing the score? A comparison of RTOG/EORTC and LENT/SOMA scores. Int J Radiat Oncol Biol Phys 2003;55(4):1013–1018.

269. Garre ML, Gandus S, Cesana B, et al. Health status of long term survivors after cancer in childhood. Am J Pediatr Hematol Oncol 1994;16:143–152.

270. Von der Weid N, Beck D, Caflisch U, Feldges A, Wyss M, Wagner HP. Standardized assessment of late effects in long term survivors of childhood cancer in Switzerland: results of a Swiss Pediatrics Oncology Group (SPOG) study. Int J Pedatr Hematol Oncol 1996;3:483–490.

271. Brown JK, Byers T, Doyle C, et al. Nutrition and physical activity during and after cancer treatment: an American Cancer Society guide for informed choices. CA Cancer J Clin 2003;53: 268–291.

272. Rock CL, Demark-Wahnefried W. Nutrition and survival after the diagnosis of breast cancer: a review of the evidence. J Clin Oncol 2002;20:3302–3316.

273. Kattlove H, Winn RJ. Ongoing care of patients after primary treatment for their cancer. CA Cancer J Clin 2003;53:172–196.

274. Robison LL. Cancer survivorship: Unique opportunities for research. Cancer Epidemiol Biomarkers Prev 2004;13:1093.

275. Eshelman D, Landier W, Sweeney T, Hester AL, Forte K, Darling J, Hudson MM. Facilitating care for childhood cancer survivors: integrating children's oncology group long-term follow-up guidelines and health links in clinical practice. J Pediatr Oncol Nurs 2004;21:271–280.

276. Oberfield SE, Sklar CA. Endocrine sequelae in survivors of childhood cancer. Adolesc Med 2002;13:161–169.

277. Green DM, Grigoriev YA, Nan B, et al. Congestive heart failure after treatment for Wilms' tumor: a report from the National Wilms' Tumor Study group. J Clin Oncol 2001;19:1926–1934.

278. Green DM, Peabody EM, Nan B, Peterson S, Kalapurakal JA, Breslow NE. Pregnancy outcome after treatment for Wilms tumor: a report from the National Wilms Tumor Study Group. J Clin Oncol 2002;20:2506–2513.

279. Michael YL, Kawachi I, Berkman LF, et al. The persistent impact of breast carcinoma on functional health status. Cancer (Phila) 2000;89:2176–2186.

280. Chirikos TN, Russell-Jacobs A, Jacobsen PB. Functional impairment and the economic consequences of female breast cancer. Women Health 2002;36:1–20.

281. Deimling GT, Schaefer ML, Kahana B, Bowman KF, Reardon J. Racial differences in the health of older adult long-term cancer survivors. Psychosoc Oncol (in press).

282. Chirikos TN, Russell-Jacobs A, Cantor AB. Indirect economic effects of long-term breast cancer survival. Cancer Pract 2002;10:248–255.

283. Ahles TA, Saykin AJ, Furstenberg CT, et al. Neuropsychologic impact of standard-dose systemic chemotherapy in long-term survivors of breast cancer and lymphoma. J Clin Oncol 2002; 20:485–493.

284. Ahles TA, Saykin AJ, Noll WW, et al. The relationship of APOE genotype to neuropsychological performance in long-term cancer survivors treated with standard dose chemotherapy. J Clin Oncol 2002;20(2):485–493.

285. Syrjala KL, Schroeder TC, Abrams JR, Atkins TZ, Sanders JE, Brown W, Heiman JR. Sexual function measurement and outcomes in cancer survivors and matched controls. J Sex Research 2000;37(3):213–225.

286. Syrjala KL, Roth SL, Abrams JR, Chapko MK, Visser S, Sanders JE. Prevalence and predictors of sexual dysfunction in long-term survivors of bone marrow transplantation. J Clin Oncol 1998; 16:3148–3157.

287. Paskett ED, Stark N. Lymphedema: knowledge, treatment, and impact among breast cancer survivors. Breast J 2000;6(6):373–378.

288. Simbre VC II, Admas MJ, Deshpande SS, Duffy SA, Miller TL, Lipshultz SE. Cardiomyopathy caused by antineoplastic therapies. Curr Treat Options Cardiovasc Med 2001;3:493–505.

289. Lipshultz SE, Lipsitz SR, Sallan SE, et al. Long-term enalapril therapy for left ventricular dysfunction in doxorubicin-treated survivors of childhood cancer. J Clin Oncol 2002;20:4517–4522.

290. Thompson SJ, Leigh L, Christensen R, et al. Immediate neurocognitive effects of methylphenidate on learning-impaired survivors of childhood cancer. J Clin Oncol 2001;19:1802–1808.

291. Longman AJ, Braden CJ, Mishel MH. Side-effects burden, psychological adjustment, and life quality in women with breast

cancer: pattern of association over time. Oncol Nurs Forum 1999;26:909–915.

292. Badger TA, Braden CJ, Mishel MH. Depression burden, self-help interventions, and side effect experience in women receiving treatment for breast cancer. Oncol Nurs Forum 2001;28(3):567–574.

293. Antoni MH, Lehman JM, Kilbourn KM, et al. Cognitive-behavioral stress management intervention decreases the prevalence of depression and enhances benefit finding among women under treatment for early-stage breast cancer. Health Psychol 2001;20:20–32.

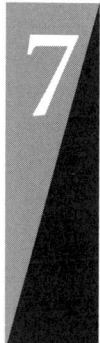

7

Medical and Psychosocial Issues in Childhood Cancer Survivors

Smita Bhatia, Wendy Landier, Jacqueline Casillas, and Lonnie Zeltzer

More than 12,000 children and adolescents younger than 20 years are diagnosed with cancer each year in the United States.[1] With the use of risk-based therapies, the overall 5-year survival rate is approaching 80%, resulting in a growing population of childhood cancer survivors.[1] In 1997, there were an estimated 270,000 survivors of childhood cancer; over two-thirds of these were older than 20 years of age.[2] This figure translates into 1 in 810 individuals under the age of 20 and 1 in 640 individuals between the ages of 20 and 39 years having successfully survived childhood cancer.

Unlike an adult, the growing child tolerates the acute side effects of therapy relatively well. However, the use of cancer therapy at an early age can produce complications that may not become apparent until years later as the child matures. The resulting complications are related to the specific therapy employed and the age of the child at the time the therapy was administered. A *late effect* is defined as a late-occurring or chronic outcome—either physical or psychologic—that persists or develops beyond 5 years from the diagnosis of cancer. These late effects include complications such as cognitive impairment, cardiopulmonary compromise, endocrine dysfunction, renal impairment, chronic hepatitis, and subsequent malignancies. As many as two-thirds of survivors experience at least one late effect as a result of treatment for cancer during childhood.[3–7] Therefore, ongoing evaluation of childhood cancer survivors is an essential component of follow-up. This chapter discusses the long-term complications that can occur among pediatric patients treated for cancer, along with recommendations for follow-up. Table 7.1 summarizes the data on the magnitude of risk and associated risk factors for select long-term outcomes.

Neurocognitive Sequelae

Neurocognitive sequelae of treatment for childhood cancer occur as a consequence of radiation to the whole brain and/or therapy with high-dose methotrexate, cytarabine, and/or intrathecal methotrexate. Children with a history of brain tumors, acute lymphoblastic leukemia (ALL), or non-Hodgkin's lymphoma (NHL) are most likely to be affected. Risk factors include increasing radiation dose, young age at the time of treatment, therapy with both cranial radiation and systemic or intrathecal chemotherapy, and female sex.[8] Severe deficits are most frequently noted in children with brain tumors, especially those who were treated with radiation therapy, and in children who were less than 5 years of age at the time of treatment.[9]

Neurocognitive deficits usually become evident within 1 to 2 years following radiation and are progressive in nature.[10] Affected children may experience information-processing deficits, resulting in academic difficulties. These children are particularly prone to problems with receptive and expressive language, attention span, and visual and perceptual motor skills. They most often experience academic difficulties in the areas of reading, language, and mathematics. Children in the younger age groups and those treated for brain tumors may experience significant drops in intelligence quotient (IQ) scores, with irradiation- or chemotherapy-induced destruction in normal white matter partially explaining intellectual and academic achievement deficits.[9,11–13]

Cardiovascular Function

Chronic cardiotoxicity usually manifests itself as cardiomyopathy, pericarditis, and congestive heart failure. The anthracyclines are well-known causes of cardiomyopathy.[14–17] The incidence of cardiomyopathy is dose dependent and may exceed 30% among patients who received cumulative doses of anthracyclines in excess of $600 \, mg/m^2$ (daunorubicin/doxorubicin equivalent).[18] With a total dose of 500 to $600 \, mg/m^2$, the incidence is 11%, falling to less than 1% for cumulative doses less than $500 \, mg/m^2$.[19] These data have formed the basis for the use of a threshold of $500 \, mg/m^2$ as the cumulative dose for cardiotoxicity. However, Kremer et al.[20] reported that a cumulative dose of anthracyclines greater than $300 \, mg/m^2$

TABLE 7.1. Clinical characteristics and risk factors for select long-term sequelae after treatment for childhood cancer.

Long-term sequelae	Cumulative probability	Risk factors
Congestive heart failure	4%–17% at 20 years (risk increasing with increasing therapeutic exposures)	• Higher cumulative dose of anthracyclines • Female sex • Younger age at exposure to anthracyclines • Black race • Presence of trisomy 21 • Radiation therapy involving the heart • Exposure to cyclophosphamide, ifosfamide, or amsacrine
Myocardial infarction	21% at 20–25 years	• Radiation therapy to the mediastinum • Dose >30 Gy • Increasing time since irradiation • Younger age at irradiation (<20 years) • Hypertension/hypercholesterolemia/DM/smoking/obesity
Ischemic stroke	12% at 15 years (among patients exposed to neck radiation)	• Radiation therapy to the head and neck • Younger age at irradiation (<20 years) • Hypertension/hypercholesterolemia/DM/smoking
Subsequent malignant neoplasms	3% at 20 years	• HD, soft tissue sarcoma, hereditary retinoblastoma • Younger age at exposure to therapeutic agents • Female sex • Radiation therapy • Exposure to alkylating agents or topoisomerase • II inhibitors

DM, diabetes mellitus; HD, Hodgkin's disease.

was associated with an increased risk of clinical heart failure (relative risk, 11.8) compared with a cumulative dose lower than 300 mg/m². Thus, a lower cumulative dose of anthracyclines may place children at increased risk for cardiac compromise.[20]

Cardiomyopathy can occur many years after completion of therapy, and the onset may be spontaneous or coincide with exertion or pregnancy. Risk factors known to be associated with anthracycline-related cardiac toxicity include mediastinal radiation;[21] uncontrolled hypertension;[17,18] exposure to other chemotherapeutic agents, especially cyclophosphamide,[18] dactinomycin,[22] mitomycin,[18] decarbazine,[23] vincristine, bleomycin, and methotrexate;[24] female sex;[25] younger age;[17,26,27] and electrolyte imbalance such as hypokalemia and hypomagnesemia.[16]

Chronic cardiac toxicity associated with radiation alone most commonly manifests as pericardial effusions or constrictive pericarditis, sometimes in association with pancarditis. Although 4,000 cGy of total heart radiation dose appears to be the usual threshold, pericarditis has been reported after as little as 1,500 cGy, even in the absence of radiomimetic chemotherapy.[28,29] Symptomatic pericarditis, which usually develops 10 to 30 months after radiation, is found in 2% to 10% of patients.[28–30] Subclinical pericardial and myocardial damage as well as valvular thickening may be common in this population,[31,32] and symptomatic pericarditis may first appear as late as 45 years after therapy.[33,34] Coronary artery disease has been reported following radiation to the mediastinum.[35]

Prevention of cardiotoxicity is a primary focus of investigation. Liposomal anthracyclines are being explored to reduce cardiotoxicity. The anthracyclines chelate iron, and the anthracycline–iron complex catalyzes the formation of extremely hydroxyl radicals. Agents such as dexrazoxane that are able to remove iron from the anthracyclines have been investigated as cardioprotectants. Clinical trials of dexrazoxane have been conducted in children, with encouraging evidence of short-term cardioprotection.[36,37] The long-term avoidance of cardiotoxicity with the use of this agent needs

to be determined.[38] Smaller doses and reduced port sizes of radiation therapy may also help in decreasing the incidence of carditis.

Pulmonary Function

Radiation-induced restrictive lung disease is seen in patients who received whole-lung radiation at a dose of 1,100 to 1,400 cGy and results primarily from a proportionate interference with the growth of both the lung and the chest wall.[39–41] Children under 3 years of age at time of therapy appear to be more susceptible to chronic toxicity. Obstructive changes are also reported after conventional radiation therapy and have been reported after 1,000 cGy total-body irradiation for hematopoietic cell transplant (HCT).[42] A cohort of 12,390 childhood cancer survivors participating in the Childhood Cancer Survivor Study (CCSS)[43] had a statistically significantly increased risk of lung fibrosis, recurrent pneumonia, chronic cough, pleurisy, use of supplemental oxygen, abnormal chest wall, exercise-induced shortness of breath, bronchitis, recurrent sinus infection, and tonsillitis when compared with sibling controls.[44] Statistically significant associations were identified for lung fibrosis and chest radiation, and for supplemental oxygen use and chest radiation, BCNU (carmustine), bleomycin, busulfan, CCNU (lomustine), and cyclophosphamide. Chest radiation was associated with a 3.5% cumulative incidence of lung fibrosis at 20 years after diagnosis.

Several chemotherapeutic agents have been associated with pulmonary disease in long-term survivors. Bleomycin toxicity is the prototype for chemotherapy-related lung injury. The chronic lung toxicity is dose dependent above a threshold cumulative dose of 400 units/m² and is exacerbated by previous or concurrent radiation therapy,[45] cyclophosphamide,[46] or subsequent oxygen therapy.[47] At doses exceeding 400 units/m², 10% of the patients experience fibrosis, and 35% to 55% suffer severe symptoms in the face of combinations of other injuries.[48] Other chemotherapeutic agents associated with chronic lung injury include BCNU,[49] busulfan, and CCNU.

Symptoms of pulmonary dysfunction include chronic cough or dyspnea, and close evaluation should be performed during yearly follow-up. All patients must be educated about the risks of smoking. The best possible approach to chronic pulmonary toxicity of anticancer therapy is preventive and includes the following: careful monitoring of pulmonary function and chest radiographs before and during bleomycin and radiation; respecting cumulative dose restrictions on bleomycin administration; and limiting radiation dosage and port sizes.

Endocrine Function

Thyroid

Hypothyroidism is the most common nonmalignant late effect involving this gland and is almost always caused by radiation of the head and neck for a nonthyroid malignancy. Laboratory evidence of primary hypothyroidism is evident in 40% to 90% of patients receiving radiation doses in excess of 1,500 cGy.[50–52] The actuarial risk of clinical hypothyroidism for subjects treated with 4,500 Gy or more is 50% at 20 years from diagnosis. Childhood brain tumor survivors were compared with siblings as part of the CCSS study, and were found to be at a 14.3-fold-increased risk of developing hypothyroidisms.[53] Risk factors associated with the development of hypothyroidism include increasing dose of radiation (higher risk associated with conventionally fractionated radiotherapy as compared with hyperfractionated radiotherapy), thyroidectomy, use of iodide-containing contrast material as in lymphangiography, older age at irradiation, and female gender.[54,55]

Hyperthyroidism has been reported in up to 5% of the survivors of Hodgkin's disease (HD) and is associated with radiation doses exceeding 3,500 cGy.[54] Thyroid nodules are observed among patients exposed to radiation. Female gender and radiation doses exceeding 2,500 cGy have been identified as risk factors.[54] The actuarial risk of female survivors of HD developing a thyroid nodule is 20% at 20 years from diagnosis. Patients with HD receiving radiation to the thyroid gland have been reported to be at an 18-fold-increased risk of developing thyroid cancer when compared with the general population.

Growth

Poor linear growth and short adult stature are common complications following successful treatment for childhood cancer.[56] Although in some children catch-up growth may occur, short stature may be permanent or even progressive. Severe growth retardation, defined as a standing height below the fifth percentile, has been observed in as many as 30% to 35% of survivors of childhood brain tumors[57–59] and 10% to 15% of patients treated for leukemia.[60,61] Whole-brain irradiation has been identified as the principal cause of short stature.[60] Compared with siblings, childhood brain tumor survivors participating in the CCSS study were at a 277.8-fold-

increased risk of developing growth hormone deficiency.[53] The effects of cranial irradiation appear to be related to age and sex, with children younger than 5 years at time of therapy and girls being more susceptible to the radiation effect.[62–64] The effects of radiation are also dose dependent, with doses exceeding 3,000 cGy associated with growth retardation in 50% of the patients.[58,59] The mechanism by which cranial irradiation induces short stature is not clear. Growth hormone deficiency and early onset of puberty in girls may contribute to loss of final height.[65] Direct inhibition of vertebral growth by spinal irradiation often contributes to short stature.

Body Mass Index

An increased prevalence of obesity has been reported among survivors of childhood ALL, with the prevalence increasing with increasing dose of cranial radiation. In a study conducted by Sklar et al.,[66] the percentage of subjects who were overweight at attainment of final height was 10.5%, 40%, and 38% for subjects treated with no cranial radiation, 18 Gy of cranial radiation, and 24 Gy of cranial radiation, respectively. This study documented that children with ALL given cranial radiation develop increases in their body mass index early on during their treatment and remain at significant risk for becoming overweight as young adults. A recent report has shown that the age-and race-adjusted odds ratio (OR) for being obese in ALL survivors treated with cranial radiation doses of 20 Gy or more in comparison with siblings was 2.6 for females and 1.9 for males.[67] Furthermore, the OR for obesity was greatest among girls diagnosed at 0 to 4 years of age and treated with radiation doses of 20 Gy or more. Thus, this study clearly demonstrated in a large cohort of ALL survivors that 20 Gy or more is associated with an increased prevalence of obesity, especially in females treated at a young age. It is therefore important for healthcare professionals to recognize this risk and to address it in the long-term follow-up of the survivors.

Gonadal Function

MALES

Male survivors of childhood cancer may experience germ cell depletion and abnormalities of gonadal endocrine function. These abnormalities may be secondary to radiation, chemotherapy, or surgery, with the effects of therapy varying depending on age at treatment. In patients who receive testicular radiation doses of 400 to 600 cGy, azoospermia may persist for 3 to 5 years, and at doses above 600 cGy, germinal loss with resulting increases in follicle-stimulating hormone (FSH) and decreases in testicular volume usually appears to be irreversible.[68,69] Prepubertal testicular germ cells also appear to be radiosensitive, although tubular damage may be difficult to assess until the patient has progressed through puberty. Radiation therapy at doses of 2,000 cGy or higher is also toxic to Leydig cells, with resulting inadequate production of testosterone.[70]

Chemotherapy can also interfere with testicular function. Alkylating agents decrease spermatogenesis in long-term survivors of cancer. The effects of cyclophosphamide and chlorambucil are dose dependent but are reversible in up to 70%

of patients after several years.[71] Among pubertal boys treated for HD with six cycles of mechlorethamine, vincristine, prednisone, and procarbazine (MOPP), azoospermia is found in 80% to 100%, and is reversible in only 20% of cases.[72] After adriamycin, bleomycin, vinblastine, and dacarbazine (ABVD), the incidence of azoospermia was 36%, with 100% recovery.[73] The effect of MOPP on Leydig cell function appears to be age related, with normal pubertal progression after therapy for patients treated before the onset of puberty, gynecomastia with low testosterone and increased luteinizing hormone (LH) in patients treated during adolescence, and compensated Leydig cell failure without gynecomastia in adults.[71]

FEMALES

Radiation therapy effects on the ovary are both age- and dose dependent. Amenorrhea develops in only 68% of prepubescent girls treated with higher doses of radiation (1,200–1,500 cGy).[74] Spinal irradiation for the treatment of ALL and brain tumors appears to result in clinically significant ovarian damage in some young women, although the majority of these women go on to experience normal puberty and menarche, generally at a slightly older age. Girls treated with whole abdominal and/or pelvic irradiation for HD or Wilm's tumor or other solid tumors are at a high risk of ovarian failure. Patients who receive HCT with total-body irradiation, both single-dose and fractionated, are at a high risk of developing permanent ovarian failure. Almost all patients who undergo HCT after the age of 10 years will develop premature ovarian failure, whereas only 50% of girls transplanted before the age of 10 years will.[75]

Ovarian failure has also been observed after chemotherapy, in particular, with alkylating agents. Toxicity is, again, dose- and age dependent. Only 30% of women and girls younger than 35 years of age at exposure to MOPP chemotherapy develop temporary amenorrhea, with irreversible ovarian failure seen in a small minority.[76] Females who receive high-dose, myeloablative therapy with alkylating agents in the context of allogeneic or autologous HCT are at high risk of developing ovarian failure.[76]

PREGNANCY OUTCOMES OF
CHILDHOOD CANCER SURVIVORS

Radiation therapy and many of the chemotherapeutic agents used in the treatment of childhood cancer could potentially be mutagenic and have an adverse effect on the health of the offspring of the survivors. Green et al.[77] evaluated the health of the offspring of partners of male childhood cancer survivors participating in the CCSS and demonstrated that the proportion of pregnancies of the partners of male survivors that ended with a liveborn infant was significantly lower than for the partners of male siblings of the survivors who served as controls. This study of male survivors did not identify adverse pregnancy outcomes for the partners of male survivors treated with most chemotherapeutic agents. A similar study focusing on offspring of the female survivors failed to identify adverse pregnancy outcomes for female survivors treated with most chemotherapeutic agents. The offspring of women who received pelvic irradiation were at risk for low birth weight.[78]

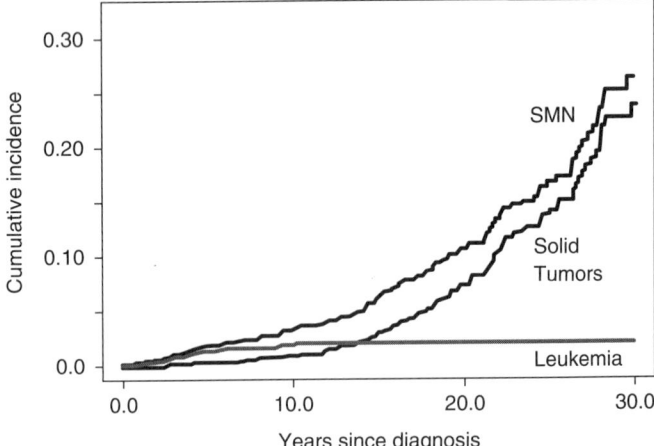

FIGURE 7.1. Cumulative incidence of subsequent malignant neoplasms after extended follow-up of Hodgkin's disease in childhood. (Adapted from Bhatia et al.,[81] by permissions of *Journal of Clinical Oncology*.)

Second Malignant Neoplasms

Several studies following large cohorts of childhood cancer survivors have reported a threefold- to sixfold-increased risk of a second cancer, when compared with the general population, and this risk continues to increase as the cohort ages[79–83] (Figure 7.1; see Chapter 17).

Late Mortality Among Childhood Cancer Survivors

Several investigators have shown a 10-fold excess in overall mortality among 5-year childhood cancer survivors when compared with the general population.[84,85] The excess mortality was due to death from primary cancer, second cancer, cardiotoxicity, and noncancer death.

Psychosocial Issues of Childhood Cancer Survivors

There is a large body of scientific literature addressing the subject of psychosocial outcomes for childhood cancer survivors. Findings are varied in part as a result of differing definitions for psychosocial outcomes among the studies. For example, in some studies the outcomes are defined in terms of psychologic health (e.g., depression, anxiety, posttraumatic stress, posttraumatic growth, and somatization). In other studies, the outcomes are defined in terms of social health (e.g., employment, education, and marriage). In addition, many pediatric cancer survivorship studies focusing on psychosocial outcomes are limited because of small sample size and/or lack of a comparison group. Many of the studies are from the health-related quality of life (HRQOL) literature because assessment of psychosocial outcomes is often included as part of a global HRQOL assessment. Notwithstanding these differences in definitions of study outcomes and study designs, the scientific literature concerning psychosocial outcomes in childhood cancer survivors is summarized in the following sections.

Psychologic Health

An emerging body of literature indicates that childhood cancer survivors are experiencing good psychologic health years after completion of their cancer treatment. One of the earliest studies, done by Teta et al.,[86] assessed the prevalence of major depression in 450 long-term childhood cancer survivors and found no difference in depression between survivors, their siblings, and general population norms. Elkin et al.,[87] using a standardized self-report measure (the Symptom Checklist-90-Revised or SCL-90-R), assessed psychologic functioning in adolescent and young adult survivors who attended a long-term follow-up clinic for pediatric cancer survivors at a single institution. Results of this study indicated that the study population was significantly psychologically healthier than age- and gender-matched norms for the general population based on SCL-90 scores. For the small percentage of survivors who displayed some psychologic symptoms, three factors were associated with an increased risk of maladjustment: older patient age at follow-up, greater number of relapses, and presence of severe functional impairment (defined as requiring frequent assistance with activities of daily living). The findings from these earlier studies were confirmed in a recently reported study by Zebrack et al.[88] on psychological outcomes in survivors of childhood leukemia and lymphoma, using data from the Childhood Cancer Survivor Study (CCSS).

Systematic literature reviews of the smaller studies published on this topic have also reported psychological well-being following treatment for childhood cancer; however, there are subgroups of survivors who may be at risk for poorer psychosocial health outcomes.[89–94] The largest and most recent of these studies to date was reported by Hudson et al.,[95] who analyzed data from the 9,535 adult survivors in the CCSS cohort compared with a randomly selected cohort of the survivors' siblings ($n = 2,916$). When compared with siblings, survivors in this study were significantly more likely to report adverse general health and moderate to severe impairment in mental health across all diagnostic groups. However, although general health was reported to be very good, with only 10.9 percent reporting fair or poor health, specific adverse effects were relatively common, as reflected by 43.6% of the cohort reporting impairment in one or more of the health domains evaluated in the study. Specifically, three

diagnostic groups (survivors of Hodgkin's disease, sarcomas, or bone tumors) were found to be at increased risk for continued cancer-related anxiety.[95] Furthermore, the authors emphasize that these three diagnoses are more common in the adolescent age group. Because adolescence is the developmental period during which abstract thinking develops, adolescents diagnosed with cancer may have a better understanding of the meaning of their diagnosis and the risks of treatment. The findings of this study confirmed the results of earlier studies[96–98] (Table 7.2). Thus, these studies suggest that there are certain at-risk groups of survivors who may be experiencing negative psychosocial sequelae and therefore may benefit from targeted psychosocial support interventions during long-term follow-up care.

The childhood cancer survivorship literature also suggests that use of a posttraumatic stress model is helpful in elucidating the long-term psychosocial sequelae for certain subsets of childhood cancer survivors[99–102] (Table 7.3). Family members, friends, and caregivers are also affected by the survivorship experience and are therefore included in the definition of survivorship.[2] It is, therefore, not surprising that there are reports of family members being affected by posttraumatic stress disorder (PTSD). Kazak et al.[94] did not find an increased prevalence of PTSD in a cohort of 133 childhood leukemia survivors when compared with a control group, but did find more PTSD symptoms in their mothers and fathers. Barakat et al.[93] found that past perceived life threat and family social support resources contributed to PTSD symptoms in both parents and survivors. All these studies suggest that the childhood cancer experience is complex and extends beyond the survivor, even years after the completion of therapy.

Social Health

Review of the childhood cancer survivorship literature indicates that overall this population is doing well in terms of social and emotional adjustment. Differences in educational needs, behavioral adjustment, employment status, and marriage rate for certain populations of childhood cancer survivors do occur. A recent longitudinal study of the social functioning of childhood cancer survivors 2 years following completion of therapy was conducted by Reiter-Purtill et al.[103] Children who completed cancer treatment were compared

TABLE 7.2. Summary of additional studies demonstrating adverse psychologic outcomes in childhood cancer survivors.

Study	Sample size	Primary disease	Comparison group	Adverse outcomes	Risk factors
Zeltzer et al.[96]	500	ALL, treated on CCG protocols	Siblings	Depression, tension, anger, and confusion	Females, minorities, unemployed
Mulhern et al.[97]	183	Any pediatric malignancy	Normative data from the general population	Deficits in social competence and behavioral abnormalities	Presence of functional impairments, older age at evaluation, treatment with cranial irradiation, residence in a single-parent household
Glover et al.[98]	555	Leukemia	Siblings	Mood disturbance	Females, nonwhite males, females with a special education history, high school dropouts with a special education history, age younger than 12.5 years of age at diagnosis, survivors with negative perceptions of current health

ALL, acute lymphoblastic leukemia; CCG, Children's Cancer Group.

TABLE 7.3. Studies supporting the posttraumatic stress model in childhood cancer survivors.

Study	Sample size	Age range	Percent with posttraumatic stress symptoms or disorder	Risk factors
Stuber et al.[99]	64	7–19 years	13%	Symptoms of increased anxiety and reexperiencing traumatic incidents, which persisted many years after the end of treatment without evidence of decrement over time
Hobbie et al.[101]	78	18–40 years	20.5%	Anxiety and other psychologic distress
Meeske et al.[102]	51	18–37 years	20%	Poorer QOL (as measured by the SF-36), increased psychologic distress

QOL, quality of life; SF-36, Short Form-36.

with children who were not chronically ill. The children's self-reports, as well as peer and teacher assessments of social functioning, were obtained while children were on therapy and then 2 years following completion of therapy. Findings of this study indicated minimal impact on the social functioning of the majority of childhood cancer survivors, but certain subpopulations were found to be vulnerable. Specifically, children who underwent high-intensity treatment were perceived by their peers as more "prosocial and less aggressive," although they had fewer nominations as "best friends." The authors hypothesized that this group of survivors may be less assertive about making and/or maintaining friendships or that their less-aggressive behavior may be due to fatigue. A study by Spirito et al.[104] reported similar findings when they compared 56 children (aged 5–12 years) to healthy controls using questionnaires assessing social adjustment, including the Self-Perception Profile. In this study, the only reported difference was of greater feelings of isolation in the childhood cancer survivors compared with the controls.

Conversely, reports of lower social competence were demonstrated by Mulhern et al.[105] In a cohort of survivors (n = 183) 2 or more years off-therapy, social competence and behavioral adjustment were assessed using a standardized questionnaire (The Child Behavior Checklist). Functional (but not cosmetic) impairments were found to increase the risk for academic and adjustment problems. Other risk factors for social and emotional problems included: older age at assessment (correlated with time since diagnosis and time since completion of therapy), treatment with cranial irradiation, and living in a single-parent household. Similarly, a study by Pendley et al.[106] found that adolescent survivors who had been off treatment for longer periods of time reported more social anxiety as well as more-negative body image and lower self-worth.

Educational attainment as an outcome of social health has also been assessed in the leukemia survivor study[107] and in the CCSS[108,109] (Table 7.4). The findings from these studies indicate that survivors are more likely to use special educational services, but overall are just as likely to graduate from high school when compared with their siblings.

Multiple studies have assessed the vocational status of childhood cancer survivors. One of the earliest studies assessing occupational status was completed by Meadows et al.[110] The cohort of survivors demonstrated no differences in educational achievement or occupational status by diagnostic group, age at diagnosis, or treatment received. Nicholson et al.[111] compared osteosarcoma and Ewing sarcoma survivors with sibling controls and found that employment status and annual income were similar in the two groups despite the physical impairments following limb amputation for many of the sarcoma survivors. Hays et al.[112] reported similar employment findings in more than 200 childhood cancer survivors. Specifically, the employment status of the survivors was similar to individually matched controls. There were, however, findings of employment discrimination for entry into the military for survivors during the initial years following completion of therapy. The authors concluded that childhood cancer survivors who were treated in the era between 1945 and 1975 had few economic sequelae that extended beyond the first decades after treatment.

TABLE 7.4. Childhood Cancer Survivor Study (CCSS) studies assessing educational attainment as an outcome measure for social health.

Study	Sample size	Primary disease	Comparison group	Educational outcome assessed	Findings	Risk factors
Mitby et al[108]	12,000	Any pediatric malignancy	3,000 siblings	Use of special education services	23% of survivors compared with 8% of siblings used special education services	Diagnosis <6 years of age; brain tumor, leukemia, and HD survivors; treatment variables of use of IT MTX and CXRT (with a positive dose–response relationship found)
Nagarajan et al.[109]	694	Osteosarcoma or Ewing's sarcoma	Age at diagnosis (≤12 years compared with >12 years), type of surgery (amputation vs. limb-sparing), and 2,667 siblings	Graduation from high school or college	No differences found between the different age or surgery groups.	More than 12 years/amputation group was less likely to graduate from high school and college compared with siblings, but there were still high rates of reports of graduation from high school in the survivors group (93%) and for those survivors older than 25 years of age, and 50% reported being a college graduate

HD, Hodgkin disease; IT MTX, intrathecal methotrexate; CXRT, cranial irradiation.

The literature regarding employment outcome for childhood cancer survivors yields mixed conclusions (see also Chapter 20). For example, a study by Novakovic et al.[113] found that although nearly 90 survivors of Ewing's sarcoma did not differ in educational achievement, they were less likely to be employed full time when compared with sibling controls. Conversely, Evans and Radford[114] assessed educational achievement and employment in a small group of survivors and found that survivors were significantly less likely to complete higher education than their siblings, but had similar rates of employment and were earning similar salaries. The differences in the findings may represent the small sample sizes in the various studies.

Marital status has also been assessed as a measure of social well-being for survivors of childhood cancer. In one of the earlier studies, Makipernaa[115] interviewed 94 survivors of solid tumors diagnosed between 1960 and 1976. When the survivor population was compared with the general Finnish population, fewer female survivors were married. Green et al.[116] found that the percentages of married male and female survivors were both significantly lower than the U.S. population norms. Byrne et al.[117] studied a much larger population of childhood cancer survivors and found that both male and female survivors were less likely to be married when compared with a sibling control group. The study also demonstrated that survivors of central nervous system (CNS) malignancies accounted for the majority of unmarried survivors, with the males in this diagnostic group having the greatest relative risk. The findings of these two earlier studies were also confirmed more recently in a large CCSS cohort. Rauck et al.[118] described the marital status of more than 10,000 childhood cancer survivors within the CCSS cohort and compared them to the U.S. population according to age-specific groups. Compared with the U.S. population, childhood cancer survivors, particularly females and Caucasians, were less likely to have ever been married. CNS tumor survivors as a subgroup, and particularly males within this group, were less likely to have ever been married and were more likely to divorce or separate when compared with childhood cancer survivors who had other diagnoses, as well as with the general U.S. population. Felder-Puig et al.[119] also found a lower incidence of marriage in survivors of bone cancer. Interestingly, survivors in this study reported staying home longer after reaching adulthood than did the control group of a similar age. The investigators postulated that the survivors would, therefore, postpone marriage for a longer time than their peers. A study by Gray et al.[120] yields further insight regarding interpersonal relationships in survivors of childhood cancer. In this study, survivors reported higher intimacy motivation, but were more likely to express dissatisfaction with important relationships, when compared with a peer group. Nonetheless, despite differences in marriage rates, studies support the fact that, overall, survivors of pediatric malignancies are doing well in terms of psychosocial functioning and that only certain subgroups are at greatest risk for adverse psychosocial sequelae.

Special Populations

Two special populations of survivors (childhood acute lymphoblastic leukemia and brain tumors) warrant special attention due to their increased risk for adverse psychosocial outcomes as a result of previous CNS treatment: Acute lymphoblastic leukemia (ALL) is the most commonly diagnosed pediatric malignancy, with an annual incidence of 3,250 children and adolescents diagnosed each year in the United States and a survival rate of approximately 85%.[1] Brain tumors are the second most commonly diagnosed pediatric malignancy, and the most common solid neoplasm. Approximately 2,200 children and adolescents under 20 years of age are diagnosed within the United States each year. The overall survival rate is approximately 68%.[1] Thus, there are rapidly growing numbers of survivors treated for both of the most commonly diagnosed pediatric malignancies.

ACUTE LYMPHOBLASTIC LEUKEMIA SURVIVORS

Improvement in the survival rates for ALL in the 1980s and 1990s has resulted in the emergence of studies focused on the neuropsychologic consequences in this population. Brown et al.[121] followed a small cohort of ALL survivors who received prophylactic chemotherapy to the CNS. Survivors, when compared with their siblings, showed impairment in right hemispheric simultaneous processing when evaluated at the off-therapy time point. These differences were not found while the patient was actively undergoing treatment for ALL, a finding that illustrates the importance of continued long-term neuropsychologic evaluation for this group of survivors, as deficits may not be evident on initial assessments. Cetingul et al.[122] studied a small sample of 5-year Turkish survivors of childhood ALL and compared them to their siblings. In this study, total IQ scores of survivors were significantly lower than the sibling control group, although small numbers limit the conclusions drawn from this study. Kingma et al.[123] also studied academic performance in a small sample of Dutch ALL survivors who were treated with cranial irradiation (18 or 25 Gy) and intrathecal methotrexate as CNS prophylaxis, and compared them to siblings. Survivors were more likely to be placed in special education programs than were siblings, although there was no effect of sex or irradiation dose. The investigators concluded that cranial irradiation and chemotherapy administered at a young age were associated with poorer academic career outcomes for survivors. Haupt et al.[107] completed a large multicenter retrospective trial of adult survivors of childhood ALL with sibling controls, assessing practical, easily understandable educational outcomes that included "enrollment in special programs, grades during high school, graduation from high school, college admission, and college graduation."[107] Similar to the findings of smaller studies, ALL survivors in this study were more likely to enter special education or learning-disabled programs when compared with siblings. Higher doses of cranial irradiation (24 Gy versus 18 Gy versus none) and young age (less than 6 years of age) at diagnosis were found to be the most important predictors for poor educational outcomes, defined as a lesser likelihood of entering college.

It should also be noted that craniospinal irradiation, used in early treatment regimens for ALL to prevent CNS leukemia, resulted in neurodevelopmental delays in children. In the early 1980s, Robison et al.[124] and Moss et al.[125] demonstrated that prophylactic treatment of the CNS with craniospinal irradiation was associated with decreased IQ scores. These early studies documenting the risk of neurocognitive late effects, coupled with the high cure rates, have led to the elimination of prophylactic craniospinal irradiation from most current ALL treatment regimens. Therefore, the importance of assessing long-term psychosocial outcomes of childhood cancer treatment cannot be overemphasized, because there may be direct and practical applications for intervention and long-term follow-up care.

BRAIN TUMOR SURVIVORS

The second special population of childhood cancer survivors who warrant further discussion regarding psychosocial outcomes are those treated for pediatric brain tumors. Roman and Sperduto[126] reviewed the literature on the neuropsychologic effects of cranial radiation. Research on low-dose whole-brain radiation (such as that used for childhood ALL patients) was compared with studies on high-dose focal or whole-brain radiation used in the treatment of brain lesions. In this review, the investigators found that the low-dose whole-brain radiation (18–24 Gy) resulted in the mild decline of IQ and that subsequent learning disabilities may be the result of poor attention and memory instead of low intellectual level. Conversely, pediatric survivors who received higher-dose radiation for the treatment of brain tumors, particularly those who received whole-brain radiation, were found to be at risk for poorer cognitive outcomes. In a subsequent study by Anderson et al.,[127] higher-dose radiation used for treatment of brain tumors (when compared with that used for other malignancies) was more often found to be associated with late cognitive effects. Further research has shown that neurocognitive deficits occurring among brain tumor survivors most commonly involve the areas of memory, attention, and academic achievement.[126,128] Whether cognitive deficits in these brain tumor survivors are primarily caused by disruption of "executive function" (ability to organize and prioritize activities to be functionally effective) is suspected but not yet proven. Data forthcoming from the CCSS will help to answer this question.

A study by Glaser et al.[129] evaluated school behavior in a small sample of brain tumor survivors compared with a control group of school-age siblings. The brain tumor survivors had good social reintegration but also had evidence of impaired cognition, emotion, and lower self-esteem. Even though they worried more than the control group, the brain tumor survivors attended school willingly and interacted with their peers normally. Zebrack et al.[88] assessed psychologic outcomes in more than 1,000 adult long-term survivors of childhood brain tumors within the CCSS cohort and compared them with almost 3,000 sibling controls and normative data from the general population. The majority of survivors and siblings reported few symptoms of psychologic distress 5 or more years after the original cancer diagnosis. The prevalence of psychologic distress was similar to that found in the general population. Yet, when accounting for significant sociodemographic, socioeconomic, and health status variables, survivors of childhood brain cancer, in aggregate, appear to report significantly higher global distress and depression scores than do siblings. Factors associated with higher levels of psychologic distress for both survivors and siblings included female sex, low household income, lower educational attainment, being unmarried, having no employment in the past 12 months, and poor physical health status. There were no diagnostic- or treatment-related variables that were associated with an increase in distress symptoms for this group of childhood brain tumor survivors.

Providing Follow-Up Care for Childhood Cancer Survivors

Essential Elements of Follow-Up Care

General agreement exists that survivors of childhood cancer require ongoing lifelong follow-up to provide early intervention for, or prevention of, potential late effects of treatment.[130–134] The Children's Oncology Group (COG) has developed systematic evidence-based, exposure-related guidelines for ongoing follow-up of pediatric cancer survivors. These guidelines allow the clinician to determine a specific follow-up plan for each survivor, tailored to risk of late effects based on therapeutic exposures. A comprehensive treatment summary (Table 7.5) is also an essential tool for providing

TABLE 7.5. Components of a comprehensive treatment summary.

Essential elements	Details
Demographics	Treating institution, treatment team
Diagnosis	Date, site(s), stage
Relapse(s)	Date(s)
Subsequent malignant neoplasms	Date(s), types
Protocol(s)	Title(s)/number(s), dates initiated and completed
Completion of therapy	Date
Chemotherapy	Names and administration routes for all agents Cumulative doses (per m²) for alkylators, anthracyclines, and bleomycin Determination of intermediate/high (≥1,000 mg/m²) dose vs. standard dose for cytarabine and methotrexate
Radiation	Dates, type, fields, total dose, number of fractions/dose per fraction
Surgical procedures	Type(s), date(s)
Hematopoietic cell transplant	Type(s), date(s), GVHD prophylaxis/treatment
Major medical events	Events with potential for residual/late effects
Adverse drug reactions/allergies	Name of drug, type of reaction

GVHD, graft-versus-host disease.

comprehensive survivorship care. The Children's Oncology Group Long-Term Follow-Up Guidelines, accompanying health education materials (known as "Health Links"), and a model comprehensive treatment summary form are available to clinicians free of charge on the Children's Oncology Group website at www.survivorshipguidelines.org.

Models of Clinical Care Delivery

In 1997, the American Academy of Pediatrics mandated that children with cancer should be treated in specialized centers for pediatric oncology care[135]; between 1989 and 1991, 94% of children diagnosed with cancer under the age of 15 in the United States were seen at an institution that was affiliated with the cooperative pediatric oncology clinical trials groups.[136] Specialized pediatric oncology centers that are members of the Children's Oncology Group are required to provide long-term follow-up services for survivors of pediatric cancer[137]; this can be accomplished in a variety of ways.[11,134,138–142]

SPECIALIZED LONG-TERM FOLLOW-UP CLINICS

In some pediatric oncology centers, the original treatment team, or a designated multidisciplinary long-term follow-up team at the treatment center, continue to provide life long follow-up to the childhood cancer survivor. Generally, the ongoing follow-up is limited to an annual comprehensive multidisciplinary health evaluation, and the survivor is encouraged to establish an ongoing relationship with a primary healthcare provider in their local community for routine healthcare needs. The long term follow-up care is often directed by a nurse practitioner specializing in healthcare for childhood cancer survivors. Benefits of this approach are that the patient remains in contact with a team that is knowledgeable and committed to long-term follow-up care, contact with the original treatment center is maintained, opportunities for research are optimized, and multidisciplinary referrals are usually available within the healthcare system (although referrals for patients who are beyond the pediatric age range may be limited in pediatric centers). Disadvantages of this approach include the unfamiliarity of the pediatric treatment team with the healthcare issues that arise as the survivor ages, reluctance of the older patient to return to a pediatric facility (especially if pediatric patients are present in the clinic/waiting room at the time of the long-term follow-up clinic), problems with reimbursement for specialized services not covered by insurance companies, and, often, problems of access due to long distances between the medical center and the survivor's residence. An example of successful implementation of this model is the Survivorship Clinic at the City of Hope National Medical Center in Duarte, California. As an NIH-designated Comprehensive Cancer Center, City of Hope provides specialized cancer-related care to patients throughout the lifespan, allowing ongoing long-term follow-up of patients with pediatric malignancies as they enter and progress through adulthood.

TRANSITION MODELS

Pediatric oncology centers, often as a result of institutional policies with an upper age limit for care, may require transition of young adult survivors to adult care providers. In some instances, institutions have established formalized transition programs with specialized long-term follow-up programs for adult survivors of childhood cancer [e.g., Children's Medical Center of Dallas transitions its survivors to the ACE (After the Cancer Experience) Program for Young Adult Survivors at the University of Texas Southwestern, and Children's Memorial Hospital in Chicago transitions its survivors to the STAR (Survivors Taking Action and Responsibility) Program for Young Adult Survivors at Northwestern University]. Transition programs often use collaborative practice models, drawing on expertise from both oncology and primary care providers, and maintain many of the benefits of the specialized long-term follow-up clinics, with the added benefit of care providers with expertise in adult medicine. Affiliation of these programs with academic institutions usually provides access to multidisciplinary referrals; however, because the setting is academic and the focus is on survivorship care, ongoing primary care is often not accessible through these specialized programs, and distance to the center may remain problematic for some survivors.

ADULT ONCOLOGY DIRECTED CARE

In this model, when the survivor reaches adulthood, the pediatric provider makes a referral to an adult oncologist for ongoing follow-up. Advantages of this system include ongoing monitoring for disease recurrence in a system designed for adult medical care, and accessibility to care in the local community. Disadvantages include the unfamiliarity of most adult oncologists with the long-term follow-up evaluations indicated for childhood cancer survivors, and the likelihood of early discharge from specialty care once there is minimal risk of disease recurrence. However, with appropriate education and collaboration, this model has been used successfully to provide ongoing long-term follow-up care for childhood cancer survivors. An example of this model is the cooperative agreement between the Children's Hospital of Philadelphia and the oncology service of the University of Pennsylvania Medical Center.

COMMUNITY-BASED CARE

In this model, follow-up care is provided by an adult primary care provider (e.g., internist, family practitioner), who ideally is in ongoing communication with the original pediatric oncology treatment team or long-term follow-up center. Advantages of this system include seamless care for the patient, who can see their local primary care provider for most healthcare services and develop an ongoing relationship with a provider who is familiar with their specialized healthcare needs. Disadvantages include the primary care provider's lack of familiarity with the potential late effects for which the survivor is at risk, the considerable effort required for the primary care provider to determine appropriate follow-up care for the survivor, the survivor's potential lack of access to multidisciplinary specialty care providers, and the potential loss of contact with the survivor. The community-based system of care has been used successfully by St. Jude Children's Research Hospital (Memphis, TN) to provide care for survivors who are more than 10 years posttreatment. In this setting, potential disadvantages of this system have been addressed by providing a dedicated staff at St. Jude to track the status of these survivors and to provide ongoing consultation with community healthcare providers as required.

Acknowledgment. Supported in part by 5 U10 CA13539-26S2.

References

1. Reis LAG, Eisner MP, Kosary CL, et al. SEER Cancer Statistics Review, 1973–1998. Bethesda, MD: National Cancer Institute, MD, 2001.

2. Hewitt M, Weiner SL, Simone JV. Childhood Cancer Survivorship: Improving Care and Quality of Life. Washington, DC: National Academies Press, 2003.

3. Sklar CA. An overview of the effects of cancer therapies: the nature, scale, and breadth of the problem. Acta Paediatr Scand Suppl 1999;433:1–4.

4. Garré ML, Gandus S, Cesana B, et al. Health status of long-term survivors after cancer in childhood. Am J Pediatr Hematol Oncol 1994;16:143–152.

5. Oeffinger KC, Eshelman DA, Tomlinson GE, et al. Grading of late effects in young adult survivors of childhood cancer followed in an ambulatory adult setting. Cancer (Phila) 2000;88:1687–1695.

6. Stevens MCG, Mahler H, Parkes S. The health status of adult survivors of cancer in childhood. Eur J Cancer 1998;34:694–698.

7. Vonderweid N, Beck D, Caflisch U, et al. Standardized assessment of late effects in long-term survivors of childhood cancer in Switzerland: results of a Swiss Pediatric Oncology Group (SPOG) pilot study. Int J Pediatr Hematol/Oncol 1996;3:483–490.

8. Brown RT, Sawyer MB, Antoniou G, et al. A 3-year follow-up of the intellectual and academic functioning of children receiving central nervous system prophylactic chemotherapy for leukemia. J Dev Behav Pediatr 196;17(6):392–398.

9. Kramer J, Moore IM. Late effects of cancer therapy on the central nervous system. Semin Oncol Nurs 1989;5:22–28.

10. Moore IM, Packer RJ, Karl D, et al. Adverse effects of cancer treatment on the central nervous system. In: Schwartz CL HW, Constine LS, Ruccione KS (eds). Survivors of Childhood Cancer: Assessment and Management. St. Louis: Mosby, 1994:81–95.

11. Fochtman D. Follow-up care for survivors of childhood cancer. Nurse Pract Forum 1996;6:194–200.

12. Packer RJ, Sutton LN, Atkins TE, et al. A prospective study of cognitive function in children receiving whole-brain radiotherapy and chemotherapy: 2-year results. J Neurosurg 1989;70:707–713.

13. Mulhern RK, Reddick WE, Palmer SL, et al. Neurocognitive deficits in medulloblastoma survivors and white matter loss. Ann Neurol 1999;46:834–841.

14. Shan K, Lincoff AM, Young JB. Anthracycline-induced cardiotoxicity. Ann Intern Med 1966;125:47–58.

15. Grenier MA, Lipshultz SE. Epidemiology of anthracycline cardiotoxicity in children and adults. Semin Oncol 1998;25:72–85.

16. Pai VB, Nahata MC. Cardiotoxicity of chemotherapeutic agents: incidence, treatment and prevention. Drug Saf 2000;22:263–302.

17. Prout MN, Richards MJS, Chung KJ, et al. Adriamycin cardiotoxicity in children. Cancer (Phila) 1977;39:62.

18. Minow RA, Benjamin RS, Gottlieb JA. Adriamycin (NSC-123127) cardiotoxicity: a clinicopathologic correlation. Cancer Chemother Rep 1975;6:195.

19. Bossi G, Lanzarini L, Laudisa ML, et al. Echocardiographic evaluation of patients cured of childhood cancer: a single center study of 117 subjects who received anthracyclines. Med Pediatr Oncol 2001;36:593–600.

20. Kremer LCM, van Dalen EC, Offringa M, et al. Anthracycline-induced clinical heart failure in a cohort of 607 children: long-term follow-up study. J Clin Oncol 2001;19:191–196.

21. Fajardo L, Stewart J, Cohn K. Morphology of radiation-induced heart disease. Arch Pathol 1968;86:512–519.

22. Kushner JR, Hansen VL, Hammar SP. Cardiomyopathy after widely separated courses of Adriamycin exacerbated by actinomycin D and mithramycin. Cancer (Phila) 1975;36:1577.

23. Smith PJ, Eckert H, Waters KD, et al. High incidence of cardiomyopathy in children treated with Adriamycin and DTIC in combination chemotherapy. Cancer Treat Rep 1977;61:1736.

24. Von Hoff D, Rozencweig M, Piccart M. The cardiotoxicity of anticancer agents. Semin Oncol 1982;9:23.

25. Lipshultz SE, Lipshultz SR, Mone SM, et al. Female sex and higher drug dose as risk factors for late cardiotoxic effects of doxorubicin therapy for childhood cancer. N Engl J Med 1995;332:1738–1743.

26. Pratt CB, Ransom JL, Evans WE. Age-related Adriamycin cardiotoxicity in children. Cancer Treat Rep 1978;62:1381.

27. Von Hoff DD, Rozencweig M, Layard M, et al. Daunomycin induced cardiotoxicity in children and adults. Am J Med 1977;62:200.

28. Martin RG, Rukdeschel JC, Chang P, et al. Radiation-related pericarditis. Am J Cardiol 1975;35:216.

29. Marks RDJ, Agarwal SK, Constable WC. Radiation induced pericarditis in Hodgkin's disease. Acta Radiol Ther Phys Biol 1973;12:305.

30. Mill WB, Baglan RJ, Kurichetz P, et al. Symptomatic radiation induced pericarditis in Hodgkin's disease. Int J Radiat Oncol Biol Phys 1984;10:2061.

31. Kadota RP, Burgert EO, Driscoll DJ, et al. Cardiopulmonary function in long-term survivors of childhood Hodgkin's lymphoma: a pilot study. Mayo Clin Proc 1988;63:362.

32. Perraut DJ, Levy M, Herman JD, et al. Echocardiac abnormalities following cardiac radiation. J Clin Oncol 1985;3:546.

33. Scott DL, Thomas RD. Late onset constrictive pericarditis after thoracic radiotherapy. Br Med J 1978;1:341.

34. Haas JM. Symptomatic constrictive pericarditis developing 45 years after radiation therapy to the mediastinum: a review of radiation pericarditis. Am Heart J 1969;77:89.

35. Boivin JF, Hutchinson GB, Lubin JH, et al. Coronary artery disease in patients treated for Hodgkin's disease. Cancer (Phila) 1992;69:1241–1247.

36. Bu'Lock FA, Gabriel HM, Oakhill A, et al. Cardioprotection by ICRF187 against high dose anthracycline toxicity in children with malignant disease. Br Heart J 1993;70:185–188.

37. Wexler L. Ameliorating anthracycline cardiotoxicity in children with cancer: clinical trials with dexrazoxane. Semin Oncol 1998;25:86–92.

38. Iarussi D, Indolfi P, Coppolino P, et al. Recent advances in the prevention of anthracycline cardiotoxocity in childhood. Curr Med Chem 2001;8:1667–1678.

39. Littman P, Meadows AT, Polgar G, et al. Pulmonary function in survivors of Wilm's tumor: patterns of impairment. Cancer (Phila) 1976;37:2773.

40. Benoit MR, Lemerle J, Jean R, et al. Effects on pulmonary function of whole lung irradiation for Wilms' tumor in children. Thorax 1982;37:175.

41. Miller RW, Fusner JE, Fink RJ, et al. Pulmonary function abnormalities in long-term survivors of childhood cancer. Med Pediatr Oncol 1986;14:202.

42. Springmeyer SC, Flourney N, Sullivan KM, et al. Pulmonary function changes in long-term survivors of allogeneic marrow transplantation. In: Gale RP (ed). Recent Advances in Bone Marrow Transplantation. New York: Liss, 1983:343.

43. Robison LL, Mertens AC, Boice JD Jr, et al. Study design and cohort characteristics of the Childhood Cancer Survivor Study:

a multi-institutional collaborative project. Med Pediatr Oncol 2002;38(4):229–339.

44. Mertens AC, Yasui Y, Liu Y, et al. Pulmonary complications in survivors of childhood and adolescent cancer. A report from the Childhood Cancer Survivor Study. Cancer (Phila) 2002;95: 2431–2441.

45. Gisberg SJ, Comis RL. The pulmonary toxicity of antineoplastic agents. Semin Oncol 1982;9:34.

46. Bauer KA, Sskarin AT, Balikian JP, et al. Pulmonary complications associated with combination chemotherapy programs containing bleomycin. Am J Med 1983;74:557.

47. Goldiner PL, Schweizer O. Hazards of anesthesia and surgery in bleomycin-treated patients. Semin Oncol 1979;6:121.

48. Samuels ML, Johnson DE, Holoye PY, et al. Large doses of bleomycin therapy and pulmonary toxicity: a possible role of prior radiotherapy. JAMA 1976;235:1117.

49. Aronin PA, Mahaley MSJ, Rudnick SA, et al. Prediction of BCNU pulmonary toxicity in patients with malignant gliomas: an assessment of risk factors. N Engl J Med 1980;303:183.

50. Hancock S, Cox R, McDougall I. Thyroid diseases after treatment of Hodgkin's disease. N Engl J Med 1991;325:599.

51. Glatstein E, McHardy-Young S, Brast N, et al. Alterations in serum thyrotropin (TSH) and thyroid function following radiotherapy in patients with malignant lymphoma. J Clin Endocrinol Metab 1971;32:833.

52. Rosenthal MB, Goldfine ID. Primary and secondary hypothyroidism in nasophanryngeal carcinoma. JAMA 1976;236:1591.

53. Gurney JG, Kadan-Lottick NS, Packer RJ, et al. Endocrine and cardiovascular late effects among adult survivors of childhood brain tumors: Childhood Cancer Survivor Study. Cancer (Phila) 2003;97:663–673.

54. Sklar C, Whitton J, Mertens A, et al. Abnormalities of the thyroid in survivors of Hodgkin's disease: data from the Childhood Cancer Survivor Study. J Clin Endocrinol Metab 2000;85: 3227–3232.

55. Chin D, Sklar C, Donahue B, et al. Thyroid dysfunction as a late effect in survivors of pediatric medulloblastoma/primitive neuroectodermal tumors: a comparison of hyperfractionated versus conventional radiotherapy. Cancer (Phila) 1997;80:798–804.

56. Sklar CA. Growth and neuroendocrine dysfunction following therapy for childhood cancer. Pediatr Clin N Am 1997;44: 489–503.

57. Danoff BF, Cowchock FS, Marquette C, et al. Assessment of the long-term effects of primary radiation therapy for brain tumors in children. Cancer (Phila) 1982;49:1580.

58. Onoyama Y, Mitsuyuki A, Takahashi M, et al. Radiation therapy of brain tumors in children. Radiology 1977;115:687.

59. Oberfield SE, Allen JC, Pollack J, et al. Long-term endocrine sequelae after treatment of medulloblastoma: prospective study of growth and thyroid function. J Pediatr 1986;108:219.

60. Oliff A, Bode U, Bercu BB, et al. Hypothalamic-pituitary dysfunction following CNS prophylaxis in acute lymphocytic leukemia: correlation with CT scan abnormalities. Med Pediatr Oncol 1979;7:141.

61. Robison LL, Nesbit ME, Sather HN, et al. Height of children successfully treated for acute lymphoblastic leukemia: a report from the late effects study committee of Children's Cancer Study Group. Med Pediatr Oncol 1985;13:14.

62. Berry DH, Elders MJ, Crist W, et al. Growth in children with acute lymphocytic leukemia: a Pediatric Oncology Group study. Med Pediatr Oncol 1983;11:39.

63. Papadakis V, Tan C, Heller G, et al. Growth and final height after treatment for childhood Hodgkin's disease. J Pediatr Hematol Oncol 1996;18:272–276.

64. Sklar C, Mertens A, Walter A, et al. Final height after treatment for childhood acute lymphoblastic leukemia: comparison of no cranial irradiation with 1800 and 2400 centigrays of cranial irradiation. J Pediatr 1993;123:59–64.

65. Blatt J, Bercu BB, Gillin JC, et al. Reduced pulsatile growth hormone secretion in children after therapy for acute lymphocytic leukemia. J Pediatr 1984;104:182.

66. Sklar CA, Mertens AC, Walter A, et al. Changes in body mass index and prevalence of overweight in survivors of childhood acute lymphoblastic leukemia: role of cranial irradiation. Med Pediatr Oncol 2000;35:91–95.

67. Oeffinger KC, Mertens AC, Sklar CA, et al. Obesity in adult survivors of childhood acute lymphoblastic leukemia: a report from the Childhood Cancer Survivor Study. J Clin Oncol 2003;21:1359–1365.

68. Cifton DK, Bremner WJ. The effect of testicular x-irradiation on spermatogenesis in man. J Androl 1983;4:387.

69. Rowley MM, Leach DR, Warner GA, et al. Effect of graded doses of ionizing radiation on the human testes. Radiat Res 1974; 59:665.

70. Blatt J, Sherins RJ, Niebrugge D, et al. Leydig cell function in boys following treatment for testicular relapse of acute lymphoblastic leukemia. J Clin Oncol 1985;3:1227.

71. Sherins RJ, DeVita VT. Effects of drug treatment for lymphoma on male reproductive capacity. Ann Intern Med 1973;79:216.

72. da Cunha MF, Meisrich ML, Fuller LM, et al. Recovery of spermatogenesis after treatment for Hodgkin's disease with limiting dose of MOPP chemotherapy. J Clin Oncol 1984;2:571.

73. Santaro A, Bonadonna G, Valagussa P, et al. Long-term results of combined chemotherapy-radiotherapy approach in Hodgkin's disease: superiority of ABVD plus radiotherapy versus MOPP plus radiotherapy. J Clin Oncol 1987;5:27.

74. Stillman RJ, Schilfeld JS, Schiff I, et al. Ovarian failure in long-term survivors of childhood malignancy. Am J Obstet Gynecol 1981;139:62.

75. Sarafoglou K, Boulad F, Gillio A, et al. Gonadal function after bone marrow transplantation for acute leukemia during childhood. J Pediatr 1997;130:210–216.

76. Sklar C. Reproductive physiology and treatment-related loss of sex hormone production. Med Pediatr Oncol 1999;33:2–8.

77. Green D, Whitton J, S M, et al. Pregnancy outcomes of partners of male survivors of childhood cancer: a report from the Childhood Cancer Survivor Study. J Clin Oncol 2003;21:716–721.

78. Green D, Whitton JA, Stovall M, et al. Pregnancy outcome of female survivors of childhood cancer: A report from the childhood cancer survivor study. Am J Obstet Gynecol 2002;187:1070–1080.

79. Neglia JP, Friedman DL, Yutaka Y, et al. Second malignant neoplasms in five-year survivors of childhood cancer: childhood cancer survivor study. J Natl Cancer Inst 2001;93:618–629.

80. Olsen JH, Garwicz S, Hertz H, et al. Second malignant neoplasms after cancer in childhood or adolescence. Nordic Society of Paediatric Haematology and Oncology Association of the Nordic Cancer Registries. BMJ 1993;307:1030–1036.

81. Bhatia S, Yasui Y, Robison LL, et al. High risk of subsequent neoplasms continues with extended follow-up of childhood Hodgkin's disease: report from the Late Effects Study Group. J Clin Oncol 2003;21:4386–4394.

82. Bhatia S, Ramsay NKC, Steinbuch M, et al. Malignant neoplasms following bone marrow transplantation. Blood 1996;87: 3633–3639.

83. Darrington DL, Vose JM, Anderson JR, et al. Incidence and characterization of secondary myelodysplastic syndrome and acute myelogenous leukemia following high-dose chemoradiotherapy and autologous stem cell transplantation for lymphoid malignancies. J Clin Oncol 1994;12:2527–2534.

84. Mertens AC, Yasui Y, Neglia JP, et al. Late mortality experience in five-year survivors of childhood and adolescent cancer: the childhood cancer survivors study. J Clin Oncol 2001;19: 3163–3172.

85. Moller TR, Garwicz S, Barlow L, et al. Decreasing late mortality among five-year survivors of cancer in childhood and

adolescence: a population-based study in the Nordic countries. J Clin Oncol 2001;19:3173–3181.

86. Teta MJ, Del Po MC, Kasl SV, et al. Psychosocial consequences of childhood and adolescent cancer survival. J Chronic Dis 1986; 39:751–759.

87. Elkin T, Phipps S, Mulhern R. Psychological functioning of adolescent and young adult survivors of pediatric malignancy. Med Pediatr Oncol 1997;29:582–588.

88. Zebrack BL, Zeltzer LK, Whitton J, et al. Psychological outcomes in long-term survivors of childhood leukemia, Hodgkin's disease, and non-Hodgkin's lymphoma: a report from the Childhood Survivor Study. Pediatrics 2002;110:42–52.

89. Eiser C, Hill J, Vance YH. Examining the psychological consequences of surviving childhood cancer: systematic review as a research method in pediatric psychology. J Pediatr Psychol 2000; 25:449–460.

90. Zeltzer LK. Cancer in adolescents and young adults psychosocial aspects. Long term survivors. Cancer (Phila) 1993;15: 3463–3468.

91. Chang PN. Psychosocial needs of long-term childhood cancer survivors: a review of the literature. Pediatrician 1991;18:20–24.

92. Fritz GK, Williams JR, Amylon MD. After treatment ends: psychosocial sequelae in pediatric cancer survivors. Am J Orthopsychiatry 1988;58:552–561.

93. Barakat LP, Kazak AE, Meadows AT, et al. Families surviving childhood cancer: a comparison of posttraumatic stress symptoms with familes of healthy children. J Pediatr Psychol 1997;22:843–859.

94. Kazak AE, Barakat LP, Meeske K, et al. Post traumatic stress, family functioning and social support in survivors of childhood leukemia and their mothers and fathers. J Consult Clin Psychol 1997;65:120–129.

95. Hudson MM, Mertens AC, Yasui Y, et al. Health status of adult long-term survivors of childhood cancer. A report from the childhood cancer survivor study. JAMA 2003;290:1583–1592.

96. Zeltzer LK, Chen E, Weiss R, et al. Comparison of psychologic outcome in adult survivors of childhood acute lymphoblastic leukemia versus sibling controls: a cooperative Children's Cancer Group and National Institutes of Health study. J Clin Oncol 1997;15:547–556.

97. Mulhern RK, Wasserman AL, Friedman AG, et al. Social competence and behavioral adjustment of children who are long-term survivors of cancer. Pediatrics 1989;83:18–25.

98. Glover DA, Byrne J, Mills JL, et al. Impact of CNS treatment on mood in adult survivors of childhood leukemia: a report from the Children's Cancer Group. J Clin Oncol 2003;21:4395–4401.

99. Stuber ML, Christakis DA, Houskamp B, et al. Posttrauma symptoms in childhood leukemia survivors and their parents. Psychosomatics 1996;37:254–261.

100. Stuber ML, Kazak AE, Meeske K, et al. Predictors of posttraumatic stress symptoms in childhood cancer survivors. Pediatrics 1997;100:958–964.

101. Hobbie WL, Stuber M, Meeske K, et al. Symptoms of posttraumatic stress in young adult survivors of childhood cancer. J Clin Oncol 2000;18:4060–4066.

102. Meeske KA, Ruccione K, Globe DR, et al. Posttraumatic stress, quality of life, and psychological distress in young adult survivors of childhood cancer. Oncol Nurs Forum 2001;28:481–489.

103. Reiter-Purtill J, Vannatta K, Gerhardt CA, et al. A controlled longitudinal study of the social functioning of children who completed treatment of cancer. J Pediatr Hematol/Oncol 2003; 25:467–473.

104. Spirito A, Stark LJ, Cobiella C, et al. Social adjustment of children successfully treated for cancer. J Pediatr Psychol 1990; 15:359–371.

105. Mulhern R, Wasserman A, Friedman A, et al. Social competence and behavioral adjustment of children who are long-term survivors of cancer. Pediatrics 1989;83:18–25.

106. Pendley JS, Dahlquist LM, Dreyer ZA. Body image and psychosocial adjustment in adolescent cancer survivors. J Pediatr Psychol 1997;22:29–43.

107. Haupt R, Fears TR, Robison LL, et al. Educational attainment in long-term survivors of childhood acute lymphoblastic leukemia. JAMA 1994;272:1134–1135.

108. Mitby PA, Robison LL, Whitton JA, et al. Utilization of special education services and educational attainment among long-term survivors of childhood cancer: a report from the Childhood Cancer Survivor Study. Cancer (Phila) 2003;97: 1115–1126.

109. Nagarajan R, Neglia JP, Clohisy DR, et al. Education, employment, insurance, and marital status among 694 survivors of pediatric lower extremity bone tumors: a report from the childhood cancer survivor study. Cancer (Phila) 2003;97: 2554–2564.

110. Meadows AT, McKee L, Kazak AE. Psychosocial status of young adult survivors of childhood cancer: a survey. Med Pediatr Oncol 1989;17:466–470.

111. Nicholson HS, Mulvihill JJ, Byrne J. Late effects of therapy in adult survivors of osteosarcoma and Ewing's sarcoma. Med Pediatr Oncol 1992;20:6–12.

112. Hays DM, Landsverk J, Sallan SE, et al. Educational, occupational, and insurance status of childhood cancer survivors in their fourth and fifth decades of life. J Clin Oncol 1992;10: 1397–1406.

113. Novakovic B, Fears TR, Horowitz ME, et al. Late effects of therapy in survivors of Ewing's sarcoma family of tumors. J Pediatr Hematol Oncol 1997;19:220–225.

114. Evans SE, Radford M. Current lifestyle of young adults treated for cancer in childhood. Arch Dis Child 1995;72:423–426.

115. Makipernaa A. Long-term quality of life and psychosocial coping after treatment of solid tumours in childhood. A population-based study of 94 patients 11–28 years after their diagnosis. Acta Paediatr Scand Suppl 1989;78:728–735.

116. Green DM, Zevon MA, Hall B. Achievement of life goals by adult survivors of modern treatment for childhood cancer. Cancer (Phila) 1991;67:206–213.

117. Byrne J, Fears TR, Steinhorn SC, et al. Marriage and divorce after childhood and adolescent cancer. JAMA 1989;262:2693–2699.

118. Rauck AM, Green DM, Yasui Y, et al. Marriage in the survivors of childhood cancer: a preliminary description from the Childhood Cancer Survivor Study. Med Pediatr Oncol 1999;33:60–63.

119. Felder-Puig R, Formann AK, Mildner A, et al. Quality of life and psychosocial adjustment of young patients after treatment of bone cancer. Cancer (Phila) 1998;83:69–75.

120. Gray RE, Doan BD, Shermer P, et al. Psychologic adaptation of survivors of childhood cancer. Cancer (Phila) 1992;70: 2713–2721.

121. Brown RT, Madan-Swain A, Pais R, et al. Cognitive status of children treated with central nervous system prophylactic chemotherapy for acute lymphocytic leukemia. Arch Clin Neuropsychol 1992;7:481–497.

122. Cetingul N, Aydinok Y, Kantar M, et al. Neuropsychologic sequelae in the long-term survivors of childhood acute lymphoblastic leukemia. Pediatr Hematol Oncol 1999;16: 213–220.

123. Kingma A, Rammeloo LAJ, van der Does-van den Berg A, et al. Academic career after treatment for acute lymphoblastic leukemia. Arch Dis Child 2000;82:353–357.

124. Robison LL, Nesbit MEJ, Sather HN, et al. Factors associated with IQ scores in long-term survivors of childhood acute lymphoblastic leukemia. Am J Pediatr Hematol Oncol 1984;6: 115–121.

125. Moss HA, Nannis ED, Poplack DG. The effects of prophylactic treatment of the central nervous system on the intellectual functioning of children with acute lymphocytic leukemia. Am J Med 1981;71:47–52.

126. Roman DD, Sperduto PW. Neuropsychological effects of cranial radiation: current knowledge and future directions. Int J Radiat Oncol Biol Phys 1995;31:983–998.

127. Anderson DM, Rennie KM, Ziegler RS, et al. Medical and neurocognitive late effects among survivors of childhood central nervous system tumors. Cancer (Phila) 2001;92:2709–2719.

128. Johnson DL, McCabe MA, Nicholson HS, et al. Quality of long-term survival in young children with Medulloblastoma. J Neurosurg 1994;80:1004–1010.

129. Glaser AW, Abdul Rashid NF, Walker DA. School behavior and health status after central nervous system tumours in childhood. Br J Cancer 1997;76:643–650.

130. Arceci RJ, Reaman GH, Cohen AR, et al. Position statement for the need to define pediatric hematology/oncology programs: a model of subspecialty care for chronic childhood diseases. Health Care Policy and Public Issues Committee of the American Society of Pediatric Hematology/Oncology. J Pediatr Hematol Oncol 1998;20:98–103.

131. Bleyer WA, Smith RA, Green DM, et al. American Cancer Society Workshop on Adolescents and Young Adults with Cancer. Workgroup #1: Long-term care and lifetime follow-up. Cancer (Phila) 1993;71:2413.

132. Masera G, Chesler M, Jankovic M, et al. SIOP Working Committee on psychosocial issues in pediatric oncology: guidelines for care of long-term survivors. Med Pediatr Oncol 1996; 27:1–2.

133. Wallace WH, Blacklay A, Eiser C, et al. Developing strategies for long term follow up of survivors of childhood cancer. BMJ 2001;323:271–274.

134. Hollen PJ, Hobbie WL. Establishing comprehensive specialty follow-up clinics for long-term survivors of cancer. Providing systematic physiological and psychosocial support. Support Care Cancer 1995;3:40–44.

135. American Academy of Pediatrics Section on Hematology/Oncology. Guidelines for the pediatric cancer center and role of such centers in diagnosis and treatment. Pediatrics 1997;99:139–141.

136. Ross JA, Severson RK, Robison LL, et al. Pediatric cancer in the United States. A preliminary report of a collaborative study of the Childrens Cancer Group and the Pediatric Oncology Group. Cancer (Phila) 1993;71:3415–3421.

137. Children's Oncology Group. Requirements for Institutional Membership. Arcadia: COG, 2001.

138. Hobbie WL, Ogle S. Transitional care for young adult survivors of childhood cancer. Semin Oncol Nurs 2001;17:268–273.

139. Konsler GK, Jones GR. Transition issues for survivors of childhood cancer and their healthcare providers. Cancer Pract 1993; 1:319–324.

140. Oeffinger KC, Eshelman DA, Tomlinson GE, et al. Programs for adult survivors of childhood cancer. J Clin Oncol 1998;16: 2864–2867.

141. Richardson RC, Nelson MB, Meeske K. Young adult survivors of childhood cancer: attending to emerging medical and psychosocial needs. J Pediatr Oncol Nurs 1999;16:136–144.

142. Rigon H, Lopes LF, do Rosario Latorre M, et al. The GEPETTO program for surveillance of long-term survivors of childhood cancer: preliminary report from a single institution in Brazil. Med Pediatr Oncol 2003;40:405–406.

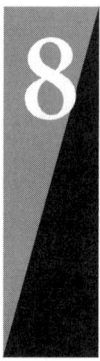

Medical and Psychosocial Issues in Hodgkin's Disease Survivors

Jon Håvard Loge and Stein Kaasa

The first attempts to treat Hodgkin's disease by radiotherapy were conducted at the beginning of the last century. The prognosis for survival was poor but slowly improved by the use of radiotherapy and some chemotherapy until 1960. For example, in 1939 a 20-year survival rate of 17% was reported.[1]

During the 1960s, the prognosis for survival vastly improved, which was mainly related to the introduction of improved staging systems, better understanding of the spread and course of the disease, improved diagnostic methods, and refined therapy. The latter included improved radiotherapy and the introduction of chemotherapeutic regimens such as the MOPP (mechlorethamine, vincristine, procarbazine, prednisone) in 1967.[2] The therapeutic pessimism turned into optimism, and the clinicians dared to speak of a cure. Cure was defined as follows: "We can speak of a cure when in time, probably a decade or so after treatment, there remains a group of disease-free survivors whose progressive *death rate* from all causes is similar to that of a normal population of the same sex and age constitution."[3,4]

This chapter is about the price of cure in terms of medical late effects and psychosocial issues related to survivorship. To speak of a price of cure first became relevant when death no longer was the predominant outcome. The improved prognosis for survival achieved during the 1960s created an increasing number of survivors, and studies of possible late effects thereby became possible. For the clinician, a patient consulting for late effects, medical or psychosocial, probably has now become a more commonly encountered clinical problem than a patient presenting with Hodgkin's disease itself.

Late effects can mainly be divided into three categories. First, there are the late medical effects, which include secondary cancers or ill effects on one or more organ systems. Second, there are the late effects in subjective health, which include symptoms such as fatigue or pain as well as psychologic phenomena such as anxiety and depression. Third, there are the late effects encountered as difficulties in returning to normal life such as resuming work or difficulties in partnership or in participation in leisure activities. The definition of a late effect is not commonly agreed upon, but it is reasonable to separate late effects from acute effects by both duration and time of debut. Some late effects such as fatigue might be traced back to the period of active disease. Other late effects such as secondary cancers might present after a shorter or longer period without symptoms or signs of disease.

Challenges in Clinics and Research

The late effects represent several challenges for the researcher as well as for the clinician. In the investigation of late effects the researcher is challenged by the complexity of the late effects, but also by the effects of aging, environment, lifestyle, behavior, etc. upon health. Consequently, it may be difficult to find causal factors related to the outcomes observed. For the clinicians (as well as for the researcher) the challenge is to understand what the needs of the survivors are. An increased understanding of long-term effects of somatic, psychologic, and social nature will, it is hoped, help healthcare providers to better deliver follow-up programs for patients and family members and to better understand their needs.

The low incidence of Hodgkin's disease generates relatively few survivors and consequently a relative scarcity of data. The social mobility in many Western countries is high, and many survivors are lost to follow-up or are even impossible to locate several years after treatment. Furthermore, the treatment regimens are under constant revision, and late effects caused by one regimen may not necessarily be caused by another type of treatment. Some late effects are relevant only for subgroups of survivors such as breast cancer affecting females irradiated by fields including their breast during their reproductive years. Such factors further add to the scarcity of data. Additionally, some late affects such as secondary cancers first become manifest many years after termination of treatment (see Chapter 17). A long latency period between active disease and debut of late effects might also generate findings, which are not necessarily related to Hodgkin's disease or its treatment. For example, is symptomatic coronary heart disease 30 years after termination of treatment to be looked upon as a late effect, as related to nutrition, smoking habits, and physical exercise, after termination of treatment, or as a combination of all these factors? To answer such a question the researcher needs large samples (i.e., statistical power), advanced medical technology, and skilled experienced clinicians to evaluate the patients, and from a design point of view, controlled groups are needed. The distinction between late effects and morbidity related to increasing age becomes increasingly blurred as the observation time increases. At present there is a scarcity of prospectively collected data, which limits the possibility of drawing valid conclusions about causality. Ideally, one should therefore have comparative data to identify the late effects of Hodgkin's disease. Lack of a comparison group is of particular concern regarding subjective outcomes such as fatigue, which is frequently found in the general population, and may be caused by a series of factors during a lifetime observation.[5] The optimal study design is a prospective follow-up of the survivors from the time of diagnoses through the treatment and into the follow-up phase for many years. In such nonrandomized designs, valid control groups are needed, which should be age- and gender matched and generated by random draws from the general population. In cross-sectional designs, subjective health outcomes from the general population may serve as valid comparisons and will definitely strengthen the conclusions, while the validity of "ad hoc-generated comparisons groups" should be questioned. Volunteer bias is an example that may represent a serious threat to the internal validity of studies with ad hocgenerated comparison groups such as relatives or hospital visitors.

The constitution of a survivor population might also be biased. For example, the patients treated at the Norwegian Radium Hospital (NRH) were assumed to be representative of the Norwegian population of Hodgkin's disease survivors. After survival of the NRH cohorts was investigated, it was concluded that patients with a better prognosis for survival were found in this sample, as compared with the national sample.[6]

The choice of outcome measures may also represent a challenge. For example, the current most commonly used measures for late effects such as psychologic distress and fatigue have limitations with regard to content, reliability, and validity. Another major limitation is the lack of standardization of outcome measures. Different outcome measures have been used to measure the same phenomenon such as fatigue and pain. On the other hand, prospective studies might *lock* the data collection to measurement techniques that become obsolete during the observation period.

Given an accumulating prevalence of late effects, content and organization of the follow-ups should be discussed and ideally investigated in research and in quality assurance programs, and an increasing emphasis on economic effects on the healthcare system should be questioned. Furthermore, it should be asked: What part of the healthcare system is best suited for conducting surveillance, what is a reasonable price for a surveillance program, and should the optimal program be individualized? Finally, how are medical students and future oncologists/radiotherapists best trained to detect and treat late effects? In sum, these challenges also raise ethical dilemmas related to what to tell the patients about late effects and the possibility of creating lifelong patients under continuous observation for possible late effects that might never even occur.

Epidemiology

Incidence of Hodgkin's Disease

The incidence of Hodgkin's disease (HD) varies across countries but is at a comparable level (approximately 2 to 3 per 100,000) in the Western countries.[7] Generally, more males than females are affected (M/F ratio, approximately 60:40). Incidence in the Western world was stable until 1980, slowly decreased during the period 1980–1990, and thereafter it has slightly increased.[8] The decreased incidence was mostly due to a decreasing number of patients above 60 years of age with non-Hodgkin's lymphomas earlier being misclassified as Hodgkin's disease.[6,8,9] More than 50% of the patients are 39 years of age or younger at time of diagnosis.[7]

Prevalence of Survivorship

A disease mainly affecting young adults combined with a good prognosis for survival (best among the younger patients) generates a population of survivors with a long life expectancy. In general, the 5-year survival for all patients with Hodgkin's disease exceeds 80%, and for patients 39 years of age or younger, more than 90% are expected to live for 5 years or more.[10,11] Consequently, the prevalence of survivorship has steadily increased over the past three to four decades. The long life expectancy of the survivors permits long-term follow-up studies but also makes control for expected diseases necessary. As indicated earlier, it is therefore urgent to design prospective and large enough follow-up studies of Hodgkin's disease survivors. Without conducting such studies our follow-up programs may not only be burdensome to the healthcare system, but many patients may be offered invalid follow-up.

The latest Norwegian data illustrate this point clearly. Although the yearly incidence of Hodgkin's disease has been around 80 new cases per year (2/100,000) during the past two decades, the number of Norwegians alive and having had Hodgkin's disease has been steadily increasing and now exceeds 1,500.[12] In 1990 the prevalence of survivorship was 1,100 in a population of about 4.5 million.[13]

Advanced disease and B symptoms in addition to age predict incomplete remission, relapse, and shortened survival after first-line treatment.[14,15] Age is at present the single most important predictor for survival. Advanced disease and relapse both increase the treatment burden. Some survivors have therefore received intensive treatment (chemotherapy and radiotherapy) in several cycles eventually supplemented with high-dose chemotherapy and bone marrow transplantation. In general, the most recent improvement in survival is therefore a consequence of more-intensive treatment. Potentially the more-intensive treatment may affect the prevalence of long-term medical and/or psychosocial effects. Subgroups of survivors might therefore be of special interest for future assessments of late effects. However, such groups must be considered relatively small, which affects whether proper follow-up studies can be performed, unless such studies are conducted as multicenter studies with a sufficient number of patients.

Medical Issues

About the Treatment

Treatment with radiotherapy has during the past decades been partly replaced and/or combined with chemotherapy. Radiotherapy as a single modality is today given only to a subgroup of patients with limited disease.

In the 1960s, fractionated large fields were irradiated with the consequence of a substantially increased survival rate. Continuous research on radiotherapy techniques has resulted in more individualized treatment, and today more often smaller fields are delivered as compared to the standard mantle fields used at the start of the radiotherapy era. To reduce radiotherapy-related acute and late toxicity, the total dose in many programs has been reduced from a standard total dose of 40 Gy treated in 3 Gy per fraction to a dose of 30 to 35 Gy with reduced single fraction to a proximately 1.75 Gy. Critical organs are sometimes included in the fields, such as lung, heart, thyroid, major blood vessel, and bone marrow, which may give rise to late effects.

Combination chemotherapy was introduced into the treatment plans of Hodgkin's disease in the mid-1960s with the so-called MOPP regimens (mechlorethamine, vincristine, procarbazine, prednisone) as the gold standard in most countries.[2] Other combinations of chemotherapy have been in use as well as various ways of escalating doses to improve survival and reduce acute toxicity and long-term morbidity.

Both treatment modalities, that is, radiotherapy and chemotherapy or combinations, can potentially give the patients medical (somatic) late side effects. Furthermore, the cancer itself may also have and will alter the biology of the host (i.e., the patient). So, consequently, either of these factors, separately or in combination, may result in late morbidity for HD survivors.

Long-Term Morbidity: General Considerations

The most frequent causes of death other than Hodgkin's disease itself are cardiac disease and secondary malignancy, while infertility, thyroid abnormalities, and pulmonary disease may cause serious late effects of various prevalences in Hodgkin's disease survivors.[16] The most commonly encountered late medical effects are presented in Table 8.1. In a recent review it was concluded that secondary malignancies and ischemic heart disease are the two most frequent causes of death.[17] However, it must be kept in mind that, in patients with good prognoses, the actual overall survival at 20 years is about 93%,[11] and that treatment-related mortality exceeds the mortality from Hodgkin's disease 12 to 15 years after the primary treatment.[18]

TABLE 8.1. **Main medical late effects of Hodgkin's lymphoma and its treatment.**

- Secondary cancers
- Cardiac disease
- Endocrine dysfunction
  —Hypothyroidism
  —Hypogonadism
- Lung damage
- Dental caries

Cardiac Late Effects

An increased incidence of coronary heart disease, specifically in patients less than 40 years of age, has been attributed to radiotherapy. The expected number of cardiovascular deaths in age- and sex-matched population was similar to the cardiovascular deaths in Hodgkin's disease populations.[19] The history of myocardial infarction was no more frequent after mantle field irradiation than in HD patients who received chemotherapy,[20] whereas others have reported an increased risk of myocardial infarction after mediastinal irradiation.[21,22] Up to a threefold increase in the relative risk of cardiac deaths has been reported.[23] In another retrospective review, coronary artery disease occurred in patients who were treated at the ages of 16, 21, 35, and 48 years with latency periods of 19, 12, 7, and 3 years, respectively.[24]

The technology used to evaluate morbidity, such as valvular dysfunction, may have major impact on the findings. Before Doppler technology was used, valvular dysfunction was considered a rare finding in survivors of Hodgkin's disease. By using Doppler echo cardiography, aortic and/or mitral valvular regurgitation and valve thickness have been observed at rates of 24% to 40% of patients treated successfully for Hodgkin's disease.[25-27] The clinical implications of these findings are at present unknown.

Endocrine Dysfunction

The prevalence of hypothyroidism varies substantially between studies. As for most of the other medical side effects as well as for the subjective ones, sample selection, definition of cases, etc. have a major influence on the results. The rate of hypothyroidism seems to be influenced by observation time, irradiation (field and amount), and the definition of hypothyroidism.[28-30] In a sample from Norway where 221 patients were observed, 55% developed biochemical hypothyroidism 3 to 23 years after treatment.[20]

In the Stanford study, the actual risk of thyroid disease was 52% after 20 years and rose to 67% after a follow-up of 26 years.[16] In this study, younger patients, women, combined-modality treatment, and time since radiation were associated with a high incidence of thyroid disease, whereas other studies from Europe have not confirmed these findings.[20,31]

Although thyroid abnormality is prevalent in HD survivors, the early use of thyroid supplementation in patients with elevated thyroid-stimulating hormone (TSH) level has greatly reduced the risk of overt clinical hypothyroidism when compared with earlier studies.[32] However, no consensus seems to have been reached with regard to when and on which indications to start hormonal substitution in patients with biochemical hypothyroidism.

Lung Damage

Dyspnea is a subjective phenomenon experienced by the patients as shortness of breath. Consequently it is recommended that dyspnea as well as other subjective symptoms should be assessed by the patients themselves by means of questionnaires or other subjective measures. Dyspnea is frequently reported in HD survivors in approximately 30% of the cases.[20] In the Norwegian study, dyspnea was not associated with sex, age, or chemotherapy.[20] Pulmonary complications after radiotherapy are first observed clinically as an acute radiation pneumonitis, followed by radiation fibrosis, which evolves over time and seems to reach a stable appearance after 9 to 12 months.[33] Pulmonary toxicity secondary to chemotherapy is rare; however, bleomycin may enhance pulmonary dysfunction when given in conjunction with radiotherapy.[34]

In one study consisting of a selected cohort of 116 patients treated with mediastinal radiotherapy alone or in combination with chemotherapy, 30% of the patients had pulmonary dysfunction and associated reductions in total lung capacity, forced vital capacity, forced expiratory volume in 1 second, and gas transfer impairment.[35] The size of the radiation fields has been found to be related to the extent of fibrosis, and the most dramatic changes were observed in patients treated simultaneously with bleomycin and anthracyclines.[35] In single cases major interindividual variations have been found with respect to the sensitivity of the lung parenchyma to develop radiation fibrosis.

In conclusion, a consistent finding is that the severity of the fibrosis is related to the volume of irradiation, the presence of parenchymal involvement in the disease itself, and the use of bleomycin and anthracyclines.

Comments

Most studies assessing medical morbidity in HD survivors have either a retrospective design and/or a cross-sectional design. The studies are performed ad hoc, with few upfront hypotheses stated, and how to define the level of morbidity and which indicators to use to define morbidity varies considerably. Scientific discussions of possible confounding factors are rarely presented, and few studies have comparison groups. Based on the findings in one of the studies including a comparison group, it has been, for example, suggested that the incidence of cardiac death is not any higher than in the matched population.[19] However, details on how these comparisons were performed were not given. A similar criticism can be raised for treatment of symptoms and biochemical findings of hypothyroidism. Most studies have an ad hoc retrospective design, and consequently it is difficult to draw valid conclusions with regard to treatment proposals.

Psychosocial Issues

Historical Perspective and General Points

The first descriptions of the psychosocial aspects of cancer survivorship were conflicting. Case observations led to the postulation of a Damocles syndrome in which the survivors lived their lives under the constant threat of a relapse.[36] The syndrome was characterized as a specific psychologic state with tension, emptiness, and lack of pleasure and direction of life. The other position, in general held by epidemiologists, stated that the cancer survivors lived well-adjusted lives and were as satisfied with their lives as the general population.[37] It is now obvious that the two concepts were equally wrong and that both positions were based on methodologic shortcomings. The epidemiologists based their statements on too-

general outcome measures and the psychologists based their postulation of a specific syndrome upon case observations without sufficient perspective on the generalizability of their observations.

From a psychiatric point of view, one can hypothesize that the psychologic burden of survivorship per se would be more of a posttraumatic stress disorder than depression. Being cured is difficult to characterize as a loss with subsequent potential for development of depression. However, reduced health status after cure, either objectively or subjectively, might represent a loss and thereby a potential for development of depression. Premorbid characteristics as well as social and psychologic support during and after the disease will always interact with the stressor (i.e., the disease and the treatment). No published studies have investigated these variables systematically.

Most published studies of psychosocial aspects of cancer survivorship have been descriptive and lacking a specific hypothesis. The study by Cella and Tross from 1986 is one exception, and three possible psychologic sequelae were proposed (anticipatory, residual, and current) and explored with generally negative findings.[38] Facing death and receiving burdensome treatment during a period of life when friends fulfill education and establish themselves in jobs and families may be regarded as a longlasting trauma, and the model of a posttraumatic stress disorder may apply for this population. Such a specific model for development of late psychosocial effects has not been tested, except for the study by Cella and Tross.[38] Generally, the studies of psychologic late effects have used self-report measures of psychologic distress as outcomes, and none has looked for specific psychiatric diagnoses. There have been several methodologic limitations, among which selection bias is probably the most serious and difficult to handle. It is reasonable to assume that late effects might increase the response rates, and this is of particular concern in cross-sectional studies relying on one single data collection. Still, it is reasonable to conclude that psychosocial late effects in survivors of Hodgkin's disease are the exception rather than the rule.

Quality of Life

Quality of life (QOL) reflects the definition of health as proposed by the World Health Organization in 1947 with emphasis on the subjective aspect of health and not only the absence of disease.[39] During the 1980s and 1990s, the concept of QOL became more directed toward health by the introduction of the term Health-Related Quality of Life. The latter operationalizes health as encompassing a social, a physical, and a mental dimension. It should be regarded as a narrowing of the concept QOL, and some therefore prefer the term subjective health. The distinction is not only of academic interest. Figure 8.1 demonstrates the responses from survivors of Hodgkin's disease and normal controls to a single question about satisfaction with life, which is close to the more global concept of QOL. More of the survivors reported being very satisfied with their lives than the normal controls, in spite of more health problems among the survivors. This is in line with findings reported by Cella and Tross.[38] In spite of the possible existential dimension of this finding, overall QOL does not seem to capture the health-related aspects of the survivors' quality of life (i.e., their subjective health status).

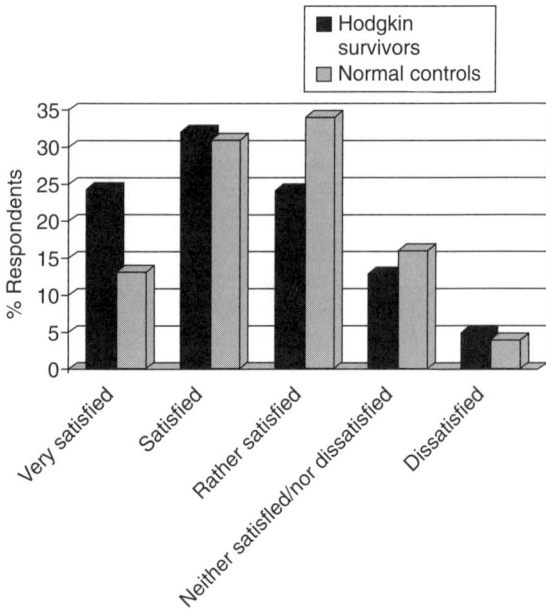

FIGURE 8.1. Satisfaction with life in Norwegian survivors of Hodgkin's disease (*n* = 453) and in normal control subjects (*n* = 2323). (Unpublished data from the authors.)

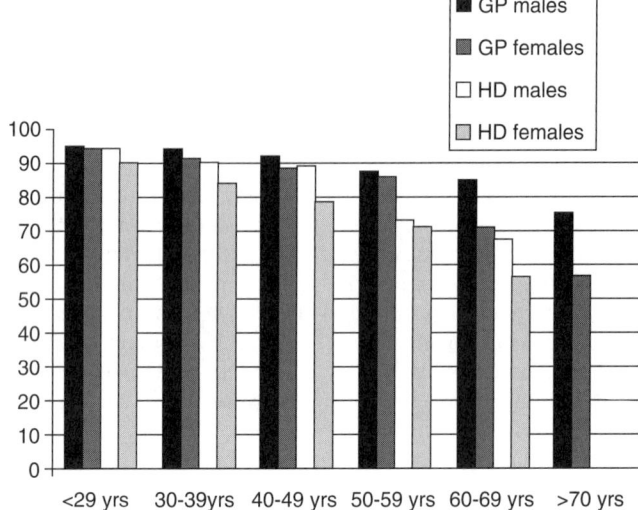

FIGURE 8.2. Physical functioning as measured by the Physical Functioning Scale of the SF-36 in the general Norwegian population (*GP*) (Norwegian norm data; *n* = 2263) and survivors of Hodgkin's disease (*HD*; *n* = 459). (Data from references 48, 49.)

Subjective Health Status: Early Findings

The first studies of subjective health status in survivors of Hodgkin's disease were published in 1986.[38,40] As demonstrated in Table 8.2, the first studies included quite different sample sizes, and the findings were inconsistent, partly reflecting different measures of subjective health. Only two studies included comparison groups. In these studies, selected cohorts of U.S. patients from controlled clinical trials were included. A minority of all U.S. cancer patients are included in clinical trials, and the generalizability of the findings can therefore be questioned.

Subjective Health Status: Physical Health

Physical health is about physical symptoms such as pain, dyspnea, and nausea in addition to physical functioning, which generally includes different physical activities commonly performed during a day. Present subjective health status measures such as the SF-36, the European Organization for Research and Treatment of Cancer Core Quality of Life Questionnaire (EORTC QLQ C-30), and the Functional Assessment of Cancer Therapy-General (FACT-G) all put a great emphasis on physical functioning, which generally is affected by somatic health events and has low correlation with mental health.[45–47] In the SF-36, 10 of 36 items are about

physical functioning.[47] However, the content of physical functioning scales varies among the instruments, and this hinders comparisons across the instruments. Physical functioning in the general population is related to age and gender (Figure 8.2).[48,49] The decline by age reflects increasing morbidity with increasing age and needs to be controlled for in studies of cancer survivors.[48]

The first studies of Hodgkin's disease survivors indicated problems with the survivors' physical health, but standardized measures were not applied.[41,50,51] Three studies from the 1990s included both standardized measures of physical functioning (the EORTC QLQ C-30 and the SF-36) and comparison groups.[42,44,49] The findings were surprisingly similar in that physical functioning was reduced by approximately 0.5 SD compared to the control groups.[42,44,49] None of the studies demonstrated any robust associations between disease characteristics, treatment, and reduced physical functioning. Some later studies have failed to replicate this finding, but the design of these studies limits the possibility of drawing firm conclusions.[52,53]

Clinicians report stiffness and pain from the musculoskeletal system as common among the survivors.[20] However, compared with healthy controls, no differences in pain level between survivors and controls have been detected.[42,44,49] Another somatic symptom, dyspnea, is included the cancer-specific instrument EORTC QLQ C30 but not in the generic instrument SF-36. Joly et al compared

TABLE 8.2. Early studies of health-related quality of life among survivors of Hodgkin's disease.

Study	Year	Country	N	Origin of sample	Mean observation period (years)	Effect stage/ treatment	Comparison group
Cella[38]	1986	USA	60	Hospital	Unknown	Yes	Yes
Fobair[40]	1986	USA	403	Clinical trials	9	Yes	No
Kornblith[41]	1992	USA	273	Advanced disease/clinical trials	6	No	No
van Tulder[42]	1994	Netherlands	81	Hospital	14	No	Yes
Norum[43]	1996	Norway	42	Hospital	4	Yes	No
Joly[44]	1996	France	93	Region	10	No	Yes

French survivors with randomly selected and matched controls and found nearly three times higher levels of dyspnea in the survivors than in the controls.[44] A Spanish study from 2003 also found higher levels of dyspnea in the survivors than in healthy controls.[54] Given the difficulties patient have in distinguishing dyspnea from fatigue and the association between fatigue and gas transfer impairment, a further elaboration on this point seems warranted.[55]

The French study by Joly et al. found very low levels of nausea and vomiting as measured by the EORTC QLQ C30 and no difference between the survivors and the age- and gender-matched healthy controls.[44] Cameron et al. also reported low levels of nausea and vomiting but pointed to the possibility of classical conditioning as the mechanism underlying persisting symptoms such as distress in the survivors.[56] By exploring and confirming a specific mechanism, this study yielded knowledge that is directly applicable in the prevention and/or treatment of persisting symptoms by use of psychologic techniques.

There are some main limitations to our present knowledge on the physical health of the survivors. On a group level their physical health is lowered, and the reduction is of clinical significance.[57] Still, the majority enjoys a physical health similar to the general population of same age. The survivors with reduced physical health have not been clearly identified, and how the survivors' physical health is affected by time since termination of primary treatment is not documented. The mechanisms underlying the survivors' reduced physical health are unknown, and this lack hinders efforts to prevent and treat. The reduced physical health might reflect the total sum of negative health events such as gas transfer impairment, muscular wasting, and hypothyroidism. Another explanation might be an association between reduced physical health and other subjective late effects such as fatigue.[58] However, none of the published studies on physical health has controlled for the level of fatigue.

Subjective Health Status: Fatigue

The first report on fatigue among Hodgkin's disease survivors was published by Fobair et al. in 1986, and fatigue was a major problem as 37% had not regained their energy.[40] Patients with self-reported energy loss were more likely to be depressed.[40] Another early study demonstrated that Hodgkin's disease survivors were more fatigued than survivors of testicular cancer.[51] A British study of lymphoma patients off treatment described mental and physical fatigue as major concerns.[59,60] However, in all the earliest studies published before 1997 fatigue was measured by single questions (i.e., not validated and reliability tested questionnaires), and such single questions have disputable validity and reliability.[61] Further, none of the early studies took into account the high prevalence of fatigue in the general population (11% to 45%).[61,62] The main studies on fatigue in the survivors are presented in Table 8.3.

Newer studies employing standardized measures and comparison groups have confirmed that fatigue is a major problem among the survivors compared to healthy subjects and more of a problem among survivors of Hodgkin's disease than among survivors of other cancer types.[63–68] The prevalence of fatigue is clearly related to the measurement technique, and the exact magnitude of this problem is therefore not known.[61]

Attempts to relate persisting fatigue to disease and treatment characteristics have yielded conflicting results. The close connection between disease burden and type of treatment also hinders analyses of separate effects of the two. However, a recent prospective study demonstrated that combined treatment yielded higher levels of fatigue only during the first year as compared to radiation therapy.[63] Thereafter, the two groups reported similar levels of fatigue, which was significantly higher than in the general population (Figure 8.3).[63]

A cross-sectional study reported an association between late pulmonary sequelae (in particular, gas transfer impairment) and fatigue.[55] A significant association between psychologic distress and fatigue has been demonstrated.[40,69] However, a review strongly supported a differentiated view on fatigue and depression in cancer patients.[70] Some authors have proposed a common mechanism underlying the symptoms of cancer and cancer treatment, namely, cytokines, which induce sickness behavior in animal models including

TABLE 8.3. Fatigue in survivors of Hodgkin's disease: Main studies.

Author	Year	Sample (N)	Main finding	Comparison group (N)	Type of measurement
Fobair[40]	1986	403	37% tired	—	Single item
Devlen[59,60]	1987	90/120[a]	30%/42% tired	—	Single item
Bloom[51]	1993	85	22% energy not returned	Testicular survivors	Single item
van Tulder[42]	1994	81	No significant difference	Healthy controls	SF-36
Loge[65b]	1999	458	24%–27% chronic fatigued	General population norms	Fatigue Questionnaire
Kornblith[64]	1998	273	More fatigued than controls	Acute leukemia survivors	POMS
Wettergren[67]	2003	121	Worries about fatigue	Healthy controls	SEIQoL-DW
Fosså[68]	2003	458	24% chronic fatigued	Testicular survivors	Fatigue Questionnaire
Ganz[63]	2003	247	Persistent fatigue > population norms	—	SF-36
Ruffer[66]	2003	836	21% higher level	Healthy controls	MFI

SF-36, Short Form 36; POMS, Profile of Mood States; SEIQoL-DW, Schedule for the Evaluation of the Individual Quality of Life-Direct Weighting.

[a] Two studies; retrospective and prospective including Hodgkin's disease and non-Hodgkin lymphomas.

[b] Identical sample of Hodgkin's disease survivors.

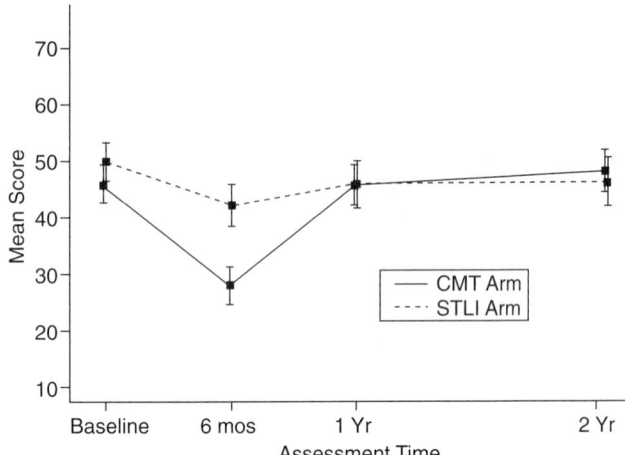

FIGURE 8.3. Average SF-36 Vitality Scale scores (mean with 95% CI) by assessment time and treatment arm. Lower scores reflect greater fatigue. *STLI*, subtotal lymphoid irradiation; *CMT*, combined-modality therapy. For healthy men aged 35 to 44 years, the mean Vitality Scale score is 65.5. For women aged 35 to 44 years, it is 59.4. (From Ganz et al.,[63] by permission of *Journal of Clinical Oncology*.)

fatigued behavior.[71] However, attempts to correlate some of the relevant cytokines to fatigue have failed.[72]

Except for the study by Ganz, all studies on fatigue in Hodgkin's disease survivors were cross-sectional, which limits the possibility of inferences about causality. No prospective longitudinal studies to investigate the course of fatigue among Hodgkin's disease survivors have been published. This lack of knowledge limits the clinician's ability to give valid and reliable information to individual patients on the expected course of their fatigue.

At present, we can therefore only hypothesize about the mechanisms underlying fatigue in the survivors. In some, as in the general population, fatigue is probably part of being psychologically distressed.[73] However, as compared to sufferers of the chronic fatigue syndrome, the survivors have significantly lower levels of psychologic distress as measured by the Hospital Anxiety and Depression Scale.[69,73] Second, fatigue might reflect the combined burden of the late complications after having had Hodgkin's disease. Fatigue is by many considered a final common endpoint that is associated with most diseases; this indicates that fatigue is an "unclean" endpoint affected by most altered health states. Third, fatigue might be a specific late effect after Hodgkin's disease and related to some specific mechanisms characteristic of this disease; this might include the cytokines, which is supported by the altered immunity found in many of the survivors. At present, none of these seems more strongly supported than the others, and given the complexity of fatigue all might be correct in subgroups of fatigued survivors.

Subjective Health Status: Mental Health

Some of the earliest studies indicated rather great psychologic problems among the survivors. For example, Kornblith et al. reported in 1992 psychologic distress one SD above that of healthy subjects, and 22% met the criterion suggested for a psychiatric diagnosis.[41] Later studies from the 1990s did not confirm this finding. Three studies used health-related

quality of life (HRQOL) measures and different comparison groups, and none reported any deviances in mental health (SF-36) or emotional functioning (EORTC QLQ C-30) between the survivors and the controls.[42,44,49] The first comparative study between Hodgkin's disease survivors and testicular cancer survivors did not find any significant difference in psychologic outcomes between the two groups of survivors.[51]

One study from the last part of the 1990s identified as many as 27% of the survivors as probable anxiety and depression cases, but no comparison group was included.[74] Previous psychiatric problems, psychiatric problems during the treatment phase, and low education were identified as risk factors. The most intensive treatment regimen was associated with increased risk for probable anxiety.[74] This study employed the Hospital Anxiety and Depression Scale (the HADS), which generally tends to produce high levels of anxiety and higher prevalences of anxiety cases than depression cases.[75] This finding was confirmed by the most recent study, which found no differences in the level of depression between Hodgkin's disease survivors, testicular cancer survivors, and the general Norwegian population.[68] The levels of anxiety in both groups of survivors (4.7 in testicular cancer survivors and 4.6 in Hodgkin's disease survivors) were slightly elevated as compared to the general population (3.9).[68] In sum, these studies indicate that the level of depressive symptoms is not elevated in the survivors, that anxiety symptoms are just slightly elevated, and that we do not know whether these symptoms are part of a specific psychiatric condition.

Some other psychologic symptoms have been assessed and reported as more prevalent than expected. Cella et al. in 1986 reported no elevated level of psychologic distress, but indication of psychosocial dysfunction in areas such as intimacy motivation, increased avoidant thinking about disease, and illness-related concerns.[38] These findings may be of clinical relevance, for example, as effectors on partnership and illness behavior but have to our knowledge not been addressed in later studies.

Social Functioning

Three aspects of social functioning have received special attention in the literature: divorce rate, difficulties in returning to ordinary work, and difficulties in getting health insurance/borrowing from banks. Additional aspects of social life such as participation in leisure activities, sexual activity, sexual interest, and reproduction have also been included in some studies.

In general, it is reasonable to state that the social consequences of survivorship from cancer are influenced by social mechanisms that may vary considerably across culturally relatively comparable nations, as is in accordance with the handicap model as proposed by the WHO.[76] For example, in the Scandinavian countries health insurance is public and granted to every citizen. Life insurance is partly private and partly public, and in sum insurance is probably of lesser relevance in these countries than in the United States. An early U.S. study demonstrated difficulties in getting health insurance.[41] The lack of a comparison group hinders estimation of the clinical significance of this possible late effect.

In general, the relationship between cancer, cancer treatment, late medical or late subjective health effects, and social consequences is complex and relatively poorly understood.

Type of treatment seems to be of lesser relevance, while subjective late effects was associated with poorer social functioning.[63,77]

Difficulties returning to an ordinary job are also affected by country-specific variables in addition to the labor market in general. The earliest U.S. studies indicated various work-related problems such as getting a job or working at a former pace.[38,40,41] The Norwegian data demonstrated that the majority of the survivors with a mean follow-up time of 12 years were in full-time work at follow-up.[77] However, about 20% were permanently disabled, compared with 10% of the general Norwegian population of similar age at the time of the follow-up study.[77] Predictors of disablement were increasing age, low education, combined-treatment modality, and high levels of anxiety, depression, and fatigue.[77] The French study by Joly et al. did not demonstrate lower proportions of survivors at work, but they had less ambitious professional plans.[44] The latter finding was replicated by the Norwegian study.[77]

Divorce is generally a common event in most Western countries. The earliest studies found divorce rates up to 32% among the survivors.[40] Among the French survivors studied by Joly et al., the divorce rate was lower among the survivors than among the controls but length of the marriage was not controlled for.[44] Generally, several methodologic aspects hinder interpretation of whether the divorce rate deviates from the general population. The age of the survivors and controls at time of data collection, the different divorce rates across different age groups, and the effect of marriage duration upon divorce rate all add to the uncertainty of the published data on divorce rates. Additionally, one could also hypothesize different mechanisms for divorce between spouses being married during the treatment phase and between spouses who marry after termination of treatment. A couple living through the treatment of Hodgkin's disease faces serious and long-lasting stressors. Generally such strain may strengthen bonds in some couples but also represent tensions that subsequently end up in divorce in others. The modern tendency to involve the family including the children during the treatment phase may have positive effects for the family as a whole, but this has not been addressed in published studies until now. On the other hand, one may also speculate that such a practice increases the total burden on the family and particularly on the healthy spouse. No studies until now have addressed the burden of disease and treatment on the family, but one might speculate that the stress on the family is affected by the quality of care which the family receives during and after the treatment phase. For example, a recent study has demonstrated much less psychologic distress among the relatives of patients included in a palliative program as compared to the relatives of patients receiving standard care.[78]

The prevalence of sexual problems among Hodgkin's disease survivors has been reported to be between 12% and 20%, whereas infertility among women and men has been reported to be less than 10% and less than 20%, respectively.[40,41,44,64,77] In the Norwegian sample, the great majority of the men reporting infertility had received treatment known to reduce fertility (chemotherapy containing an alkylating agent and procarbazine). One single study reported difficulties in participation in leisure activities, and this was related to fatigue.[37]

Treatment

Medical Late Effects

Treatment of late medical effects after curative treatment of Hodgkin's disease has, to our knowledge, not been systematically investigated. For patients with symptoms from heart, lung, and/or thyroid gland, general guidelines on how to treat or relieve symptoms have been followed. For patients with hypothyroidism, general international accepted treatment guidelines seem advisable to follow. Similar approaches have also been used by cardiologists and lung physicians. However, it is reasonable to assume that the pathophysiology for these conditions in many cases is different in Hodgkin's disease survivors than in other groups of patients. If these assumptions are correct, one may argue that at least patients need to be followed systematically and prospectively after treatment is initiated to evaluate both immediate and long-term effects of the intervention. Furthermore, one may also expect that the condition itself, for example, cardiac sequelae after radiotherapy, may have a different "natural cause" than what is expected in patients with the same condition, but with other causes. Additionally, one may also expect that in many patients with Hodgkin's disease a combination of factors may cause the condition itself.

For patients with no symptoms, but with pathologic blood markers, X-rays, or physiologic tests, no clear treatment guidelines are established to our knowledge. For these patients one may possibly overtreat some patients who are nonsymptomatic if the treatment itself does not prevent the development of the disease or undertreat patients if the treatment itself is effective to prevent the development of symptoms.

Taking all these uncertainties under consideration, we therefore argue that multicenter treatment studies are needed to establish sufficient knowledge so it may become possible to establish international guidelines, not only on the diagnostic level in this cohort of patients, but also on the treatment level.

Subjective Late Effects

Generally, specific treatment studies of subjective late effects have not been published and the clinician must therefore rely on general knowledge from other fields of medicine. An open pilot study on the effects of physical exercise upon fatigue in survivors supported the findings of a meta-analysis on the treatment of the chronic fatigue syndrome (CFS).[79,80] The fatigue level was reduced by 50% after an intervention of 12 weeks duration.[79] CFS differs from chronic fatigue in the survivors on several variables, including level of psychologic distress,[69] but physical exercise has multiple effects including lowered anxiety, depression, and fatigue levels. The exact mechanism for this effect in the survivors and in other patient groups is not known. The other type of therapy with effect on CFS, cognitive behavioral therapy, has not been tested on survivors specifically. However, it is reasonable to assume that physical exercise also has cognitive effects, that is, the subjects gain other cognitions about their physical capacity during such a training period. Oldervoll et al. also demonstrated that aerobic exercise improved subjective physical functioning and aerobic capacity.[79]

The high prevalence of hypothyroidism among the survivors and the tendency to substitute with thyroxine yield many survivors on thyroxine substitution therapy for long periods. It is reasonable to assume that fatigue is a central symptom when substitution is started. However, the clinical effect of such substitution is questionable, at least in terms of reduced fatigue-level. Knobel et al. demonstrated a significant higher level of fatigue among patients receiving thyroxine substitution than among unsubstituted patients with biochemical hypothyroidism.[55]

Anecdotally, fatigued survivors are offered antidepressants. In sufferers of the CFS, antidepressants have no effect unless fatigue is part of a depressive disorder.[80] A recent study of the effects of an antidepressant upon fatigue and depression in cancer patients demonstrated that fatigue was not improved (i.e., serotonin was not the mediator of fatigue in cancer patients) while depressive symptoms improved.[81] In sum, these findings indicate that fatigue in the survivors should not be treated with antidepressants unless fatigue is part of a depressive condition characterized by lowered mood and other depressive symptoms.

Treatment of psychologic symptoms should be based on a psychiatric diagnosis (see Chapter 18). Conditioned responses are best treated by unconditioning if the symptoms need to be treated. Whether to treat such symptoms depends on the subjects' wishes and the symptom burden. Conditioned responses only experienced at the sight of the hospital are probably less burdensome than responses triggered by food or beverages.[56] Anxiety may reflect quite different disorders: posttraumatic stress disorder (PTSD), panic disorder, or generalized anxiety disorder. Both pharmacologic and psychotherapeutic interventions differ among the three, and treatment must follow the general outlines for treatment of these conditions. For example, PTSD can be treated with exposure therapy, cognitive therapy, selective seratonin reuptake inhibitors (SSRIs), or combinations of the three.[82] Treatment of depression in somatically ill patients principally equals treatment of depression in "pure" psychiatric patients, although the presence of other somatic symptoms such as nausea can be of importance for the patients' compliance with the treatment.[83]

Conclusions

Present Level of Knowledge

Our present level of knowledge on late medical effects is characterized by uncertainties regarding prevalence and clinical significance of reported findings. The distinction between late effects and age- and lifestyle-related morbidity is unclear and generally is not properly controlled for. However, there is an increased risk for secondary cancers and particularly breast cancer in women irradiated by fields involving their breast during their reproductive years. Fatigue seem to be the most consistently reported subjective late effect, and survivors of Hodgkin's disease seem to be at particular risk for this late effect compared to other cancer survivors.

Treatment of late effects generally follows the general guidelines for treatment of the specific condition at stake, and the need for specific treatment studies may seem disputable. Some special considerations regarding volume of irradiation might indicate a need for specialized studies of optimal adju-

vant treatment of breast cancer, for example. Given the prevalence of persisting fatigue and the uncertainty related to the treatment of fatigue, there seems to be a need for controlled trials on the treatment of this symptom.

Future

Future research on late effects should ideally be based upon larger data sets collected prospectively as part of multicenter studies, and the data collection should ideally start when treatment starts. Smaller or medium-sized cross-sectionally designed studies with retrospective data collection without specified hypotheses have been dominating until now, and such studies will probably be of lesser relevance in the future. There is also a need for representative comparison groups that make it possible to specifically estimate if there is an increase in specific disorders and symptoms. At present the cancer registers have this function regarding the secondary cancers, and this advantage has made the prevalence estimates of secondary cancers the most reliable among the reported late medical effects. An optimal strategy can be establishment of surveillance programs for the most prevalent and/or disabling late effects. There is also a definite need for improvement of measurement techniques for subjective late effects, but this is not a challenge for studies of cancer survivors in particular but rather a general challenge for the assessment of subjective health status. A better understanding of biologic mechanisms related to late subjective effects and particularly fatigue is warranted. Such knowledge can improve prevention as well as therapy.

In sum, the ideal goal should be to have sufficient knowledge to identify which patients are at risk for developing which late effects so that preventive measures can be taken at the earliest possible time or that optimal treatment can be offered before the late effects become a health problem of significant magnitude.

References

1. Gilbert R. Radiotherapy in Hodgkin's disease (malignant granulomatosis): anatomic and clinical foundations, governing principles, results. Am J Roentgenol 1939;41:198–241.
2. De Vita VT, Serpick AA, Carbone PP. Combination chemotherapy in the treatment of advanced Hodgkin's disease. Ann Intern Med 1970;73:881–895.
3. Easson EC, Russel MH. The cure of Hodgkin's disease. Br Med J 1963;1:1704–1707.
4. Easson EC. Possibilities for the cure of Hodgkin's disease. Cancer (Phila) 1966;19:345–350.
5. Wessely S, Hotopf M, Sharpe M. Chronic fatigue and its syndromes. Oxford: Oxford University Press, 1999.
6. Foss AA, Egeland T, Hansen S, Langholm R, Holte H, Kvaloy S. Hodgkin's disease in a national and hospital population: trends over 20 years. Eur J Cancer 1997;33(14):2380–2383.
7. Thomas RK, Re D, Zander T, Wolf J, Diehl V. Epidemiology and etiology of Hodgkin's lymphoma. Ann Oncol 2002;13(suppl 4): 147–152.
8. Glaser SL, Swartz WG. Time trends in Hodgkin's disease incidence. The role of diagnostic accuracy. Cancer (Phila) 1990; 66(10):2196–2204.
9. Glaser SL. Recent incidence and secular trends in Hodgkin's disease and its histologic subtypes. J Chronic Dis 1986;39(10): 789–798.

10. Aleman BM, van den Belt-Dusebout AW, Klokman WJ, Van't Veer MB, Bartelink H, van Leeuwen FE. Long-term cause-specific mortality of patients treated for Hodgkin's disease. J Clin Oncol 2003;21(18):3431–3439.

11. Vaughan HB, Vaughan HG, Linch DC, Anderson L. Late mortality in young BNLI patients cured of Hodgkin's disease. Ann Oncol 1994;5(suppl 2)0:65–66.

12. The Cancer Registry of Norway. Cancer in Norway 2001. Oslo: The Cancer Registry of Norway, 2004.

13. The Cancer Registry of Norway. Cancer in Norway 1992. Oslo: The Cancer Registry of Norway, 1992.

14. Canellos GP. Primary treatment of Hodgkin's disease. Ann Oncol 2002;13(suppl 4):153–158.

15. Josting A, Engert A, Diehl V, Canellos GP. Prognostic factors and treatment outcome in patients with primary progressive and relapsed Hodgkin's disease. Ann Oncol 2002;13(suppl 1): 112–116.

16. Donaldson SS, Hancock SL, Hoppe RT. The Janeway lecture. Hodgkin's disease: finding the balance between cure and late effects. Cancer J Sci Am 1999;5(6):325–333.

17. Yung L, Linch D. Hodgkin's lymphoma. Lancet 2003;361(9361): 943–951.

18. Ng AK, Bernardo MP, Weller E, et al. Long-term survival and competing causes of death in patients with early-stage Hodgkin's disease treated at age 50 or younger. J Clin Oncol 2002;20(8): 2101–2108.

19. van Rijswijk RE, Verbeek J, Haanen C, Dekker AW, van Daal WA, van Peperzeel HA. Major complications and causes of death in patients treated for Hodgkin's disease. J Clin Oncol 1987;5(10):1624–1633.

20. Abrahamsen AF, Loge JH, Hannisdal E, et al. Late medical sequelae after therapy for supradiaphragmatic Hodgkin's disease. Acta Oncol 1999;38(4):511–515.

21. Boivin JF, Hutchison GB, Lubin JH, Mauch P. Coronary artery disease mortality in patients treated for Hodgkin's disease. Cancer (Phila) 1992;69(5):1241–1247.

22. Cosset JM, Henry-Amar M, Pellae-Cosset B, et al. Pericarditis and myocardial infarctions after Hodgkin's disease therapy. Int J Radiat Oncol Biol Phys 1991;21(2):447–449.

23. Hancock SL, Tucker MA, Hoppe RT. Factors affecting late mortality from heart disease after treatment of Hodgkin's disease. JAMA 1993;270(16):1949–1955.

24. Sears JD, Greven KM, Ferree CR, D'Agostino RB Jr. Definitive irradiation in the treatment of Hodgkin's disease. Analysis of outcome, prognostic factors, and long-term complications. Cancer (Phila) 1997;79(1):145–151.

25. Lund MB, Ihlen H, Voss BM, et al. Increased risk of heart valve regurgitation after mediastinal radiation for Hodgkin's disease: an echocardiographic study. Heart 1996;75(6):591–595.

26. Gustavsson A, Eskilsson J, Landberg T, et al. Late cardiac effects after mantle radiotherapy in patients with Hodgkin's disease. Ann Oncol 1990;1(5):355–363.

27. Glanzmann C, Huguenin P, Lutolf UM, Maire R, Jenni R, Gumppenberg V. Cardiac lesions after mediastinal irradiation for Hodgkin's disease. Radiother Oncol 1994;30(1):43–54.

28. Hancock SL, Cox RS, McDougall IR. Thyroid diseases after treatment of Hodgkin's disease. N Engl J Med 1991;325(9): 599–605.

29. Peerboom PF, Hassink EA, Melkert R, DeWit L, Nooijen WJ, Bruning PF. Thyroid function 10–18 years after mantle field irradiation for Hodgkin's disease. Eur J Cancer 1992;28A(10): 1716–1718.

30. Brierley JD, Rathmell AJ, Gospodarowicz MK, et al. Late effects of treatment for early-stage Hodgkin's disease. Br J Cancer 1998; 77(8):1300–1310.

31. Bethge W, Guggenberger D, Bamberg M, Kanz L, Bokemeyer C. Thyroid toxicity of treatment for Hodgkin's disease. Ann Hematol 2000;79(3):114–118.

32. Mauch P, Tarbell N, Weinstein H, et al. Stage IA and IIA supradiaphragmatic Hodgkin's disease: prognostic factors in surgically staged patients treated with mantle and paraaortic irradiation. J Clin Oncol 1988;6(10):1576–1583.

33. Hassink EA, Souren TS, Boersma LJ, et al. Pulmonary morbidity 10–18 years after irradiation for Hodgkin's disease. Eur J Cancer 1993;29A(3):343–347.

34. Loyer E, Fuller L, Libshitz HI, Palmer JL. Radiographic appearance of the chest following therapy for Hodgkin disease. Eur J Radiol 2000;35(2):136–148.

35. Lund MB, Kongerud J, Nome O, et al. Lung function impairment in long-term survivors of Hodgkin's disease. Ann Oncol 1995;6(5):495–501.

36. Koocher G, O'Malley J. The Damocles Syndrome: Psychosocial Consequences of Surviving Childhood Cancer. New York: McGraw-Hill, 1981.

37. Tross S, Holland JC. Psychological sequelae in cancer survivors. In: Holland JC, Rowland JH (eds). Handbook of Psychooncology. London: Oxford University Press, 1990:101–116.

38. Cella DF, Tross S. Psychological adjustment to survival from Hodgkin's disease. J Consult Clin Psychol 1986;54(5):616–622.

39. The Constitution of the World Health Organisation. WHO Chronicle 1947;29.

40. Fobair P, Hoppe RT, Bloom J, Cox R, Varghese A, Spiegel D. Psychosocial problems among survivors of Hodgkin's disease. J Clin Oncol 1986;4(5):805–814.

41. Kornblith AB, Anderson J, Cella DF, et al. Hodgkin disease survivors at increased risk for problems in psychosocial adaptation. The Cancer and Leukemia Group B. Cancer (Phila) 1992;70(8): 2214–2224.

42. van Tulder MW, Aaronson NK, Bruning PF. The quality of life of long-term survivors of Hodgkin's disease. Ann Oncol 1994; 5(2):153–158.

43. Norum J, Wist EA. Quality of life in survivors of Hodgkin's disease. Qual Life Res 1996;5(3):367–374.

44. Joly F, Henry-Amar M, Arveux P, et al. Late psychosocial sequelae in Hodgkin's disease survivors: a French population-based case-control study. J Clin Oncol 1996;14(9):2444–2453.

45. Aaronson NK, Cull A, Kaasa S. The EORTC modular approach to quality of life assessment in oncology. Int J Ment Health 1994;23:75–96.

46. Cella DF, Tulsky DS, Gray G, et al. The Functional Assessment of Cancer Therapy scale: development and validation of the general measure. J Clin Oncol 1993;11(3):570–579.

47. Ware JE. The SF-36 health survey. In: Spilker B (ed). Quality of Life and Pharmaeconomics in Clinical Trials. Philadelphia: Lippincott-Raven, 1996:337–346.

48. Loge JH, Kaasa S. Short form 36 (SF-36) health survey: normative data from the general Norwegian population. Scand J Soc Med 1998;26(4):250–258.

49. Loge JH, Abrahamsen AF, Ekeberg O, Kaasa S. Reduced health-related quality of life among Hodgkin's disease survivors: a comparative study with general population norms. Ann Oncol 1999;10(1):71–77.

50. Bloom JR, Gorsky RD, Fobair P, et al. Physical performance at work and at leisure: validation of a measure of biological energy in survivors of Hodgkin's disease. J Psychosocial Oncol 1990; 8(1):49–63.

51. Bloom JR, Fobair P, Gritz E, et al. Psychosocial outcomes of cancer: a comparative analysis of Hodgkin's disease and testicular cancer. J Clin Oncol 1993;11(5):979–988.

52. Greil R, Holzner B, Kemmler G, et al. Retrospective assessment of quality of life and treatment outcome in patients with Hodgkin's disease from 1969 to 1994. Eur J Cancer 1999;35(5): 698–706.

53. Olweny CL, Juttner CA, Rofe P, et al. Long-term effects of cancer treatment and consequences of cure: cancer survivors enjoy

quality of life similar to their neighbours. Eur J Cancer 1993; 29A(6):826–830.

54. Gil-Fernandez J, Ramos C, Tamayo T, et al. Quality of life and psychological well-being in Spanish long-term survivors of Hodgkin's disease: results of a controlled pilot study. Ann Hematol 2003;82(1):14–18.

55. Knobel H, Havard LJ, Brit LM, Forfang K, Nome O, Kaasa S. Late medical complications and fatigue in Hodgkin's disease survivors. J Clin Oncol 2001;19(13):3226–3233.

56. Cameron CL, Cella D, Herndon JE, et al. Persistent symptoms among survivors of Hodgkin's disease: an explanatory model based on classical conditioning. Health Psychol 2001;20(1): 71–75.

57. Osoba D, Rodrigues G, Myles J, Zee B, Pater J. Interpreting the significance of changes in health-related quality-of-life scores. J Clin Oncol 1998;16(1):139–144.

58. Lee JQ, Simmonds MJ, Wang XS, Novy DM. Differences in physical performance between men and women with and without lymphoma. Arch Phys Med Rehabil 2003;84(12): 1747–1752.

59. Devlen J, Maguire P, Phillips P, Crowther D. Psychological problems associated with diagnosis and treatment of lymphomas. II: Prospective study. Br Med J (Clin Res Ed) 1987;295(6604): 955–957.

60. Devlen J, Maguire P, Phillips P, Crowther D, Chambers H. Psychological problems associated with diagnosis and treatment of lymphomas. I: Retrospective study. Br Med J (Clin Res Ed) 1987; 295(6604):953–954.

61. Lewis G, Wessely S. The epidemiology of fatigue: more questions than answers. J Epidemiol Community Health 1992;46(2): 92–97.

62. Pawlikowska T, Chalder T, Hirsch SR, Wallace P, Wright DJ, Wessely SC. Population based study of fatigue and psychological distress [see comments]. BMJ 1994;308(6931):763–766.

63. Ganz PA, Moinpour CM, Pauler DK, et al. Health status and quality of life in patients with early-stage Hodgkin's disease treated on Southwest Oncology Group Study 9133. J Clin Oncol 2003;21(18):3512–3519.

64. Kornblith AB, Herndon JE, Zuckerman E, et al. Comparison of psychosocial adaptation of advanced stage Hodgkin's disease and acute leukemia survivors. Cancer and Leukemia Group B. Ann Oncol 1998;9(3):297–306.

65. Loge JH, Abrahamsen AF, Ekeberg O, Kaasa S. Hodgkin's disease survivors more fatigued than the general population. J Clin Oncol 1999;17(1):253–261.

66. Ruffer JU, Flechtner H, Tralls P, et al. Fatigue in long-term survivors of Hodgkin's lymphoma: a report from the German Hodgkin Lymphoma Study Group (GHSG). Eur J Cancer 2003; 39(15):2179–2186.

67. Wettergren L, Bjorkholm M, Axdorph U, Bowling A, Langius-Eklof A. Individual quality of life in long-term survivors of Hodgkin's lymphoma: a comparative study. Qual Life Res 2003; 12(5):545–554.

68. Fossa SD, Dahl AA, Loge JH. Fatigue, anxiety and depression and mental health in long-term survivors of testicular cancer. J Clin Oncol 2003;21:1249–1254.

69. Loge JH, Abrahamsen AF, Ekeberg, Kaasa S. Fatigue and psychiatric morbidity among Hodgkin's disease survivors. J Pain Symptom Manag 2000;19(2):91–99.

70. Visser MR, Smets EM. Fatigue, depression and quality of life in cancer patients: how are they related? Support Care Cancer 1998;6(2):101–108.

71. Cleeland CS, Bennett GJ, Dantzer R, et al. Are the symptoms of cancer and cancer treatment due to a shared biologic mechanism? A cytokine-immunologic model of cancer symptoms. Cancer (Phila) 2003;97(11):2919–2925.

72. Knobel H, Loge JH, Nordoy T, et al. High level of fatigue in lymphoma patients treated with high dose therapy. J Pain Symptom Manag 2000;19(6):446–456.

73. Wessely S, Chalder T, Hirsch S, Wallace P, Wright D. Psychological symptoms, somatic symptoms, and psychiatric disorder in chronic fatigue and chronic fatigue syndrome: a prospective study in the primary care setting. Am J Psychiatry 1996;153(8): 1050–1059.

74. Loge JH, Abrahamsen AF, Ekeberg O, Hannisdal E, Kaasa S. Psychological distress after cancer cure: a survey of 459 Hodgkin's disease survivors. Br J Cancer 1997;76(6):791–796.

75. Herrmann C. International experiences with the Hospital Anxiety and Depression Scale: a review of validation data and clinical results. J Psychosom Res 1997;42(1):17–41.

76. Minaire P. Disease, illness and health: theoretical models of the disablement process. Bull WHO 1992;70(3):373–379.

77. Abrahamsen AF, Loge JH, Hannisdal E, Holte H, Kvaloy S. Sociomedical situation for long-term survivors of Hodgkin's disease: a survey of 459 patients treated at one institution. Eur J Cancer 1998;34(12):1865–1870.

78. Ringdal GI, Ringdal K, Jordhoy MS, Ahlner-Elmqvist M, Jannert M, Kaasa S. Health-related quality of life (HRQOL) in family members of cancer victims: results from a longitudinal intervention study in Norway and Sweden. Palliat Med 2004;18(2): 108–120.

79. Oldervoll LM, Kaasa S, Knobel H, Loge JH. Exercise reduces fatigue in chronic fatigued Hodgkin's disease survivors: results from a pilot study. Eur J Cancer 2003;39(1):57–63.

80. Whiting P, Bagnall AM, Sowden AJ, Cornell JE, Mulrow CD, Ramirez G. Interventions for the treatment and management of chronic fatigue syndrome: a systematic review. JAMA 2001; 286(11):1360–1368.

81. Morrow GR, Hickok JT, Roscoe JA, et al. Differential effects of paroxetine on fatigue and depression: a randomized, double-blind trial from the University of Rochester Cancer Center community clinical oncology program. J Clin Oncol 2003;21(24): 4635–4641.

82. Yehuda R. Post-traumatic stress disorder. N Engl J Med 2002; 346(2):108–114.

83. Gill D, Hatcher S. Antidepressants for depression in people with physical illness. Cochrane Database Syst Rev 2000;2:CD001312.

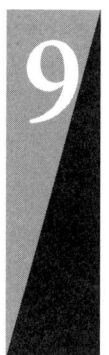

Medical and Psychosocial Issues in Testicular Cancer Survivors

Sophie D. Fosså, Lois B. Travis, and Alvin A. Dahl

Testicular cancer (TC) is the most frequent malignancy in men between 20 and 40 years of age, and the annual incidence rates are continuously increasing in the Western world.[1] Since the introduction of cisplatin-based chemotherapy, at least 90% of the patients are cured,[2] and testicular cancer survivors (TCSs) currently have a life expectancy similar to that of age-matched normal men, with posttreatment life spans of 30 to 50 years. Thus, an increasing number of TCSs experience survivorship problems related to the malignancy, its treatment, or both.

Treatment

Unilateral orchiectomy is the primary treatment of TC and yields the histologic diagnosis of seminoma and nonseminoma with equal frequency. Modern post-orchiectomy therapy of TC is based on the histologic type and the extent of disease. Risk-adapted treatment is based on a balance between malignancy-related risk factors, expected side effects, the likelihood of regular follow-up, and, not least, the patient's preference. As effective chemotherapy is available to salvage most of the patients who relapse, today's clinicians tend to administer the least toxic treatment schedule to both low-risk patients without metastases and to the good prognosis metastatic group.[3]

In patients with nonmetastatic seminoma, the standard adjuvant radiotherapy field currently comprises the intra-diaphragmatic paraaortic lymph nodes,[4] which are irradiated to 20 Gy.[5] Surveillance[6] is a valid alternative, or the use of one cycle of chemotherapy.[7] *Surveillance* is also the standard policy in patients with nonmetastatic, nonseminomatous germ cell tumors,[8] with nerve-sparing retroperitoneal lymph node dissection (RPLND), or two cycles of chemotherapy as alternatives in selected patients.[9,10] In patients with metastatic disease, the standard *chemotherapy* regimen is cisplatin based, most often containing etoposide and bleomycin,[11,12] eventually modified by ifosfamide[13] or taxol in high-risk patients or used as salvage chemotherapy.[14] In patients with metastatic disease, induction chemotherapy is frequently followed by surgical resection of residual masses.[15]

Each of the foregoing principal therapeutic modalities (surgery, radiotherapy, chemotherapy) leads to transient short-term (less than 1 year) and long-term (1 year or more) side effects, and their severity often increases with combined treatment. Previous cross-sectional studies on long-term side effects in TCSs have predominantly examined the side effects within the first 5 years posttreatment. Relatively few studies have follow-up times beyond 5 years.

Not all long-term sequelae in TCSs are caused by treatment. Impaired posttreatment endocrine and exocrine gonadal function, for example, is related both to the germ cell malignancy itself and to its treatment. The development of a contralateral testicular tumor is treatment independent and represents primary germ cell carcinogenesis at another site. The diagnosis of a second, possibly treatment-related, malignancy must be clearly separated from a late relapse with non-germ cell differentiation. Leukemia in patients with mediastinal germ cell tumor may thus be treatment related or may arise on the background of the extragonadal germ cell malignancy,[16] recognizable by modern molecular biologic techniques.[17]

Second Malignancies

Solid Tumors

The most serious late toxicity of therapy for TC is the development of a non-germ cell malignancy, for simplicity referred to as second cancer. Although several investigations[18,19] have evaluated the risk of second cancers among patients with TC, few studies have estimated long-term risks among large numbers of TCSs, taking into consideration both histology and initial treatment. The largest study to date comprised more than 28,000 1-year TCSs (1935–1993) reported to population-based cancer registries in North America and Europe.[18] Second cancers were diagnosed in 1,406 patients [observed to expected ratio (O/E), 1.43; 95% confidence interval (CI), 1.36–1.51; absolute excess risk, 16 excess cancers per 10,000 men per year]. Second cancer risk was similar following seminomas (O/E, 1.4) and nonseminomatous tumors (O/E, 1.5).

TABLE 9.1. Relative risk of second malignancies following treatment of testicular cancer.

	Number of second cancers	Relative risk		
		All	Seminoma	Nonseminoma
All second cancers	1,406	1.43	1.42	1.50
All solid tumours	1,251	1.35	1.35	1.36
Stomach	93	1.95	1.73	2.95
Small intestine	12	3.18	4.35	—
Colon	105	1.27	1.30	1.32*
Rectum	77	1.41	1.58	0.92*
Pancreas	66	2.21	2.35	1.85*
Kidney	55	1.50	1.50	1.41*
Bladder	154	2.02	2.12	1.85
Melanoma	58	1.69	1.57	1.74
Thyroid	19	2.92	2.61	3.82
Connective tissue	22	3.16	3.46	2.40*
Non-Hodgkin's lymphoma	68	1.88	1.83	2.09
All leukemias**	64	2.13	1.92	2.78

*Nonsignificant.

**Statistical significance restricted to acute leukemia.

Source: Modified from Travis et al,[18] by permission of *Journal of the Naional Cancer Institute,* with emphasis on statistically significant (*P* < 0.05) observations.

Among all TCSs, significantly increased risks were observed for all malignancies taken together: malignant melanoma, acute lymphoblastic leukemia, acute nonlymphocytic leukemia, non-Hodgkin's lymphoma, and cancers of the stomach, colon, rectum, pancreas, kidney, bladder, thyroid, and connective tissue (Table 9.1). The risk of solid tumors increased with follow-up time since the diagnosis of TC and reached 1.5 after two decades (*P* trend, 0.00002). Twenty-year survivors of TC remained at significantly increased risk for cancers of stomach (O/E, 2.3), colon (O/E, 1.7), pancreas (O/E, 3.2), kidney (O/E, 2.3), bladder (O/E, 2.8), and connective tissue (O/E, 4.7). The cumulative risk of any second cancer 25 years after TC diagnosis was 15.7% (Figure 9.1, Table 9.2). The larger risk for seminoma patients (18.2%; 95% CI,

16.8–19.6) than for those with nonseminomatous tumors (11.1%; 95% CI, 9.3–12.9) most likely reflects the older mean age of the former group (39.2 years versus 29.8 years), given the similarity in the excess cumulative risks. The temporal distribution of increased risks and apportionment between treatment groups were consistent with the late sequelae of radiation for cancers of stomach, bladder, and possibly pancreas. These findings were thus consistent with the location of these organs in the infradiaphragmatic radiotherapy fields administered for TC. Although information on radiotherapy fields and dose are not registered in cancer registry records, Travis et al.[18] provided estimates of the average radiation doses received by stomach (mean, 13–26 Gy), bladder (mean, 22.4–45 Gy), and pancreas (mean, 16.7–33.8 Gy) at treatment doses of 25 and 50 Gy for seminomas and nonseminomatous germ cell cancer, respectively, using standard anteroposterior (AP)/posteroanterior paraaortic or inguinal iliac fields.[4]

Previous clinical series have found significantly eightfold-increased risks of stomach cancer (*n* = 2) following infra- and supradiaphragmatic irradiation for testicular tumors[20] and a four- to fivefold risk with abdominal radiotherapy (*n* = 10).[21] There are few data, however, that quantify the relationship between radiation dose and the risk of gastric cancer.[22] In particular, the precise impact of radiation field size and/or dose is not clearly defined for current infradiaphragmatic adjuvant

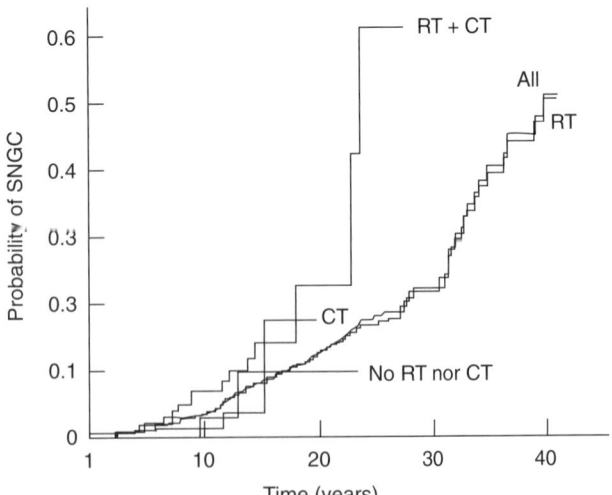

FIGURE 9.1. Cumulative risk of any second non-germ cell cancer by time from primary diagnosis for different treatment groups. (See Table 9.2.) *RT,* radiotherapy; *CT,* chemotherapy. (From Hoff Wanderas et al,[23] by permission of *European Journal of Cancer.*)

TABLE 9.2. Patients at risk at start of interval.[a]

Time from diagnosis (years)	Treatment category (n)				
	RT	CT	RT + CT	No RT or CT	All
1–9	1,194	346	277	189	2,006
10–19	827	112	83	59	1,081
20–29	365	2	7	5	379
30–39	92	—	—	—	92

[a] See Figure 9.1 for further information and definitions.

radiotherapy. Therefore, the NCRI (National Cancer Research Institute, UK) Testis Cancer Clinical Studies Group has initiated a long-term follow-up study of 2,500 patients with stage I TC treated between 1962 and 1994 with infradiaphragmatic radiotherapy, recording the individual target fields and doses, and any salvage treatment as predictors of development of second cancer.

Before the use of cisplatin in TC therapy, few patients treated with chemotherapy only lived long enough to develop a secondary malignancy. To date, modern chemotherapy alone (e.g., bleomycin, etoposide, and cisplatin, or BEP) has not, to our knowledge, been associated with an increased risk of secondary solid tumors. The number of patients observed for more than 10 years after cisplatin-based chemotherapy is limited, however, and further follow-up will be required.

There is also little information on whether TC patients treated with both radiotherapy and chemotherapy are at greater risk of solid tumors than those who received radiation alone. Van Leeuwen et al.[21] found that the risk of all gastrointestinal cancers following radiotherapy alone (O/E, 2.9; 95% CI, 1.8–4.4; observed, 22) did not differ significantly from the risk (O/E, 5.5; 95% CI 1.1–15.9; observed, 3) in patients given both radiotherapy and chemotherapy, but low numbers in the latter group limit the statistical power to detect any difference.

Hoff Wanderas et al.[23] showed that the risk of all second non-germ cell cancers following radiotherapy alone (O/E, 1.58; 95% CI, 1.3–1.9; observed, 130) was significantly larger than the risk (O/E, 3.54; 95% CI, 2.0–5.8; observed, 15) after radiotherapy plus chemotherapy, but also pointed out that patients in the latter group frequently received multiple irradiation fields and larger doses. Further, many patients who received combined-modality therapy also received chemotherapy regimens that included doxorubicin.[23] Breslow and colleagues[24] reported that children (n = 234) given doxorubicin and more than 35 Gy of abdominal radiation for Wilm's tumor were at 36-fold risk (95% CI, 16–72; observed, 8) of second solid tumors, compared with no second tumors observed among children (n = 291) given doxorubicin alone.[24] These investigators[24] hypothesized that doxorubicin might inhibit the repair of radiation-induced damage, perhaps through its effects on topo-isomerase II. Evidence with regard to the human carcinogenicity of doxorubicin itself remains conflicting.[20]

Leukemias

TCS patients are at increased risk of leukemia[18,21,25–29]; however, there are few analytical studies that characterize in detail the contribution of both radiotherapy and chemotherapy to these cancers (see also Chapter 17). Travis and colleagues[16] conducted an international case-control investigation of secondary myelodysplastic syndrome or leukemia within a cohort of 18,567 1-year TCSs survivors of TC diagnosed between 1970 and 1993 and reported to eight population-based cancer registries in North America and Europe. For all patients (36 cases, 106 controls), detailed information on all treatment was gathered for chemotherapy drugs including cumulative dose and duration of chemotherapy. External-beam radiotherapy, usually to paraaortic and pelvic regions, was administered to 101 patients. Radiotherapy for 17 patients (restricted to 1970–1980) included mediastinal

irradiation (mean dose, 35.0 Gy), in addition to abdominal and pelvic fields; 3 additional patients were given extended-field (abdomen/pelvis/chest) radiotherapy and alkylating agent chemotherapy. For patients who received radiation limited to abdomen and pelvis without alkylating agents, larger mean treatment doses were used for nonseminomatous tumors (35.4 Gy) than for seminomas (30.7 Gy). Daily radiotherapy logs for each patient were used to calculate an average dose to the active bone marrow.

For all TC patients, leukemia risk increased with increasing radiation dose to active bone marrow (P = 0.02), with patients given chest radiotherapy in addition to abdominal/pelvic fields accounting for much of the risk at higher doses.[16] A nonsignificant 3-fold-increased relative risk of leukemia was demonstrated after pelvic-abdominal radiotherapy (mean dose to bone marrow, 10.9 Gy) without alkylating agent chemotherapy; for patients who received additional supradiaphragmatic irradiation (mean dose to bone marrow 19.5 Gy), a significantly increased 11-fold risk was apparent. For patients given radiotherapy limited to abdomen and pelvis, the estimated relative risk (RR) of leukemia associated with a treatment dose of 25, 30, and 35 Gy was 2.2, 2.5, and 2.9, respectively; none of these estimates was statistically significant.

Radiation dose to active bone marrow and cumulative dose of cisplatin to treat TC were both predictive of elevated risks of leukemia (P = 0.001) in a statistical model that took into account all treatment parameters.[16] The highly significant dose–response relationship observed for total amount of cisplatin and leukemia risk was in accord with results in a study of women treated with platinum-based chemotherapy for ovarian cancer.[30]

Although the cumulative dose of etoposide used to treat TC did not contribute to leukemia risk when doses of cisplatin and radiation were taken into account, patients given etoposide also received larger amounts of cisplatin, making it difficult to tease apart any individual contributions to leukemia risk.[16] The predicted risk of leukemia associated with a cumulative cisplatin dose of 650 mg was 3.2 (95% CI, 1.5–8.4); larger cumulative doses (1,000 mg cisplatin) were associated with significantly increased sixfold risks. In terms of absolute risk, Travis et al.[16] estimated that of 10,000 testicular cancer patients treated with cisplatin-based chemotherapy with a cumulative cisplatin dose of about 650 mg and followed for 15 years, 16 excess leukemias might result.

Based on small numbers, prior studies have linked etoposide and cisplatin for TC with excess leukemias,[26–29] usually at high cumulative doses of etoposide (3,000 mg/m²)[26] in contrast to the lower total doses administered in the study by Travis et al.,[30] which are similar to the dose of less than 2,000 mg/m² (33) used today. Smith et al.[31] reported that the 6-year cumulative risk of secondary leukemia among patients who received 1,500 to 2,999 mg/m² etoposide was small (0.7%), based on a survey of clinical trials. In a recent review of the literature, Kollmannsberger et al.[32] concluded that the cumulative incidence of leukemia for TC patients given etoposide at cumulative doses of less than 2,000 mg/m² and more than 2,000 mg/m² was 0.5% and 2% at a median of 5 years follow-up.

Whether combined radiochemotherapy for TC results in a larger risk of leukemia than chemotherapy alone has not been well-studied. Van Leeuwen et al.[21] found no significant difference between the risk of leukemia following chemotherapy alone (one case) and combined modality therapy (two cases), but the small numbers precluded any opportunity to detect a difference. Similarly, in the case-control study by Travis et al.,[16] only a small number of patients were given combined-modality therapy (two cases and four controls), and the risk of leukemia (fivefold) was nearly identical for all investigated patients.

Contralateral TC

Three percent to 5% of the patients with unilateral TC develop a germ cell malignancy of the contralateral testicle.[33] The increased risk of contralateral TC in men with TC has generally been thought to reflect shared etiologic influences.[34] Few large studies,[33,35] however, have provided estimates of the risk for contralateral TC. The largest investigation[35] to date, based on 60 cases occurring in 2,201 men diagnosed with a first primary germ cell cancer (1953–1990), reported that the cumulative risk of a contralateral testicular cancer at 15 years of follow-up was 3.9% (95% CI, 2.8%–5.0%). The investigators also concluded that the risk was not significantly altered by treatment of the first cancer. Patients with a contralateral testicular cancer usually undergo a second orchiectomy with the subsequent need of lifelong androgen substitution.

Patients with extragonadal germ cell tumors (EGCT) are at a significantly elevated risk for subsequently developing TC, most probably based on the existence of carcinoma in situ in one or both testicles.[36,37] In a large, international study of 635 patients with EGCT conducted by Hartmann and colleagues,[36] the cumulative risk of developing a metachronous TC was 10.3% at 10 years. The treatment follows the risk-adapted strategies as for TC with principally the same long-term sequelae.

Based on the increased risk of developing a new gonadal germ cell tumor, TCSs and patients with a cured extragonadal tumor are recommended to perform regular testicular self-examination.

Gonadal Toxicity

Spermatogenesis and Leydig Cell Function

According to today's most relevant hypothesis, germ cell carcinogenesis starts in the primordial cells during the 8th week of embryonic life.[38] Deleterious environmental influences may result in aberrant gonadal development that subsequently manifests as testicular maldescent, testicular atrophy, reduced Lydig cell function, impaired spermatogenesis, or even germ cell malignancy. These etiologic factors together with tumor-related influences are the reasons why about 60% of unilaterally orchiectomized patients with newly diagnosed TC have impaired spermatogenesis before any additional treatment.[39–43] Impaired Leydig cell function and reduced sperm cell production may be found even in patients with TC before orchiectomy of the affected testicle.[41–43] Further, this etiologic hypothesis also explains why 10% to 15% of TCSs have permanently reduced exocrine and endocrine gonadal function even without having received chemotherapy or radiotherapy.[44,45]

The exocrine long-term gonadal function in TCSs has been extensively studied, although the available investigations do not clearly differentiate between cisplatin-based chemotherapy containing vinblastine from those containing etoposide or ifosfamide. Carboplatin seems to be less gonadotoxic than cisplatin.[46] Standard cisplatin-based chemotherapy (four cycles) and infradiaphragmatic radiotherapy (36 Gy or less) transiently reduces or abolishes spermatogenesis (low sperm counts; high serum follicle-stimulating hormone, FSH) with recovery starting 6 to 8 months after treatment discontinuation. These effects are dependent on the type of the radiation target field as well as types of cytotoxic drugs, number of cycles, and cumulative doses[4,39,40,42,47–59] (Figure 9.2, Table 9.3). Age above 35 years and reduced pretreatment gonadal function reduce the ability for such recovery.[52]

The Leydig cell function is affected by radiotherapy or chemotherapy at a lesser degree than spermatogenesis, but Nord et al.[45] demonstrated an increasing number of hypogonadal long-term TCSs in relation to treatment type and treatment intensity. According to this study 16% of the long-term TCSs are hypogonadal, most often subclinically, but 25% of these TCSs need androgen substitution.

There is no effective treatment available for TCSs who have become oligo- or azospermic as a result of cytotoxic treatment. Moreover, treatment with luteinizing hormone-releasing hormone (LH-RH) analogues together with chemotherapy has not shown sufficient gonadal protection either.[60] Pretreatment cryopreservation of sperm cells[61] and exogenous androgen substitution[62] thus remain the only means to ameliorate gonadotoxic long-term sequelae.

Somatic Aspects of Fertility

Posttreatment fertility is threatened by ejaculatory dysfunction, permanent azospermia, or high-grade oligospermia, and psychosocial distress.

After bilateral radical template RPLND[63,64] almost all TCSs have to face infertility problems as a result of postoperative "dry ejaculation." The introduction of unilateral and/or nerve-sparing procedures[10] has reduced this proportion to 10% to 15% even when the operation is performed following chemotherapy.[65] However, even though statistical analyses have proven that fertility-saving strategies have been successful in groups of patients prediction of posttreatment fertility is difficult in the *individual patient*. It is, therefore,

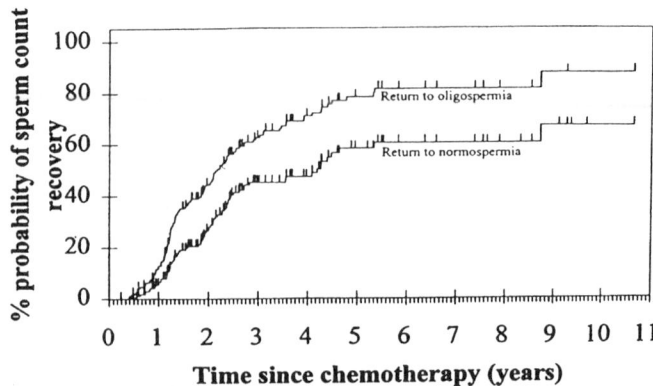

FIGURE 9.2. Recovery to oligospermia and normospermia in 178 patients after chemotherapy for testicular cancer. (From Lampe et al,[47] by permission of *Journal of Clinical Oncology*.)

TABLE 9.3. Long-term gonadal function in testicular cancer survivors.[a]

Author		Number of patients	Observation time (months)	Sperm count (10⁶/mL)	Azospermia	Elevated		Sub-normal testosterone
						LH	FSH	
Surgery only								
Aass (1991)		33	24–48b	20[c] (0–222)[b]	11/24	1	8	5
Jacobsen (2000)		60	63	37 (0–243)			10	
Radiotherapy								
Aass (1991)		36	24–48	11 (0–76)	9/22	2	13	4
Jacobsen (1997)								
Dog-leg		44	12	20 ± 14, 0[d]				
Paraaortic		24	12	49 ± 35, 6[d]				
Fosså (1999)								
Dog-leg		48	18		17/48			
Paraaortic		54	18		6/54			
Chemotherapy								
Cisplatin-based								
Standard								
Aass (1991)		42	24–48	65	5/17	5	17	6
Petersen (1994)		33	79	(0–166)	5/27	8	8	1
Stephenson (1995)		30	>24	6 (0–83)	6/30			
Palmieri (1996)		28	37	35 (0–90)	6/28	4	11	3
High dose or combined with radiotherapy	Aass (1991)	19	24–48			3	12	4
	Peterson (1994)	21	58	0 (0–70)	8/17	8	22	2
	Palmieri (1996)	10	36	8 (0–18)	3/10	6	8	2
Carboplatin	Reiter (1998)	22	48	(35–128)				
	Lampe (1999)	59	30		12/59			
Not specified	Bokemeyer (1996)	63	58			21	40	6
	Lampe (1999)	119	30		50/119			
	Strumberg (2002)	30	15			13	22	2

Blank spaces indicate that information is not provided.

[a] Limited to reports published after 1990.

[b] Range.

[c] Median.

[d] Mean ± standard deviation (only patients with pretreatment sperm count ≥10).

recommended that sperm banking[61] with the possibility of assisted fertilization[66] is offered to all patients with newly diagnosed TC who do not explicitly exclude future fatherhood (see also Chapter 19).

Gonadal Long-Term Effects of Treatment for Bilateral TC

Testicular radiotherapy (18–20 Gy) usually prevents the development of an invasive cancer in TCSs with cancer in situ in the contralateral testicle,[67] although with an increased risk of hypogonadism. Surgical testicle-saving strategies are recommended in case of small tumors.[68]

Neurologic Morbidity

Peripheral Neurotoxicity

Cisplatin-based chemotherapy leads to dose-dependent peripheral sensory neuropathy (paraesthesiae, pain) with a peak occurrence about 6 months after treatment initiation and a slight decrease thereafter.[53,69–73] Vinblastine displays an at least additive effect, whereas VP-16 is less neurotoxic.[11] About 20% of TCSs report peripheral sensory neuropathy

("quite a bit," "very much") 2 years after three or four cycles of BEP chemotherapy,[73] although objective measurements reveal persistent peripheral neuropathy in 70% to 80% of the patients.[74] The long-term peripheral sensory neuropathy is, however, only rarely handicapping, and most TCSs have "become used" to this problem at long-term follow-up.

Ototoxicity

Ototoxicity represents a specific long-term sequela in TCSs after cisplatin-containing chemotherapy,[53,57,69,73,75,76] with tinnitus and hearing loss in about 25% and 20% of the patients, respectively.[53,69,73] Audiograms indicate that cisplatin mostly decreases the auditory acuity above 4,000 Hz.[57] To decrease long-term ototoxicity, each cycle of standard chemotherapy (BEP) should be given during 5 days, in particular if more than three cycles are planned.[73]

Autonomic Neuropathy

The resection of sympathetic nerve fibers may lead to considerable persistent disturbance of blood flow and temperature sense in the legs.[77] The possibility exists that chemotherapy-induced long-term autonomic neurotoxicity contributes to vascular dysfunction.[78,79]

Because no effective treatment exists for cisplatin-induced peripheral neuropathy or ototoxicity, prevention of these late effects is essential by adequate hydration during drug administration and possibly by the supportive use of amifosfine.[80]

Nephrotoxicity

Cisplatin is highly nephrotoxic if sufficient hydration and diuresis are not provided during the drug's administration. Even then, four cycles of standard BEP may lead to chronic dose-dependent, though often subclinical, decrease of the glomerular function.[81]

Several authors have described persistent low serum magnesium and/or low phosphate levels after standard chemotherapy,[53,69] although not all investigators have been able to confirm these findings.[81,82] Carboplatin is less nephrotoxic than cisplatin, but doses of 1,500 mg/m^2 or more given over 3 days have a comparable effect as cisplatin 50 mg/m^2 applied on 1 day.[83]

Radiation target fields always include parts of the renal arteries, with the risk of postradiation subintimal fibrosis and reduction of the arterial flow. Fosså et al.[81] showed that infradiaphragmatic radiotherapy (30–40 Gy) leads to subclinical nephrotoxicity after a mean observation time of 11 years, in particular if combined with chemotherapy.

Cardiovascular Toxicity

Raynaud's Phenomenon

About 20% to 30% of TCSs report the development of Raynaud-like phenomenon after standard BEP chemotherapy that peak at 6 months after chemotherapy and subsequently slightly decrease to a persistent pathologic level.[53,56,73,76,84] These side effects are related to disturbance of autonomic innervation as well as thickening of the intima in small arteries with reduction of the blood vessel volume. Most studies point to bleomycin as an important etiological agent.[69] Interestingly, TCSs complaining of postchemotherapy Raynaud's phenomenon display an increased risk for erectile dysfunction.[78]

Cardiovascular Risk Factors and Major Events

Increased risk of postchemotherapy cardiovascular morbidity in TCSs as compared with TCSs on surveillance or men from the general population is evidenced in several studies[53,85–87] (Tables 9.4, 9.5). Today's chemotherapy for TC may even represent a high-risk factor for the development of a "metabolic syndrome" (diabetes mellitus, hypertension, hypercholesterolemia, obesity) and myocardial infarction.[86,88]

Huddart et al.[82] point out the possibility that partial heart irradiation during adjuvant radiotherapy may increase the risk of life-threatening cardiac events, as portions of the heart receive radiation doses of 30 to 90 cGy during current routine radiotherapy. TCSs having received former times mediastinal radiotherapy (30–40 Gy) for stage II or III TC represent a high-risk group for cardiac events and should be monitored accordingly.[89] These observations are in line with the findings of Fosså et al.[90] of an increased relative risk of cardiovascular mortality in TCSs treated from 1962 to 1993, most of them having received radiotherapy.

TABLE 9.4. Cardiovascular risk factors in TCSs.

Author	Number of patients	Observation time (years)[a]	High cholesterol[b]	Reduced renal function[c]	Low Mg[c]	Hypertension[b]	Abnormal body mass index (BMI) increase
Surgery only							
Meinardi (2002)	40	8	58%			8%	28%
Fosså (2003)	14	11		14%	7%		
Huddart (2003)	24	10	1%	8%	0%	9%	
Radiotherapy							
Fosså (2003)	18	11		28%	0%		
Huddard (2003)	230	10	3%	13%	0%	12%	
Chemotherapy							
Boyer (1992)	497			8–43%			
Osanto (1992)	43	4		15%			
Bokemeyer (2000)	63	5	32%	19%	18%	15%	32%
Meinardi (2000)	62	8	79%	31%	8%	39%	21%
Strumberg (2002)	32	15	81%			25%	48%
Fosså (2003)	44	11		30%	5%		
Huddard (2003)	390	10	2%	14%	0%	21%	
Chemotherapy + Radiotherapy							
Fosså (2003)	9	11		56%	0%		
Huddard (2003)	130	10	0%	27%	2%	13%	

[a] Median.

[b] Above.

[c] Below the institution's normal range.

TABLE 9.5. Cardiovascular events in TCSs: angina pectoris, myocardial infarction, cerebrovascular hemorrhage, cardiovascular death.

Author	Number of patients	Median observation time (years)	Number of events	Age-adjusted RR
Chemotherapy				
Boyer (1992)[a]	480	≥1	23	
Bokemeyer (1996)	63	5	2	
Meinardi (2000)[86]	62	8	5	7.1 (1.9–18.3)[c]
Strumberg (2002)	32	15	1	
Cardiovascular mortality				
Huddart (2003)[b82]	992	10	68	
All treatment	242		9	Reference
Surgery only	230		22	2.40 (1.04–5.49)
Radiotherapy	390		26	2.59 (1.15–5.84)
Chemotherapy	130		11	2.78 (1.09–7.07)
Chemotherapy + radiotherapy				
Lagars (2004)	211	>15	23	1.95 (1.24–2.94)
Fosså (2004)[d90]				
Not specified	3,378	1962–1997	107	1.2 (1.0–1.5)

[a] Review.

[b] Mono-institutional.

[c] Numbers in parentheses, 95% confidence interval.

[d] Cancer Registry based.

Gastrointestinal Toxicity

With the target doses and target fields administered today,[4,91] the prevalence of slight gastrointestinal (GI) symptoms among TCSs[70,91,92] is only marginally above the proportion reported by the general population.[93] Major long-term GI problems such as peptic ulcer are observed in only 3% to 5% of the TCSs.[94,95] Target doses of 36 Gy or more or the combination of radiotherapy with radiosensitizing cytostatic drugs (adriamycin, cisplatin) increase the risk of persistent diarrhea and malabsorption.[70,96] Increased retroperitoneal fibrosis has occasionally been observed causing ureteric or biliary stenosis[97] or mimicking pancreatic cancer.[98]

Other Long-Term Toxicities

The typical acute toxicities of bleomycin of the skin and the lungs do not, in general, remain as long-term morbidities, whereas corticosteroid-related aseptic osteonecrosis represents a rare long-term complication in TCSs.[99]

Psychosocial and Quality-of-Life Issues

Introduction

Psychologic distress, health-related quality of life, as well as sexual dysfunction and paternity distress, have all been the focus for several quantitative and a few qualitative investigations in TCSs. Hardly any of these studies have randomized controlled designs.

TC involves an organ intrinsically associated with reproduction, sexuality, and masculine self-image, issues of importance to ill and healthy men alike. Global health-related quality of life (HRQoL) as assessed by available instruments does not cover these functions. The only available TC module[100] has not been completely validated. Paternity issues are regularly rated with unvalidated questions, whereas mental health and issues of sexuality have been studied by psychometrically validated and nonvalidated forms.

TCSs, similar to men in the general population, may have significant pretreatment problems such as unemployment, economical worries, mental disorders, relational problems, and other physical illnesses. The influence of such pretreatment issues on posttreatment adaptation is not well known because of the lack of prospective studies with sufficient sample sizes. Sociocultural differences in relationship to masculinity, sexuality, fertility, and employment should also be kept in mind when findings are compared across studies. Long-term TCSs also have problems in common with cancer patients in general, such as fear of recurrence and death. Coping ability has not been studied in either short- or long-term TCSs.

The overall conclusion so far is that long-term TCSs in general show good psychosocial adaptation; the mean HRQoL is at the level of the general male population. However, TCSs show a higher prevalence of anxiety disorders and some sexual dysfunctions.

Partnered Relationship in TCSs

In most studies, the majority of TCSs (70% to 90%) were in partnered relationships when TC was diagnosed. The rate of divorce and broken relationships for TCSs is 5% to 10% in most follow-up studies. Those couples that did separate saw the cancer as a significant factor in their breakup.[101,102]

Few wives found their husbands less attractive or masculine as TCSs, and in the few studies of wives, the majority found their sexual satisfaction unchanged.[103] The main concern of the wives was to have children, particularly if the couple had not achieved parenthood before the TC was diagnosed. Moynihan[104] found that 22% of partners had psychiatric morbidity, mainly anxiety and fertility worries.

Changes in Body Image

The studies published so far do not confirm any devastating effects on body image or feelings of masculinity as suggested by van Basten et al.[105] However, Gritz et al.[103] reported that 23% of patients perceived a permanent decrease in overall attractiveness. Rudberg et al.[84] reported that 15% of Swedish TCSs felt less attractive, whereas 33% was found in a sample from Japan.[106] No negative impact of orchidectomy was reported in a Scottish[107] and in an Italian sample.[108] These differences could reflect different cultural attitudes toward orchiectomy.

Health-Related Quality of Life

Posttreatment HRQoL is not identical to therapy-related psychologic or somatic morbidity, but relates to the patient's overall perception of physical and psychosocial well-being, including family life, leisure activity, and occupational situation. Older studies found that TCSs generally were strong, fit, and satisfied compared with controls.[103,109–111] Newer studies with validated instruments have confirmed that HRQoL generally is as good in TCSs as in the general male population.[112,113] Data from Norwegian TCSs ($n = 1,409$) with a mean follow-up age of 11 years show minimal differences on the eight dimensions of Short Form 36 (SF-36) compared with the general male population ($n = 2673$)[114] (Figure 9.3).

The influence of treatment modalities on HRQoL is still unsettled, mostly due to small samples with lack of statistical power. Joly et al.[113] found no differences ($n = 71$), while Rudberg et al.[112] ($n = 277$) found that those treated with intensive chemotherapy scored less favorably concerning HRQoL. In initially metastatic patients postchemotherapy RPLND did not worsen HRQoL as compared with chemotherapy alone.[115] Recently, Fosså et al.[73] reported that 2 years after chemotherapy, 36% of TCSs displayed improved and 13% deteriorated HRQoL, compared with baseline.

Mental Health

Most studies report a higher level of anxiety symptoms and higher prevalence of anxiety disorders among TCSs (20%)

compared with controls and in the general population.[104,116,117] There is indication that a considerable proportion of TCSs live with a low feeling of safety.[117] It is unclear if there is more mental morbidity associated with the more-intensive treatment regimens. If the prevalence of depression is increased, it is also unsettled due to considerable overlap between depression and fatigue. The level of fatigue, but not of depression, was reported to be higher than in the general population, but lower than among male patients with Hodgkin's disease.[117] Fatigue was considered a major problem by many TCSs.[118]

During recent years, increasing attention has been paid to postchemotherapy cognitive mental disturbances in cancer patients.[119,120] In the European experience about 20% of the TCSs report decreased cognitive functions 2 years after four cycles of BEP.[73] In the future, prospective studies are highly needed to assess changes of cognitive functions in TCSs.

Social Functioning

The continuation of planned education and professional life after treatment obviously is of great importance for TCSs, but only few reports have dealt with this issue. Studies indicate that most TCSs continue in work.[105,108] Kaasa et al.[116] reported even greater work satisfaction in TCSs in general than in an age-matched population sample. There appears to be little change in relation to friends and social contacts.[112]

Obtaining bank loans and life insurance is a common problem for TCSs,[113] although national policies vary considerably.

Sexual Dysfunctions

Two systematic reviews of sexual functioning in TCSs[121,122] emphasize the considerable methodologic problems in the field. TC treatment can result in both physiologic changes in sexual functioning and trigger emotional reactions (e.g., sexual performance anxiety, fear of loss of control, uncertainty about the future). Fatigue and general malaise can have profound effect on libido, as can hair loss and weight loss. Emotional factors such as uncertainty about the future, anxiety, and loss of control may also inhibit libido. Generally,

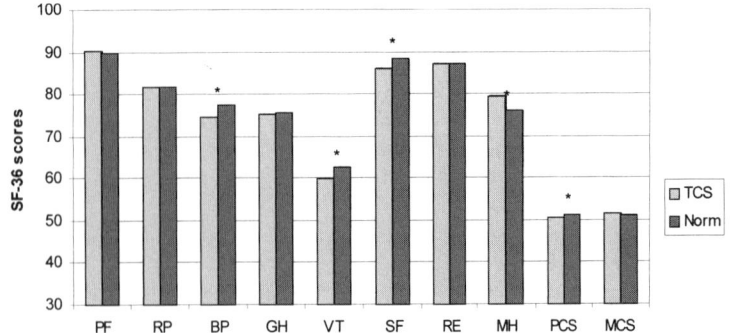

FIGURE 9.3. Health-related quality of life (SF-36) in testicular cancer survivors (TCSs) versus age-matched men from the general population. PF, physical functioning; RP, role physical; BP, bodily pain; GH, general health; VT, vitality; SF, social functioning; RE, role emotional; MH, mental health; PCS, physical composite score; MCS, mental composite score. Norm data are age adjusted to mach the TCS. *P less than 0.05. (From A MyKletun et al,[114] by permission of *Journal of Clinical Oncology*.)

TABLE 9.6. Future directions.

Healthcare professionals	Patients
Clinical routine	1. Psychologic acceptance of being a TCS, sometimes with unavoidable side effects
1. Thorough pretreatment counseling and information on expected unavoidable side effects	2. Adoption of a healthy lifestyle (nonsmoking, weight control, physical activity)
2. Use of risk-adapted therapy	3. Testicular self-examination
3. Organization of long-term follow-up	
4. Evidence-based treatment of side effects, including psychosocial support, and structured intervention trials	
Research	
1. Prospective studies	
2. Biochemical pharmacokinetic and pharmacogenetic analyses	
3. Epidemiologic investigations comparing TCSs with other cancer survivors and the general population	

there seems to be a high correlation between sexual functioning before and after treatment for TC, whereas the relation to treatment modality is less clear.[123–125] Findings must be considered in relation to age[123] and to the prevalence in the general population.[126] Erectile dysfunction is, for example, reported at the same level as in the general population (approximately 10%).[127]

Thirty per cent to 50% of TCSs report a decrease in sexual functioning compared with before treatment for TC.[112,123–125,127] Two-thirds reported decreased sexual activity, and one-third was dissatisfied with their sexual functioning.[127]

Psychologic and behavioral features such as desire, orgasmic pleasure, sexual activity, and satisfaction are affected by all treatment modalities, even surveillance. Reduction or loss of orgasm, loss of desire, and sexual dissatisfaction all show a prevalence of approximately 20%, which is significantly higher than in the general population.[127] Even in the surveillance group, 25% of TCSs report negative changes, which is the same proportion as in the radiation group, whereas those with chemotherapy reported more dysfunctions.[122] Psychologic functioning plays a strong role for these sexual dysfunctions.[128,129]

Fertility Issues

Biologic inability to father a child presents a serious challenge to a man's perception of his masculinity, to his self-esteem, and to his intimate relations, although the inability to achieve paternity evokes different responses at various points in a man's life.

Rieker et al.[130] found that fertility distress was common, but was a major problem only among those childless and those with ejaculatory dysfunction. No significant relationship was, however, found between TC-related infertility and marital separation.[101,104]

Psychologic Interventions

A randomized controlled trial of psychologic support in relation to primary treatment of TC showed an effectiveness that hardly differed from that of nonintervention.[131] Treatment for sexual dysfunctions in TCSs has been scarcely described, but seems to follow general principles for such dysfunctions.

Summary and Future Directions

The introduction of cisplatin-based chemotherapy into the treatment of testicular cancer has been one of the largest successes during the past three decades in oncology. Both oncologists and TCSs, however, must accept that long-term toxicity cannot completely be avoided: 10% to 20% of TCSs develop long-term health problems, most of them only slightly interfering with the patients' quality of life.

To minimize treatment-induced side effects, oncologists should follow evidence-based risk-adapted therapeutic guidelines, thus avoiding over- and undertreatment (Table 9.6). Furthermore, TCSs must be educated about the importance of adopting a healthy lifestyle (smoking cessation, weight control, physical activity) to minimize life-threatening side effects such as cardiovascular toxicity. They should be offered long-term follow-up in specialized multidisciplinary cancer survivor clinics that follow structured clinical and research programs with the aim at an early phase to recognize side effects and, if possible, to intervene (for example, testosterone substitution in hypogonal TCSs). Such long-term follow-up of TCSs and other cancer survivors will enable large-scale comparative epidemiologic investigations. Avoiding unnecessary anxiety, a former TC patient should also be made aware of his increased risk of tumor development in the contralateral testicle, warranting regular self-examination. Only rarely the oncologist will have to discuss the excess risk of subsequent non-germ cell cancer, although this risk should always be considered by healthcare professionals seeing TCSs with "unusual" symptoms.

Many of the reports on TCSs' long-term toxicity rely on the patients' responses to questionnaires. However, during recent years clinical investigators increasingly have validated these responses by objective measures, such as clinical examinations and organ-specific functional tests.[45,79,82,86] Interestingly, such studies have demonstrated that, for example, cisplatin or cisplatin adducts are retained in the human body (plasma, liver, muscle) for at least 20 years.[132,133] Whether an association exists between such cisplatin retention and long-term toxicity should be studied in future analyses, which should also take into account pharmacogenetic and molecular biologic parameters. The results of such investigations will increase our understanding of the considerable variability of physical and psychosocial long-term toxicity and will assist the identification of risk groups.

So far, the medical literature on long-term survivorship in TC patients almost exclusively contains cross-sectional studies. Prospective investigations are needed to identify premorbid risk factors of physical and psychosocial long-term toxicity.

References

1. Engeland A, Haldorsen T, Tretli S, et al. Prediction of cancer incidence in the Nordic countries up to the years 2000 and 2010. A Collaborative Study of the Five Nordic Cancer Registries. APMIS 1993;101(suppl 38):1–124.

2. Einhorn LH, Williams SD, Loehrer PJ, et al. Evaluation of optimal duration of chemotherapy in favorable-prognosis disseminated germ cell tumours: a Southeastern Cancer Study Group protocol. J Clin Oncol 1989;7:387–391.

3. International Germ Cell Cancer Collaborative Group (IGCCCG). The International Germ Cell Consensus Classification: a prognostic factor-based staging system for metastatic germ cell cancers. J Clin Oncol 1997;15:594–603.

4. Fosså SD, Horwich A, Russell JM, et al. Optimal planning target volume for stage I testicular seminoma: A Medical Research Council Testicular Tumour Working Group. J Clin Oncol 1999; 17:1146–1154.

5. Fosså SD, Jones WG, Stenning SP, for the TE18 Collaborators; MRC Clinical Trials Unit, London. Quality of life (QL) after radiotherapy (RT) for stage I seminoma: results from a randomised trial of two RT schedules (MRC TE18). Proc Am Soc Clin Oncol 2002;21:188.

6. Warde P, Specht L, Horwich A, et al. Prognostic factors for relapse in stage I Seminoma managed by surveillance: a pooled analysis. J Clin Oncol 2002;20:4448–4452.

7. Oliver RTD, Edmonds PM, Ong JYH, et al. Pilot studies of 2 and 1 course carboplatin as adjuvant for stage I seminoma: should it be tested in a randomized trial against radiotherapy? Int J Radiat Oncol Biol Phys 1994;29:3–8.

8. Read G, Stenning SP, Cullen MH, et al. Medical Research Council Prospective study of surveillance for stage I testicular teratoma. J Clin Oncol 1992;10:1762–1768.

9. Cullen MH, Stenning SP, Parkinson MC, et al. for the Medical Research Council Testicular Tumour Working Party. Short-course adjuvant chemotherapy in high-risk stage I nonseminomatous germ cell tumors of the testis: a Medical Research Council report. J Clin Oncol 1996;14:1106–1113.

10. Donohue JP, Foster RS, Rowland RG, et al. Nerve-sparing retroperitoneal lymphadenectomy with preservation of ejaculation. J Urol 1990;144:287–292.

11. Williams SD, Birch R, Einhorn LH, et al. Treatment of disseminated germ-cell tumours with cisplatin, bleomycin, and either vinblastin or etoposide. N Engl J Med 1987;316:1435–1440.

12. de Wit R, Roberts JT, Wilkinson PM, et al. Equivalence of three or four cycles of bleomycin, etoposide, and cisplatin chemotherapy and of a 3- or 5-day schedule in good-prognosis germ cell cancer: a randomized study of the European Organization for Research and Treatment of Cancer Genitourinary Tract Cancer Cooperative Group and the Medical Research Council. J Clin Oncol 2001;19:1629–1640.

13. Nichols CR, Catalano PJ, Crawford ED, et al. Randomized comparison of cisplatin and etoposide and either bleomycin or ifosfamide in treatment of advanced disseminated germ cell tumours: an Eastern Cooperative Oncology Group, Southwest Oncology Group, and Cancer and Leukemia Group B Study. J Clin Oncol 1998;16:1287–1293.

14. Motzer RJ, Sheinfeld J, Mazumdar M, et al. Paclitaxel, ifosfamide and cisplatin second-line therapy for patients with relapsed testicular germ cell cancer. J Clin Oncol 2000;18:2413–2418.

15. Toner G, Panicek D, Heelan R, et al. Adjuvant surgery after chemotherapy for nonseminomatous germ cell tumors: recommendations for patient selection. J Clin Oncol 1990;8: 1683–1694.

16. Travis LB, Andersson M, Gospodarowicz M, et al. Treatment-associated leukemia following testicular cancer. J Natl Cancer Inst 2000;92:1165–1171.

17. Bosl GJ, Ilson DH, Rodriguez E, et al. Clinical relevance of the i(12P) marker chromosome in germ cell tumours. J Natl Cancer Inst 1994;86:349–355.

18. Travis LB, Curtis RE, Storm H, et al. Risk of second malignant neoplasms among long-term survivors of testicular cancer. J Natl Cancer Inst 1997;89:1429–1439.

19. Van Leeuwen FE, Travis LB. Second cancers. In: Devitz VT, et al. (eds). Cancer: Principles and Practice of Oncology, 6th ed. Philadelphia: Lippincott Williams & Wilkins, 2001:2939–2964.

20. Fosså SD, Langmark F, Aass N, et al. Second non-germ cell malignancies after radiotherapy of testicular cancer with or without chemotherapy. Br J Cancer 1990;61:639–643.

21. Van Leeuwen FE, Stiggelbout AM, van den Belt-Dusebout AW, et al. Second cancer risk following testicular cancer: a follow-up study of 1,909 patients. J Clin Oncol 1993;11:415–424.

22. United Nations Scientific Committee on the Effects of Atomic Radiation (UNSCEAR). Report to the General Assembly, with Scientific Annexes. Sources and Effects of Ionizing Radiation, UNSCEAR. New York: United Nations, 2000.

23. Hoff Wanderas E, Fosså SD, Tretli S. Risk of subsequent non-germ cell cancer after treatment of germ cell cancer in 2006 Norwegian male patients. Eur J Cancer 1997;33:253–262.

24. Breslow NE, Takashima JR, Whitton JA, et al. Second malignant neoplasms following treatment for Wilm's tumor: a report from the National Wilms' Tumor Study Group. J Clin Oncol 1995; 13:1851–1859.

25. Redman JR, Vugrin D, Arlin ZA, et al. Leukemia following treatment of germ cell tumors in men. J Clin Oncol 1984;2: 1080–1087.

26. Pedersen-Bjergaard J, Daugaard G, et al. Increased risk of myelodysplasia and leukaemia after etoposide, cisplatin, and bleomycin for germ-cell tumours. Lancet 1991;338:359–363.

27. Nichols CR, Breeden ES, Loehrer PJ, et al. Secondary leukemia associated with a conventional dose of etoposide: review of serial germ cell tumor protocols. J Natl Cancer Inst 1993;85: 36–40.

28. Bokemeyer C, Schmoll HJ, Kuczyk MA, et al. Risk of secondary leukemia following high cumulative doses of etoposide during chemotherapy for testicular cancer (letter). J Natl Cancer Inst 1995;87:58–60.

29. Boshoff C, Begent RH, Oliver RT, et al. Secondary tumours following etoposide containing therapy for germ cell cancer. Ann Oncol 1995;6:35–40.

30. Travis LB, Holowaty E, Hall P, et al. Risk of leukemia following platinum-based chemotherapy for ovarian cancer. N Engl J Med 1999;340:351–357.

31. Smith MA, Rubinstein L, Anderson JR, et al. Secondary leukemia or myeloodysplastic syndrome after treatment with epipodophyllotoxins. J Clin Oncol 1999;17:569–577.

32. Kollmannsberger C, Hartmann JT, Kanz L, et al. Therapy-related malignancies following treatment of germ cell cancer. Int J Cancer 1999;83:860–863.

33. von der Maase H, Rørth M, Walbom-Jørgensen S, et al. Carcinoma in situ of contralateral testis in patients with testicular germ cell cancer: study of 27 cases in 500 patients. Br Med J 1986;293:1398–1401.

34. Sokal M, Peckham MJ, Hendry WF. Bilateral germ cell tumours of the testis. Br J Urol 1980;52:158–162.

35. Hoff Wanderas E, Fosså SD, Tretli S. Risk of a second germ cell cancer after treatment of a primary germ cell cancer in 2201 Norwegian male patients. Eur J Cancer 1997;33:244–252.

36. Hartmann JG, Fosså SD, Nichols CR, et al. Incidence of metachronous testicular cancer in patients with extragonadal germ cell tumors. J Natl Cancer Inst 2001;93:1733–1738.

37. Fosså SD, Aass N, Heilo A, et al. Testicular carcinoma in situ in patients with extragonadal germ cell tumours: the clinical role of pre-treatment biopsy. Ann Oncol 2003;14:1412–1418.

38. Oosterhuis JW, Looijenga LHJ. The biology of human germ cell tumours: retrospective speculations and new prospectives. Eur Urol 1993;23:245–250.

39. Fosså SD, Åbyholm T, Aakvaag A. Spermatogenesis and hormonal status after orchiectomy for cancer and before supplementary treatment. Eur Urol 1984;10:173–177.

40. Hansen PV, Trykker H, Andersen J, et al. Germ cell function and hormonal status in patients with testicular cancer. Cancer (Phila) 1989;64:956–961.

41. Petersen PM, Skakkebaek NE, Vistisen K, et al. Semen quality and reproductive hormones before orchiectomy in men with testicular cancer. J Clin Oncol 1999;17:941–947.

42. Petersen PM, Skakkebæk NE, Rørth M, et al. Semen quality and reproductive hormones before and after orchiectomy in men with testicular cancer. J Urol 1999;161:822–826.

43. Carroll PR, Whitmore Jr WF, Herr HW, et al. Endocrine and exocrine profiles of men with testicular tumours before orchiectomy, J Urol 1987;137:420–423.

44. Jacobsen KD, Theodorsen L, Fosså SD. Spermatogenesis after unilateral orchiectomy for testicular cancer in patients following surveillance policy. J Urol 2001;165:93–96.

45. Nord C, Bjøro T, Ellingsen D, et al. Gonadal hormones in long-term survivors 10 years after treatment for unilateral testicular cancer. Eur Urol 2003;44:322–328.

46. Reiter WJ, Kratzik C, Brodowicz T, et al. Sperm analysis and serum follicle-stimulating hormone levels before and after adjuvant single-agent carboplatin therapy for clinical stage I seminoma. Urol 1998;52:117–119.

47. Lampe H, Horwich A, Norman A, et al. Fertility after chemotherapy for testicular germ cell cancers. J Clin Oncol 1997;15:239–245.

48. Drasga RE, Einhorn LH, Williams SD, et al. Fertility after chemotherapy for testicular cancer. J Clin Oncol 1983;1:179–183.

49. Taksey J, Bissada NK, Chaudhary UB. Fertility after chemotherapy for testicular cancer. Arch Androl 2003;49:389–395.

50. Petersen PM, Skakkebæk NE, Giwercman A. Gonadal function in men with testicular cancer: biological and clinical aspects. APMIS 1998;106:24–36.

51. Palmieri G, Lotrecchiano G, Ricci G, et al. Gonadal function after multimodality treatment in men with testicular germ cell cancer. Eur J Endocrinol 1996;134:431–436.

52. Aass N, Fosså SD, Theodorsen L, et al. Prediction of long-term gonadal toxicity after standard treatment for testicular cancer. Eur J Cancer 1991;27:1087–1091.

53. Bokemeyer C, Berger CC, Kuczyk MA, et al. Evaluation of long-term toxicity after chemotherapy for testicular cancer. J Clin Oncol 1996;14:2923–2932.

54. Fosså SD, Ous S, Abyholm T, et al. Post-treatment fertility in patients with testicular cancer. II. Influence of cisplatin-based combination chemotherapy and of retroperitoneal surgery on hormone and sperm cell production. Br J Urol 1985;57:210–214.

55. Petersen PM, Hansen SW, Giwercman A, et al. Dose-dependent impairment of testicular function in patients treated with cisplatin-based chemotherapy for germ cell cancer. Ann Oncol 1994;5:355–358.

56. Stephenson WT, Poirier SM, Rubin L, et al. Evaluation of reproductive capacity in germ cell tumor patients following treatment with cisplatin, etoposide, and bleomycin. J Clin Oncol 1995;13:2278–2280.

57. Strumberg D, Brügge S, Korn MW, et al. Evaluation of long-term toxicity in patients after cisplatin-based chemotherapy for non-seminomatous testicular cancer. Ann Oncol 2002;13:229–236.

58. Jacobsen KD, Olsen DR, Fosså K, et al. External beam abdominal radiotherapy in patients with seminoma stage I: field type, testicular dose, and spermatogenesis. Int J Radiat Oncol Biol Phys 1997;38:95–102.

59. Hansen PV, Trykker H, Svennekjær IL, et al. Long-term recovery of spermatogenesis after radiotherapy in patients with testicular cancer. Radiat Oncol 1990;18:117–125.

60. Kreuser ED, Klingmüller D, Thiel E. The role of LHRH-Analogues in protecting gonadal function during chemotherapy and irradiation. Eur Urol 1993;23:157–164.

61. Hallak J, Hendin BN, Thomas AJ, et al. Investigation of fertilizing capacity of cryopreserved spermatozoa from patients with cancer. J Urol 1998;159:1217–1220.

62. Fosså SD, Opjordsmoen S, Haug E. Androgen replacement and quality of life in patients treated for bilateral testicular cancer. Eur J Cancer 1999;35:1220–1225.

63. Whitmore WE Jr. Surgical treatment of adult germinal testis tumours. Semin Oncol 1979;6:55–68.

64. Nijman JM, Jager S, Boer PW, et al. The treatment of ejaculation disorders after retroperitoneal lymph node dissection. Cancer (Phila) 1982;50:2967–2971.

65. Jacobsen KD, Ous S, Wæhre H, et al. Ejaculation in testicular cancer patients after post-chemotherapy retroperitoneal lymph node dissection. Br J Cancer 1999;80:249–255.

66. Jacobsen KD, Fosså SD. Fatherhood in testicular cancer patients with carcinoma in situ in the contralateral testicle. Eur Urol 2000;38:725–727.

67. Giwercman A, von der Maase H, Berthelsen JG, et al. Localized irradiation of testis with carcinoma in situ: effects on Leydig cell function and eradication of malignant germ cell in 20 patients. J Clin Endocrinol Metab 1991;73:596–603.

68. Heidenreich A, Weizbach L, Höltl W, et al. Organ sparing surgery for malignant germ cell tumor of the testis. J Urol 2001;166:2161–2165.

69. Boyer M, Raghavan D. Toxicity of treatment of germ cell tumours. Semin Oncol 1992;19:128–142.

70. Aass N, Kaasa S, Lund E, et al. Long-term somatic side-effects and morbidity in testicular cancer patients. Br J Cancer 1990;61:151–155.

71. Petersen PM, Hansen SW. The course of long-term toxicity in patients treated with cisplatin-based chemotherapy for non-seminomatous germ-cell cancer. Ann Oncol 1999;10:1475–1483.

72. von Schlippe M, Fowler CJ, Harland SJ. Cisplatin neurotoxicity in the treatment of metastatic germ-cell tumour: time course and prognosis. Br J Cancer 2001;85:823–826.

73. Fosså SD, de Wit R, Roberts T, et al. Quality of life in good prognosis patients with metastatic germ cell cancer: a prospective study of the European Organization for Research and Treatment of Cancer Genitourinary Group/Medical Research Council Testicular Cancer Study Group (30941/TE20). J Clin Oncol 2003;21:1107–1118.

74. Hansen SW, Helweg-Larsen S, Trojaborg W. Long-term neurotoxicity in patients treated with cisplatin, vinblastine, and bleomycin for metastatic germ cell cancer. J Clin Oncol 1989;7:1457–1461.

75. Osanto S, Bukman A, van Hoek F, et al. Long-term effects of chemotherapy in patients with testicular cancer. J Clin Oncol 1992;10:574–579.

76. Stoter G, Koopman A, Vendrik CPJ, et al. Ten-year survival and late sequelae in testicular cancer patients treated with cisplatin, vinblastine and bleomycin. J Clin Oncol 1989;7:1099–1104.

77. Skard Heier M, Aass N, Ous S, et al. Asymmetrical autonomic dysfunction of the feet after retroperitoneal surgery in patients with testicular cancer: 2 case reports. J Urol 1992;147:470–471.

78. van Basten JP, Hoekstra HJ, van Driel MF, et al. Sexual dysfunction in nonseminoma testicular cancer patients is related to chemotherapy-induced angiopathy. J Clin Oncol 1997;15:2442–2448.

79. Hansen SW. Autonomic neuropathy after treatment with cisplatin, vinblastin, and bleomycin for germ cell cancer. Br Med J 1990;3000:511–512.

80. Koukourakis MI. Amifostine in clinical oncology: current use and future applications. Anti-Cancer Drugs 2002;13:181–209.

81. Fosså SD, Aass N, Winderen M, et al. Long-term renal function after treatment for malignant germ cell tumours. Ann Oncol 2002;13:222–228.

82. Huddart RA, Norman A, Shahidi M, et al. Cardiovascular disease as a long-term complication of treatment for testicular cancer. J Clin Oncol 2003;21:1513–1523.

83. Kollmannsberger C, Kuzcyk M, Mayer F, et al. Late toxicity following curative treatment of testicular cancer. Semin Surg Oncol 1999;17:275–281.

84. Rudberg L, Carlsson M, Nilsson S, et al. Self-perceived physical, psychologic, and general symptoms in survivors of testicular cancer 3 to 13 years after treatment. Cancer Nurs 2002;25:187–195.

85. Fosså SD, Lehne G, Heimdal K, et al. Clinical and biochemical long-term toxicity after postoperative cisplatin-based chemotherapy in patients with low-stage testicular cancer. Oncology 1995;52:300–305.

86. Meinardi MT, Gietema JA, van der Graaf WTA, et al. Cardiovascular morbidity in long-term survivors of metastatic testicular cancer. J Clin Oncol 2000;18:1725–1732.

87. Raghavan D, Cox K, Childs A, et al. Hypercholesterolemia after chemotherapy for testis cancer. J Clin Oncol 1992;10:1386–1389.

88. Nord C, Fosså SD, Egeland T. Excessive annual BMI increase after chemotherapy among young survivors of testicular cancer. Br J Cancer 2003;88:36–41.

89. Zagars GK, Ballo MT, Lee AK, Strom SS. Mortality after cure of testicular seminoma. J Clin Oncol 2004;22:640–647.

90. Fosså SD, Aass N, Harvei S, et al. Increased mortality rates in young and middle-aged patients with malignant germ cell tumours. Br J Cancer 2004;90:607–612.

91. Bamberg M, Schmidberger H, Meisner C, et al. Radiotherapy for stages I and IIA/B testicular seminoma. Int J Cancer 1999;83:823–827.

92. Yeoh E, Horowitz M, Russo A, et al. The effects of abdominal irradiation for seminoma of the testis on gastrointestinal function. J Gastroenterol Hepatol 1995;10:125–130.

93. Haug TT, Mykletun A, Dahl AA. Are anxiety and depression related to gastrointestinal symptoms in the general population? Scand J Gastroenterol 2002;37:294–298.

94. Fosså SD, Aass N, Kaalhus O. Radiotherapy for testicular seminoma stage I: treatment results and long-term post-irradiation morbidity in 365 patients. Int J Radiat Oncol Biol Phys 1989;16:383–388.

95. Hamilton CR, Horwich A, Bliss JM, et al. Gastrointestinal morbidity of adjuvant radiotherapy in stage I malignant teratoma of the testis. Radiother Oncol 1987;10:85–90.

96. Hoff Wanderås E, Fosså SD, Tretl, S, Klepp O. Toxicity in long-term survivors after adriamycin containing chemotherapy of malignant germ cell tumours. Int J Oncol 1994;4:681–688.

97. Moul JW. Retroperitoneal fibrosis following radiotherapy for stage I testicular seminoma. J Urol 1992;147:124–126.

98. Stensvold E, Aass N, Gladhaug I, et al. Erroneous diagnosis of pancreatic cancer: a possible pitfall after radiotherapy of testicular cancer. Eur J Surg Oncol 2004;30:352–355.

99. Winquist EW, Bauman GS, Balogh J. Nontraumatic osteonecrosis after chemotherapy for testicular cancer systematic review. Am J Clin Oncol 2001;24:603–606.

100. Fosså SD, Moynihan C, Serbouti S. Patients' and doctors' perception of long-term morbidity in patients with testicular cancer clinical stage I. A descriptive pilot study. Support Care Cancer 1996;4:118–128.

101. Schover LR, von Eschenbach AC. Sexual and marital relationships after treatment for nonseminomatous testicular cancer. Urology 1985;25:251–255.

102. Rieker PP, Edbril SD, Garnick MB. Curative testis cancer therapy: psychosocial sequelae. J Clin Oncol 1985;3:1117–1126.

103. Gritz ER, Wellisch DK, Wang H-J, et al. Long-term effects of testicular cancer on sexual functioning in married couples. Cancer (Phila) 1989;64:1560–1567.

104. Moynihan C. Testicular cancer: the psychosocial problems of patients and their relatives. Cancer Surv 1987;6:477–510.

105. van Basten JP, Jonker-Pool G, van Driel MF, et al. Fantasies and facts of the testes. Br J Urol 1996;78:756–762.

106. Arai Y, Kawakita M, Hida S, et al. Psychosocial aspects in long-term survivors of testicular cancer. J Urol 1996;155:574–578.

107. Blackmore C. The impact of orchiectomy upon the sexuality of the man with testicular cancer. Cancer Nurs 1988;11:33–40.

108. Caffo O, Amichetti M. Evaluation of sexual life after orchidectomy followed by radiotherapy for early stage seminoma of the testis. BJU Int 1999;83:462–468.

109. Fosså SD, Aass N, Kaalhus O. Testicular cancer in young Norwegians. J Surg Oncol 1988;39:43–63.

110. Fosså SD, Aass N, Ous S, et al. Long-term morbidity and quality of life in testicular cancer patients. Scand J Urol Nephrol 1991;138(suppl):241–246.

111. Douchez J, Droz JP, Desclaux B, et al. Quality of life in long-term survivors of nonseminomatous germ cell testicular tumors. J Urol 1993;149:498–501.

112. Rudberg L, Nilsson S, Wikblad K. Health-related quality of life in survivors of testicular cancer 3 to 13 years after treatment. J Psychosoc Oncol 2000;18:19–31.

113. Joly F, Héron JF, Kalusinski L, et al. Quality of life in long-term survivors of testicular cancer: a population-based case-control study. J Clin Oncol 2002;20:73–80.

114. Mykletun A, Dahl AA, Haaland CF, et al. Side-effects and cancer-related stress determine quality of life on long-term survivors of testicular cancer. J Clin Oncol 2005;23(13):3061–3068.

115. Weissbach L, Bussar-Maatz R, Flechtner H, et al. RPLND or primary chemotherapy in clinical stage IIA/B non-seminomatous germ cell tumours. Eur Urol 2000;37:582–594.

116. Kaasa S, Aass N, Mastekaasa A, et al. Psychosocial well-being in testicular cancer patients. Eur J Cancer 1991;27:1091–1095.

117. Fosså SD, Dahl AA, Loge JH. Fatigue, anxiety, and depression in long-term survivors of testicular cancer. J Clin Oncol 2003;21:1249–1254.

118. Jones GY, Payne S. Searching for safety signals: the experience of medical surveillance among men with testicular teratomas. Psycho-Oncology 2000;9:385–394.

119. Ozen H, Sahin A, Toklu C, et al. Psychosocial adjustment after testicular cancer treatment. J Urol 1998;159:1947–1950.

120. Schagen SB, Muller MJ, Boogerd W, et al. Late effects of adjuvant chemotherapy on cognitive function: a follow-up study in breast cancer patients. Ann Oncol 2002;13:1387–1397.

121. Nazareth I, Lewin J, King M. Sexual dysfunction after treatment for testicular cancer: a systematic review. J Psychosom Res 2001;51:735–743.

122. Jonker-Pool G, Van de Wiel HBM, Hoekstra HJ, et al. Sexual functioning after treatment for testicular cancer: review and meta-analysis of 36 empirical studies between 1975 and 2000. Arch Sex Behav 2001;30:55–74.

123. Aass N, Grünfeld B, Kaalhus O, et al. Pre- and posttreatment sexual life in testicular cancer patients: a descriptive investigation. Br J Cancer 1993;67:1113–1117.

124. Tinkler SD, Howard GCW, Kerr GR. Sexual morbidity following radiotherapy for germ cell tumours of the testis. Radiat Oncol 1992;25:207–212.

125. Incrocci L, Hop WCJ, Wijnmaalen A, et al. Treatment outcome, body image, and sexual functioning after orchiectomy and radio-

therapy for stage I-II testicular seminoma. Int J Radiat Oncol Biol Phys 2002;53:1165–1173.

126. Laumann EO, Paik A, Rosen RC. Sexual dysfunction in the United States. Prevalence and predictors. JAMA 1999;281:537–544.

127. Jonker-Pool G, van Basten JP, Hoekstra HJ, et al. Sexual functioning after treatment for testicular cancer. Cancer (Phila) 1997;80:454–464.

128. van Basten JPA, van Driel HJ, Hoekstra D, et al. Objective and subjective effects of treatment for testicular cancer on sexual function. BJU Int 1999;84:671–678.

129. Schover LR, von Eschenbach AC. Sexual and marital counselling in men treated for testicular cancer. J Sex Marit Ther 1984;10: 29–40.

130. Rieker PP, Fitzgerald EM, Kalish LA. Adaptive behavioral responses to potential infertility among survivors of testis cancer. J Clin Oncol 1990;8:347–355.

131. Moynihan C, Bliss JM, Davidson J, et al. Evaluation of adjuvant psychosocial therapy in patients with testicular cancer: randomised controlled trial. BMJ 1998;316:429–435.

132. Gerl A, Schierl R. Urinary excretion of platinum in chemotherapy-treated long-term survivors of testicular cancer. Acta Oncol 2000;39:519–522.

133. Gelevert T, Messerschmidt J, Meinardi MT, et al. Adsorptive Voltametry to determine platinum levels in plasma from testicular cancer patients treated with cisplatin. Ther Drug Monit 2001;23:169–173.

10

Medical and Psychosocial Issues in Gynecologic Cancer Survivors

Karen Basen-Engquist and Diane C. Bodurka

An emerging body of research has documented the quality of life of women with gynecologic cancer around the time of diagnosis and during treatment. However, we know much less about the quality of life and psychosocial and medical needs of gynecologic cancer survivors after treatment.[1,2] In particular, there are very few studies documenting the risk of possible late medical effects of gynecologic cancer treatment such as osteoporosis and second primary cancers. More is known about self-reported symptoms and psychosocial sequelae, such as sexual functioning and psychologic distress, but even these studies rarely focus on survivors more than 5 years after diagnosis. Additionally, much of the extant research has limitations such as small sample sizes, nonstandardized measures, and cross-sectional designs, often without appropriate comparison groups. Finally, there is a dearth of research testing interventions to ameliorate problems experienced by gynecologic cancer survivors. While in some areas additional research is needed to better describe the sequelae and determine who is at risk for adverse late effects, in others areas (e.g., sexual functioning), adequate data describing the problem are available, and a stronger focus on treatment interventions is needed (see also Chapter 19).

The shortage of research contributes to several clinical challenges in the health care of gynecologic cancer survivors. Without adequate research on the long-term late effects of gynecologic cancer, appropriate follow-up care is difficult to establish. For example, should screening tests for other cancers or for conditions such as osteoporosis be started at an earlier age or done on a different schedule? The lack of an evidence base from which to make such decisions hampers effective health care for long-term survivors. We also have limited data on potential interventions for ameliorating certain late effects. For example, the data to support clinician and patient decision making about hormone replacement therapy for gynecologic cancer survivors do not exist, particularly for those who are premenopausal at diagnosis. This situation forces providers and survivors to extrapolate data on the risks and benefits of hormone replacement in healthy post-menopausal women to women who experience premature menopause as a result of cancer treatment.

A further challenge in the care of long-term survivors of gynecologic cancer is to identify not only what the healthcare system can provide to help survivors maintain their health but what they themselves can do. Research on improving health behaviors in cancer survivors, for example, increasing physical activity, is in its infancy. Early studies show that exercise benefits quality of life and functional capacity in breast cancer survivors[3,4] and decreases fatigue in prostate cancer survivors.[5] There have been no trials in the gynecologic cancer survivor population to test the effects of changes in health behaviors such as diet, exercise, and smoking cessation on potential late effects such as chronic fatigue, osteoporosis, second primary cancers, or recurrence. Such interventions could also benefit women with comorbid conditions that are either coincidental to their cancer or risk factors for the development of gynecologic cancer, such as the obesity, hypertension, and diabetes that are prevalent among endometrial cancer survivors.[6–8]

Characteristics of Gynecologic Cancer Survivors

The three major gynecologic cancers (endometrial, cervical, ovarian) differ in terms of their risk factors, median age at diagnosis, ethnic distribution, type of treatment, and survival probability. The characteristics of survivors, therefore, vary as a function of these factors as well. Table 10.1 provides information about the three diseases that impact the characteristics of the survivor population.

Endometrial cancer is the most common gynecologic cancer in the United States, followed by ovarian and cervical.[9,10] By contrast, however, cervical cancer is more common in developing countries; worldwide it is the second most common cancer among women.[11] Despite the fact that ovarian cancer is a more common diagnosis in the United States than cervical cancer, there are more cervical cancer survivors because ovarian cancer has a relatively low overall

TABLE 10.1. Variables related to gynecologic cancers that influence the characteristics of the survivor population.

	Endometrial	Ovarian	Cervical
Projected number of cases in U.S. in 2006[9]	41,200	20,180	9,710
Percentage diagnosed with localized disease[10]	73%	29%	54%
Average 5-year survival[10]	84%	53%	71%
Median age at diagnosis[10]	65	59	47
Number of survivors in U.S.[10]	556,640	202,949	231,064
Percentage of survivors within 10 years of diagnosis[10]	44%	55%	37%
Ethnic distribution of survivors within 10 years of diagnosis[a][10]			
• White	92%	89%	77%
• African-American	5%	7%	14%
• Asian/Pacific Islander	2%	3%	4%
• Hispanic[b]	4%	6%	16%
Risk factors[6–8,13–17,63–65]	Obesity Diabetes (among obese women) Hypertension Nulliparity	Family history Nulliparity Use of talc Oral Contraceptives (protective) Tubal ligation and hysterectomy (protective)	Early initiation of sexual intercourse More than four sexual partners Smoking

[a] Information on ethnicity of survivors is available only for those diagnosed in past 10 years.

[b] Percentages total to more than 100 because the ethnic group Hispanic is not mutually exclusive of the other racial/ethnic categories.

survival. On average, cervical cancer is diagnosed at a younger age than ovarian and endometrial cancer, so survivors of cervical cancer are more likely to be dealing with family and work responsibilities in addition to cancer survivorship issues.

The ethnic distribution of each survivorship group also varies, with endometrial and ovarian cancer survivors being predominantly white. Among cervical cancer survivors, the proportion of minority ethnicity women is higher.[10] Because many cases of invasive cervical cancer are prevented by screening and treatment of preinvasive lesions, a number of invasive cervical cancers arise in women who have not had adequate screening,[12] either by choice or because of lack of access. Thus, women of lower socioeconomic status, who have poorer access to health care, may be overrepresented among cervical cancer patients and survivors.

The behavioral risk factors for the gynecologic cancer differ, and many of these behaviors may be continued after diagnosis and treatment, putting survivors at additional risk of second primaries or other comorbid conditions. Smoking, for example, is a risk factor for cervical cancer,[13–15] and one study has found that few cervical cancer survivors quit smoking after diagnosis.[16] Obesity is a risk factor for endometrial cancer,[6,7,17] indicating relatively low levels of physical activity relative to calorie consumption before diagnosis. Data are emerging that indicate endometrial cancer survivors also have low levels of physical activity.[18,19]

Medical Issues

Survivors of gynecologic cancer report lingering symptoms and treatment side effects even after treatment has concluded. Most studies of medical sequelae are limited to sur-

vivor self-report of symptoms, rather than medical evaluations. Although the self-report data are valuable, more data are needed on conditions that may not cause immediately observable symptoms, such as osteoporosis, second cancers, and cardiovascular disease.

Gastrointestinal Symptoms

Gynecologic cancer survivors, particularly those who are treated with pelvic radiation, report more gastrointestinal symptoms than women from the general population, even several years after treatment. Li et al.[18] studied 61 five-year endometrial cancer survivors (47% of whom received radiation therapy) and found that they reported more gastrointestinal symptoms (stomach ache, diarrhea, and nausea) than a comparison group of women of comparable age. A similar study of 46 cervical cancer survivors (who had not received radiation) found that they reported a similar degree of gastrointestinal distress to the same comparison group.[20] Klee and Machin also found that endometrial[21] and cervical[22] cancer survivors treated with radiation therapy reported more diarrhea than population-based controls matched for age and partner status; the group differences in diarrhea were present out to the final evaluation point, 24 months from diagnosis, although levels of diarrhea were low (average score between "not at all" and "a little"). Bye studied 79 survivors of endometrial and cervical cancer who were 3 to 4 years from their radiation treatment and found that diarrhea was their most common symptom. They reported more diarrhea than the general population, and experiencing frequent diarrhea was associated with higher fatigue and poorer social functioning.[23] Acute bowel toxicity during radiation treatment increases the probability of late bowel toxicity,[24] indicating that effective interventions to reduce bowel toxicity may have beneficial long-term effects as well.[23]

Neurotoxicity

Women with advanced cervical and endometrial cancer and most ovarian cancer patients receive neurotoxic chemotherapy regimens.[25] Although in many cases neurotoxicity remits after the conclusion of treatment, some survivors continue to experience neurotoxic effects. A study of 49 early-stage ovarian cancer survivors who were between 5 and 10 years from diagnosis found that a significant proportion still reported symptoms of neurotoxicity: numbness in the hands was reported by 10%; trouble walking, 16%, discomfort in hands, 23%; ringing in ears, 29%, discomfort in feet, 29%; trouble hearing, 35%; and muscle cramps, 39%.[26] Neurotoxicity symptoms were associated with poor physical and psychologic well-being, depression, sexual discomfort, and low confidence for managing cancer.

Pain

Approximately half of the 200 ovarian cancer survivors (no evidence of disease, 2 or more years from diagnosis) in one study reported pain or discomfort that they attributed to ovarian cancer or its treatment. Pain was located mainly in the bowel, pelvis, bladder, or groin. Of those who reported pain, 46% rated it as mild, 21.1% as severe. Approximately half of those with pain reported that it had a low impact on their lives.[27] Various somatic pains (e.g., headache, leg and back pain) were reported by 30% to 50% of cervical cancer survivors[20]; however, several studies found that pain levels of endometrial and cervical cancer survivors are similar to, or even lower than, those of controls.[18,20–23] Continued pain naturally has an impact on overall quality of life; Bye et al.[23] found that pain in endometrial cancer survivors 3 to 4 years after treatment was associated with lower quality of life and higher fatigue.

Menopausal Symptoms

Women who are premenopausal when diagnosed with gynecologic cancer often suffer a loss of ovarian function and experience premature menopause. Andersen's study of gynecologic cancer survivors in the year after diagnosis indicates that menopausal symptoms among the survivors remain higher than those of healthy controls up to 12 months from diagnosis.[28] Other studies of endometrial and cervical cancer survivors have also noted significant problems with menopausal symptoms (e.g., hot flashes, vaginal dryness/irritation[18,20,21]). However, two studies of cervical cancer survivors did not find the prevalence of hot flashes to be higher than that of a comparison group, possibly because of the use of hormone replacement therapy.[20,22] Among endometrial survivors, younger women report more hot flashes and other menopausal symptoms than older survivors.[18] In a study of ovarian cancer survivors, Carmack Taylor et al.[29] found that those who were off treatment reported less vaginal dryness and pain during intercourse than patients receiving treatment, but more than breast cancer survivors or women who had not had cancer.

Another implication of early ovarian failure, especially for younger survivors, is the increased risk of osteoporosis. This problem has not been well studied in gynecologic cancer patients, to determine either the prevalence of the problem or effective strategies to treat and/or prevent osteoporosis. One pilot study of 27 breast cancer survivors found that those who became permanently amenorrheic after chemotherapy had a 14% lower bone mineral density than breast cancer survivors who maintained or resumed menses.[30] Although this is a potentially serious problem, particularly for those survivors who have their ovaries removed or experience ovarian failure at a young age, many healthcare providers do not routinely recommend screening for osteoporosis in this population. A survey of outpatient oncology nurses indicated that bone mineral density testing is one of the least frequently performed screening tests for cancer survivors.[31]

Fatigue

Fatigue is a significant problem for many cancer patients during treatment, and it can last beyond the acute treatment phase.[32] In a longitudinal study of gynecologic patients in the year after diagnosis, Lutgendorf et al.[33] found that most aspects of survivors' mood were similar to healthy individuals, but that fatigue was elevated above norms for survivors of both early-stage and advanced disease. The study by Ersek and colleagues[32] of ovarian cancer survivors found that fatigue was the most severe physical symptom experienced by the sample. Qualitative data indicated that fatigue interfered with general activities, employment, relationships, and ability to enjoy life. Li et al.[18] found that their sample of 5-year endometrial cancer survivors reported less energy, poorer memory, and less patience than age-matched population controls, whereas Klee and Machin[21,22] found no differences in the level of tiredness between controls and survivors of endometrial and cervical cancer, and Bye et al.[23] found higher levels of fatigue in controls than survivors.

Psychosocial Issues

Despite losses inherent in gynecologic cancer and treatment, reports of overall quality of life are good.[34] The psychosocial issues that have been most frequently studied in gynecologic cancer survivors are psychologic distress and sexuality.

Psychologic Distress

Although the reported prevalence of psychologic distress among gynecologic cancer survivors varies depending on the population and the measure used, several studies have followed survivors longitudinally from diagnosis and have found that the distress experienced by gynecologic cancer survivors after diagnosis and during treatment abates over time.[21,33,35–37] A study that followed women with gynecologic cancer for 1 year after diagnosis found that their mood disturbance was not significantly different from that of women receiving surgical intervention for benign gynecologic conditions or healthy women 8 and 12 months posttreatment.[35] The majority of cross-sectional studies have found that long-term survivors report levels of psychologic distress that are comparable to women who have not had cancer,[26,33,38–41] although one study reported elevated levels of distress for survivors.[42] Wenzel's study of long-term survivors of early-stage ovarian cancer found that only 6% scored above the cutpoint for the Center for Epidemiologic Studies—Depression (CESD)

Scale.[26] Bodurka-Bevers et al.[38] found that 15% of posttreatment survivors were above the CESD cutpoint (compared to 15%–19%) for the healthy population[43,44] and that only 22% were above the 75th percentile for anxiety.[45] Congruent with findings of lower psychologic distress for long-term survivors, they also appear to be less interested in psychologic services, particularly individual counseling.[46] One study indicated that anxiety may be a bigger problems for gynecology cancer survivors than depression. Paraskevaidis et al.[47] found, in a sample of gynecologic cancer survivors (median time since diagnosis, 25 months), that 21% had clinically significant anxiety while 4% reported high levels of depression.

Psychologic concerns can persist for gynecologic cancer survivors, however, particularly those who are at high risk for recurrence or suffer lingering physical problems as a result of the cancer or its treatment. While not reporting a high prevalence of major psychiatric disorder, survivors do describe continued distress related to fears of second cancers, recurrence, and diagnostic tests.[2,26,32,39,42] This distress has been labeled the Damocles syndrome, referring to the story of Damocles, first told by Cicero, who must enjoy a grand banquet with a sword hanging by a single horsehair over his head. Cancer survivors, particularly those who have survived advanced disease, often report feeling that they have the 'sword' of recurrence hanging above them. Survivors who are at increased risk of recurrent or persistent disease, such as those with advanced gynecologic cancer, have been reported to experience higher levels of anxiety and depression.[33] Ovarian cancer, in particular, has a high risk of recurrence, and the diagnosis of persistent disease after conventional treatment appears to be more stressful than the initial diagnosis.[48]

Some studies report that younger survivors experience more severe psychologic symptoms than those who are older.[20,38] One study of long-term cervical cancer survivors of childbearing age found that while their overall quality of life was good, they were more likely to be in the lowest quartile on general health, vitality, and mental health subscales than expected based on normative data. They reported more problems with social and emotional well-being, sexual discomfort, and gynecologic symptoms compared to women who have had gestational trophoblastic disease or lymphoma.[49]

Sexual Functioning

Gynecologic cancer and its treatment often has serious, long-term effects on the sexual functioning of survivors. In 1962, Decker and Schwartzman noted that "The deprivation of sexual function may have serious sequelae . . . it appears that little attention has been given to the problem of sexual function following treatment for cervical carcinoma".[50] These authors studied 78 patients at one point in time 6 to 10 years after treatment and noted that 31% experienced partial or complete loss of sexual function. In one study that prospectively assessed sexual functioning in women with gynecologic cancer, women having surgery for benign gynecologic conditions, and healthy women, Andersen et al.[28] found numerous sexual difficulties among gynecologic cancer survivors in the year after diagnosis. Cancer survivors reported greater difficulty with sexual desire, excitement, orgasm, and resolution. Although the women who received surgery for benign conditions also reported some sexual functioning problems, they were less severe than those reported by the cancer survivors.

Carmack Taylor and colleagues[29] found lower levels of sexual activity and sexual pleasure, and higher sexual discomfort, among 248 ovarian cancer patients and survivors as compared to data from samples of healthy women and breast cancer survivors reported in other studies using the same questionnaire. Ovarian cancer survivors were also less likely to be sexually active than healthy women, regardless of whether the healthy women were pre- or postmenopausal, or on hormone replacement therapy. Patients and survivors were more likely to be sexually active if they were married, happy with their body's appearance, younger, and not on active treatment. In two additional cross-sectional studies of long-term ovarian cancer survivors, problems in sexual functioning emerged as a major concern. In a study of long-term survivors of early-stage ovarian cancer, respondents reported difficulties with decreased libido (37%) and arousal (28%), problems with orgasm (13%), and difficulty with intercourse as a result of treatment (20%). Only 12 of 49 survivors were sexually active (25%), although 51% were married.[26] Stewart and colleagues[27] reported that a significant number of the 200 ovarian cancer survivors who responded to their survey had problems with sexuality; these reports were highest among women who were treated with radiation therapy. Over half of the survivors reported that their sex lives had been negatively affected by cancer and/or its treatment. Although 64% reported that their sex lives were average to excellent before diagnosis, only 25% reported average to excellent sex lives currently. Before cancer, 36% reported their sex lives were poor to adequate, whereas now 75% rated their sex lives as poor to adequate. However, only about 20% of the sample reported a moderate to great sense of loss associated with the decline in their sexual functioning.

Survivors of cervical and endometrial cancer also experience declines in sexual functioning, and those who receive radiation therapy report more sexual difficulties.[51,52] A study of 221 indigent women treated with radiation therapy for invasive cervix cancer reported an 88% incidence of vaginal stenosis; however, sexual functioning was not evaluated in this study.[53] A decrease in sexual function in irradiated patients was reported by Seibel et al., who compared 22 patients radiated for cervical cancer versus 20 patients undergoing hysterectomy for preinvasive disease 1 year posttreatment.[54]

Schover et al.[52] conducted the first prospective evaluation of sexual function, frequency, and behavior, as well as marital happiness and psychologic distress, in 61 patients treated for early-stage cervical cancer in the United States. Although the surgical and radiation treatment groups appeared similar posttreatment and at 6-month follow-up, by 1-year women treated with radiation had more dyspareunia and problems with sexual desire and arousal than women who underwent radical hysterectomy. Pelvic examinations were performed, and a rating scale used to assess vaginal atrophy correlated with women's reports of dyspareunia, but no specific vaginal measurements were obtained. This study remains one of the few to compare the specific sexual impact of surgery versus radiation therapy.

Bruner et al evaluated vaginal stenosis, sexual activity, and satisfaction in 90 patients treated with intracavitary radiation for endometrial or cervical cancer.[55] The authors noted a correlation between decrease in vaginal length and decrease in sexual satisfaction, but a cause-and-effect relationship was not demonstrated. Most recently, Bergmark and colleagues studied vaginal changes and sexuality in Swedish women 4 or more years after completion of treatment for cervical cancer. When compared to controls, patients with a history of cervical cancer noted similar frequency of sexual intercourse, but reported decreased vaginal lubrication and a reduction in perceived vaginal length and elasticity during intercourse. A large proportion of these women also reported that they were distressed by these changes and their effects on sexual function.[56] Although this study was described as one focusing on the impact of radical hysterectomy, the majority of women had also had radiation therapy, a likely confounding variable.

Women treated for vulvar cancer may have the most severe sexual functioning problems because of the radical surgery they often receive. A cross-sectional study of 105 survivors of vulvar and cervical cancer (average of 28 months from diagnosis)[39] found that most women who were sexually active before cancer diagnosis had resumed sexual intercourse, with the exception of older women who had received radical vulvectomies and the 3 women who received pelvic exenterations. Frequency of sexual intercourse was reduced, however. Approximately three-fourths of the women experienced sexual problems during the year following diagnosis, and 66% reported continued problems. In a study of 42 women treated for in situ vulvar cancer, Andersen and colleagues found that these women experienced more disruption in sexual functioning compared to healthy women, and that these disruptions increased over time. In addition, increasing numbers of survivors discontinued sexual activity over time. Degree of sexual dysfunction was related to the extensiveness of the treatment.[57]

Interventions

The literature includes no published trials of interventions to address late psychosocial or medical effects of gynecology cancer and its treatment. There is a small number of studies testing interventions delivered during cancer treatment that may influence long-term sequelae in survivors. These studies are reviewed here to provide information regarding what interventions might benefit gynecologic cancer survivors. Several of the studies assess outcomes 12 months or more from diagnosis. We focus on these longer-term outcomes where available (Table 10.2).

Psychosocial Issues

Four studies were identified that evaluated interventions to improve psychosocial functioning of gynecologic cancer survivors. Three of these focused primarily on sexuality[58–60] and one was concerned with a broader range of psychosocial issues.[61] All four programs used fairly standard psychoeducational approaches, providing information and opportunities for emotional expression and problem solving. Two of the studies used group interventions.[60,61] The treatments focusing

on sexuality appear to have some positive effects on sexual functioning, including resuming sexual activity,[58] returning to usual frequency of sexual activity,[59] decreasing sexual fears,[60] and increasing dilator use (among younger women).[60] The intervention with the broader psychosocial focus decreased psychologic distress and improved adjustment to cancer.[61] These results indicate that psychoeducational interventions can be helpful to gynecologic cancer survivors up to a year from diagnosis and may provide benefits beyond that point. Studies by Wenzel et al[26,49] indicated that a high percentage of long-term (greater than 5 years) ovarian (43%) and cervical (60%) cancer survivors would be interested in participating in programs offering psychosocial support. Given that sexual dysfunction seems to be a very prevalent problem for long-term gynecologic cancer survivors, interventions that focus on sexuality are particularly appropriate. More research is needed to refine interventions such as those tested in these studies to produce programs that can be disseminated and implemented by physician extenders and/or survivor organizations.

Medical Issues

Only one study was identified that tested an intervention for its ability to reduce late medical effects of gynecologic cancer. Bye et al.[23,62] tested a dietary intervention to reduce diarrhea in cervical and endometrial cancer patients receiving radiation therapy. The intervention (recommendation of a low-fat, low-lactose diet during radiation therapy and for 6 weeks after treatment) was effective during treatment[62]; 3 to 4 years after treatment some positive effects were still present.[23] While these results are intriguing, more research is needed to replicate this finding.

Emerging Areas

It is critical that the study of cancer survivorship in gynecology advance beyond small descriptive studies of the sequelae of gynecologic cancer. The field needs more carefully controlled longitudinal studies of late effects, using standardized measures, triangulation of self-report measures with clinical evaluation, and adequate sample sizes. Additionally, input from survivors themselves is needed to determine what sequelae and late effects of cancer are salient to them. For example, although the prevalence of clinically significant psychologic distress appears to be fairly low in gynecologic cancer survivors, some studies indicate that long-term survivors feel they would benefit from additional psychosocial services.[26,49]

Additional research data would guide clinical care of long-term cancer survivors and would identify areas in which interventions are needed. The existing research base indicates that treatment to address menopausal symptoms, sexual functioning, anxiety about recurrence and follow-up visits, fatigue, pain, gastrointestinal symptoms, and health behaviors such as physical activity and smoking cessation would be helpful to gynecologic cancer survivors. More careful longitudinal research would identify which survivors need intervention and elucidate optimal timing for providing assistance in these areas.

TABLE 10.2. Studies evaluating interventions for gynecologic cancer survivors.

Author	Year	Intervention focus	Type of trial	Number of participants	Type of participants	Type of treatment	Length of follow-up	Results
Lamont et al[58]	1978	Psychosexual rehabilitation after pelvic exenteration	Case series	12	Gynecologic cancer patients receiving pelvic exenteration	Team approach to treatment including sex therapist meetings with patient and partner before surgery, in hospital, and after discharge as needed Provides information and counseling	6 months	Of the 12 women receiving treatment with the team approach, 8 were thought to have good adjustment before surgery. Six of these women resumed sexual activity. Seven were having orgasms within 6 months; the 7th was still recovering from surgery at the time of article publication. Decreased sexual desire and difficulty using dilators was a common concern.
Capone et al[59]	1980	Psychosocial rehabilitation and sexuality (for sexually active patients)	Quasi-experimental	97	Gynecologic cancer patients	Counseling by psychologist during initial hospitalization, minimum of four sessions	12 months	Women in experimental group more likely to have returned to usual frequency of sexual activity at 12 months than women in control group. Experimental group twice as likely to have returned to work at 12 months, but differences not significant. No significant differences between groups in emotional functioning at 12 months.
Cain et al[61]	1986	Individual and group counseling	Randomized	80 (60 with 1-year follow-up)	Gynecologic cancer patients	Patients randomized to group or individual counseling, or standard care Counseling consisted of eight weekly sessions focusing on predetermined themes Techniques included providing information, emotional expression, problem-solving, and relaxation	12 months	Survivors in both the individual and group counseling conditions had less anxiety and depression and better adjustment to their illness than the standard care group at the final (12-month) assessment.
Robinson et al[60]	1999	Sexuality and use of vaginal dilators	Randomized	32	Cervix and endometrial cancer patients receiving radiotherapy	Two 1.5-hour group sessions presented information about sexuality and cancer, promoted the idea that sex is pleasurable, and taught behavioral skills in communication about sexuality, using dilators and lubricants, and performing Kegel exercises	12 months	No impact on Sexual History Form scores (overall sexual functioning); intervention group had significantly lower scores on scale measuring sexual fears, intervention improved knowledge in older group but not younger group. Intervention increased dilator use in younger group but not older group.
Bye et al[23]	2000	Diet to reduce diarrhea during radiation treatment	Randomized	143 in initial trial, 79 (43 intervention, 36 control) in 3- to 4-year follow-up	Cervix and endometrial cancer patients receiving radiation therapy	Low-fat, low-lactose diet during radiation therapy and for 6 weeks after the end of treatment	3–4 years	7% of the intervention group and 22% of the control group reported diarrhea at follow-up ($P = 0.05$), although difference in diarrhea score was not statistically significant (Intervention group, M = 19.4; Control group, M = 29.6; $P = 0.09$). In original study, 23% of intervention group and 48% of control group reported diarrhea during radiation therapy. Diarrhea during radiation was associated with diarrhea at follow-up for the control group only. There were no differences at follow-up in quality of life.

References

1. Anderson B, Lutgendorf S. Quality of life in gynecologic cancer survivors. CA Cancer J Clin 1997;47:218–225.

2. Auchincloss SS. After treatment: psychosocial issues in gynecologic cancer survivorship. Cancer (Phila) 1995;76(suppl 10): 2117–2124.

3. Segal R, Evans W, Johnson D, et al. Structured exercise improves physical functioning in women with stage I and II breast cancer: results of a randomized controlled trial. J Clin Oncol 2001;19: 657–665.

4. Courneya KS, Mackey JR, Bell GJ, Jones LW, Field CJ, Fairey AS. Randomized controlled trial of exercise training in postmenopausal breast cancer survivors: Cardiopulmonary and quality of life outcomes. J Clin Oncol 2003;21:1660–1668.

5. Segal RJ, Reid RD, Courneya KS, et al. Resistance exercise in men receiving androgen deprivation therapy for prostate cancer. J Clin Oncol 2003;21:1653–1659.

6. Kaaks R, Lukanova A, Kurzer MS. Obesity, endogenous hormones, and endometrial cancer risk: a synthetic review. Cancer Epidemiol Biomarkers Prev 2002;11:1531–1543.

7. Goodman MT, Hankin JH, Wilkens LR, et al. Diet, body size, physical activity, and the risk of endometrial cancer. Cancer Res 1997;57:5077–5085.

8. Bristow RE. Endometrial cancer. Curr Opin Oncol 1999;11: 388–393.

9. Jemal A, Siegel R, Ward E, Murray T, Xu J, Smigal C, Thun MJ. Cancer statistics, 2006. CA Cancer J Clin 2006;56:106–130.

10. Ries LAG, Eisner MP, Kosary CL, et al. SEER Cancer Statistics Review, 1975–2000. Bethesda, MD: National Cancer Institute, 2003.

11. Waggoner SE. Cervical cancer. Lancet 2003;361:2217–2225.

12. Sung HY, Kearney KA, Miller M, Kinney W, Sawaya GF, Hiatt RA. Papanicolaou smear history and diagnosis of invasive cervical carcinoma among members of a large prepaid health plan. Cancer (Phila) 2000;88:2283–2289.

13. Kjaer SK, Engholm G, Dahl C, Bock JE. Case-control study of risk factors for cervical squamous cell neoplasia in Denmark. IV: Role of smoking habits. Eur J Cancer Prev 1996;5:359–365.

14. Wilkenstein W. Smoking and cervical cancer—current status: a review. J Epidemiol 1990;131:945–957.

15. Daling JR, Madeleine MM, McKnight B, et al. The relationship of human papillomavirus-related cervical tumors to cigarette smoking, oral contraceptive use, and prior herpes simplex virus type 2 infection. Cancer Epidemiol Biomarkers Prev 1996;5: 541–548.

16. Waggoner S, Fuhrman B, Monk B, et al. Influence of smoking on progression-free and overall survival in stage II-B, III-B and IV-A cervical carcinoma: a gynecologic or (GOG) study. Society of Gynecologic Oncologists, New Orleans, LA, January 31 to February 4 2003.

17. Furberg AS, Thune I. Metabolic abnormalities (hypertension, hyperglycemia and overweight), lifestyle (high energy intake and physical inactivity) and endometrial cancer risk in a Norwegian cohort. Int J Cancer 2003;104:669–676.

18. Li C, Samsioe G, Iosif C. Quality of life in endometrial cancer survivors. Maturitas 1999;31:227–236.

19. Scruggs S, Carmack Taylor C, Jhingran A, et al. Obesity and physical functioning in endometrial cancer survivors. Presented at the Annual Meeting of the Society of Behavioral Medicine, Baltimore, MD, 2004.

20. Li C, Samsioe G, Iosif C. Quality of life in long-term survivors of cervical cancer. Maturitas 1999;32:95–102.

21. Klee M, Machin D. Health-related quality of life of patients with endometrial cancer who are disease-free following external irradiation. Acta Oncol 2001;40:816–824.

22. Klee M, Thranov I, Machin D. The patients' perspective on physical symptoms after radiotherapy for cervical cancer. Gynecol Oncol 2000;76:14–23.

23. Bye A, Trope C, Loge JH, Hjermstad M, Kaasa S. Health-related quality of life occurrence of intestinal side effects after pelvic radiotherapy. Evaluation of long-term effects of diagnosis and treatment. Acta Oncol 2000;39:173–180.

24. Jereczek-Fossa BA. Postoperative irradiation in endometrial cancer: still a matter of controversy. Cancer Treat Rev 2001; 27:19–33.

25. DiSaia PJ, Creasman WT. Clinical Gynecologic Oncology. St. Louis: Mosby, 2002:675.

26. Wenzel LB, Donnelly JP, Fowler JM, et al. Resilience, reflection, and residual stress in ovarian cancer survivorship: a gynecologic oncology group study. Psycho-Oncology 2002;11:142–153.

27. Stewart DE, Wong F, Duff S, Melancon CH, Cheung AM. "What doesn't kill you makes you stronger": an ovarian cancer survivor survey. Gynecol Oncol 2001;83:537–542.

28. Andersen BL, Anderson B, deProsse C. Controlled prospective longitudinal study of women with cancer: I. Sexual functioning outcomes. J Consult Clin Psychol 1989;57:683–691.

29. Carmack Taylor C, Basen-Engquist K, Shinn EH, Bodurka DC. Predictors of sexual functioning in ovarian cancer patients. J Clin Oncol 2004;22:881–889.

30. Headley JA, Theriault RL, LeBlanc AD, Vassilopoulou-Sellin R, Hortobagyi GN. Pilot study of bone mineral density in breast cancer patients treated with adjuvant chemotherapy. Cancer Invest 1998;16:6–11.

31. Mahon SM, Williams MT, Spies MA. Screening for second cancers and osteoporosis in long-term survivors. Cancer Pract 2000;8:282–290.

32. Ersek M, Ferrell BR, Dow KH, Melancon CH. Quality of life in women with ovarian cancer. West J Nurs Res 1997;19:334–350.

33. Lutgendorf SK, Anderson B, Ullrich P, et al. Quality of life and mood in women with gynecologic cancer: a one year prospective study. Cancer (Phila) 2002;94:131–140.

34. McCartney CF, Larson DB. Quality of life in patients with gynecologic cancer. Cancer (Phila) 1987;60:2129–2136.

35. Andersen BL, Anderson B, deProsse C. Controlled prospective longitudinal study of women with cancer: II. Psychological outcomes. J Consult Clin Psychol 1989;57:692–697.

36. Klee M, Thranov I, Machin D. Life after radiotherapy: the psychological and social effects experienced by women treated for advanced stages of cervical cancer. Gynecol Oncol 2000;76: 5–13.

37. Greimel E, Thiel I, Peintinger F, Cegnar I, Pongratz E. Prospective assessment of quality of life of female cancer patients. Gynecol Oncol 2002;85:140–147.

38. Bodurka-Bevers D, Basen-Engquist K, Carmack CL, et al. Depression, anxiety and quality of life in patients with epithelial ovarian cancer. Gynecol Oncol 2000;78:302–308.

39. Corney RH, Everett H, Howells A, Crowther ME. Psychosocial adjustment following major gynaecological surgery for carcinoma of the cervix and vulva. J Psychosom Res 1992;36:561–568.

40. Andersen BL, Hacker NF. Psychosexual adjustment after vulvar surgery. Obstet Gynecol 1983;62:457.

41. Miller BE, Pittman B, Case D, McQuellon RP. Quality of life after treatment for gynecologic malignancies: A pilot study in an outpatient clinic. Gynecol Oncol 2002;87:178–184.

42. Cull A, Cowie VJ, Farquharson DI, Livingstone JR, Smart GE, Elton RA. Early stage cervical cancer: psychosocial and sexual outcomes of treatment. Br J Cancer 1993;68:1216–1220.

43. Radloff LS. The CES-D scale: a self-report depression scale for research in the general population. Appl Psychol Measure 1977; 1:385–401.

44. Roberts RE, Vernon SW. The center for epidemiologic studies depression scale: its use in a community sample. Am J Psychiatry 1983;140:41–46.

45. Spielberger CD, Gorsuch RL, Lushene R, Vagg PR, Jacobs GA. State-Trait Anxiety Inventory for Adults: Sampler Set Manual, Test, Scoring Key, vol 1. Palo Alto, CA: Consulting Psychologists Press, 1983:70.

46. Pistrang N, Winchurst C. Gynaecological cancer patients' attitudes towards psychological services. Psychol Health Med 1997; 2:135–147.

47. Paraskevaidis E, Kitchener HC, Walker LG. Doctor-patient communcation and subsequent mental health in women with gynaecological cancer. Psycho-Oncology 1993;2:195–200.

48. Guidozzi F. Living with ovarian cancer. Gynecol Oncol 1993; 50:202–207.

49. Basen-Engquist K, Paskett ED, Buzaglo J, et al. Cervical cancer: behavioral factors related to screening, diagnosis, and survivors' quality of life. Cancer (Suppl) 2003;98:2009–2014.

50. Decker WH, Schwartzman E. Sexual function following treatment for carcinoma of the cervix. Am J Obstet Gynecol 1962; 83:401–405.

51. Juraskova I, Butow P, Robertson R, Sharpe L, McLeod C, Hacker N. Post-treatment sexual adjustment following cervical and endometrial cancer: a qualitative insight. Psycho-Oncology 2003;12:267–279.

52. Schover LR, Fife M, Gershenson DM. Sexual dysfunction and treatment for early stage cervical cancer. Cancer (Phila) 1989; 63:204–212.

53. Hartman P, Diddle AW. Vaginal stenosis following irradiation therapy for carcinoma of the cervix uteri. Cancer (Phila) 1972; 30:426–429.

54. Seibel MM, Freeman MG, Graves WL. Carcinoma of the cervix and sexual function. Obstet Gynecol 1980;55:484–487.

55. Bruner DW, Lanciano R, Keegan M, Corn B, Martin E, Hanks GE. Vaginal stenosis and sexual function following intracavitary radiation for the treatment of cervical and endometrial carcinoma. Int J Radiat Oncol Biol Phys 1993;27:825–830.

56. Bergmark K, Avall-Lundqvist E, Dickman PW, Henningsohn L, Steineck G. Vaginal changes and sexuality in women with a history of cervical cancer. N Engl J Med 1999;340:1383–1389.

57. Andersen BL, Turnquist, Dawn, et al. Sexual functioning after treatment of in situ vulvar cancer: preliminary report. Obstet Gynecol 1988;71:15–19.

58. Lamont JA, De Petrillo AD, Sargeant EJ. Psychosexual rehabilitation and exenterative surgery. Gynecol Oncol 1978;6:236–242.

59. Capone MA, Good RS, Westie KS, Jacobson AF. Psychosocial rehabilitation of gynecologic oncology patients. Arch Phys Med Rehabil 1980;61:128–132.

60. Robinson JW, Faris PD, Scott CB. Psychoeducational group increases vaginal dilation for younger women and reduces sexual fears for women of all ages with gynecological carcinoma treated with radiotherapy. Int J Radiat Oncol Biol Phys 1999;44:497–506.

61. Cain EN, Kohorn EI, Quinlan DM, Latimer K, Schwartz PE. Psychosocial benefits of a cancer support group. Cancer (Phila) 1986;57:183–189.

62. Bye A, Kaasa S, Ose T, Sundfor K, Trope C. The influence of low-fat, low lactose diet on radiation induced diarrhoea. Clin Nutr 1992;11:147–153.

63. Brekelmans CT. Risk factors and risk reduction of breast and ovarian cancer. Curr Opin Obstet Gynecol 2003;15:63–68.

64. Gershenson DA, Tortolero-Luna G, Malpica A, et al. Ovarian intraepithelial neoplasia and ovarian cancer. Gynecol Cancer Prev 1996;23:475–543.

65. Edmondson RJ, Monaghan JM. The epidemiology of ovarian cancer. Int J Gynecol Cancer 2001;11:423–429.

11

Medical, Psychosocial, and Health-Related Quality of Life Issues in Breast Cancer Survivors

Julie Lemieux, Louise J. Bordeleau, and
Pamela J. Goodwin

Women with breast cancer account for the largest group of female cancer survivors. It is estimated that there are currently 10.5 million cancer survivors in the United States; 40% of the female survivors are breast cancer survivors.[1] The growing number of breast cancer survivors reflects increasing incidence of the disease, diagnosis at earlier stages when outcome is better, and widespread adoption of effective adjuvant treatment.

Methodologic Issues in Survivorship Research

The Office of Cancer Survivorship of the National Cancer Institute (U.S.) defines a survivor as follows: "An individual is considered a cancer survivor from the time of cancer diagnosis, through the balance of his or her life. Family members, friends and caregivers are also impacted by the survivorship experience and are therefore included in this definition."[1] This is a very broad definition; most survivorship research in breast cancer focuses on the experience of individuals with cancer after they have completed their primary therapy, usually while they are free of recurrent disease. Some studies have focused on women who are 1, 3, 5, or more years post-diagnosis. In breast cancer, where long-term survival is becoming increasingly common, this variable definition may account for some of the inconsistencies in the literature. In this chapter, we have not adopted a single definition of survivorship but have tried to relate results to the definition used in each study.

Definition, recruitment, and identification of study populations are among the most challenging aspects of breast cancer survivorship research. Ideally, if the objective is to examine long-term outcomes, an inception cohort identified at a uniform time early in the course of the disease should be assembled (e.g., women with locoregional breast cancer in the immediate postoperative period, before adjuvant therapy). Prospective recruitment of a sample such as this is costly and time consuming. An alternative approach involves the use of administrative databases (including tumor registries) that retrospectively identify women diagnosed years earlier; however, careful attention must be paid to refusers and nonresponders, who may differ in important ways from responders. Investigators often conducted cross-sectional surveys of breast cancer patients attending follow-up clinics, or in a community. The populations thus assembled may not be representative of all breast cancer survivors, particularly when response rates are low, or well women have been discharged from follow-up clinics. Convenience samples, drawn from breast cancer advocacy groups or other sources, were recruited in some studies. This approach may lead to systematic overestimation or underestimation of the long-term impact of breast cancer and its treatment, because participation of women in these groups may be related to their survivorship experience.

Inclusion of a control population without cancer should be considered in breast cancer survivorship research. This condition allows the effects of aging and comorbid conditions to be differentiated from those of prior breast cancer and its treatment, important for many of the medical concerns of breast cancer survivors (e.g., menopause, osteoporosis, heart disease). Although inclusion of a noncancer control group is often desirable, it increases costs and complexity of research. Instead, investigators may opt to use measurement instruments for which population-based norms are available, comparing the results obtained in the breast cancer survivors with published results in age-matched controls.

Breast cancer survivorship studies often examine a broad variety of attributes: medical status, psychosocial issues, health-related quality of life (HRQOL), and sexuality, for example. Some of these attributes are readily measurable (e.g., bone density after chemotherapy-induced early menopause) while others are not (e.g., the social impact of breast cancer diagnosis). It is important that measurement instruments be valid and reliable and that they measure key areas of interest. A wide variety of standardized, validated instruments are available to measure many of the important psychosocial issues and health-related quality of life (HRQOL) in breast cancer survivors. When valid instruments are not available for key attributes, such as body image postmastectomy, investigators may need to develop new instruments and validate these instruments during the course of the research. In selecting questionnaires, investigators should avoid overburdening respondents.

It is likely that not all salient issues in breast cancer survivors have been identified. Recent evidence that cognitive dysfunction may occur in women receiving adjuvant chemotherapy is a prime example. Investigators should be aware of new and ongoing research and be prepared to examine newly emerging concepts.

Statistical analysis should include the use of appropriate statistical tests, with adjustment for the effects of age because it could be an important confounder. The use of baseline information, which allows evaluation of change over time, can provide valuable insights into the breast cancer survivorship process. As noted previously, comparison of study data with population-based norms also provides insight into the impact of aging versus the impact of prior breast cancer diagnosis.

In the remainder of this chapter, we review the survivorship literature in breast cancer, first as it relates to medical status and then as it relates to psychosocial status and HRQOL. This separation is somewhat artificial; there is overlap between the sections. Because most studies are observational, grading of evidence regarding efficacy of interventions is usually not possible.

Medical Status

Arm Symptoms/Upper Body Function

Treatment for breast cancer can be associated with a number of localized physical sequelae including arm edema (AE), impaired shoulder mobility, pain, neurologic deficits, and reduced upper body function. The literature assessing arm symptoms and limitations is summarized in Table 11.1.

There are three approaches to arm measurement: (1) circumference at various points (with bony landmarks as references), (2) volumetric measurements using limb submersion in water, and (3) skin and soft tissue tonometry.[2] Tape-measured circumference (10 cm above and below the olecranon or the lateral epicondyle) has been the traditional method but can be imprecise. Volumetric measurements are more accurate but have limited availability. Tonometry is not used clinically.

The occurrence of, and risk factors for, AE have been reviewed by Erickson et al.[3] The reported incidence of AE has ranged from 0% after partial or total mastectomy with sentinel node biopsy to 56% after modified radical mastectomy (MRM) or breast-conserving surgery (BCS) with both axillary lymph node dissection (ALND) and axillary radiation therapy

(XRT).[4,5] Werner et al.[6] reported that the median time to development of AE in patients treated with BCS, ALND (almost one-third had level 3 ALND), and breast XRT (with or without axillary XRT) was 14 months (range, 2–92 months); 97% of those who developed AE did so by 4 years.

The association between the extent of breast surgery and AE is less clear. Tasmuth et al. reported AE to be significantly more frequent in a prospective cohort study of 93 women treated with MRM versus BCS; however, women undergoing MRM had axillary XRT (also associated with AE) more commonly than those undergoing BCS.[7] Paci et al.[8] reported the odds ratio of chronic AE to be slightly, but not significantly, higher after MRM [odds ratio (OR), 1.62; 95% confidence interval (CI), 0.91–2.88] than after BCS (XRT was not examined). In a randomized trial comparing MRM to BCS with XRT to the breast and internal mammary and supraclavicular nodes, Gerber et al. reported the rate of AE did not differ between the two groups; however, axillary XRT (given if the dissection was inadequate or there was extracapsular extension) was not considered in the analysis.[5]

The risk of AE increases with the extent of axillary dissection. Yeoh et al.[9] reported frequency of AE to be 25% with no axillary surgery, 50% after axillary sampling, and 84% after ALND. The risk of AE was higher with an increasing number of axillary lymph nodes resected (more than 15 nodes[10]; more than 40 nodes[11]) in two studies. Schrenk et al. reported AE did not occur in a small cohort of patients undergoing sentinel lymph node dissection.[4] In a prospective randomized trial of sector resection and ALND with or without breast XRT, young age [relative risk (RR), 0.93 per year of increasing age; 95% CI, 0.91–0.97] and number of lymph nodes resected (RR, 1.11 per lymph node resected; 95% CI, 1.05–1.18) were significantly associated with any arm symptoms (not necessarily AE).[12]

Axillary XRT has been associated with AE. Senofsky et al., in a cohort of 264 patients treated with total ALND, found AE to occur in 6% of those not treated with XRT, 14.7% of those receiving XRT to the breast only, and 29.6% of those receiving XRT to the breast and regional nodes.[13] Furthermore, Keramopoulos et al. reported AE to be significantly more frequent when XRT was delayed (6 months postoperatively) than when it was given immediately postoperatively (4% versus 27%).[11]

The combination of XRT and ALND further increases the risk of AE. Kissin et al.[14] reported AE in 8.3% of women treated with breast surgery and axillary XRT, 9.1% undergoing axillary sampling and XRT, and 7.4% undergoing ALND only (7.4%). However, AE occurred in 38.3% of women undergoing both ALND and axillary XRT. In a randomized trial comparing ALND to axillary sampling, a significant increase in arm volume was experienced in 14 (12 of whom received axillary XRT) of 47 (29.8%) patients treated with ALND.[15] None of the 48 patients undergoing axillary sampling experienced AE (regardless of XRT).

The occurrence of other reduced upper body function, pain, neurologic deficits, and restricted shoulder mobility has also been evaluated. In a prospective cohort study, decline in upper body function was substantially higher during the first year after MRM or BCS with or without XRT than in the subsequent 4 years.[16] Cardiopulmonary comorbidity significantly increased the risk of decline in upper body function at 5 months (OR, 2.8; 95% CI, 1.3–5.7). Cardiopulmonary

TABLE 11.1. Arm symptoms in treatment for breast cancer.

Reference	Primary objective(s)	Study population and follow-up (years)	Number of patients	Type of local treatment	Instruments	Response rate	Results and conclusions
Kissin et al. 1986[14]	Compare the incidence of AE by subjective and objective methods; identify independent risk for late AE; compare the incidence of AE after different treatments	Cohort (clinic) diagnosed at least 1 year prior	200 patients	BCS or MRM with no axillary surgery, sampling or ALND	• Subjective: graded as no difference, moderate AE, or severe AE (patient + observer) • Objective: (1) arm circumference measured 15 cm above and 10 cm below the lateral epicondyle, (2) volume measured by water immersion		Objective AE more frequent (25.5%) than subjective AE (14%). Subjective AE was significantly more common after ALND with XRT (38.3%), axillary XRT alone (8.3%), axillary sampling with XRT (9.1%), and ALND alone (7.4%).
Yeoh et al. 1986[9]	Assess the complications following surgery and postoperative XRT	Cohort assessed median F/U of 1.7–3.24 years	187 patients	Surgical management of the axilla: none, sampling, or ALND with three different XRT dose fractionation	• Physical exam: (1) arm circumference measured 7.5 cm above the olecranon process, (2) shoulder movement and degree of restriction		Complication rates similar with three different XRT schedules. AE ± restriction of shoulder movements were different at 30 months with no surgery (25%), sampling (50%), and ALND (84%).
Borup Christensen et al. 1989[15]	Compare the sequelae of ALND vs. axillary sampling ± XRT	Prospective randomized trial with assessment at 14 days, 3, 6, and 12 months postoperative	100 patients	BCS or MRM ± XRT, randomization to ALND vs. axillary sampling	• Physical exam: (1) arm volume (measured by water displacement and corrected for changes in body weight), (2) shoulder mobility using 360 scale • Questionnaire re: arm swelling, shoulder mobility, and loss of sensibility.		AE (≥10% volume increase) in 14pts (all with ALND), 12 received XRT. Impairment of shoulder mobility was more frequent after axillary XRT ($P = 0.07$).

Study	Objective	Design	Sample	Treatment	Measures	Response	Results
Satariano et al. 1990[138]	Assess physical functioning	Case control (3 and 12 months post diagnosis) [Metropolitan Detroit Cancer Surveillance System]	571 cases (breast cancer) 647 controls (no breast cancer)	Not mentioned	Structured interview with items from (1) Massachusetts Health Care Panel Study, (2) Framingham Disability Study, and (3) the National Institute on Aging EPESE	Cases: 81.1% 3 months, 95.1% 12 months Controls: 83.3% 3 months, 90.9% 12 months	At 3 months, cases age 55–74 had greater difficulty completing tasks requiring upper body strength. At 12 months, upper body strength remained diminished in cases aged 65–74, more so than cases aged 55–64.
Senofsky G.M. et al. 1991[13]	Assess the effects of TAL	Prospective cohort, median follow-up of 41 months	264 patients	BSC or MRM + TAL ± XRT	• Medical records review • Clinical examination: AE graded I–IV (method of measurement not stated).		AE in 9.4% of patients. Breast and nodal XRT significantly associated with AE. Breast edema associated with XRT.
Segerstrom et al. 1991[18]	Study the natural history of pain and functional impairment after surgery and XRT	Prospective cohort assessed at 1–23 months and 1 week–24 months after exam 1	100 patients	MRM + ALND + high-dose XRT (±XRT to axilla)	• Questionnaire • Physical exam: (1) arm edema (water displacement method); (2) ROM (inspection)	93 patients (93%)	AE observed in 43% of patients; AE disappeared in 8 patients at follow-up [all had slight to moderate edema]. Stiffness and edema good predictors of subjective functional impairment.
Werner et al. 1991[6]	Assess predictors of AE	Cohort of patients receiving XRT, median F/U of 37 months	282 patients	BCS + ALND (30.5% had level I, II, and III dissected) + XRT	• Arm circumference measured 13 cm above and 10 cm below the olecranon on both arms		Transient AE in 7.4%, chronic arm edema in 12.1%. Persistent AE at 5 years in 16%. Body mass index strongly associated with AE.
Sneeuw et al. 1992[139]	Assess the cosmetic and functional outcomes of BCS and relationship to psychosocial functioning	Cohort, mean 4 years (2–11 years)	160 patients eligible	BCS + XRT; most patients had ALND	• In-home interview: GHQ, QOL • Physical exam	76 (47.5%) patients	High levels of psychologic distress, disturbance of body image, and decreased sexual functioning ~25%. Patient ratings of overall cosmesis and AE significantly associated with body image.
Gerber et al. 1992[5]	To compare pain, motion, and edema after MRM vs. BCS with ALND and XRT	Prospective randomized trial, annual evaluation	247 patients	MRM vs. BCS + XRT with ALND	• Physical exam: (1) functional ROM (goniometry), (2) chest wall tenderness, (3) arm circumference at ulnar styloid, olecranon, and 35 cm proximal to the ulnar styloid, (4) cosmetic outcome	165 patients (66.8%) had pre-op and post-op ROM, 131 (53%) patients had pre-op and 1 yr post-op arm circumference	Greater chest wall tenderness post-XRT. Slower recovery of pre-operative ROM post MRM. No difference in arm circumference.

(continued)

TABLE 11.1. Arm symptoms in treatment for breast cancer. (*continued*)

Reference	Primary objective(s)	Study population and follow-up (years)	Number of patients	Type of local treatment	Instruments	Response rate	Results and conclusions
Lin et al. 1993[19]	Assess impact of ALND	Retrospective review	283 patients	BCS or MRM + ALND	• Chart review • Physical examination 1 year: arm circumference, ROM, numbness, and pain.		Arm swelling (≥2 cm) in 16% of women, ≥15 degrees of restriction in 17%, numbness in the distribution of the intercostals brachial nerve in 78%, and numbness and pain in 22%.
Keramopoulos et al. 1993[11]	Assess arm morbidity following treatment	Clinic population over a 6-month window	104 patients	BCS or MRM with ALND	• Interview • Physical examination: arm circumference measured at 15 cm above and 10 cm below the lateral epicondyles in both hands.		Late AE (>3 months postsurgery) occurred in 17%; more frequent when XRT <6 months postoperative or >40 LN resected. Limb pain was more frequent >60 years old or after MRM.
Kiel et al. 1996[10]	Incidence of AE after BCS and XRT	Cohort q 6 mo for up to 3 years	402 women	BCS + XRT (±AND)	• Physical examination: arm circumference measured 15 cm above and 10 cm below the olecranon process.	183 included in the study	Axillary dissection (>15 LN) and age (>55 years) are predictors of AE.
Paci et al. 1996[8]	Assess long-term sequelae of breast cancer surgery	Cohort of 5-year survivors	346 survivors	BCS or MRM	• Interview • Physical exam: arm circumference measured at six points	238 women (68.8%)	30.2% had a chronic lymphedema and 18.9% a shoulder deficit. Chronic lymphedema greater after MRM vs. BCS. Early lymphedema more frequent after BCS.
Tasmuth et al. 1996[7]	Assess physical symptoms and anxiety/depression	Prospective cohort day—1, 1 month, 6 months, and 1 year after surgery	105 women	MRM vs. BCS with ALND ± XRT	• Interview • Neurologic examination • Grip strength • Arm circumference • STAI + 2 additional questions re depression	93 women (89%)	Incidence of chronic posttreatment pain higher after BCS vs. MRM. Phantom sensations in 25%. Psychologic morbidity highest before surgery and decreased with time.

Study	Objective	Design	Sample	Surgery	Measures	Results	Conclusions
Liliegren et al. 1997[12]	Assess arm morbidity after sector resection and ALND ± XRT	Prospective randomized trial 3, 12, 24, and 36 months after surgery	381 women	Sector resection and ALND ± XRT	• Arm circumference 10cm above and below the elbow on both arms • Subjective arm symptoms (graded as none, moderate, or severe)	Arm circumference: 273pts at 3–12 mo., 270pts at 13–36mo., <50pts at >36 mo. Arm symptoms: 368 pts at 3–12 mo., 335 pts at 13–36 mo., 115 pts >36 mo.	Extent of surgical procedure and young age are determinants of arm morbidity. Arm symptoms are most common during the first year.
Silliman et al. 1999[17]	To identify risk factors for decline in upper body function	Cross-sectional observational study 3–5 months postoperative	300 women	BCS or MRM ± XRT	• Review of medical records • Telephone interview	213 women (71%)	Extent and type of primary therapy and cardiopulmonary comorbidity associated with a decline in upper body function.
Schrenk et al. 2000[4]	Assess postoperative morbidity of the operated arm	Prospective cohort 15–17 months F/U	35 women	BCS or MRM ± XRT with ALND or SN dissection	• Physical exam: arm circumference (15cm above and 10cm below the lateral epicondyle), numbness, mobility, strength, stiffness • Interview	35 patients (100%)	SN associated with negligible morbidity compared with ALND.
Lash et al. 2000[16]	Assess the effect of patient characteristics and therapy on self-reported upper-body function and discomfort	Prospective cohort 5 and 21 months postoperative	388 invited, 303 interviewed	MRM or BCS ± XRT	• Review of medical records • Computer-assisted telephone interviews		Cardiopulmonary comorbidity associated with decline at 5-month interview (OR 2.8, 95% CI 1.3–5.7). ALND associated with axillary numbness, pain.
Lash et al. 2002[140]	Characterize the incidence and predictors of upper body function decline and recovery	Cohort for 5 years	303 women	BCS ± XRT or MRM	• Review of medical records • Telephone interviews • SF-36	82 met case definition for upper-body function decline. 32 met the definition for recovery.	The incidence of decline in the first year was substantially higher than in the subsequent 4 years. Women with less than a high school education had an increased risk of decline (HR 2.3). Recovery was higher for women followed by breast cancer specialist.

BCS, breast-conserving surgery; XRT, radiation therapy; HR, hazard ratio; OR, odds ratio; ALND, axillary lymph node dissection; SN, sentinel node dissection; AE, arm edema; F/U, follow-up; TAL, total axillary lymphadenectomy; EPESE, Established Populations for the Epidemiological Study of the Elderly; GHQ, General Health Questionnaire; STAI, State Trait Anxiety Inventory; SF-36, Medical Outcomes Study Short Form—36 Items.

morbidity was an independent predictor of upper body function decline [P = 0.006] in a second study[17]; mastectomy and XRT were also associated with significant declines in upper body function. Women treated with an ALND were more likely to report numbness or pain in the axilla (OR, 6.4; 95% CI, 0.2–33).[16]

In a prospective cohort study, Segerstrom et al.[18] reported 35 of 93 (37.6%) patients had restricted shoulder range of motion during the first 2 years after surgery; this increased to 49.5% up to 2 years later. Paci et al.[8] reported that 18.9% of patients experienced shoulder deficit as assessed by physical examination performed 5 or more years after diagnosis. Lin et al.[19] reported 15° or greater loss of ROM in 17% of the patients and 30° or more loss in 4% at 1 or more years after ALND. In contrast, Gerber et al.[5] found no significant loss in functional ROM (assessed using goniometry) 1 year postoperatively; however, patients undergoing MRM reached their preoperative ROM more slowly than those undergoing BCS.[5] Pain and chest wall tenderness have been reported following breast surgery.[5,7,11] Pain was more frequent after BCS in one study[7] and after mastectomy in another.[11]

Arm symptoms have been associated with psychologic, social, sexual, and functional morbidity.[20] In two case-control studies, women experiencing AE after treatment for breast cancer showed greater psychologic morbidity and greater impact of illness measured using the Psychosocial Adjustment to Illness Scale (PAIS), effects that remained stable over a 6-month period, even if AE was being treated.[21,22] Maunsell et al. also reported the proportion of women experiencing psychological distress as measured by the Psychiatric Symptom Index (PSI) increased significantly with an increased number of problems in the affected arm.[23]

In summary, significant physical and functional sequelae in the arm and upper body may occur as a result of local therapy, especially ALND and axillary XRT. Prospective, population-based studies that include an assessment of patient demographics, risk factors, stage, and treatment coupled with outcome evaluation that involves standardized, blinded assessment of arm symptoms and function preoperatively and during long-term follow-up would expand available information; intervention research to identify effective management approaches is urgently needed.

Menopause

Women with breast cancer may experience early menopause as a result of their treatment. They report a higher frequency of menopausal symptoms than women in the general population.[24] The high frequency of menopausal symptoms in breast cancer survivors is caused by several factors[25]: (1) age at diagnosis (frequently over 50 years), (2) abrupt discontinuation of hormone replacement therapy (HRT) at the time of breast cancer diagnosis, (3) induction of premature menopause by therapy (i.e., chemotherapy and ovarian ablation), and (4) induction of estrogen deficiency symptoms by therapy (e.g., tamoxifen and aromatase inhibitors) (Table 11.2). Chemotherapy is frequently associated with either temporary or permanent amenorrhea. The incidence of amenorrhea is related to the type of chemotherapy regimen, the cumulative dose (particularly cyclophosphamide), and the age of the patient.[26,27] Surgically induced menopause and premature menopause have been associated with more severe symptoms than natural menopause.[28,29] The health consequences of menopause can be divided into four categories: vasomotor symptoms, genitourinary signs and symptoms, skeletal effects, and cardiovascular effects.[30] In a survey of 190 breast cancer survivors, the most common symptoms experienced were hot flashes (65%), night sweats (44%), vaginal dryness (44%), difficulty sleeping (44%), depression (44%), and dyspareunia (26%).[31] Hot flashes (HF) are more frequent, severe, distressing, and of greater duration in breast cancer survivors compared with controls without breast cancer.[32]

Before 2002, HRT was frequently prescribed to healthy women for the control of menopausal symptoms and primary prevention of disease (i.e., cardiovascular disease and osteoporosis). In 2002, the Women's Health Initiative (WHI), a large randomized trial of HRT versus placebo in healthy women, was stopped early because overall health risks of combined estrogen plus progesterone exceeded benefits at an average 5.2-year follow-up.[33] Risks of coronary heart disease, stroke, pulmonary embolism, and invasive breast cancer were increased, whereas risks of colon cancer and hip fracture were minimally decreased. Results for estrogen alone versus placebo did not show an increased risk for breast cancer.[33a]

The use of HRT in breast cancer survivors has been controversial.[34,35] Four case series,[36–39] three case-control studies,[40–43] and one cohort study[44] failed to identify an increased risk in women who chose to take HRT; two additional studies reported a lower risk of recurrence and death when HRT was used.[42,43] The studies are susceptible to selection bias, particularly in view of the reluctance of many breast cancer survivors to accept HRT.[45,46] One randomized clinical trial of HRT in 434 breast cancer survivors was recently stopped for safety reasons because of an unacceptably high risk of breast cancer events [hazard ratio (HR), 3.5; 95% CI, 1.5–8.1] in women receiving HRT.[47] Women on HRT were advised to discontinue the treatment. Current guidelines[34,48] that recommend postmenopausal breast cancer survivors be encouraged to consider alternatives to HRT but state that minimal HRT use may be considered in a well-informed patient with severe symptoms will likely be modified in view of these results, with a greater focus on recommending nonhormonal approaches to symptom management.

Vasomotor symptoms are the most common complaint of perimenopausal and postmenopausal women. More than 60% of postmenopausal women experience hot flashes, and one-third of those find them nearly intolerable.[49] HRT relieves HF in 80% to 90% of women who initiate treatment.[50–52]

Progestational agents (e.g., megestrol acetate, medroxyprogesterone acetate, and depo-Provera) decrease HF by 85%.[53–57] Herbal remedies, including soy products and black cohosh, have been reported to minimally decrease HF or have no effect. Vitamin E (800 IU/day) minimally decreases HF (i.e., one fewer HF/day). Clonidine is modestly active in reducing hot flashes. Selective serotonin reuptake inhibitors (SSRIs) such as venlafaxine and paroxetine have also been shown to significantly reduce HF. Possible interactions between SSRIs and selective estrogen receptor modulators (SERMS) are being evaluated. Gabapentin (widely used in neurologic disorders) has been recently reported to reduce HF scores.[58] Most of these trials have evaluated the short-term effect (e.g., 4–12 weeks); long-term effects have not been addressed.

Severe symptoms of urogenital atrophy occur in nearly half of postmenopausal women surviving breast cancer.

Lubricants and moisturizers have been shown to be helpful but do not completely relieve symptoms. Very low dose vaginal estrogen creams can reverse atrophy but systemic absorption of estrogen may occur. Newer methods of estrogen delivery include a ring device (Estring; Pfizer, New York, NY). This device provides almost complete relief of symptoms and minimal systemic absorption[48]; however, recent evidence that lipid levels may be altered[59] raises concerns about its use.

One randomized trial[60] evaluated the use of a comprehensive menopause assessment program in breast cancer survivors; the intervention (which did not involve use of estrogen but permitted megestrol acetate and nonhormonal agents such as clonidine) reduced menopausal symptoms and improved sexual functioning when compared with a control arm.

Bone loss occurs at a rate of 1% to 5% per year and is greatest during the first 5 years after natural menopause.[61] Chemotherapy-induced ovarian failure causes more rapid and significant bone loss.[62] Tamoxifen in premenopausal, but not postmenopausal, women and aromatase inhibitors have also been associated with increased bone loss. Bone density should be monitored in survivors.[63] Preventive measures such as proper intake of vitamin D and calcium, regular exercise, and counseling about the relationship between cigarette smoking, alcohol, and bone loss should be initiated in all patients. Pharmacologic approaches currently recommended for survivors include (1) bisphosphonates (alendronate, risedronate), (2) SERMs (raloxifene), and (3) calcitonin.

The risk of coronary heart disease increases with increasing age.[64,65] HRT in the primary and secondary prevention of coronary heart disease has not been shown to reduce cardiac events in four large randomized clinical trials.[33,66,67] Management of known risk factors and encouragement of lifestyle modification are warranted.[68]

Pregnancy

Limited data exist on the effect of pregnancy on breast cancer outcome. Based on the experience at major institutions[68–71] and population-based registries,[68,72,73] women who become pregnant after a diagnosis of breast cancer appear to have similar breast cancer outcomes to those who do not. Selection biases may be responsible for these results. Prior chemotherapy does not appear to have teratogenic effects in future pregnancies[74,75]; however, local breast cancer treatment (i.e., surgery and XRT) may affect the ability to lactate after BCS.[68,76,77] Breast cancer and pregnancy have been recently reviewed.[78,79]

Fatigue

Fatigue is often experienced during, and shortly after, cancer treatment. The level of fatigue in a large survey of breast cancer survivors (1–5 years after initial diagnosis) was comparable with that of age-matched controls using the RAND-36 questionnaire.[80,81] However, severe and persistent fatigue was experienced in a subgroup of survivors and was related to depression and pain. In a second smaller cohort study, fatigue (measured using a number of fatigue questionnaires including the RAND-36) was more common in breast cancer survivors than in age-matched controls.[81,82]

Second Malignancies

Second malignancies (e.g., angiosarcoma, sarcoma, and skin cancer) at the site of previous local treatment for breast cancer occur in less than 1% of survivors (see Chapter 17).[68]

Cardiac Toxicity

The most common form of anthracycline-induced cardiotoxicity is chronic cardiomyopathy.[83] The risk of cardiomyopathy is principally dependent on the cumulative anthracycline dose and may occur years after therapy.[84] Prospective monitoring of signs and symptoms of congestive heart failure (CHF) revealed a 9% risk of CHF after 450 mg/m^2 doxorubicin and 25% after 500 mg/m^2 [85]; this risk may be higher when doxorubicin is used in combination with paclitaxel.[86] Prospective cardiac monitoring using MUGA scans has been included in more recent clinical trials of breast cancer treatment including anthracyclines, taxanes, and herceptin. Based on a recent randomized trial,[87] cardiotoxicity is particularly pronounced when herceptin is combined with either adriamycin or epirubicin plus cyclophosphamide (any cardiotoxicity = 27%, grade 3–4 cardiotoxicity = 10%). Bradycardia has been reported with the use of paclitaxel alone.

Surveillance

Evidence-based surveillance strategies for breast cancer survivors have been established.[63] There are sufficient data to recommend monthly breast self-examination, annual mammography of the preserved and contralateral breast, as well as a careful history and physical examination every 3 to 6 months for 3 years, then every 6 to 12 months for 2 years, then annually. Data are not sufficient to recommend routine radiologic investigations or blood work (including tumor markers). Primary care of breast cancer survivors has also been reviewed.[68] Grunfeld et al.[88] conducted a large randomized trial of specialist versus general practitioner care in Great Britain; patients were more satisfied with care provided by the latter, with no differences in medical outcomes being observed, although only a small number of medical events were reported.

Psychosocial Status and HRQOL

Breast cancer is a stressful event that can perturb psychologic equilibrium and reduce HRQOL in the short-term[89–92]; recent survivorship research has evaluated long-term sequelae. Early studies involved mainly small convenience samples (maximum, 61 survivors), descriptive designs, and interview-based measurements.[93–97] Key results of these studies include observations that the majority of survivors are fairly to very satisfied with their lives 8 years after diagnosis despite thoughts of recurrence reported by 50%[93]; that survivors have a positive perception of life and attach less importance to trivial stressors even though fear of recurrence is a major concern[94]; and that the majority of survivors thrive despite experiencing problems related to breast cancer and its treatment.[95] Several ongoing issues were identified in a focus group of 10-year survivors: integration of disease into current life, change in relationship with others, restructuring life perspective, and unresolved issues.[96]

TABLE 11.2. Menopause in breast cancer survivors.

Reference	Primary objective(s)	Study population and follow-up (years)	Number of patients	Instruments	Response rate	Results and conclusions
Guidozzi et al. 1999[141]	Determine whether ERT adversely affects outcome of survivors	Prospective descriptive study of women 8–91 months postdiagnosis treated with oral continuous opposed ERT observed for 24–44 months	24	• History and physical exam 3×/year • Mammogram yearly. • BSE taught to the patient. • Appointment with surgeon annually.		No recurrences.
Brewster et al. 1999[142]	Evaluate the outcome of patients who elected ERT	Convenience sample treated with oral continuous ERT for at least 3 months starting 41 months (range 0–401 months) postdiagnosis; median F/U 30 months	145	• Routine surveillance by an oncologist	145/168	13 recurrences (9%).
Vassilopoulou-Sellin et al. 1999[144]	Determine whether ERT alters the development of new or recurrent breast cancer	Prospective randomized study of ERT, cohort of nonpartipicants	319	• Monitor clinical outcome for new or recurrent cancer	319/331	ERT does not seem to increase events. Events during follow-up: 20/280 in controls vs. 1/39 in ERT group.
Ganz et al. 1999[45]	Assess willingness to undergo HRT in survivors	Sample of survivors from a previous survey an average of 3.1 years postdiagnosis	39	• Interview • Standardized health-related instruments including the RAND Health Survey • Decision analysis interview.		Older survivors are reluctant to take estrogen. Increased willingness to consider therapy if multiple symptoms coexisted and the risk of recurrence was small.
Ganz et al. 2000[60]	Assess the efficacy of a comprehensive menopausal assessment (CMA) intervention program in achieving relief of symptoms, improvement in QOL, and sexual functioning in survivors	Randomized controlled design of postmenopausal breast cancer survivors (8 months to 5 years after diagnosis)	72	• Menopausal symptom scale score adapted from the Breast Cancer Prevention Trial Symptom Checklist • Vitality Scale from the RAND Health Survey 1.0 • Sexual Summary Scale from the Cancer Rehabilitation Evaluation System.	72/197	A clinical assessment and intervention program for menopausal symptom management is feasible and acceptable to patients, leading to reduction in symptoms and improvement in sexual functioning.
Peters et al. 2001[143]	Define the prevalence of ERT usage, identify risks	Cohort of survivors (ER+ in 74%), median disease-free 46.7 months (range, 0–448 months), followed for ≥60 months, treated with ERT	56	• Review of medical records Routine surveillance by an oncologist including history and physical examinations every 3–6 months, annual mammograms and CXR, and evaluation of liver chemistries at each visit.	56/607 interviewed	Use of ERT was not associated with increased events.

Study	Objective	Study design/sample	N	Methods / Data source	Response	Results
O'Meara et al. 2001[43]	Evaluate the impact of HRT on recurrence and mortality	Record-based study of women 35–74 years identified in the SEER records (1977–1994) (1 user matched to 4 nonusers) (48% of users/59% of nonusers ER+)	2,755	Data obtained from: • The Cancer Surveillance System • Group Health Cooperative pharmacy • Medical records		Lower risks of recurrence and mortality observed with HRT.
Harris et al. 2002[24]	Assess the burden of menopausal symptoms, HRT use, and alternative treatments in recent survivors	Population-based, case-control study of survivors (8–11 months postdiagnosis) and age-matched controls	183	• Standardized telephone questionnaire • F/U 10-minute telephone questionnaire on HRT and menopause	93% cases, 95% controls	Cases more likely to experience menopausal symptoms, less likely to use HRT, more likely to use alternative therapies (soy, vitamin E, and herbal remedies).
Durna et al. 2002[144]	Compare the QOL of survivors who received HRT and those who did not	Nonrandomized qualitative study of women from a cancer registry. QOL was compared for 3 groups based on the time since diagnosis: <4 years, 4–8 years and >8 years	123	Questionnaires including: • Demographic data • QOL Breast Cancer version Questionnaire • QOL Self Evaluation Questionnaire	123/190 (64.8%)	No significant difference between users and nonusers. Near-normal QOL after a 4-year adjustment period.
Carpenter et al. 2002[32]	Compare the HF symptom experience and related outcomes between survivors and healthy women	Descriptive, cross-sectional, comparative study of survivors (mean of 39 months postdiagnosis) and age-matched healthy female volunteers	69 survivors/ 63 age-matched	Questionnaires: • Demographic and disease/treatment information • Gynecologic and reproductive history form • Hot flash questionnaire and diary • POMS-SF • PANAS • HFRDIS	69/207 survivors	Hot flashes are a significant problem for survivors. Survivors with severe hot flashes reported significantly greater mood disturbance, higher negative affect, more interference with daily activities (sleep, concentration, and sexuality), and decreased QOL.
Biglia et al. 2003[46]	Determine the prevalence of menopausal symptoms, explore attitudes toward HRT or other treatments and the willingness to take estrogen	Convenience sample (early breast cancer) Mean F/U not stated	250	• 35-item questionnaire formulated for this study	Not stated	Survivors are interested in treatments that may improve their QOL, but fear of HRT persists among survivors and their doctors.
Holmberg 2004[47]	To examine impact of HRT on events in survivors	RCT of HRT vs. no therapy in survivors	434	• Clinical examination, mammography	345 had ≥1 follow-up	RCT stopped early because of excess events in survivors treated with HRT (relative hazard 3.5, 95% CI 1.5–8.1).

HRT, hormone replacement therapy; ERT, estrogen replacement therapy; RCT, randomized clinical trial; F/U, follow-up; POMS-SF, Profile of Mood States-Short Form; PANAS, Positive and Negative Affect Scale; HFRDIS, Hot Flash-Related Daily Interference Scale; BSE, breast self-examination; QOL, quality of life.

Second-generation studies used stronger designs, more standardized measurement approaches, and larger sample sizes. They were more often population based and/or used control groups of women without breast cancer. They frequently used generic instruments (applicable to healthy and medically ill individuals) for which normative data are available. One generic instrument that has been widely used in survivorship research is the Medical Outcomes Study Short Form—36 (MOS SF-36), a reliable and valid measure of HRQOL. It has 36 items rated on a 5-point Likert scale. There are eight subscales grouped in two composite scales: Physical Component Summary (PCS) and Mental Component Summary (MCS). Cancer-specific instruments, which measure attributes that are specific or unique to cancer patients, were also used in a large number of studies. Due to their nature, normative data for the general population are not available for these instruments. Nonetheless, they provide data that can be used to describe groups of survivors, evaluate change in their status over time, or compare different groups of survivors. Specific examples of these instruments are discussed.

Psychologic Status and Overall HRQOL

Many studies have examined psychosocial status and HRQOL in breast cancer survivors as a single group. Results of these studies are reviewed first, followed by a discussion of the status of defined subgroups of survivors.

Several cross-sectional, case-control, and cohort studies using the MOS SF-36 have reported scores on the Mental Component Summary scale or one of its subscales in breast cancer survivors 2 to 8 years postdiagnosis to be comparable with, or better than, scores obtained from either the general population or individuals with other chronic illnesses[80,98–102] (Table 11.3). Dorval et al.[103] used the Psychiatric Symptom Index (PSI), another generic instrument that measures the presence and intensity of four psychologic dimensions (depression, anxiety, cognitive impairment, and irritability) in a case-control study; no difference was found between 8-year survivors and controls randomly matched for age and residence. Studies using the generic measure of mood, the Profile of Mood States (POMS), reported women with breast cancer who were 2 years postdiagnosis to have scores comparable to published norms[80] or to a control group.[104] Taken together, these observations using generic instruments provide little evidence of impaired long-term HRQOL or psychologic status in breast cancer survivors compared to the general population.

A cancer-specific instrument, the QOL Cancer Survivors Tool (QOL-CS), yielded psychologic subscale scores that were worse than those for the social, spiritual well-being, and physical subscales 5.7 years postdiagnosis.[105] The inclusion of specific questions related to fear of recurrence of the cancer, which are not explicitly evaluated in generic questionnaires, and the specific population studied (members of the National Coalition for Cancer Survivorship) may have contributed to this result. Mosconi et al.[102] used the European Organization for Research and Treatment of Cancer Quality of Life Questionnaire Core-30 (EORTC QLQ-C30), a multidimensional cancer-specific questionnaire, to study Italian breast and colon cancer survivors. Overall HRQOL was reported to be

good, and scores for emotional functioning did not differ between the two groups of survivors.

Physical Functioning

Earlier, we discussed specific physical symptoms in breast cancer survivors. The MOS SF-36 has been employed to measure general physical functioning. Physical functioning scores in survivors have been reported to be similar to,[102] or better than, published norms for individuals with other chronic illnesses[80,106] or the general population.[106] However, some studies[98,99,101] reported physical functioning scores in survivors that were lower than norms for the general population. A modest decline in physical functioning over time (mean, 6.3 years) has been reported by Ganz et al.[99]; the magnitude of the decline was small and was thought to be related to aging. Dow et al.[105] studied members of the National Coalition for Cancer Survivorship, a group that may not be representative of all cancer survivors. Overall physical well-being scores were good compared with other domains (e.g. psychologic); however, problems with components of physical well-being (i.e., pain, energy) were identified.

Thus, evaluation of general physical functioning in breast cancer survivors has yielded inconsistent results in comparison with published norms for the general population. However, differences from general population norms are small and may be due to effects of age.

Sexual Functioning

Breast cancer diagnosis and treatment can adversely affect sexuality. Surgical treatment of the primary tumor can affect body image, while systemic therapy can cause premature menopause or vaginal dryness. Measurement of the impact of breast cancer and its treatment on sexual functioning is challenging because few instruments specifically address this aspect of HRQOL. These measurement challenges may be compounded by a reporting bias if survivors are reluctant to respond to questions about sexual functioning. The use of specific questionnaires (e.g., the Sexual Activity Questionnaire, SAQ) in recent studies permits a more detailed assessment than is possible using more general multidimensional questionnaires.

Matthews et al.[98] administered the Satisfaction with Life Domains Scale for Cancer (SLDS-C) to breast cancer survivors (American Cancer Society Reach to Recovery volunteers) a mean of 8.6 years postdiagnosis. Scores for sexual functioning were worse than for other aspects of functioning. Dow et al.[105] also reported that satisfaction with sex life was the worst of all domains on the Functional Assessment of Cancer Therapy—General (FACT-G) in 294 survivors taking part in a peer-support group 5.7 years postdiagnosis. In contrast, Kurtz et al.[107] reported 5- to 10-year breast cancer survivors had high levels of sexual satisfaction on the Long Term Quality of Life Instrument.

Ganz et al.[99,106] used questionnaires that specifically address sexual functioning in two recent studies. In a cross-sectional study of 864 women,[106] use of the Watts Sexual Functioning Questionnaire identified modest increases in sexual dysfunction with aging but use of the Cancer

TABLE 11.3. Psychosocial status and health-related quality of life (HRQOL) overall associations in breast cancer survivors.

Reference	Primary objective(s)	Study population and follow-up (years)	Number of subjects	Instrument(s)	Response rate	Results and conclusions
Vinokur et al. 1989[120]	To assess the effect of age, time since diagnosis and disease severity	Case-control (population-based screening program) 53% > 5 years	178 survivors 176 controls	• HSC • PM • SE • ICO • PQOL • PREF • SC • Others	91%	Comparable QOL (physical, mental, health, and emotional well-being) in survivors and controls. Severity and recency of diagnosis were independent predictors of adverse effects on mental and physical well-being in survivors. Younger survivors with recent diagnosis have psychosocial concerns. Older with recent diagnosis have physical concerns.
Ellman et al. 1995[145]	To measure anxiety and depression	Case-control (screening clinic registry) 13 years	331 survivors 584 controls	• HADS	76% (survivors) 75% (controls)	Significantly more cases of depression and anxiety in controls. Time since diagnosis did not affect depression or anxiety except for the first anniversary.
Kurtz et al. 1995[107]	To explore six aspects of QOL	Hospital based tumor registry >5 years	191	• LTQL • CARES	55%	Best scores on psychologic domain and sexual satisfaction. Good psychologic state highly correlated with low somatic concerns and sexual satisfaction. Middle-aged: more positive philosophical/spiritual outlook.
Ganz et al. 1996[80]	To describe psychosocial concerns and QOL among survivors	Participants in rehabilitation RCT 2–3 years	139 (12 had recurrence)	• FLIC • CARES • SF-36 • POMS	77%	FLIC-POMS: no difference at 2–3 years versus 1 year. CARES: decline in global QOL, sexual and marital functioning at 3 vs. 1 year. Sexual functioning difficulties persisted from diagnosis to 3 years. Arms symptoms persist. Maximum recovery in QOL 1 year after treatment.
Dow et al. 1996[105]	To describe QOL in survivors including positive and negative outcomes	Convenience sample (mailed questionnaire to national coalition for cancer survivorship-peer support) 5.7 years	294 BCS (56 had recurrence)	• QOL-CS • FACT-G	56%	Fatigue, aches, sleep problems, fear of recurrence, family distress, sex life problems persisted over time. Physical QOL better than emotional/social QOL.
Saleeba et al. 1996[146]	To compare emotional status of survivors to screening population	Case-control (MDACC, screening clinic) >5 years	Survivors = 52 Control = 88	• BDI • STAI	Not stated	Mean depression score higher in survivors (within normal range). Survivors seek more frequent counseling (29% vs. 16%).
Weitzner et al. 1997[147]	To compare mood and QOL of survivors to screening population	Case-control, clinic samples >5 years	Survivors = 60 Controls = 93	• BDI • STAI • FPQLI	Not stated	No difference between cases and controls. Worse mood score correlated with lower QOL in survivors.
Lee 1997[148]	To examine social support, type of surgery, geographic location, and QOL	Convenience sample (Reach for Recovery volunteers) 14.1 years	100	• FPQLI	88%	QOL not associated with number of support persons, mental status, time from surgery, or type of surgery.
Ganz et al. 1998[106]	To describe survivorship in relation to age, menopausal status, treatment	Cross-sectional (random selection from two large metropolitan areas; tumor registry, clinics, hospitals) 3.1 years	864	• SF-36 • CES-D • DAS • CARES • WSFQ • Others	39%	Survivors had more frequent physical symptoms. Worse sexual functioning in survivors with chemo, menopause. and age <50, but no difference in sexual satisfaction and marital/partner adjustment. Unpartnered women have concerns about dating. Body image worse with MT.

(continued)

TABLE 11.3. Psychosocial status and health-related quality of life (HRQOL) overall associations in breast cancer survivors. *(continued)*

Reference	Primary objective(s)	Study population and follow-up (years)	Number of subjects	Instrument(s)	Response rate	Results and conclusions
Ganz et al. 1998[100]	To describe QOL related to adjuvant treatment	Cross-sectional (mailed survey, tumor registry, clinics, hospitals) 2.7–3.1 years	1,098	• SF36 • CES-D • CARES • LLS • Others	35%	No difference in mental-psychologic (SF-36, CES-D) and global QOL according to treatment. Physical and sexual: worse functioning in adjuvant therapy. Small adverse impact of adjuvant treatment on physical functioning but no impact on overall QOL.
Dorval et al. 1998[103]	To compare QOL in 8-year survivors	Survivors cohort assembled from seven hospitals, random digit dialing age-matched control, random digit dialing age-matched control 8.8 years	124 survivors (26 had new events) 427 controls	• PSI • LWMAT • MOS SSS • Others	96% (survivors) 61% (controls)	No difference in QOL. Arm problems and sexual satisfaction worse in survivors.
Dorval et al. 1999[108]	To examine marital breakdown	Survivors cohort assembled from seven hospitals 3 months–8 years	366	• SLES • LWMA • Others	89%–95%	Marital breakdown similar in survivors and controls. Marital satisfaction: predictor of marital breakdown in both groups.
Joly et al. 2000[135]	To evaluate long-term QOL in relation to chemo	Inception cohort (from a RCT on chemo) 9.6 years	119	• EORTC QLQ-C30 • Others	68%	No difference in functioning scales, body image, sex life, breast symptoms, social or professional life; trend for poorer cognitive functioning in CMF.
Montazeri et al. 2001[149]	To assess QOL at two time points	Members of the three support groups 1–5 years (54%)	56	• HADS	100%	29% and 14% scored above "case" cutpoint for anxiety and depression at baseline; significant improvement at 1 year.
Holzner et al. 2001[136]	To evaluate the effect of time on QOL	Convenience sample (outpatient)	87	• EORTC QLQ-C30 • FACT-B	Not stated	Worse emotional, cognitive, sexual functioning, global QOL >5 years vs. 2–5 years posttreatment. Better global QOL, social, emotional functioning >5 years vs. 1–2 years post Rx. Highest QOL in the period between 2–5 year post Rx.
Matthews et al. 2002[98]	To compare health status, life satisfaction, and QOL	Convenience sample (peer support-volunteers) 8.6 years	586	• SF-36 • SLDS-C	63%	Survivors reported higher emotional well-being, social functioning, and vitality but lower physical functioning compared to population-based norms. Worse sexual satisfaction, body image, physical strength for survivors. Younger women had better physical functioning but lower emotional well-being and vitality.
Tomich et al. 2002[101]	To compare QOL and psychologic well-being in BCS and controls	Survivors from RCT of peer and education groups; neighborhood controls >5.5 years	BCS = 164 Control = 164	• WAS • SWBS • FACI • SF-36 • PANAS	61%	Overall HRQOL similar in survivors and controls; no-intervention survivors had worse physical functioning. Poor QOL associated with beliefs of lasting harmful effect of treatment, low level of personal control, lack of sense of purpose in life.

Study	Purpose	Sample	N	Instruments	Response rate	Findings
Kessler et al. 2002[137]	To assess HRQOL	Convenience sample (ACS Reach for Recovery program) Mean 3.5 years (<0.1 to >10 years)	148 (23 had metastasis)	• PANAS • QOLM (Selby and Boyd) • Others	71%	QOL improved with increasing time from diagnosis and less extensive disease. More positive and less negative affect associated with better QOL.
Mosconi et al. 2002[102]	To assess long-term HRQOL of survivors	Survivors in a RCT of F/U testing (colon cancer survivors also studied) 8.3 years	433	• SF-36 • EORTC QLQ-C30	52%	Long-term survivors have HRQOL comparable to age/sex-matched norms. HRQOL lower with comorbidities or chemo. Physical functioning lower in breast vs. colon survivors.
Cimprich et al. 2002[121]	To assess age, duration of survival, and QOL	Tumor registry of Midwestern comprehensive cancer center 11.5 years	105	• QOL-CS	54%	Lower QOL on physical domain in older survivors. Lower QOL on social domain in younger survivors. Best QOL (overall and physical) in middle-aged survivors.
Ganz et al. 2002[99]	To evaluate long-term survivorship	5- to 10-year F/U of earlier cohort (population-based tumor registries, clinics, and hospitals) 6.3 years	817 (*54 had recurrence and were excluded)	• SF-36 • LLS • CES-D$ • PANAS • RDAS • SAQ • CARES • MOS-SSS • Others	61%	Excellent physical and emotional well-being (minimal declines reflected expected age-related changes). No change in sexual interest but sexual activities declined. Stable energy level and social functioning. Some symptoms improved; others worsened. Survivors not receiving chemo had better overall QOL, physical functioning, less sexual discomfort.
Ganz et al. 2003[122]	To evaluate QOL and reproductive health in younger survivors	Cohort (two hospitals tumor registries) 5.9 years	577	• SF-36 • LLS • CES-D • PANAS • SAQ • Others	56%	High level of physical functioning. Youngest: Decrement in vitality, lowest score in social and emotional functioning, more depressive symptomatology, lower positive affect, and more negative affect. Amenorrhea frequent in women age ≥40 and associated with poorer health perception.
Ganz et al. 2003[123]	To examine HRQOL in older survivors	Cohort (identified through pathology reports, tumor registries) 3–5, 6–8, and 15–17 months	691	• PF10 • MHI-5 • CARES-SF-36 • MOS-SSS • Others	43%	Physical and mental health score decreased significantly at 15 months (SF-36). Improvement at 15 months in CARES.

Response rate: as stated in the paper or if not, the percentage of eligible patients who completed the study.

*, Valid and reliable instruments.

QOL, quality of life; BC, breast cancer; F/U, follow-up; Rx, treatment; ACS, American Cancer Society; HSC, Hopkins Symptom Checklist*; PM, positive morale, based from Bradburn's positive affect scale*; SE, self-esteem: based on Rosenberg's scale of self esteem; ICO, internal control orientation, based on Rotter's scale; PQOL, perceived QOL, based on scale developed by Andrews and Withey; PREF, perceived role and emotional functioning, SC, social contacts, from Berkman's Social Network Index; HADS, Hospital Anxiety and Depression Scale*; LTQL, long-term quality of life*; CARES, Cancer Rehabilitation Evaluation System*; FLIC, Functional Living Index–Cancer*; SF-36, RAND or MOS Short-Form-36*; POMS, Profile of Mood States*; QOL-CS, Quality of Life–Cancer Survivors*; FACT, Functional Assessment of Cancer Therapy*; BDI, Beck Depression Inventory*; STAI, State-Trait Anxiety Inventory*; FPQLI, Ferrans and Powers Quality of Life Index*; CES-D, Center of Epidemiologic Studies–Depression Scale*; DAS, Dyadic Adjustment Scale*; WSFQ, Watts Sexual Function Questionnaire*; PSI, Psychiatric Symptom Index*; LWMAT, Locke-Wallace Marital Adjustment Test*; MOS SSS, MOS Social Support Survey*; SLES, Stressful Life Event Scale*; EORTC-QLQ C-30, European Organization for Research and Treatment of Cancer–Quality of Life Questionnaire C-30*; SLDS-C, Satisfaction with Life Domains Scales for Cancer; WAS, Words Assumption Scale; SWBS, Spiritual Well-Being Scale of FACI (Functional Assessment of Chronic Illness therapy); PANAS, Positive and Negative Affect Schedule*; QOLM, WOL Measurement, Selby and Boyd*; RDAS, Revised Dyadic Adjustment Scale*; SAQ, Sexual Activity Questionnaire*; LLS, Ladder of Life scale*; PF-10, 10-item functioning scale from SF-36; MHI-5, Mental Health Inventory, from the SF-36.

135

Rehabilitation Evaluation System (CARES) identified no impairment in sexual satisfaction. Sexual functioning was significantly worse in those who received chemotherapy (but not tamoxifen), particularly in women who were menopausal (either naturally or secondary to treatment) and in women under 50 years of age. Using the SAQ in their cohort study of 763 long-term breast cancer survivors, this group also reported sexual discomfort to be greatest in women who received chemotherapy but identified no differences in sexual pleasure or sexual habits.[99] In summary, sexual functioning appears to be adversely impacted in breast cancer survivors, particularly in younger women who receive adjuvant chemotherapy.

Social Functioning and Marital Status

Studies evaluating social functioning in breast cancer survivors have usually shown little evidence of impairment. The social functioning subscale of the MOS SF-36 has yielded similar scores in breast cancer survivors and in the general population in the majority of studies.[80,98–102] Use of the EORTC QLQ-C30 has also demonstrated high level of social functioning in breast cancer survivors.[102] Use of the MOS Social Support Measure also showed no difference between breast cancer patients with a control population[99,103] and no change according to time elapsed since diagnosis.[99]

In a cohort of 763 survivors, there was no significant change in marital status over 5 years of follow-up.[99] In another cohort followed for 8 years, no difference in divorce or separation rates at 12 months, 18 months, and 8 years after diagnosis was identified in survivors compared to age-/residence-matched women.[108] In survivors, low marital satisfaction at 3 months predicted future marital difficulties (16.7% divorced at 1 year versus 2.1% in those with high marital satisfaction; $P = 0.02$). Women not in a partnered relationship expressed concerns about dating, telling about cancer, and fear of initiating sexual relationship.[80,106]

Finally, in their follow-up of 817 long-term breast cancer survivors, Ganz et al. reported more than two-thirds had stable household income and 20% had increased income (versus 12% who had decreased income) since diagnosis.[99] Eighty percent reported no change in employment status; a minority moved from full- to part-time work or retired. Marital status did not change. In a separate study, this group reported that 90% of survivors had health insurance 2 or 3 years postdiagnosis, although some had their premiums increased or had switched to a spouse's plan.[80] Most (65%) were working or doing volunteer work.

Thus, there is little evidence that social or marital functioning or employment is adversely affected in survivors. Specific concerns about dating have been reported, especially in young, unpartnered women.

Cognitive Functioning

In 1995, Wieneke and Dienst[109] published the first report of cognitive dysfunction in women with breast cancer (Table 11.4). To date, four reports have evaluated cognitive functioning during and within the first 2 years postchemotherapy using a battery of neuropsychologic tests[109–111] or the High

Sensitivity Cognitive Screen,[104] a valid reliable instrument that predicts overall qualitative results of formal neuropsychologic testing. All four studies identified significantly lower cognitive functioning in women receiving adjuvant chemotherapy (with or without anthracyclines) compared with those not receiving chemotherapy or to a control group without breast cancer. Cognitive dysfunction was more prevalent in women who received high-dose chemotherapy in one study.[111] Interestingly, there appears to be little correlation between cognitive functioning as assessed by the test battery and self-reported by the patient.[110,111]

Studies evaluating cognitive dysfunction beyond 2 years have yielded conflicting results. Schagen et al.[112] reported improvement in performance in all chemotherapy groups between 2 and 4 years posttreatment. Ahles et al.[113] reported patients who had been diagnosed at least 5 years earlier had greater cognitive impairment on a battery of neuropsychologic tests and were more likely to report memory problems on the Squire Memory Self-Rating Questionnaire if they had received adjuvant chemotherapy.

Cognitive dysfunction in women receiving adjuvant chemotherapy is an emerging area of interest in survivorship research. Future research should identify risk factors for this complication and evaluate potential interventions to minimize its impact.

Spirituality

Spirituality is often poorly addressed in multidimensional questionnaires. Based on the holistic Ferrell[114] model of QOL in breast cancer survivors (physical, psychologic, social, spiritual), Wyatt et al. developed the Long-Term Quality of Life (LTQL) instrument, which includes a philosophical/spiritual view dimension.[115] Kurtz et al.,[107] using this instrument in long-term (more than 5 years) survivors, reported a positive spiritual outlook to be associated with good health habits and an increased likelihood of being supportive of others. In their cohort of long-term survivors (6.3 years), Ganz et al.[99] reported a positive impact of breast cancer on religious beliefs and activities, an effect that tended to be more pronounced in young survivors. Dow et al.[105] used the QOL-CS to evaluate spiritual well-being in members of the National Coalition for Cancer Survivorship. Although fears about future cancer and uncertainty about the future were identified as important concerns, beneficial spiritual outcomes including hopefulness and having a purpose in life as well as positive and spiritual change were also reported. Further research is needed to confirm these early observations, using population-based controls as a comparison group.

Diet and Complementary and Alternative Medicine

Maunsell et al.[116] evaluated diet during the first year after breast cancer diagnosis in a group of 250 women who were surveyed with a standardized interview about diet changes. Forty-one percent of women reported a change in their diet; these changes were positive (i.e., healthy) in over 90%. Women under 50 years and those who were more distressed

TABLE 11.4. QOL and cognitive dysfunction in breast cancer survivors.

Reference	Primary objective(s)	Study population and follow-up (years)	Number of subjects	Instruments	Response rate	Results and conclusions
Wieneke et al. 1995[109]	To evaluate cognitive functioning after adjuvant chemo	Convenience sample (clinic) 6.6 months post chemo	28	• Neuropsychologic tests	84%	Cognitive deficit related to tests norms (adjusted for age, education, gender) in 5 of 7 domains assessed. 75% had moderate impairment on at least 1 test. Level of impairment unrelated to depression, type of chemo, time since treatment; positively related to the length of chemo.
van Dam et al. 1998[111]	To assess the prevalence of cognitive deficit after adjuvant chemo	RCT of high-dose vs. standard dose chemo Control group were BCS who did not received chemo 2 years	34 high dose 36 standard dose 34 no chemo	• Neuropsychologic tests • Semistructured interview for self-reported cognitive functioning • EORTC QLQ-C30 • HSCL-25	84%–85% (chemo treated) 68% (controls)	Lower global QOL and higher score on depression subscale with high dose. Cognitive impairment: 32% high dose, 17% standard dose, 9% no chemo ($P = 0.043$).
Schagen et al. 1999[110]	To assess neuropsychologic functioning following CMF vs. no chemo	Consecutive series 2 years	39 chemo 34 control	• Neuropsychologic test • Semistructured interview • EORTC QLQ-C30 • HSCL-25	78% (chemo) 68% (control)	Higher IQ at baseline in CMF group. Neuropsychologic tests: 28% of patients in chemo cognitively impaired vs. 12% in control. Self-reported problems: in chemo group, more problems with concentration and memory. No relation between reported complaints and neuropsychologic testing. Chemo: lower QOL (physical, cognitive), greater depression.
Brezden et al. 2000[104]	To assess cognitive function in chemo vs. control patients	Convenience sample (two academic hospitals) 2.1 years for the group post chemo	Chemo: 31 Postchemo: 40 Controls: 36	• HSCS • POMS	Not stated	More patients with cognitive impairment during or after chemo vs. controls. No difference in mood status in the three groups.
Schagen et al. 2002[112]	To assess long-term neuropsychologic sequelae following chemo	Follow-up of earlier cohort[120,121] 4 years	103	• Neuropsychologic tests • EORTC QLQC30 • HSCL	84%–96%	Improvement in performance in all chemo group (FEC, high-dose, CMF) and a slight deterioration in controls. Cognitive dysfunction following adjuvant chemo may be transient.
Ahles et al. 2002[113]	To compare neuropsychologic functioning of long-term survivors	Tumor registry 9.7 years for BC	BC = 70 Lymphoma = 58	• Neuropsychologic tests • SMSRQ • CES-D • STAI • FSI	75%	Neuropsychologic test and SMSRQ: chemo group score lower than local therapy group (adjusted for age and education). No other differences.

Response rate: as stated in the paper or if not, the percentage of eligible patients who completed the study.

[*] Valid and reliable instruments.

CMF, cyclophosphamide, methotrexate, 5-fluouracil; Chemo, chemotherapy; RCT, randomized controlled trial; FEC, 5-fluouracil, epirubicin, cyclophosphamide; BC, breast cancer; neuropsychologic tests, a battery of tests were used, Cf. see reference for more details; EORTC-QLQC-30, European Organization for Research and Treatment of Cancer-Quality of Life Questionnaire C-30[*]; HSCL, Hopkins Symptom Checklist-25; HSCS, High Sensitivity Cognitive Screen[*]; POMS, Profile of Mood States[*]; SMSRQ, Squire Memory Self-Rating Questionnaire; CES-D, Center for Epidemiological Study-Depression[*]; STAI, State-Trait Anxiety Inventory[*]; FSI, Fatigue Symptom Inventory[*].

at diagnosis were most likely to change their diets ($P = 0.0001$).

Burstein et al.[117] evaluated complementary and alternative medicine (CAM) use during the first 12 months after breast cancer diagnosis. Twenty-eight percent of 480 women began an alternative therapy after diagnosis; these women tended to be younger and more educated. Ganz et al.[99] reported vitamins and herbal preparations were used by 86.6% and 49.3% of breast cancer survivors, respectively. More than half (60.7%) altered diet or used dietary supplements. Few women were using psychosocial or counseling therapies (13%) or attending a cancer support group (5.5%). More than one-third reported enhanced physical activity postdiagnosis. Lee et al.[118] conducted telephone interviews in 379 women (black, Chinese, Latino, white) 3 to 6 years after breast cancer diagnosis. At least one alternative therapy was used by 48.3%. Most common approaches therapies were dietary change (26.6%), herbal/homeopathic medication (13.5%), psychologic or spiritual healing (30.1%), and physical approaches such as yoga or acupuncture (14.2%). Therapies were used for brief periods, usually for 3 to 6 months. Women who used alternative therapies were younger and more educated.

Thus, more than one-third of breast cancer survivors use at least one kind of alternative therapy. Nonpharmacologic supplements appear to be most commonly used. Further research is needed to evaluate duration of use and changes over time in use of CAMS, comparing survivors to healthy controls.

Psychosocial Status and HRQOL in Defined Subgroups

Consideration of breast cancer survivors as a group may mask important differences in subgroups and over time. In this section we summarize research examining subgroups defined by age, ethnicity, and treatment (surgery, adjuvant therapy) and according to time elapsed since diagnosis.

Age at Diagnosis

Age at diagnosis appears to be an important determinant of the survivorship experience. This may be due, in part, to treatment: women who receive chemotherapy, many of whom are younger, experience greater long-term physical and sexual sequelae (see following discussion); psychosocial effects of mastectomy may also differ with age, especially in the short term.[119] However, Ganz et al.[106] reported poorer sexual functioning in younger survivors who became menopausal, regardless of whether they received chemotherapy. Vinokur et al.[120] compared survivors (50% of whom were followed more than 5 years) to controls participating in a breast cancer screening program; younger survivors had more problems in psychosocial adjustment while older survivors had more physical difficulties. Cimprich et al.[121] reported similar findings in 105 survivors using the QOL-CS. Women over 65 at diagnosis had worse scores in the physical domain while those diagnosed before 44 years of age had poorer scores in the social domain. Women diagnosed between 45 and 65 years of age had the best overall HRQOL. Two pivotal studies examining survivorship issues in younger[122] and older women[123] have been reported

recently. In the first of these, a cohort of 577 patients diagnosed at age 50 or younger was assembled for the Cancer and Menopause Study a mean of 5.9 years postdiagnosis.[122] Most had received adjuvant chemotherapy. Physical functioning was good. The youngest women reported poor mental health, less vitality, and poorer social and emotional functioning (MOS SF36). In the second study, 691 women aged 65 years of age or more at diagnosis were evaluated 3, 6, and 15 months after surgery.[123] Physical and mental functioning (MOS SF-36) showed significant declines during the year of follow-up. Declines in the former were associated with greater comorbidity and receipt of adjuvant chemotherapy. In contrast, the CARES Psychosocial Summary and Medical Interaction Scales showed significant improvement over time. Social support was lowest in women over 75 years. The discrepant results obtained with the MOS SF-36 Mental Health Inventory and the CARES Psychosocial Summary Scale were explored: the former appeared to be influenced to a greater extent by declines in physical functioning and the latter appeared to reflect adaptation and adjustment to cancer-specific concerns. In summary, younger age is associated with lower mental and emotional well-being. Older women experience more physical problems, partly the result of aging.

Ethnicity

The impact of ethnicity on survivorship has been poorly studied. Ashing-Giwa et al.[124] investigated HRQOL in white and African-American survivors. Response rate among African-Americans was significantly lower than among whites (44% versus 65%). The former were more often single, had a lower income, and lower HRQOL. Multivariate analyses revealed that 45% of the variance in HRQOL was accounted for by general health perception, life stress, partnership status, and income; ethnicity was not a significant contributor. The authors concluded that African-American and white breast cancer survivors report favorable overall QOL; differences are secondary to life burden and socioeconomic factors but not to ethnicity per se.

Primary Surgical Procedure

The primary surgical procedure performed also appears to impact survivorship (Table 11.5). Maunsell et al.[119] reported that psychologic distress (measured using the PSI) at 3 months was worse in women undergoing BCS; this difference was not present at 18 months. Age modified this effect; the greater psychologic distress at 3 months was not present in women under 40 years. Follow-up 8 years after diagnosis found that psychologic distress declined over time and was similar to that in the general population.[125] Ganz et al.,[126] using a battery of general questionnaires, reported few differences in HRQOL with respect to type of surgery; however, women undergoing mastectomy had more problems with clothing and body image than those undergoing BCS. Mosconi et al.[102] found none of the EORTC QLQ C-30 domains to be affected by the type of surgery. Janni et al.[127] studied 76 pairs of patients who had undergone either a mastectomy or BCS a mean of 3.8 years earlier; women undergoing mastectomy were significantly less satisfied with their cosmetic result and change in appearance and were twice as likely to be stressed by their physical appearance secondary to the surgery. No

TABLE 11.5. Survivorship and surgery in breast cancer survivors.

Reference	Primary objective(s)	Study population and follow-up (in years)	Number of subjects	Instruments	Response rate	Results and conclusions
Schain et al. 1983[130]	To compare QOL after MRM vs. BCS	RCT of MRM vs. BCS 11.3 months	38	• Others	97%	No difference in psychosocial outcomes, except greater concerns about seeing oneself naked in MRM. 69% of BCS vs. 28% of MT had limited arm motion.
Meyer et al. 1989[131]	To compare long-term psychosocial and sexual adaptation after MRM vs. BCS	Convenience sample (one center) 5 years	58	• Interview	68%	No differences in psychiatric state, marital adjustment, fear of recurrence. BCS preserves female identity and acceptance of body image.
Maunsell et al. 1989[119]	To describe psychologic distress after MRM vs. BCS	Cohort (consecutive cases from seven hospitals) 3 and 18 months	227 at 3 months and 205 at 18 months	• PSI • LES (modified) • DSI • Others	97%	At 3 months, greater psychologic distress (PSI) in BCS vs. MRM but no difference at 18 months. Age modified the relation: BCS was protective for women <40 years of age.
Ganz et al. 1992[126]	To evaluate QOL and psychologic adjustment after MRM vs. BCS	RCT testing (two rehabilitation programs) 1 year	109	• FLIC • CARES • Karnofsky (PS) • POMS • GAIS	44%	No difference in mood disturbance, QOL, performance status, global adjustment. MRM associated with more difficulties with clothing and body image.
Mock 1993[150]	To compare body image with MRM, MRM + delayed R, MRM + immediate R, BCS	Clinical sample from four hospitals 14 months	257	• BIS • TSCS • BIVAS	57%	Body image was more positive after BCS (when measured by BIVAS but not by BIS). No difference in self-concept.
Omne-Pontén et al. 1994[128]	To assess psychosocial adjustment after MRM vs. BCS	Consecutive clinic patients 6 years	66	• Interview • Others	80% (of the first study)	No impact of the surgery on psychosocial adjustment.
Dorval et al. 1998[125]	To assess psychosocial adjustment after MRM vs. BCS	Cohort (seven hospitals) 3 months, 18 months, 8 years	235 at 3 months 211 at 18 months 124 at 8 years	• PSI • MOS-SSS • LES • LWMAT	97% 3 months 97% 18 months 96% 8 years	At 8 years no difference in QOL. BCS protected women against distress if they were <50 years of age at diagnosis (short and long term).
Curran et al. 1998[129]	To describe QOL after MRM vs. BCS	Sample from EORTC trial 10801 2 years	278	• Newly constructed questionnaire	14%–64% (between different countries)	BCS gives a better body image with no increase in fear of recurrence. Cosmetic results: patient rating superior to the surgeon.
Rowland et al. 2000[133]	To evaluate women's adaptation to different types of surgery	Two cohorts (from two large metropolitan areas) 2.7 and 3.2 years	1,957	• SF-36 • MOS SSS • CES-D • RDAS • WSFQ • CARES	54%	Fewer problems with body image and sexual attractiveness after BCS vs. MRM ± R. MT + R: report more negative impacts on sex life. MRM ± R vs. BCS: more physical symptom and discomfort at the surgical site. No difference in emotional, social, role function (CES-D, SF-36).
Janni et al. 2001[127]	To compare impact of BCS vs. MRM	Convenience sample (one hospital) 3.8 years	152 pairmatched patients	• EORTC QLQ C-30 • Other	Not stated	No difference for QOL between the two groups. MRM women had less satisfaction with cosmetic results, appearance, and were more emotionally distressed by these issues.
Nissen et al. 2001[134]	To compare QOL after BCS, MRM, MRM ± R	RCT of effect of advanced practice nursing 2 years	198	• MUIS • POMS • FACT-B	94%	BCS vs. MRM: no difference in well-being. More mood disturbance and poorer well-being in MRM + R vs. MRM alone.

Response rate: reported by the author or calculated as the percentage of eligible patients who completed the study.

*, Valid and reliable instruments.

MRM, modified radical mastectomy; BCS, breast-conserving surgery; R, reconstruction; PSI, Psychiatric Symptom Index*; LES, Life Events Schedule*; FLIC, Functional Living Index–Cancer*; CARES, Cancer Rehabilitation Evaluation System*; POMS, Profile of Mood States*; GAIS, Global Adjustment to Illness Scale*; SBAS, Social Behaviour Assessment Schedule*; BIS, Body Image Scale*; TSCS, Tennessee Self-Concept Scale*; BIVAS, Body Image Visual Analogue Scale; MOS-SSS, MOS Social Support Survey*; LES, Life Experience Survey*; LWMAT, Locke-Wallace Marital Adjustment Test*; SF-36, RAND or MOS Short-Form-36*; CES-D, Center of Epidemiologic Studies–Depression Scale*; RDAS, Revised Dyadic Adjustment Scale*; WSFQ, Watts Sexual Function Questionnaire*; EORTC-QLQ C-30, European Organization for Research and Treatment of Cancer–Quality of Life Questionnaire C-30*; MUIS, Mishel Uncertainty in Illness Scale*; FACT, Functional Assessment of Cancer Therapy*.

differences were seen in EORTC QLQ-C30 scores. Psychosocial adjustment measured using the Social Adjustment Scale was similar in the mastectomy and BCS treatment groups; however, women undergoing mastectomy felt mutilated and less attractive.[128] A companion study to EORTC trial 10801 comparing mastectomy to BCS and radiotherapy surveyed 278 patients 2 years after treatment.[129] Body image and satisfaction with treatment were better in the BCS. There was no difference in fear of recurrence. Patients considered their cosmetic results to be more acceptable than the surgeon did at several time points. Other studies have reported beneficial effects of BCS on body image.[130,131] In summary, BCS leads to enhanced body image and, in younger women (less than 40), it may protect against psychologic distress. No differences in depression were identified in one study of spouses of women undergoing mastectomy or BCS.[132]

Breast Reconstruction

Breast reconstruction is offered to reduce the adverse impact of mastectomy. Rowland et al.[133] studied a cohort of 1,957 long-term (1 to 5 years) survivors in Los Angeles and Washington. Women undergoing mastectomy had more physical symptoms related to the surgery regardless of whether they had reconstruction. No differences in overall HRQOL or worry about cancer returning were identified in women undergoing BCS, mastectomy alone, or mastectomy with reconstruction. Body image and feelings of sexual attractiveness were significantly better after BCS compared with mastectomy with or without reconstruction. Women who had reconstruction were younger and better educated than those in the other two groups. They also expressed greater concern that their cancer had a negative impact on their sex life. Nissen et al.[134] reported that women who had a mastectomy with reconstruction had greater mood disturbance and poorer well-being 18 months after surgery compared with those who did not undergo reconstruction.

Adjuvant Therapy

There is growing evidence that adjuvant therapy adversely affects survivors' HRQOL. In a cross-sectional survey, Ganz et al.[100] reported global HRQOL (measured using the Ladder of Life and the MOS SF-36) to be similar 1 to 5 years postdiagnosis in women who received chemotherapy and/or tamoxifen compared with those who received no adjuvant therapy. However, physical and sexual functioning were worse in women receiving adjuvant therapy. A mean of 6.3 years postdiagnosis, the no-adjuvant treatment group reported more favorable scores for global HRQOL (Ladder of Life) and most domains of the MOS SF-36 than those who received adjuvant therapy.[99] There were no differences in emotional functioning (MOS SF-36, Center for Epidemiology Study—Depression). The sexual discomfort scale (SAQ) and sexual functioning (CARES) were significantly worse in women who received adjuvant chemotherapy compared to those who received either tamoxifen or no therapy. Mosconi et al.[102] reported slightly better HRQOL (EORTC QLQ-C30) in women treated with tamoxifen versus those who received either chemotherapy or no adjuvant therapy. In contrast, participants of an adjuvant trial of chemotherapy versus no treatment who were 9.6 years postdiagnosis reported no differences in sexual functioning/enjoyment according to treatment arm.[135] Small sample size (119 patients) and the long interval after diagnosis may account for these results. In summary, the majority of studies have identified long-term adverse effects of adjuvant therapy, notably chemotherapy.

Time Elapsed Since Diagnosis

The status of survivors also varies according to time elapsed since diagnosis. Ganz et al.[99] re-evaluated a cross-sectional sample of survivors who had been recruited 1 to 5 years postdiagnosis when they were a mean of 6.3 (minimum, 5) years postdiagnosis. Small decreases in physical functioning, role functioning-physical, bodily pain, and general health (MOS SF-36) over time were thought to be related to aging. Sexual activity with a partner declined significantly and specific symptoms persisted, especially in women receiving chemotherapy. In an earlier cohort study, Ganz et al.[80] compared HRQOL measured using the POMS and Functional Living Index for Cancer at 2 and 3 years after surgery to that between 1 month and 1 year after surgery. Most scores improved between 1 month and 1 year,[126] but there was no subsequent improvement. This might reflect ongoing rehabilitation problems, as most CARES scores worsened between 1 and 3 years postdiagnosis. Holzner et al.[136] evaluated 87 breast cancer survivors using two cancer-specific questionnaires. Women who were more than 5 years postdiagnosis had significantly worse global QOL, role functioning, sexual functioning, and enjoyment than those 1 to 2 or 2 to 5 years postdiagnosis. However, women more than 5 years postdiagnosis were slightly older than those 1 to 2 and 2 to 5 years postdiagnosis (55.1 years old versus 52.9 and 52.5 years old, respectively). Women 2 to 5 years postdiagnosis had less impairment in emotional and social functioning than those diagnosed earlier or later. In contrast, Kessler et al.,[137] studying a convenience sample of 148 breast cancer survivors 0.3 to 19 years postdiagnosis, reported that overall QOL and life satisfaction were high and that greater time since diagnosis and lesser extent of disease were associated with improved global QOL. Thus, HRQOL and most aspects of physical and psychosocial functioning improve during the first few years after breast cancer diagnosis. However, specific treatment-related problems and symptoms persist long term, and there is some evidence of HRQOL decline 2 to 5 years after diagnosis, possibly related to aging.

Conclusions

Long-term survivors have a high level of functioning and good HRQOL, often comparable to that of the general population. However, many survivors experience physical symptoms (notably arm symptoms and early menopause) and reduced sexual functioning related to their diagnosis and treatment. Young women, those receiving chemotherapy, and those with comorbidity may be at greatest risk. Younger women experience greater psychologic distress. Cognitive dysfunction has recently been identified in women receiving adjuvant chemotherapy. BCS leads to enhanced body image; however, reconstruction does not add a major benefit in terms of QOL. Quality of survivorship in different ethnic groups has been inadequately investigated.

A considerable body of observational research has been conducted in breast cancer survivors. Although there are knowledge gaps that should be addressed in further observational research, there is also a need for research to develop and evaluate interventions that will reduce the adverse impact of breast cancer diagnosis and treatment which has been identified in research to date. Primary areas for intervention research include psychologic distress and sexual dysfunction in younger women; cognitive dysfunction, sexual dysfunction, and fatigue in women receiving chemotherapy; and body image in women undergoing mastectomy with or without reconstruction.

References

1. http://dccps.nci.gov/ocs/prevalence/prevalence.html survivor, accessed October 1, 2006.
2. Gerber LH. A review of measures of lymphedema. Cancer (Phila) 1998;83:2803–2804.
3. Erickson VS, Pearson ML, Ganz PA, Adams J, Kahn KL. Arm edema in breast cancer patients. J Natl Cancer Inst 2001;93:96–111.
4. Schrenk P, Rieger R, Shamiyeh A, Wayand W. Morbidity following sentinel lymph node biopsy versus axillary lymph node dissection for patients with breast carcinoma. Cancer (Phila) 2000;88:608–614.
5. Gerber L, Lampert M, Wood C, et al. Comparison of pain, motion, and edema after modified radical mastectomy vs. local excision with axillary dissection and radiation. Breast Cancer Res Treat 1992;21:139–145.
6. Werner RS, McCormick B, Petrek J, et al. Arm edema in conservatively managed breast cancer: obesity is a major predictive factor. Radiology 1991;180:177–184.
7. Tasmuth T, von Smitten K, Kalso E. Pain and other symptoms during the first year after radical and conservative surgery for breast cancer. Br J Cancer 1996;74:2024–2031.
8. Paci E, Cariddi A, Barchielli A, et al. Long-term sequelae of breast cancer surgery. Tumori 1996;82:321–324.
9. Yeoh EK, Denham JW, Davies SA, Spittle MF. Primary breast cancer. Complications of axillary management. Acta Radiol Oncol 1986;25:105–108.
10. Kiel KD, Rademacker AW. Early-stage breast cancer: arm edema after wide excision and breast irradiation. Radiology 1996;198:279–283.
11. Keramopoulos A, Tsionou C, Minaretzis D, Michalas S, Aravantinos D. Arm morbidity following treatment of breast cancer with total axillary dissection: a multivariated approach. Oncology 1993;50:445–449.
12. Liljegren G, Holmberg L. Arm morbidity after sector resection and axillary dissection with or without postoperative radiotherapy in breast cancer stage I. Results from a randomised trial. Uppsala-Orebro Breast Cancer Study Group. Eur J Cancer 1997;33:193–199.
13. Senofsky GM, Moffat FL Jr, Davis K, et al. Total axillary lymphadenectomy in the management of breast cancer. Arch Surg 1991;126:1336–1341; discussion 1341–1342.
14. Kissin MW, Querci della Rovere G, Easton D, Westbury G. Risk of lymphoedema following the treatment of breast cancer. Br J Surg 1986;73:580–584.
15. Borup Christensen S, Lundgren E. Sequelae of axillary dissection vs. axillary sampling with or without irradiation for breast cancer. A randomized trial. Acta Chir Scand 1989;155:515–519.
16. Lash TL, Silliman RA. Patient characteristics and treatments associated with a decline in upper-body function following breast cancer therapy. J Clin Epidemiol 2000;53:615–622.
17. Silliman RA, Prout MN, Field T, Kalish SC, Colton T. Risk factors for a decline in upper body function following treatment

for early stage breast cancer. Breast Cancer Res Treat 1999; 54:25–30.
18. Segerstrom K, Bjerle P, Nystrom A. Importance of time in assessing arm and hand function after treatment of breast cancer. Scand J Plast Reconstr Surg Hand Surg 1991;25:241–244.
19. Lin PP, Allison DC, Wainstock J, et al. Impact of axillary lymph node dissection on the therapy of breast cancer patients. J Clin Oncol 1993;11:1536–1544.
20. Passik SD, McDonald MV. Psychosocial aspects of upper extremity lymphedema in women treated for breast carcinoma. Cancer (Phila) 1998;83:2817–2820.
21. Woods M, Tobin M, Mortimer P. The psychosocial morbidity of breast cancer patients with lymphoedema. Cancer Nurs 1995;18:467–471.
22. Tobin MB, Lacey HJ, Meyer L, Mortimer PS. The psychological morbidity of breast cancer-related arm swelling. Psychological morbidity of lymphoedema. Cancer (Phila) 1993;72:3248–3252.
23. Maunsell E, Brisson J, Deschenes L. Arm problems and psychological distress after surgery for breast cancer. Can J Surg 1993; 36:315–320.
24. Harris PF, Remington PL, Trentham-Dietz A, Allen CI, Newcomb PA. Prevalence and treatment of menopausal symptoms among breast cancer survivors. J Pain Symptom Manag 2002;23:501–509.
25. Ganz PA. Menopause and breast cancer: symptoms, late effects, and their management. Semin Oncol 2001;28:274–283.
26. Goodwin PJ, Ennis M, Pritchard KI, Trudeau M, Hood N. Risk of menopause during the first year after breast cancer diagnosis. J Clin Oncol 1999;17:2365–2370.
27. Bines J, Oleske DM, Cobleigh MA. Ovarian function in premenopausal women treated with adjuvant chemotherapy for breast cancer. J Clin Oncol 1996;14:1718–1729.
28. Bachmann GA. Vasomotor flushes in menopausal women. Am J Obstet Gynecol 1999;180:S312–S316.
29. Schwingl PJ, Hulka BS, Harlow SD. Risk factors for menopausal hot flashes. Obstet Gynecol 1994;84:29–34.
30. Theriault RL, Sellin RV. Estrogen-replacement therapy in younger women with breast cancer. J Natl Cancer Inst Monogr 1994;16:149–152.
31. Mortimer JE. Hormone replacement therapy and beyond. The clinical challenge of menopausal symptoms in breast cancer survivors. Geriatrics 2002;57:25–31.
32. Carpenter JS, Johnson D, Wagner L, Andrykowski M. Hot flashes and related outcomes in breast cancer survivors and matched comparison women. Oncol Nurs Forum 2002;29: E16–E25.
33. Rossouw JE, Anderson GL, Prentice RL, et al. Risks and benefits of estrogen plus progestin in healthy postmenopausal women: principal results. From the Women's Health Initiative randomized controlled trial. JAMA 2002;288:321–333; and 33a. Stefanick ML, Anderson GL, Margolis KL, Hendrix SL, Rodabough RJ, Paskett ED, Lane DS, Hubbell FA, Assaf AR, Sarto GE, Schenken RS, Yasmeen S, Lessin L, Chlebowski RT. Effects of conjugated equine estrogens on breast cancer and mammography screening in postmenopausal women with hysterectomy. JAMA 2006;295:1647–1657.
34. Pritchard KI, Khan H, Levine M. Clinical practice guidelines for the care and treatment of breast cancer: 14. The role of hormone replacement therapy in women with a previous diagnosis of breast cancer. Can Med Assoc J 2002;166:1017–1022.
35. Marsden J. Hormone-replacement therapy and breast cancer. Lancet Oncol 2002;3:303–311.
36. DiSaia PJ, Grosen EA, Kurosaki T, Gildea M, Cowan B, Anton-Culver H. Hormone replacement therapy in breast cancer survivors: a cohort study. Am J Obstet Gynecol 1996;174:1494–1498.
37. Decker D, Cox T, Burdakin J. Hormone replacement therapy (HRT) in breast cancer survivors. Proc Am Soc Clin Oncol 1996;15:209.

38. Bluming AZ, Waisman JR, Dosik GM. Hormone replacement therapy (HRT) in women with previously treated breast cancer, update IV. Proc Am Soc Clin Oncol 1998;17:496.

39. Powles TJ, Hickish T, Casey S, O'Brien M. Hormone replacement after breast cancer. Lancet 1993;342:60–61.

40. Wile AG, Opfell RW, Margileth DA. Hormone replacement therapy does not affect breast cancer outcome. Proc Am Soc Clin Oncol 1991;10:58.

41. Wile AG, Opfell RW, Margileth DA. Hormone replacement therapy in previously treated breast cancer patients. Am J Surg 1993;165:372–375.

42. Eden JA, Wren BG, Dew J. Hormone replacement therapy after breast cancer. Educational book. Alexandria (VA): American Society of Clinical Oncology, 1996:187–189.

43. O'Meara ES, Rossing MA, Daling JR, Elmore JG, Barlow WE, Weiss NS. Hormone replacement therapy after a diagnosis of breast cancer in relation to recurrence and mortality. J Natl Cancer Inst 2001;93:754–762.

44. Vassilopoulou-Sellin R, Asmar L, Hortobagyi GN, et al. Estrogen replacement therapy after localized breast cancer: clinical outcome of 319 women followed prospectively. J Clin Oncol 1999;17:1482–1487.

45. Ganz PA, Greendale GA, Kahn B, O'Leary JF, Desmond KA. Are older breast carcinoma survivors willing to take hormone replacement therapy? Cancer (Phila) 1999;86:814–820.

46. Biglia N, Cozzarella M, Cacciari F, et al. Menopause after breast cancer: a survey on breast cancer survivors. Maturitas 2003;45:29–38.

47. Holmberg L, Anderson H. HABITS (hormonal replacement therapy after breast cancer—is it safe?): a randomised comparison: trial stopped. Lancet 2004;363:453–455.

48. Treatment of estrogen deficiency symptoms in women surviving breast cancer. Part 6: Executive summary and consensus statement. Proceedings of a conference held at Boar's Head Inn, Charlottesville, Virginia, September 21–23, 1997. Oncology (Huntingt) 1999;13:859–861, 865–866, 871–872 passim.

49. Kronenberg F. Hot flashes: epidemiology and physiology. Ann N Y Acad Sci 1990;592:52–86; discussion 123–133.

50. Notelovitz M, Lenihan JP, McDermott M, Kerber IJ, Nanavati N, Arce J. Initial 17beta-estradiol dose for treating vasomotor symptoms. Obstet Gynecol 2000;95:726–731.

51. Rabin DS, Cipparrone N, Linn ES, Moen M. Why menopausal women do not want to take hormone replacement therapy. Menopause 1999;6:61–67.

52. Stearns V, Hayes DF. Approach to menopausal symptoms in women with breast cancer. Curr Treat Options Oncol 2002;3:179–190.

53. Loprinzi CL, Michalak JC, Quella SK, et al. Megestrol acetate for the prevention of hot flashes. N Engl J Med 1994;331:347–352.

54. Bullock JL, Massey FM, Gambrell RD Jr. Use of medroxyprogesterone acetate to prevent menopausal symptoms. Obstet Gynecol 1975;46:165–168.

55. Morrison JC, Martin DC, Blair RA, et al. The use of medroxyprogesterone acetate for relief of climacteric symptoms. Am J Obstet Gynecol 1980;138:99–104.

56. Schiff I, Tulchinsky D, Cramer D, Ryan KJ. Oral medroxyprogesterone in the treatment of postmenopausal symptoms. JAMA 1980;244:1443–1445.

57. Bertelli G, Venturini M, Del Mastro L, et al. Intramuscular depot medroxyprogesterone versus oral megestrol for the control of postmenopausal hot flashes in breast cancer patients: a randomized study. Ann Oncol 2002;13:883–888.

58. Guttuso T Jr, Kurlan R, McDermott MP, Kieburtz K. Gabapentin's effects on hot flashes in postmenopausal women: a randomized controlled trial. Obstet Gynecol 2003;101:337–345.

59. Naessen T, Rodriguez-Macias K, Lithell H. Serum lipid profile improved by ultra-low doses of 17 beta-estradiol in elderly women. J Clin Endocrinol Metab 2001;86:2757–2762.

60. Ganz PA, Greendale GA, Petersen L, Zibecchi L, Kahn B, Belin TR. Managing menopausal symptoms in breast cancer survivors: results of a randomized controlled trial. J Natl Cancer Inst 2000;92:1054–1064.

61. Basil JB, Mutch DG. Role of hormone replacement therapy in cancer survivors. Clin Obstet Gynecol 2001;44:464–477.

62. Shapiro CL, Manola J, Leboff M. Ovarian failure after adjuvant chemotherapy is associated with rapid bone loss in women with early-stage breast cancer. J Clin Oncol 2001;19:3306–3311.

63. Recommended breast cancer surveillance guidelines. American Society of Clinical Oncology. J Clin Oncol 1997;15:2149–2156.

64. Barrett-Connor E, Bush TL. Estrogen and coronary heart disease in women. JAMA 1991;265:1861–1867.

65. Colditz GA, Willett WC, Stampfer MJ, Rosner B, Speizer FE, Hennekens CH. Menopause and the risk of coronary heart disease in women. N Engl J Med 1987;316:1105–1110.

66. Effects of estrogen or estrogen/progestin regimens on heart disease risk factors in postmenopausal women. The Postmenopausal Estrogen/Progestin Interventions (PEPI) Trial. The Writing Group for the PEPI Trial. JAMA 1995;273:199–208.

67. Hulley S, Grady D, Bush T, et al. Randomized trial of estrogen plus progestin for secondary prevention of coronary heart disease in postmenopausal women. Heart and Estrogen/progestin Replacement Study (HERS) Research Group. JAMA 1998;280:605–613.

68. Burstein HJ, Winer EP. Primary care for survivors of breast cancer. N Engl J Med 2000;343:1086–1094.

69. Surbone A, Petrek JA. Childbearing issues in breast carcinoma survivors. Cancer (Phila) 1997;79:1271–1278.

70. Collichio FA, Agnello R, Staltzer J. Pregnancy after breast cancer: from psychosocial issues through conception. Oncology (Huntingt) 1998;12:759–765, 769; discussion 770, 773–775.

71. Blakely LJ, Buzdar AU, Lozada JA, et al. Effects of pregnancy after treatment for breast carcinoma on survival and risk of recurrence. Cancer (Phila) 2004;100:465–469.

72. Kroman N, Jensen MB, Melbye M, Wohlfahrt J, Mouridsen HT. Should women be advised against pregnancy after breast-cancer treatment? Lancet 1997;350:319–322.

73. Velentgas P, Daling JR, Malone KE, et al. Pregnancy after breast carcinoma: outcomes and influence on mortality. Cancer (Phila) 1999;85:2424–2432.

74. Sutton R, Buzdar AU, Hortobagyi GN. Pregnancy and offspring after adjuvant chemotherapy in breast cancer patients. Cancer (Phila) 1990;65:847–850.

75. Mulvihill JJ, McKeen EA, Rosner F, Zarrabi MH. Pregnancy outcome in cancer patients. Experience in a large cooperative group. Cancer (Phila) 1987;60:1143–1150.

76. Higgins S, Haffty BG. Pregnancy and lactation after breast-conserving therapy for early stage breast cancer. Cancer (Phila) 1994;73:2175–2180.

77. Tralins AH. Lactation after conservative breast surgery combined with radiation therapy. Am J Clin Oncol 1995;18:40–43.

78. Moore HC, Foster RS Jr. Breast cancer and pregnancy. Semin Oncol 2000;27:646–653.

79. Rosner D, Yeh J. Breast cancer and related pregnancy: suggested management according to stages of the disease and gestational stages. J Med 2002;33:23–62.

80. Ganz PA, Coscarelli A, Fred C, Kahn B, Polinsky ML, Petersen L. Breast cancer survivors: psychosocial concerns and quality of life. Breast Cancer Res Treat 1996;38:183–199.

81. Bower JE, Ganz PA, Desmond KA, Rowland JH, Meyerowitz BE, Belin TR. Fatigue in breast cancer survivors: occurrence, correlates, and impact on quality of life. J Clin Oncol 2000;18:743–753.

82. Andrykowski MA, Curran SL, Lightner R. Off-treatment fatigue in breast cancer survivors: a controlled comparison. J Behav Med 1998;21:1–18.

83. Hochster H, Wasserheit C, Speyer J. Cardiotoxicity and cardioprotection during chemotherapy. Curr Opin Oncol 1995;7:304–309.

84. Steinherz LJ, Steinherz PG, Tan CT, Heller G, Murphy ML. Cardiac toxicity 4 to 20 years after completing anthracycline therapy. JAMA 1991;266:1672–1677.

85. Swain SM. Adult multicenter trials using dexrazoxane to protect against cardiac toxicity. Semin Oncol 1998;25:43–47.

86. Sparano JA. Doxorubicin/taxane combinations: cardiac toxicity and pharmacokinetics. Semin Oncol 1999;3(suppl 9):14–19.

87. Slamon DJ, Leyland-Jones B, Shak S, et al. Use of chemotherapy plus a monoclonal antibody against HER2 for metastatic breast cancer that overexpresses HER2. N Engl J Med 2001;344:783–792.

88. Grunfeld E, Fitzpatrick R, Mant D, et al. Comparison of breast cancer patient satisfaction with follow-up in primary care versus specialist care: results from a randomized controlled trial. Br J Gen Pract 1999;49:705–710.

89. Zabora J, BrintzenhofeSzoc K, Curbow B, Hooker C, Piantadosi S. The prevalence of psychological distress by cancer site. Psycho-Oncology 2001;10:19–28.

90. Gallagher J, Parle M, Cairns D. Appraisal and psychological distress six months after diagnosis of breast cancer. Br J Health Psychol 2002;7:365–376.

91. Kissane DW, Clarke DM, Ikin J, et al. Psychological morbidity and quality of life in Australian women with early-stage breast cancer: a cross-sectional survey. Med J Aust 1998;169:192–196.

92. Aragona M, Muscatello MR, Mesiti M. Depressive mood disorders in patients with operable breast cancer. J Exp Clin Cancer Res 1997;16:111–118.

93. Halttunen A, Hietanen P, Jallinoja P, Lonnqvist J. Getting free of breast cancer. An eight-year perspective of the relapse-free patients. Acta Oncol 1992;31:307–310.

94. Fredette SL. Breast cancer survivors: concerns and coping. Cancer Nurs 1995;18:35–46.

95. Ferrans CE. Quality of life through the eyes of survivors of breast cancer. Oncol Nurs Forum 1994;21:1645–1651.

96. Wyatt G, Kurtz ME, Liken M. Breast cancer survivors: an exploration of quality of life issues. Cancer Nurs 1993;16:440–448.

97. Carter BJ. Long-term survivors of breast cancer. A qualitative descriptive study. Cancer Nurs 1993;16:354–361.

98. Matthews BA, Baker F, Hann DM, Denniston M, Smith TG. Health status and life satisfaction among breast cancer survivor peer support volunteers. Psycho-Oncology 2002;11:199–211.

99. Ganz PA, Desmond KA, Leedham B, Rowland JH, Meyerowitz BE, Belin TR. Quality of life in long-term, disease-free survivors of breast cancer: a follow-up study. J Natl Cancer Inst 2002;94:39–49.

100. Ganz PA, Rowland JH, Meyerowitz BE, Desmond KA. Impact of different adjuvant therapy strategies on quality of life in breast cancer survivors. Recent Results Cancer Res 1998;152:396–411.

101. Tomich PL, Helgeson VS. Five years later: a cross-sectional comparison of breast cancer survivors with healthy women. Psycho-Oncology 2002;11:154–169.

102. Mosconi P, Apolone G, Barni S, Secondino S, Sbanotto A, Filiberti A. Quality of life in breast and colon cancer long-term survivors: an assessment with the EORTC QLQ-C30 and SF-36 questionnaires. Tumori 2002;88:110–116.

103. Dorval M, Maunsell E, Deschenes L, Brisson J, Masse B. Long-term quality of life after breast cancer: comparison of 8-year survivors with population controls. J Clin Oncol 1998;16:487–494.

104. Brezden CB, Phillips KA, Abdolell M, Bunston T, Tannock IF. Cognitive function in breast cancer patients receiving adjuvant chemotherapy. J Clin Oncol 2000;18:2695–2701.

105. Dow KH, Ferrell BR, Leigh S, Ly J, Gulasekaram P. An evaluation of the quality of life among long-term survivors of breast cancer. Breast Cancer Res Treat 1996;39:261–273.

106. Ganz PA, Rowland JH, Desmond K, Meyerowitz BE, Wyatt GE. Life after breast cancer: understanding women's health-related quality of life and sexual functioning. J Clin Oncol 1998;16:501–514.

107. Kurtz ME, Wyatt G, Kurtz JC. Psychological and sexual well-being, philosophical/spiritual views, and health habits of long-term cancer survivors. Health Care Women Int 1995;16:253–262.

108. Dorval M, Maunsell E, Taylor-Brown J, Kilpatrick M. Marital stability after breast cancer. J Natl Cancer Inst 1999;91:54–59.

109. Wieneke MH, Dienst ER. Neuropsychological assessment of cognitive functioning following chemotherapy for breast cancer. Psycho-Oncology 1995;4:61–66.

110. Schagen SB, van Dam FS, Muller MJ, Boogerd W, Lindeboom J, Bruning PF. Cognitive deficits after postoperative adjuvant chemotherapy for breast carcinoma. Cancer (Phila) 1999;85:640–650.

111. van Dam FS, Schagen SB, Muller MJ, et al. Impairment of cognitive function in women receiving adjuvant treatment for high-risk breast cancer: high-dose versus standard-dose chemotherapy. J Natl Cancer Inst 1998;90:210–218.

112. Schagen SB, Muller MJ, Boogerd W, et al. Late effects of adjuvant chemotherapy on cognitive function: a follow-up study in breast cancer patients. Ann Oncol 2002;13:1387–1397.

113. Ahles TA, Saykin AJ, Furstenberg CT, et al. Neuropsychologic impact of standard-dose systemic chemotherapy in long-term survivors of breast cancer and lymphoma. J Clin Oncol 2002;20:485–493.

114. Ferrell BR. Overview of breast cancer: quality of life. Oncology Patient Care 1993;3:7–8.

115. Wyatt G, Kurtz ME, Friedman LL, Given B, Given CW. Preliminary testing of the Long-Term Quality of Life (LTQL) instrument for female cancer survivors. J Nurs Meas 1996;4:153–170.

116. Maunsell E, Drolet M, Brisson J, Robert J, Deschenes L. Dietary change after breast cancer: extent, predictors, and relation with psychological distress. J Clin Oncol 2002;20:1017–1025.

117. Burstein HJ, Gelber S, Guadagnoli E, Weeks JC. Use of alternative medicine by women with early-stage breast cancer. N Engl J Med 1999;340:1733–1739.

118. Lee MM, Lin SS, Wrensch MR, Adler SR, Eisenberg D. Alternative therapies used by women with breast cancer in four ethnic populations. J Natl Cancer Inst 2000;92:42–47.

119. Maunsell E, Brisson J, Deschenes L. Psychological distress after initial treatment for breast cancer: a comparison of partial and total mastectomy. J Clin Epidemiol 1989;42:765–771.

120. Vinokur AD, Threatt BA, Caplan RD, Zimmerman BL. Physical and psychosocial functioning and adjustment to breast cancer. Long-term follow-up of a screening population. Cancer (Phila) 1989;63:394–405.

121. Cimprich B, Ronis DL, Martinez-Ramos G. Age at diagnosis and quality of life in breast cancer survivors. Cancer Pract 2002;10:85–93.

122. Ganz PA, Greendale GA, Petersen L, Kahn B, Bower JE. Breast cancer in younger women: reproductive and late health effects of treatment. J Clin Oncol 2003;21:4184–4193.

123. Ganz PA, Guadagnoli E, Landrum MB, Lash TL, Rakowski W, Silliman RA. Breast cancer in older women: quality of life and psychosocial adjustment in the 15 months after diagnosis. J Clin Oncol 2003;21:4027–4033.

124. Ashing-Giwa K, Ganz PA, Petersen L. Quality of life of African-American and white long term breast carcinoma survivors. Cancer (Phila) 1999;85:418–426.

125. Dorval M, Maunsell E, Deschenes L, Brisson J. Type of mastectomy and quality of life for long term breast carcinoma survivors. Cancer (Phila) 1998;83:2130–2138.

126. Ganz PA, Schag AC, Lee JJ, Polinsky ML, Tan SJ. Breast conservation versus mastectomy. Is there a difference in psychological adjustment or quality of life in the year after surgery? Cancer (Phila) 1992;69:1729–1738.

127. Janni W, Rjosk D, Dimpfl TH, et al. Quality of life influenced by primary surgical treatment for stage I-III breast cancer-long-term follow-up of a matched-pair analysis. Ann Surg Oncol 2001;8:542–548.

128. Omne-Ponten M, Holmberg L, Sjoden PO. Psychosocial adjustment among women with breast cancer stages I and II: six-year follow-up of consecutive patients. J Clin Oncol 1994;12:1778–1782.

129. Curran D, van Dongen JP, Aaronson NK, et al. Quality of life of early-stage breast cancer patients treated with radical mastectomy or breast-conserving procedures: results of EORTC Trial 10801. The European Organization for Research and Treatment of Cancer (EORTC), Breast Cancer Co-operative Group (BCCG). Eur J Cancer 1998;34:307–314.

130. Schain W, Edwards BK, Gorrell CR, et al. Psychosocial and physical outcomes of primary breast cancer therapy: mastectomy vs excisional biopsy and irradiation. Breast Cancer Res Treat 1983;3:377–382.

131. Meyer L, Aspegren K. Long-term psychological sequelae of mastectomy and breast conserving treatment for breast cancer. Acta Oncol 1989;28:13–18.

132. Omne-Ponten M, Holmberg L, Bergstrom R, Sjoden PO, Burns T. Psychosocial adjustment among husbands of women treated for breast cancer; mastectomy vs. breast-conserving surgery. Eur J Cancer 1993;29A:1393–1397.

133. Rowland JH, Desmond KA, Meyerowitz BE, Belin TR, Wyatt GE, Ganz PA. Role of breast reconstructive surgery in physical and emotional outcomes among breast cancer survivors. J Natl Cancer Inst 2000;92:1422–1429.

134. Nissen MJ, Swenson KK, Ritz LJ, Farrell JB, Sladek ML, Lally RM. Quality of life after breast carcinoma surgery: a comparison of three surgical procedures. Cancer (Phila) 2001;91:1238–1246.

135. Joly F, Espie M, Marty M, Heron JF, Henry-Amar M. Long-term quality of life in premenopausal women with node-negative localized breast cancer treated with or without adjuvant chemotherapy. Br J Cancer 2000;83:577–582.

136. Holzner B, Kemmler G, Kopp M, et al. Quality of life in breast cancer patients—not enough attention for long-term survivors? Psychosomatics 2001;42:117–123.

137. Kessler TA. Contextual variables, emotional state, and current and expected quality of life in breast cancer survivors. Oncol Nurs Forum 2002;29:1109–1116.

138. Satariano WA, Ragheb NE, Branch LG, Swanson GM. Difficulties in physical functioning reported by middle-aged and elderly women with breast cancer: a case-control comparison. J Gerontol 1990;45:M3–M11.

139. Sneeuw KC, Aaronson NK, Yarnold JR, et al. Cosmetic and functional outcomes of breast conserving treatment for early stage breast cancer. 2. Relationship with psychosocial functioning. Radiother Oncol 1992;25:160–166.

140. Lash TL, Silliman RA. Long-term follow-up of upper-body function among breast cancer survivors. Breast J 2002;8:28–33.

141. Guidozzi F. Estrogen replacement therapy in breast cancer survivors. Int J Gynaecol Obstet 1999;64:59–63.

142. Brewster WR, DiSaia PJ, Grosen EA, McGonigle KF, Kuykendall JL, Creasman WT. An experience with estrogen replacement therapy in breast cancer survivors. Int J Fertil Womens Med 1999;44:186–192.

143. Peters GN, Fodera T, Sabol J, Jones S, Euhus D. Estrogen replacement therapy after breast cancer: a 12-year follow-up. Ann Surg Oncol 2001;8:828–832.

144. Durna EM, Crowe SM, Leader LR, Eden JA. Quality of life of breast cancer survivors: the impact of hormonal replacement therapy. Climacteric 2002;5:266–276.

145. Ellman R, Thomas BA. Is psychological wellbeing impaired in long-term survivors of breast cancer? J Med Screen 1995;2:5–9.

146. Saleeba AK, Weitzner MA, Meyers CA. Subclinical psychological distress in long-term survivors of breat cancer: a preliminary communication. J Psychosocial Oncol 1996;14:83–93.

147. Weitzner MA, Meyers CA, Stuebing KK, Saleeba AK. Relationship between quality of life and mood in long-term survivors of breast cancer treated with mastectomy. Support Care Cancer 1997;5:241–248.

148. Lee CO. Quality of life and breast cancer survivors. Psychosocial and treatment issues. Cancer Pract 1997;5:309–316.

149. Montazeri A, Jarvandi S, Haghighat S, et al. Anxiety and depression in breast cancer patients before and after participation in a cancer support group. Patient Educ Couns 2001;45:195–198.

150. Mock V. Body image in women treated for breast cancer. Nurs Res 1993;42:153–157.

Medical and Psychosocial Issues in Prostate Cancer Survivors

Tracey L. Krupski and Mark S. Litwin

O f the more than 200,000 men diagnosed each year with prostate cancer in the United States,[1] most live with their disease or the effects of treatment for many years.[2] Although many men remain asymptomatic throughout their lives, others face a multitude of physical and psychosocial challenges. Because the duration of survival is typically long, patients and their families are particularly interested in optimizing their quality of life. At the generic level, health-related quality of life (HRQOL) encompasses an individual's perceptions of his or her own health and ability to function in the physical, emotional, and social domains.[3,4] In prostate cancer survivors, the medical outcomes of urinary, bowel, and sexual impairments that result from treatment will influence the rest of the patient's life. The psychosocial aspects of HRQOL are impacted by the intimate nature of these medical side effects. Urinary leakage and erectile dysfunction may cause both private and public social embarrassment. In addition, such treatment-related complications may be compounded by the additional stressors associated with aging, such as retirement or death of peers.[5] Nearly one-third of men diagnosed with prostate cancer in a genitourinary clinic had levels of psychologic distress that met criteria for anxiety disorder.[6]

This chapter examines the medical and psychosocial issues impacting men with early- and late-stage prostate cancer. Late-stage patients are included because the course of prostate cancer recurrence is often indolent. Therefore, men with prostate cancer typically "survive" to require secondary treatments that compound existing medical problems. For men with early-stage tumors, the focus is on the repercussions of treatment decision on medical outcomes, the partner, decisional regret, and fear of recurrence. For men with advanced disease, the focus is on these issues with the addition of end-of-life decisions. The chapter concludes with emerging research challenges.

Early-Stage Medical Issues

Survivor Demographics

The strongest risk factors for prostate cancer are age and positive family history.[7,8] When survival rates are compared without controlling for stage, Caucasian men have improved survival rate compared to African-American, Hispanic, and American Indian men.[9–11] Survival rates are favorably influenced by higher socioeconomic status and the presence of a spouse or partner.[12,13] African American and Hispanic men bear a disproportionately high prostate cancer burden when compared to Caucasians.[14] Numerous studies have confirmed that both African-American and Hispanic men present with more-advanced [higher initial prostate-specific antigen (PSA) and T stage] prostate cancer than do non-Hispanic white men.[1,10,15–17] Debate exists as to whether this is a function of underlying differences in biology or disparities in access to health care. Ross et al.[18] found African-American men to have testosterone levels that were 15% higher than white men, suggesting a possible endocrine explanation for their increased risk. Because access to the healthcare system is influenced by socioeconomic parameters such as income and insurance status, African-American and Hispanic men often lack consistent high-quality medical care.[19,20]

Treatment Decision Making and the Effect on Survivorship

The impact of treatment effects on HRQOL is the major issue affecting posttreatment psychosocial quality of survivorship. Since the advent of prostate-specific antigen (PSA) screening in the early 1990s, most men present with early-stage disease, leading them to consider a variety of issues related to treatment. Those diagnosed with early-stage prostate cancer are challenged to choose among several treatment options (radical prostatectomy, radiation therapy, or watchful waiting) because studies have not yet proven an overall survival benefit of one treatment option over another.[21,22] The cure rates, defined as no evidence of biochemical (PSA) recurrence, for early-stage disease following radiation therapy or surgery range from 70% to 94%.[23–26] However, the medical outcomes do differ among these treatment options.

Medical Outcomes

Prostate cancer survivors face three long-term medical problems following primary treatment: incontinence, erectile dysfunction, and recurrence. The likelihood of these side effects will vary depending on the primary treatment chosen, stage of disease, and need for additional treatments. However, to date, no randomized controlled trials evaluating brachytherapy versus prostatectomy have been performed. The American College of Surgeons Oncology Group initiated such a trial but it was closed in 2004 for lack of enrollment. Cancer control outcomes and complication rates are inferred from predominantly retrospective, single-institution studies using different endpoints.

POSTSURGICAL INCONTINENCE

Even with improved surgical technique, urinary leakage after operative intervention persists (Table 12.1). Centers of excellence often report high rates of continence and potency whereas community-based outcomes may be different.[27–30] Causative factors for disparate outcomes include differences in patient selection, surgical volume, surgical skill, and definitions used for particular outcomes.[30–34] Further, the reporting of symptoms has been shown to be most accurate when elicited with written, confidential surveys that are self-administered and submitted to third parties, rather than by physician assessment.[35,36]

Time to recovery varies for each condition and may continue for at least 2 years after therapy.[37–39] Talcott et al.[40–42] reported that 12 months after prostatectomy 35% of patients were wearing pads, whereas Walsh et al.[40–42] reported this rate to be only 7%, despite using what appears to be the same definition and time point. These differences could be due to surgical technique, but the disparity is striking. Using yet another definition, Catalona and colleagues[43] also reported at 12 months that 45% of men under 70 years old claimed total

urinary continence. Indeed, several authors have found that the definition itself influences continence rates. Wei[41] reported continence rates that varied from 43% to 84% depending on whether the definition was total urinary control or zero to one pad per day. Similarly, Krupski et al. found that among men claiming total urinary control, 98% also claimed no pads; however, among those reporting no pads, only 47% reported total control. Hence, total control is the stricter definition.[44] By 2 years postsurgery, further improvement in urinary control is unlikely. Therefore, men must learn to adapt with any residual incontinence for the rest of their lives. Table 12.1 depicts surgical rates of incontinence.

MANAGEMENT

Posttreatment incontinence may be secondary to bladder dysfunction or sphincteric insufficiency.[45] The former of these is treated with anticholinergic therapy, timed voiding, and fluid restriction in the evening.[46] If the etiology of the incontinence is from an incompetent sphincter, bulking agents may be attempted, although long-term results have been mixed at best. Collagen and Durasphere are agents that, if injected in the periuretheral space, will increase sphincter competence.[47] Smith et al.[48] treated 62 postprostatectomy patients with multiple collagen injections, and one-third achieved social continence. Patients experiencing minimal incontinence (fewer than three pads/day) have the greatest chance of benefiting from a bulking agent.[49] The definitive therapy for patients with severe incontinence is an artificial urinary sphincter (AUS). After placement of an AUS, 76% were dry.[50] Appropriate patient selection is important, as mechanical failure, infection, and erosion are known complications.[51]

POSTSURGICAL POTENCY

All surgical series have demonstrated that men undergoing radical prostatectomy have more sexual impairment than do age-matched controls.[43,52,53] The spectrum of reported potency using a similar definition, erections sufficient for intercourse, ranges from 87% to 21% to 14%[40,54,55] (Table 12.2).

Because the cavernosal nerves provide the innervation required for erections, the logical assumption would be that preservation of both sets of nerves would lead to higher potency rates. As familiarity and acceptance of nerve-sparing techniques developed, potency rates increased. A community-based urologist employed chart review techniques and reported 71% potency rates after bilateral nerve-sparing

TABLE 12.1. Postsurgical continence.

	N	Definition of incontinence	% incontinent	Time from procedure
Assessment of treating physician				
Zincke et al. 1994[128]	1,728	Uses three or more pads/day	5	5 years
Eastham et al. 1996[28]	581	Leaks with moderate activity	9	2 years
Murphy et al. 1994[176]	1,796	Requires a pad	19	
		Complete incontinence	4	
Survey data				
Talcott et al. 1998[177]	279	Wears an absorptive pad	35	1 year
Stanford et al. 2000[178]	1,291	Requires a pad	21	1.5 years
		Severe leaking	8.4	1.5 years
Smith et al. 2000[43]	941	Less than total urinary control	65	1 year
		Occasional dribbling	14	1 year
Walsh et al. 2000[40]	64	Using pads	7	1.5 years
Potosky et al. 2000[115]	1,156	Wearing a pad	9	2 years

TABLE 12.2. Postsurgical potency.

	N	*Definition of potency*	*% potent*	*Time from procedure*
Cohn et al. 2002[a][55]	199	Erections rigid enough for vaginal penetration	71	1.5 years
Murphy et al. 1994[a][176]	1059	Capable of full erection	35	1 year
Smith et al. 2000[43]	941	Sufficient for intercourse, <70 years old	25	1 year
Walsh et al. 2000[40]	64	Unassisted intercourse ± phosphodiesterase (PDE) inhibitor	86	1.5 years
Moul et al. 1998[54]	374	Full erections when stimulated	13	10 months
Potosky et al. 2000[115]	1156	Erection sufficient for intercourse	20	2 years

[a]Assessment by treating physician.

prostatectomy, which is similar to the 86% reported by centers of excellence.[40,55]

MANAGEMENT

The treatment of erectile dysfunction consists of a stepwise approach beginning with the least invasive therapies progressing to surgical options. The type 5 phosphodiesterase inhibitors (PDEs) constitute the first line of therapy because they are an oral medication. The largest body of evidence surrounds sildenafil, as it has been marketed the longest, and suggests that PDEs increase penile nitric oxide, leading to cavernosal smooth muscle dilation and engorgement.[56] Younger men who have undergone unilateral or bilateral nerve sparing appear to benefit the most.[57] Zagaja et al.[58] found that postprostatectomy patients enjoyed an increasing response rate with highest satisfaction 18 to 24 months after surgery. Local medical therapies require an intraurethral suppository or needle injection into the cavernosal bodies (ICI). The success rate of the intraurethral suppository as measured by successful intercourse at home is reported at 40%.[59] ICI in postsurgical patients results in 60% to 90% of men developing an erection, but many patients conceptually have difficulty undertaking this therapy.[60,61] Third-line therapy is a vacuum device; an external vacuum device generates negative pressure, leading to penile engorgement. Soderdahl et al.[62] randomized groups of men to ICI or an external vacuum device and found a statistical difference in preference for ICI (50%) compared to the vacuum device (27%). Last, a penile prosthesis can result in an active sex life. Although no data specifically relate to postsurgical patients, general function and satisfaction have been reported as around 85%.[63] An industry-sponsored multicenter trial demonstrated 5- and 10-year reliability rates of 85% and 71%, respectively.[64]

URETHRAL STRICTURE

Anastomotic stricture has been reported in 0.5% to 10% of patients following surgical treatment of prostate cancer.[65] Patients will typically present with a decreased force of urinary stream. If left untreated, urinary obstruction and urinary retention may result. Gentle dilation in the clinic is often sufficient, but for more-severe strictures an endoscopic operative procedure is necessary.[66]

External-Beam Radiation

For prostate cancer, the traditional target radiation dose with a four-field box is 70 Gy. The advent of three-dimensional (3-D) conformal therapy allowed radiation oncologists to increase the dose to 78 Gy. However, several studies documented that morbidity is both dose- and volume dependent.[67] Although the higher dose results in improved biochemical recurrence for men with high-risk disease, increased complications are also seen.[67,68] The late complications (2–5 years postprocedure) associated with such dosing follow: persistent incontinence, 29%; grade 2 to 3 bladder toxicity, 9% to 20%; grade 2 or higher rectal toxicity, 14% to 26%; and only 51% retained erections adequate for intercourse.[67,69,70] Ensuring that less than 25% of the rectum receives the higher dose minimizes these complications. Fowler et al.[30] assessed complication rates in Medicare beneficiaries treated with external-beam radiation and compared these rates to a previously published sample of Medicare surgery patients. They noted that radiation patients experienced less incontinence (7% versus 32%), more erections (77% versus 44%), and greater bowel dysfunction (10% versus 4%). Tables 12.3 through 12.5 summarize the complication rates by radiation type. An additional side effect of external radiation not seen with

TABLE 12.3. Postradiation bladder complications.

	N	*Definition of bladder symptom*	*% affected*	*Time from procedure*
Brachytherapy				
Wallner et al. 2002[73]	380	Grade 1–2 toxicity	19	1 year
Talcott et al. 2001[93]	105	Daily leakage	11	5 years
		Wearing a pad	16	
External beam				
Fowler et al. 1996[30]	621	Pads for wetness	7	5 years
Potosky et al. 2000[115]	435	Wearing a pad	3	2 years
Storey et al. 2000[70] (70 Gy vs. 78 Gy)	189	Grade 2 or higher	20 and 9	5 years
External beam + brachytherapy				
Ghaly et al. 2003[94]	51	Grade 1–2	7	6 months
Zeitlin et al. 1998[86]	212	Any leakage of urine	4	2 years

TABLE 12.4. Postradiation potency.

	N	Definition of potency	% potent	Time from procedure
Brachytherapy				
Stutz et al. 2003[83]	148	Score of 22 on Sexual Health Inventory	69	2 years
Raina et al. 2003[85]	79	Erections sufficient for vaginal penetration – PDE	29	4 years
		Erections sufficient for vaginal penetration + PDE	70	
Potters et al. 2001[82]	482	Erection suitable for intercourse + PDE	76	3 years
External beam				
Fowler et al. 1996[30]	621	Ability to achieve erection	77	5 years
Potosky et al. 2000[115]	435	Erection sufficient for intercourse	39	2 years
External beam + brachytherapy				
Potters et al. 2001[82]	482	Erection suitable for intercourse + PDE	56	3 years
Zeitlin et al. 1998[86]	212	Ability to have satisfactory vaginal intercourse	62	2 years

surgery is fatigue. Immediately after initiation of radiotherapy, patients experience increasing symptoms of fatigue. Longer follow-up reveals the fatigue is temporary, with most men returning to baseline by 6 months.[71,72]

Brachytherapy

Brachytherapy (BT) is touted as having a very low rate of acute or long-term complications. In the initial 6 months all patients suffer from obstructive or irritative symptoms as a consequence of the radiation prostatitis. A randomized prospective comparison of iodine-125 (^{125}I) and palladium-103 (^{103}Pd) found that American Urologic Association symptom scores (now called the International Prostate Symptom Score, IPSS) peaked at 1 month and were generally higher in the ^{125}I patients. ^{125}I patients also experienced slightly higher grade 1 and grade 2 urinary and rectal morbidity.[73] The literature, in general, suggests that 2% to 18% of patients experience grade 2 or 3 urinary or rectal morbidity. Examples of such complications include stricture, urethritis, cystitis, proctitis, and rectal ulceration.[74–79] Urinary retention has been reported at 10% and incontinence was as high as 6% in the Medicare population.[80,81] Potency with implants alone is 69% to 76% at 1 to 3 years after implantation.[82,83] Because even the longest modern BT series span only 12 to 15 years, very little literature exists on long-term complications from BT. Merrick et al. commented that long-term urinary morbidity is restricted to patients having a prior transurethral resection of the prostate. Long-term erectile dysfunction ranges from as low

as 29% without use of a phosphodiesterase inhibitor to as high as 70% at 5 years. The most serious and difficult to treat of the reported complications is a prostatourethral–rectal fistula.[84–88]

External-Beam Therapy Combined with Brachytherapy

Controversy still exists over the role for combined radiotherapy in prostate cancer.[76] Patients at low risk for extracapsular disease (Gleason less than 7, PSA less than 10 ng/dL, clinical stage less than T2b) are excellent candidates for brachytherapy monotherapy.[89,90] However, patients at intermediate or high risk for extracapsular disease may be better served by combined radiotherapy or either form of radiotherapy with the addition of androgen ablation.[24,91,92] The Radiation Therapy Oncology Group has initiated trial P-0232 [external-beam radiation therapy (EBRT) + BT versus BT] to assess these issues.[93,94]

Management

Following EBRT or BT, patients are started prophylactically on alpha-blockers to decrease the expected side effects of dysuria and frequency that result from radiation prostatitis. Select patients may stay on the alpha-blocker for 6 to 12 months. Nonsteroidals and antiinflammatory suppositories are used to treat proctitis. For a patient with a large prostate gland (more than 50 mm³), androgen deprivation therapy is

TABLE 12.5. Postradiation bowel complications.

	N	Definition of bowel toxicity	% affected	Time from procedure
Brachytherapy				
Wallner et al. 2002[73]	380	Grade 1	20	1 year
Talcott et al. 2001[93]	105	Diarrhea or watery stool several times/week	6	
External beam				
Potosky et al. 2000[115]	435	Bowel urgency	36	2 years
Storey et al. 2000[70] (70 Gy vs. 78 Gy)	189	Grade 2 or 3	14 and 21	5 years
Kuban et al. 2003[67] (70 Gy vs. 78 Gy)	1,087	Grade 2 or 3	12 and 26	5 years
External beam + brachytherapy				
Zeitlin et al. 1998[86]	212	Blood per rectum (proctitis)	21	2 years

employed to "downsize" the prostate, facilitating BT.[95] The added benefit of androgen deprivation therapy is to decrease the risk of postoperative urinary retention. Sacco et al. have also demonstrated that dexamethasone (4 mg twice daily for 1 week then 2 mg twice daily) instead of androgen ablation also decreases the risk of retention in these patients.[96] Erectile dysfunction is treated in the same manner as for postsurgical patients as already described.

Prostate-Specific Health-Related Quality of Life

Several cross-sectional surveys have compared health-related quality of life outcomes after brachytherapy, external-beam radiation, and radical prostatectomy. Two studies reported that overall HRQOL was similar between brachytherapy and radical prostatectomy patients, with those undergoing brachytherapy having better urinary control but similar bother.[97,98] However, in a study of 1,400 patients, Wei et al.[99] found that men receiving brachytherapy experienced worse outcomes in the areas of urinary, bowel, and sexual HRQOL than did those undergoing either of the other two treatments. This finding contrasts with that of Eton et al.,[100] who reported that brachytherapy patients had the least sexual dysfunction and the best physical functioning of all treatment groups, and with that of Davis et al.[101] who reported that bowel bother was worst after external-beam therapy. Direct comparison of such studies is difficult because demographic characteristics, clinical factors, and measurement instruments vary from one investigator to another. Van Andel et al.[102] reported that radiation patients, on average, are 7.9 years older, have lower socioeconomic status, and more often have a higher tumor stage. They also found that radiation patients reported more pain and fatigue, lower overall HRQOL, and worse sexual function than men undergoing surgery.

Early-Stage Psychosocial Issues

Partners

Cancer affects family members as well as patients. Prostate cancer, more so than other malignancies, has been labeled a "relationship disease" because it so profoundly impacts both partners.[103,104] In fact, studies have found that psychologic distress is equivalent in the prostate cancer patient and his partner.[105] Clearly, once the cancer is discovered, both partners experience increased levels of anxiety compared with healthy couples.[106]

Although there is evidence that marital status impacts prostate cancer outcomes, the direction of the effect is mixed. The diagnosis of prostate cancer may evoke anxiety or depression in both partners. The response to this stress can nurture or undermine the relationship. A good relationship can foster healthy coping skills, alleviate distress, and encourage optimism. Increased optimism has been shown to correlate with improved cancer outcomes and survival.[107]

Depression/Distress

Being diagnosed with cancer naturally evokes a sense of sadness.[108] The difficulty is to distinguish the normal response from a clinical disorder. Symptoms indicative of a clinical disorder include a sense of failure, social withdrawal, suicidal ideation, and indecision.[109–111] Few studies have examined depression in patients with early-stage disease. Kornblith et al. studied 163 men with localized prostate cancer and found that 29% reported "worry" and 21% complained of depression. Patients and spouses both had frequent intrusive thoughts and images.[112]

Psychologic distress is complicated in prostate cancer because of the dual implications of treatment and distress. Prostate cancer treatment may itself induce sexual dysfunction, which adds further to such distress. Studying traumatic distress in men newly diagnosed with early-stage disease, Bisson et al.[113] found very few depressive symptoms. Instead, patients demonstrated higher anxiety and traumatic stress symptoms. The authors postulated that older men may be more likely to use denial as a defense mechanism. A more-holistic approach by the physician, incorporating attention to both psychologic and physical needs, benefits the patient and his spouse. Emotional support allows both members of the couple to target their energies on preparing for the treatment process.

Regret

Decisional regret relates to the notion that another treatment might have been preferable. Davison et al.[114] undertook a study to assess how factors such as HRQOL and level of patient involvement in medical decision making impact decisional regret. Higher regret scores did correlate with poorer emotional and urinary function. Although not a direct measure of decisional regret, the Prostate Cancer Outcomes Study that found 92% of patients who chose surgery or radiation would do so again.[115] In contrast, Hu et al.[116] used the two-item Clark regret scale[117,118] and discerned that 16% of men with localized prostate cancer experienced decisional regret. College education and worse HRQOL appeared to foster regret, but treatment type did not have an effect.

Fear of Recurrence

Using the CaPSURE database, Mehta et al.[119] identified more than 500 men with pre- and posttreatment questionnaires to measure fear of recurrence. All patients, regardless of treatment type, reported the most severe fear of recurrence before treatment. Their levels of fear improved after treatment and remained constant over the next 2 years. Another study utilized the Profile of Mood States (POMS)[120] in men with and without biochemical recurrence. Urinary tract symptoms were associated with increased cancer fear, but biochemical recurrence alone was not associated. However, men with both urinary tract symptoms and biochemical recurrence reported the highest level of cancer fear.[121] In an attempt to elucidate better the problems faced by men with prostate cancer, Roth et al. developed a new scale to measure anxiety in prostate cancer patients. The Memorial Anxiety Scale for Prostate Cancer (MAX-PC)[122] comprises three subsections including a prostate cancer anxiety scale, PSA anxiety scale, and fear of recurrence scale. The authors identify the prostate cancer anxiety subscale as being most specific to cancer anxiety while the fear of recurrence captures general distress. Loneliness and general uncertainty about the future heighten anxiety in prostate cancer survivors. Men who have elected to undergo no treatment (watchful waiting) also experience PSA anxiety. Wallace[123] identified 19 men on watchful waiting and found they experienced heightened uncertainty, leading to a higher perception of danger, which impaired their quality of life. Discussions with other men facing similar clinical scenarios promote positive coping skill and diminish anxiety. National and local support groups can help meet the emotional and educational needs of patients concerned with facing a recurrence.[124,125]

Late-Stage Medical Issues

Demographics

African-American men have a significantly higher mortality rate from prostate cancer than do non-Hispanic white men.[126] However, the traditional 5-year survival rates are almost irrelevant to men with prostate cancer, given that this rate approaches 100%, regardless of treatment.[2] This figure includes the 15% to 35% of men who will experience biochemical progression within 10 years of treatment.[25,127,128] The natural history of disease recurrence following radical prostatectomy was characterized by Pound et al.,[23] who showed that the median time to development of metastatic disease was 8 years and death followed at a median of 5 additional years. The risk factors for progression were time to biochemical progression, Gleason score, and PSA doubling time. The earlier the PSA recurrence, the higher the Gleason score, and the faster the doubling time, the worse the prognosis. No patients placed on early hormone ablation were included in the study.

Definition of Recurrence

After a radical retropubic prostatectomy, PSA levels should be undetectable. Original assays utilized a threshold level of 0.2 ng/dL, and values less than this constituted freedom from disease. Although more-recent assays have lowered this threshold, the PSA should still be undetectable. A detectable PSA preceded clinical recurrence by 6 to 8 years.[129,130] The definition of recurrence after radiation therapy is three successive rises in PSA based on American Society for Therapeutic Radiology and Oncology (ASTRO) criteria.[131] However, because recurrent patients after either treatment will survive for many years, secondary treatment in the form of hormonal therapy results in additional medical problems.

Androgen Ablation

Medical induction of castration can be obtained through drugs affecting the production of luteinizing hormone-releasing hormone (LHRH), blocking the peripheral effects of androgens (steroidal and nonsteroidal antiandrogens), eliminating all steroid hormone production, and estrogens. The luteinizing hormone-releasing hormone agonists (which paradoxically lower LHRH levels) are typically administered by injection every 3 to 4 months whereas peripheral blocking agents are taken orally every day. However, once androgens are ablated, the prostate cancer begins an inexorable change to hormone independence.[132] Once a hormone refractory state

has developed, few effective treatment options exist. Therefore, questions arise regarding the timing of androgen ablation and which agents to use.

Hormonal Complications

The predominant treatments are LHRH agonists and non-steroidal antiandrogens, but these are not without side effects. LHRH agonists cause hot flashes, loss of libido and potency, anemia, fatigue, weight gain, depression, and decreased bone mineral density.[133,134] Antiandrogens maintain potency in a subset of patients but lead to gynecomastia and nipple tenderness.[135] Controversy remains over whether these agents are as effective when used alone as when used in combination with LHRH agonists. Two large trials demonstrated prolonged time to progression (by 2 months) in patients with modest disease; however, meta-analysis and other small studies have failed to demonstrate a significant advantage to combined androgen blockade.[136–138] Once metastatic bone deposits develop, LHRH agonists appear to be the most cost-effective, efficacious treatment.[139] However, men with high-risk disease or rising PSA are often started on hormone ablation.[140,141] To decrease the side effects, intermittent hormone ablation is increasingly being utilized.

Bone Complications

Hypogonadal men are at risk for potentially debilitating bone complications such as osteoporosis and hip fractures.[142,143] In patients with prostate cancer on androgen ablation, Hatano et al. reported a 6% nonpathologic fracture rate while Townsend et al. found a 9% overall fracture rate.[144,145] A smaller retrospective studies found even higher fracture rates of 40% after 15 years in 161 men after bilateral orchiectomy.[146] Daniell analyzed 59 men who had undergone bilateral orchiectomy for prostate cancer and found 8 (13.6%) with osteoporotic fractures of the femur or vertebra. However, when he analyzed the 17 patients still alive 5 to 12 years later, he noted that 38% had had one or more osteoporotic fractures.[147]

According to the World Health Organization, osteopenia denotes a bone mineral density between 1.0 and 2.5 standard deviations below the mean for young adults and osteoporosis is greater than 2.5 standard deviations below the mean.[148] Using this definition, Finkelstein et al. documented cortical bone density loss at least 2 standard deviations below normal in men with isolated gonadotropin-releasing hormone deficiency.[149] These changes in bone mineral density have been confirmed in men with therapeutic hypogonadism from prostate cancer treatment.[150,151] Smith et al. reported that trabecular bone mineral density of the spine decreased by 8.6% during the first year of androgen-deprivation therapy (ADT) for nonmetastatic prostate cancer.[151] With aging itself leading to decreased bone mineral density, the addition of ADT further places these men at risk.[152,153]

Management

The agents used in the treatment of osteoporosis and osteopenia depend on whether the etiology of the bone loss is from a benign or malignant process. Disease of benign etiology has been successfully treated with calcitonin, oral bisphosphonates, and a combination of vitamin D and calcium.[154,155]

However, the bone loss associated with prostate cancer and androgen deprivation therapy is accelerated, requiring additional therapeutic options.[153,156,157] A prospective randomized controlled trial revealed that intravenous bisphosphonate was effective in increasing bone mineral density in men on androgen deprivation therapy for prostate cancer.[158] Therefore, men with D0 disease as well as metastatic prostate cancer on ADT are candidates for intravenous bisphosphonates.

Fatigue

Throughout the disease trajectory, cancer patients experience fatigue, which is recognized to have a significant impact on quality of life.[159] Indeed, clinical experience with fatigue in hypogonadal men indicates that androgen deprivation therapy should lead to some degree of fatigue.[160] Stone et al.[161] used the Fatigue Severity Scale[162] to follow patients before and after treatment with goserelin and cyproterone. Fatigue worsened in 66% of patients after 3 months of androgen deprivation therapy. All patients responded to the therapy with decreasing PSA levels, eliminating disease progression as a possible source of fatigue. On multivariate analysis, only depression remained a significant predictor of fatigue.[163] The depression literature supports this association.[164] This study did not find any association with anemia, but others suggest that fatigue in prostate cancer patients on androgen deprivation therapy may be because of anemia, a well-known side effect of therapeutic hypogonadism.[165] Patients on androgen deprivation therapy experience not only the expected physical side effects such as hot flashes, loss of libido and potency, weight gain, and anemia but also the psychosocial changes of depression and fatigue. Close monitoring of all these parameters is critical.

Health-Related Quality of Life

The clinical rationale for selecting the method and agent for androgen ablation is controversial. Therefore, the physician must engage the patient in a discussion to decide what balance of side effects, cost, and risk of progression is optimal. Because the patient will likely survive for many years before developing bone metastasis or other evidence of clinical progression, the potential cost in quality of life may be great. Additionally, when the physical side effects of fatigue, sexual dysfunction, and weight are considered, deferment of this potentially emotionally debilitating therapy may promote HRQOL in men living daily with prostate cancer.

Late-Stage Psychosocial Issues

Partners

Researchers have used focus groups to describe the impact of prostate cancer on the couple as a unit. Both patients and partners feel unprepared to manage treatment- and prostate-related changes as they arise. The spousal role is increasingly difficult as the cancer progresses. Often the role shifts to that of a caregiver focusing on three major areas of concern. Caregivers contend with fear of cancer and its spread, helping patients respond to the emotional ramifications of the disease, and managing the disruptions caused by cancer.[166] For survivors of prostate cancer with late-stage disease, uncertainty prevails. Men with partners may benefit from physical assistance from their partner but bear additional emotional weight from their sense of being a burden. Men without partners experience more of a physical decline and loneliness.[166–168]

Depression

The concept that depression is linked to testosterone has been explored in the psychiatric literature. Studies have examined the treatment of elderly males with major depressive disorders with testosterone replacement. The therapy appears to be effective in men with late-onset depression.[169] Therefore, older men receiving androgen deprivation therapy for prostate cancer are an at-risk population. Among 45 men receiving androgen deprivation therapy (ADT) as prostate cancer treatment, the prevalence of major depressive disorder was eight times the national rate.[170] Although cancer progression was not the primary cause of the depression, history of depression was a strong risk factor. Involving experts in depression and palliative care can provide social support and help patients confront end-of-life issues.

Regret

Regret has been evaluated in men who developed metastasis and had initiated androgen deprivation therapy. Almost one-fourth of these men expressed regret. The demographics and time since diagnosis with metastatic disease were similar between men who were and were not regretful; however, men who had undergone orchiectomy were more likely to express regret.[119] Clark et al.[118] did find that men expressing regret were more likely to have poorer quality of life, particularly in the role and emotional limitations subscales. These men did not have more treatment-induced side effects, yet they perceived themselves as having worse functional status.

End of Life

Quality of life steadily descends in the final months of life.[171] Marriage appears to protect men from rapid decline in the physical domains but surprisingly does not offer protection in the emotional domains. Single men may feel the persistent effects of loneliness, while married men may sense being a burden. Higher socioeconomic status has been associated with a slower decline in physical domains but a more acute decline in the emotional domains.[172] Other studies in terminally ill cancer patients have found accelerated HRQOL declines at 1 to 3 weeks before death.[173] Because prostate cancer death can be so delayed, patients, family, and physicians often neglect to address end-of-life planning issues. Steinhauser et al.[174] evaluated factors considered important for a "good death," emphasizing that this is highly idiosyncratic. Control of symptoms, preparation for death, opportunity for closure, and good relationship with healthcare professionals were factors considered crucial to easing the end-of-life transition for patients and families. One responsibility of the physician is to consider what the patient and caregiver need emotionally and psychologically. This need includes assessing what interventions might be used for long-

or short-term gain or discussing transfer to a hospice or palliative care program. When these issues are adequately addressed, terminally ill patients feel more prepared for death and are better able to live to the fullest degree possible.[175]

Conclusion

The high prevalence of prostate cancer and the impact on the partner make the psychosocial aspects of prostate cancer particularly relevant to long-term survivorship. A man's masculinity is intricately intertwined with his personal identity. Therefore, the intimate nature of the treatment-related side effects of early- or late-stage prostate cancer may have far-reaching emotional consequences for these men. They are at risk for anxiety, depression, distress, fatigue, and bone complications at many stages of the disease trajectory. The most effective tool against these sequelae is awareness on the part of physicians and other health professionals in identifying psychosocial needs and directing patients to the appropriate resources.

References

1. Jemal A, Siegel R, Ward E, Murray T, Xu J, Smigal C, Thun MJ. Cancer statistics, 2006. CA Cancer J Clin 2006;56:106–130.
2. Greenlee RT, Murray T, Bolden S, Wingo PA. Cancer statistics, 2000. CA Cancer J Clin 2000;50(1):7–33.
3. Osoba D. Measuring the effect of cancer on quality of life. In: Osoba D (ed). Effect of Cancer on Quality of Life. Boca Raton: CRC Press, 1991:25–40.
4. Penson DF, Litwin MS. The Impact of Urologic Complications on Quality of Life. In: Taneja SS, Smith RB, Ehrlich RM, (eds). Complications of Urologic Surgery, 3rd edition. Philadelphia PA: WB Saunders and Co., 2000:56–66.
5. Roth AJ, Kornblith AB, Batel-Copel L, Peabody E, Scher HI, Holland JC. Rapid screening for psychologic distress in men with prostate carcinoma: a pilot study. Cancer (Phila) 1998;82(10):1904–1908.
6. Roth A, Scher H. Genitourinary malignancies. In: Holland JC (ed). Psycho-oncology. New York: Oxford University Press, 1998:39–358.
7. Spitz MR, Currier RD, Fueger JJ, Babaian RJ, Newell GR. Familial patterns of prostate cancer: a case-control analysis. J Urol 1991;146(5):1305–1307.
8. Parker SL, Tong T, Bolden S, Wingo PA. Cancer statistics, 1996. CA Cancer J Clin 1996;46(1):5–27.
9. Gilliland FD, Key CR. Prostate cancer in American Indians, New Mexico, 1969 to 1994. J Urol 1998;159(3):893–897; discussion 897–898.
10. Hoffman RM, Gilliland FD, Eley JW, et al. Racial and ethnic differences in advanced-stage prostate cancer: the Prostate Cancer Outcomes Study. J Natl Cancer Inst 2001;93(5):388–395.
11. Underwood W, De Monner S, Ubel P, Fagerlin A, Sanda MG, Wei JT. Racial/ethnic disparities in the treatment of localized/regional prostate cancer. J Urol 2004;171(4):1504–1507.
12. Nayeri K, Pitaro G, Feldman JG. Marital status and stage at diagnosis in cancer. N Y State J Med 1992;92(1):8–11.
13. Harvei S, Kravdal O. The importance of marital and socioeconomic status in incidence and survival of prostate cancer. An analysis of complete Norwegian birth cohorts. Prev Med 1997;26(5 pt 1):623–632.
14. ACS. Cancer Facts and Figures. Washington, DC: American Cancer Society, 2003.
15. Zietman A, Moughan J, Owen J, Hanks G. The Patterns of Care Survey of radiation therapy in localized prostate cancer: similarities between the practice nationally and in minority-rich areas. Int J Radiat Oncol Biol Phys 2001;50(1):75–80.
16. Ries LA, Wingo PA, Miller DS, et al. The annual report to the nation on the status of cancer, 1973–1997, with a special section on colorectal cancer. Cancer (Phila) 2000;88(10):2398–2424.
17. Hankey BF, Ries LA, Edwards BK. The surveillance, epidemiology, and end results program: a national resource. Cancer Epidemiol Biomarkers Prev 1999;8(12):1117–1121.
18. Ross R, Bernstein L, Judd H, Hanisch R, Pike M, Henderson B. Serum testosterone levels in healthy young black and white men. J Natl Cancer Inst 1986;76(1):45–48.
19. Hargraves JL, Hadley J. The contribution of insurance coverage and community resources to reducing racial/ethnic disparities in access to care. Health Serv Res 2003;38(3):809–829.
20. Cunningham PJ, Kemper P. The uninsured getting care: where you live matters. Issue Brief Cent Stud Health Syst Change 1998(15):1–6.
21. D'Amico AV, Whittington R, Malkowicz SB, et al. Biochemical outcome after radical prostatectomy, external beam radiation therapy, or interstitial radiation therapy for clinically localized prostate cancer. JAMA 1998;280(11):969–974.
22. Holmberg L, Bill-Axelson A, Helgesen F, et al. A randomized trial comparing radical prostatectomy with watchful waiting in early prostate cancer. N Engl J Med 2002;347(11):781–789.
23. Pound CR, Partin AW, Eisenberger MA, Chan DW, Pearson JD, Walsh PC. Natural history of progression after PSA elevation following radical prostatectomy. JAMA 1999;281(17):1591–1597.
24. D'Amico AV, Moul J, Carroll PR, Sun L, Lubeck D, Chen MH. Cancer-specific mortality after surgery or radiation for patients with clinically localized prostate cancer managed during the prostate-specific antigen era. J Clin Oncol 2003;21(11):2163–2172.
25. Catalona WJ, Smith DS. 5-year tumor recurrence rates after anatomical radical retropubic prostatectomy for prostate cancer. J Urol 1994;152(5 pt 2):1837–1842.
26. Sylvester JE, Blasko JC, Grimm PD, Meier R, Malmgren JA. Ten-year biochemical relapse-free survival after external beam radiation and brachytherapy for localized prostate cancer: the Seattle experience. Int J Radiat Oncol Biol Phys 2003;57(4):944–952.
27. Catalona WJ, Ramos CG, Carvalhal GF. Contemporary results of anatomic radical prostatectomy. CA Cancer J Clin 1999;49(5):282–296.
28. Eastham JA, Kattan MW, Rogers E, et al. Risk factors for urinary incontinence after radical prostatectomy. J Urol 1996;156(5):1707–1713.
29. Walsh PC, Partin AW, Epstein JI. Cancer control and quality of life following anatomical radical retropubic prostatectomy: results at 10 years. J Urol 1994;152(5 pt 2):1831–1836.
30. Fowler FJ Jr, Barry MJ, Lu-Yao G, Wasson JH, Bin L. Outcomes of external-beam radiation therapy for prostate cancer: a study of Medicare beneficiaries in three surveillance, epidemiology, and end results areas. J Clin Oncol 1996;14(8):2258–2265.
31. Begg CB, Riedel ER, Bach PB, et al. Variations in morbidity after radical prostatectomy. N Engl J Med 2002;346(15):1138–1144.
32. Hu JC, Gold KF, Pashos CL, Mehta SS, Litwin MS. Role of surgeon volume in radical prostatectomy outcomes. J Clin Oncol 2003;21(3):401–405.
33. Walsh PC, Partin AW. Treatment of early stage prostate cancer: radical prostatectomy. Important Adv Oncol 1994:211–223.
34. Wei JT, Montie JE. Comparison of patients' and physicians' rating of urinary incontinence following radical prostatectomy. Semin Urol Oncol 2000;18(1):76–80.
35. Litwin MS, McGuigan KA. Accuracy of recall in health-related quality-of-life assessment among men treated for prostate cancer. J Clin Oncol 1999;17(9):2882–2888.
36. Litwin MS, Lubeck DP, Henning JM, Carroll PR. Differences in urologist and patient assessments of health related quality of life in men with prostate cancer: results of the CaPSURE database. J Urol 1998;159(6):1988–1992.

37. Litwin MS, Flanders SC, Pasta DJ, Stoddard ML, Lubeck DP, Henning JM. Sexual function and bother after radical prostatectomy or radiation for prostate cancer: multivariate quality-of-life analysis from CaPSURE. Cancer of the Prostate Strategic Urologic Research Endeavor. Urology 1999;54(3):503–508.

38. Litwin MS, Pasta DJ, Yu J, Stoddard ML, Flanders SC. Urinary function and bother after radical prostatectomy or radiation for prostate cancer: a longitudinal, multivariate quality of life analysis from the Cancer of the Prostate Strategic Urologic Research Endeavor. J Urol 2000;164(6):1973–1977.

39. Fulmer BR, Bissonette EA, Petroni GR, Theodorescu D. Prospective assessment of voiding and sexual function after treatment for localized prostate carcinoma: comparison of radical prostatectomy to hormonobrachytherapy with and without external beam radiotherapy. Cancer (Phila) 2001;91(11):2046–2055.

40. Walsh PC, Marschke P, Ricker D, Burnett AL. Patient-reported urinary continence and sexual function after anatomic radical prostatectomy. Urology 2000;55(1):58–61.

41. Wei JT, Dunn RL, Marcovish R, et al. Prospective assessment of patient reported urinary continence after radical prostatectomy. J Urol 2000;164(3):744–748.

42. Talcott JA, Rieker P, Propert KJ, et al. Patient-reported impotence and incontinence after nerve-sparing radical prostatectomy. J Natl Cancer Inst 1997;89(15):1117–1123.

43. Smith DS, Carvalhal GF, Schneider K, Krygiel J, Yan Y, Catalona WJ. Quality-of-life outcomes for men with prostate carcinoma detected by screening. Cancer (Phila) 2000;88(6):1454–1463.

44. Krupski TL, Saigal CS, Litwin MS. Variation in continence and potency by definition. J Urol 2003;170(4 pt 1):1291–1294.

45. Leach GE, Trockman B, Wong A, Hamilton J, Haab F, Zimmern PE. Post-prostatectomy incontinence: urodynamic findings and treatment outcomes. J Urol 1996;155(4):1256–1259.

46. Haab F, Yamaguchi R, Leach GE. Postprostatectomy incontinence. Urol Clin N Am 1996;23(3):447–457.

47. Lightner DJ. Review of the available urethral bulking agents. Curr Opin Urol 2002;12(4):333–338.

48. Smith DN, Appell RA, Rackley RR, Winters JC. Collagen injection therapy for post-prostatectomy incontinence. J Urol 1998;160(2):364–367.

49. Cross CA, English SF, Cespedes RD, McGuire EJ. A follow-up on transurethral collagen injection therapy for urinary incontinence. J Urol 1998;159(1):106–108.

50. Montague DK, Angermeier KW. Postprostatectomy urinary incontinence: the case for artificial urinary sphincter implantation. Urology 2000;55(1):2–4.

51. Montague DK, Angermeier KW. Artificial urinary sphincter troubleshooting. Urology 2001;58(5):779–782.

52. Litwin MS, Hays RD, Fink A, et al. Quality-of-life outcomes in men treated for localized prostate cancer. JAMA 1995;273(2):129–135.

53. Fowler FJ Jr, Barry MJ, Lu-Yao G, Roman A, Wasson J, Wennberg JE. Patient-reported complications and follow-up treatment after radical prostatectomy. The National Medicare Experience: 1988–1990 (updated June 1993). Urology 1993;42(6):622–629.

54. Moul JW, Mooneyhan RM, Kao TC, McLeod DG, Cruess DF. Preoperative and operative factors to predict incontinence, impotence and stricture after radical prostatectomy. Prostate Cancer Prostatic Dis 1998;1(5):242–249.

55. Cohn JH, El-Galley R. Radical prostatectomy in a community practice. J Urol 2002;167(1):224–228.

56. Uckert S, Hedlund P, Waldkirch E, et al. Interactions between cGMP- and cAMP-pathways are involved in the regulation of penile smooth muscle tone. World J Urol 2004;22(4):261–266.

57. Zippe CD, Jhaveri FM, Klein EA, et al. Role of Viagra after radical prostatectomy. Urology 2000;55(2):241–245.

58. Zagaja GP, Mhoon DA, Aikens JE, Brendler CB. Sildenafil in the treatment of erectile dysfunction after radical prostatectomy. Urology 2000;56(4):631–634.

59. Costabile RA, Spevak M, Fishman IJ, et al. Efficacy and safety of transurethral alprostadil in patients with erectile dysfunction following radical prostatectomy. J Urol 1998;160(4):1325–1328.

60. Rodriguez VGI, Bona, AA, Benejam GJ, Cuesta P, Jioja Sanz LA. Erectile dysfunction after radical prostatectomy etiopathology and treatment. Acta Urol Esp 1997;21:909–921.

61. Fallon B. Intracavernous injection therapy for male erectile dysfunction. Urol Clin N Am 1995;22(4):833–845.

62. Soderdahl DW, Thrasher JB, Hansberry KL. Intracavernosal drug-induced erection therapy versus external vacuum devices in the treatment of erectile dysfunction. Br J Urol 1997;79(6):952–957.

63. Meuleman EJ, Mulders PF. Erectile function after radical prostatectomy: a review. Eur Urol 2003;43(2):95–101; discussion 101–102.

64. Carson CC, Mulcahy JJ, Govier FE. Efficacy, safety and patient satisfaction outcomes of the AMS 700CX inflatable penile prosthesis: results of a long-term multicenter study. AMS 700CX Study Group. J Urol 2000;164(2):376–380.

65. Geary ES, Dendinger TE, Freiha FS, Stamey TA. Incontinence and vesical neck strictures following radical retropubic prostatectomy. Urology 1995;45(6):1000–1006.

66. Kochakarn W, Ratana-Olarn K, Viseshsindh V. Vesicourethral strictures after radical prostatectomy: review of treatment and outcome. J Med Assoc Thai 2002;85(1):63–66.

67. Kuban D, Pollack A, Huang E, et al. Hazards of dose escalation in prostate cancer radiotherapy. Int J Radiat Oncol Biol Phys 2003;57(5):1260–1268.

68. Dale E, Olsen DR, Fossa SD. Normal tissue complication probabilities correlated with late effects in the rectum after prostate conformal radiotherapy. Int J Radiat Oncol Biol Phys 1999;43(2):385–391.

69. Nguyen LN, Pollack A, Zagars GK. Late effects after radiotherapy for prostate cancer in a randomized dose-response study: results of a self-assessment questionnaire. Urology 1998;51(6):991–997.

70. Storey MR, Pollack A, Zagars G, Smith L, Antolak J, Rosen I. Complications from radiotherapy dose escalation in prostate cancer: preliminary results of a randomized trial. Int J Radiat Oncol Biol Phys 2000;48(3):635–642.

71. Jereczek-Fossa BA, Marsiglia HR, Orecchia R. Radiotherapy-related fatigue: how to assess and how to treat the symptom. A commentary. Tumori 2001;87(3):147–151.

72. Janda M, Gerstner N, Obermair A, et al. Quality of life changes during conformal radiation therapy for prostate carcinoma. Cancer 2000;89(6):1322–1328.

73. Wallner K, Merrick G, True L, Cavanagh W, Simpson C, Butler W. I-125 versus Pd-103 for low-risk prostate cancer: morbidity outcomes from a prospective randomized multicenter trial. Cancer J 2002;8(1):67–73.

74. Stone NN, Stock RG. Complications following permanent prostate brachytherapy. Eur Urol 2002;41(4):427–433.

75. Peschel RE, Chen Z, Roberts K, Nath R. Long-term complications with prostate implants: iodine-125 vs. palladium-103. Radiat Oncol Invest 1999;7(5):278–288.

76. Peschel RE, Colberg JW. Surgery, brachytherapy, and external-beam radiotherapy for early prostate cancer. Lancet Oncol 2003;4(4):233–241.

77. Gelblum DY, Potters L, Ashley R, Waldbaum R, Wang XH, Leibel S. Urinary morbidity following ultrasound-guided transperineal prostate seed implantation. Int J Radiat Oncol Biol Phys 1999;45(1):59–67.

78. Gelblum DY, Potters L. Rectal complications associated with transperineal interstitial brachytherapy for prostate cancer. Int J Radiat Oncol Biol Phys 2000;48(1):119–124.

79. Snyder KM, Stock RG, Hong SM, Lo YC, Stone NN. Defining the risk of developing grade 2 proctitis following ^{125}I prostate brachytherapy using a rectal dose-volume histogram analysis. Int J Radiat Oncol Biol Phys 2001;50(2):335–341.

80. Merrick GS, Butler WM, Tollenaar BG, Galbreath RW, Lief JH. The dosimetry of prostate brachytherapy-induced urethral strictures. Int J Radiat Oncol Biol Phys 2002;52(2):461–468.

81. Benoit RM, Naslund MJ, Cohen JK. Complications after prostate brachytherapy in the Medicare population. Urology 2000;55(1):91–96.

82. Potters L, Torre T, Fearn PA, Leibel SA, Kattan MW. Potency after permanent prostate brachytherapy for localized prostate cancer. Int J Radiat Oncol Biol Phys 2001;50(5):1235–1242.

83. Stutz MA, Gurel MH, Moran BJ. Potency preservation after prostate brachytherapy. Int J Radiat Oncol Biol Phys 2003;57(suppl 2):S393–S394.

84. Merrick GS, Butler WM, Lief JH, Dorsey AT. Is brachytherapy comparable with radical prostatectomy and external-beam radiation for clinically localized prostate cancer? Tech Urol 2001;7(1):12–19.

85. Raina R, Agarwal A, Goyal KK, et al. Long-term potency after iodine-125 radiotherapy for prostate cancer and role of sildenafil citrate. Urology 2003;62(6):1103–1108.

86. Zeitlin SI, Sherman J, Raboy A, Lederman G, Albert P. High dose combination radiotherapy for the treatment of localized prostate cancer. J Urol 1998;160(1):91–95; discussion 95–96.

87. Jordan GH, Lynch DF, Warden SS, McCraw JD, Hoffman GC, Schellhammer PF. Major rectal complications following interstitial implantation of ^{125}iodine for carcinoma of the prostate. J Urol 1985;134(6):1212–1214.

88. Theodorescu D, Gillenwater JY, Koutrouvelis PG. Prosta-tourethral-rectal fistula after prostate brachytherapy. Cancer 2000;89(10):2085–2091.

89. Blasko JC, Grimm PD, Sylsvester JE, Cavanagh W. The role of external beam radiotherapy with I-125/Pd-103 brachytherapy for prostate carcinoma. Radiother Oncol 2000;57(3):273–278.

90. D'Amico AV, Whittington R, Malkowicz SB, et al. Biochemical outcome after radical prostatectomy or external beam radiation therapy for patients with clinically localized prostate carcinoma in the prostate specific antigen era. Cancer (Phila) 2002;95(2):281–286.

91. D'Amico AV, Schultz D, Loffredo M, et al. Biochemical outcome following external beam radiation therapy with or without androgen suppression therapy for clinically localized prostate cancer. JAMA 2000;284(10):1280–1283.

92. D'Amico AV, Schultz D, Schneider L, Hurwitz M, Kantoff PW, Richie JP. Comparing prostate specific antigen outcomes after different types of radiotherapy management of clinically localized prostate cancer highlights the importance of controlling for established prognostic factors. J Urol 2000;163(6):1797–1801.

93. Talcott JA, Clark JA, Stark PC, Mitchell SP. Long-term treatment related complications of brachytherapy for early prostate cancer: a survey of patients previously treated. J Urol 2001;166(2):494–499.

94. Ghaly M, Wallner K, Merrick G, et al. The effect of supplemental beam radiation on prostate brachytherapy-related morbidity: morbidity outcomes from two prospective randomized multicenter trials. Int J Radiat Oncol Biol Phys 2003;55(5):1288–1293.

95. Wang H, Wallner K, Sutlief S, Blasko J, Russell K, Ellis W. Transperineal brachytherapy in patients with large prostate glands. Int J Cancer 2000;90(4):199–205.

96. Sacco DE, Daller M, Grocela JA, Babayan RK, Zietman AL. Corticosteroid use after prostate brachytherapy reduces the risk of acute urinary retention. BJU Int 2003;91(4):345–349.

97. Krupski T, Petroni GR, Bissonette EA, Theodorescu D. Quality of life comparison of radical prostatectomy and interstitial brachytherapy in the treatment of clinically localized prostate cancer. Prostate Cancer Prostatic Dis 1999;2(S3):S32.

98. Downs TM, Sadetsky N, Pasta DJ, et al. Health related quality of life patterns in patients treated with interstitial prostate brachytherapy for localized prostate cancer: data from CaPSURE. J Urol 2003;170(5):1822–1827.

99. Wei JT, Dunn RL, Sandler HM, et al. Comprehensive comparison of health-related quality of life after contemporary therapies for localized prostate cancer. J Clin Oncol 2002;20(2):557–566.

100. Eton DT, Lepore SJ, Helgeson VS. Early quality of life in patients with localized prostate carcinoma: an examination of treatment-related, demographic, and psychosocial factors. Cancer (Phila) 2001;92(6):1451–1459.

101. Davis JW, Kuban DA, Lynch DF, Schellhammer PF. Quality of life after treatment for localized prostate cancer: differences based on treatment modality. J Urol 2001;166(3):947–952.

102. Van Andel G, Visser AP, Hulshof MC, Horenblas S, Kurth KH. Health-related quality of life and psychosocial factors in patients with prostate cancer scheduled for radical prostatectomy or external radiation therapy. BJU Int 2003;92(3):217–222.

103. Saigal CS, Gornbein J, Reid K, Litwin MS. Stability of time trade-off utilities for health states associated with the treatment of prostate cancer. Qual Life Res 2002;11(5):405–414.

104. Gray RE, Fitch MI, Phillips C, Labrecque M, Klotz L. Presurgery experiences of prostate cancer patients and their spouses. Cancer Pract 1999;7(3):130–135.

105. Baider L, Walach N, Perry S, Kaplan De-Nour A. Cancer in married couples: higher or lower distress? J Psychosom Res 1998;45(3):239–248.

106. Hagedoorn M, Buunk BP, Kuijer RG, Wobbes T, Sanderman R. Couples dealing with cancer: role and gender differences regarding psychological distress and quality of life. Psycho-Oncology 2000;9(3):232–242.

107. Funch DP, Marshall J. The role of stress, social support and age in survival from breast cancer. J Psychosom Res 1983;27(1):77–83.

108. Greer S, Watson M. Towards a psychobiological model of cancer: psychological considerations. Soc Sci Med 1985;20(8):773–777.

109. Massie MJ, Shakin EJ. Management of depression and anxiety in the cancer patient. In: Breitbart W, Holland JC (eds). Psychiatric Aspects of Symptoms Management in Cancer Patients. Washington, DC: American Psychiatric Press, 1993:1–21.

110. McDaniel JS, Musselman DL, Porter MR, Reed DA, Nemeroff CB. Depression in patients with cancer. Diagnosis, biology, and treatment. Arch Gen Psychiatry 1995;52(2):89–99.

111. Bukberg J, Penman D, Holland JC. Depression in hospitalized cancer patients. Psychosom Med 1984;46(3):199–212.

112. Kornblith AB, Herr HW, Ofman US, Scher HI, Holland JC. Quality of life of patients with prostate cancer and their spouses. The value of a data base in clinical care. Cancer (Phila) 1994;73(11):2791–2802.

113. Bisson JI, Chubb HL, Bennett S, Mason M, Jones D, Kynaston H. The prevalence and predictors of psychological distress in patients with early localized prostate cancer. BJU Int 2002;90(1):56–61.

114. Davison BJ, Goldenberg SL. Decisional regret and quality of life after participating in medical decision-making for early-stage prostate cancer. BJU Int 2003;91(1):14–17.

115. Potosky AL, Legler J, Albertsen PC, et al. Health outcomes after prostatectomy or radiotherapy for prostate cancer: results from the Prostate Cancer Outcomes Study. J Natl Cancer Inst 2000;92(19):1582–1592.

116. Hu JC, Kwan L, Saigal CS, Litwin MS. Regret in men treated for localized prostate cancer. J Urol 2003;169(6):2279–2283.

117. Clark JA, Wray NP, Ashton CM. Living with treatment decisions: regrets and quality of life among men treated for metastatic prostate cancer. J Clin Oncol 2001;19(1):72–80.

118. Clark JA, Wray N, Brody B, Ashton C, Giesler B, Watkins H. Dimensions of quality of life expressed by men treated for metastatic prostate cancer. Soc Sci Med 1997;45(8):1299–1309.

119. Mehta SS, Lubeck DP, Pasta DJ, Litwin MS. Fear of cancer recurrence in patients undergoing definitive treatment for prostate cancer: results from CaPSURE. J Urol 2003;170(5):1931–1933.

120. McNair DM, Lorr M, Droppleman CF. Manual: Profile of Mood States, 2nd ed. San Diego: Educational and Industrial Testing Service, 1981.

121. Ullrich PM, Carson MR, Lutgendorf SK, Williams RD. Cancer fear and mood disturbance after radical prostatectomy: consequences of biochemical evidence of recurrence. J Urol 2003; 169(4):1449–1452.

122. Roth AJ, Rosenfeld B, Kornblith AB, et al. The memorial anxiety scale for prostate cancer: validation of a new scale to measure anxiety in men with prostate cancer. Cancer (Phila) 2003; 97(11):2910–2918.

123. Wallace M. Uncertainty and quality of life of older men who undergo watchful waiting for prostate cancer. Oncol Nurs Forum 2003;30(2):303–309.

124. Kaps EC. The role of the support group, "Us Too". Cancer (Phila) 1994;74(suppl 7):2188–2189.

125. Kunkel EJ, Bakker JR, Myers RE, Oyesanmi O, Gomella LG. Biopsychosocial aspects of prostate cancer. Psychosomatics 2000;41(2):85–94.

126. Austin JP, Aziz H, Potters L, et al. Diminished survival of young blacks with adenocarcinoma of the prostate. Am J Clin Oncol 1990;13(6):465–469.

127. Trapasso JG, deKernion JB, Smith RB, Dorey F. The incidence and significance of detectable levels of serum prostate specific antigen after radical prostatectomy. J Urol 1994;152(5 pt 2): 1821–1825.

128. Zincke H, Oesterling JE, Blute ML, Bergstralh EJ, Myers RP, Barrett DM. Long-term (15 years) results after radical prostatectomy for clinically localized (stage T2c or lower) prostate cancer. J Urol 1994;152(5 pt 2):1850–1857.

129. Abi-Aad AS, Macfarlane MT, Stein A, deKernion JB. Detection of local recurrence after radical prostatectomy by prostate specific antigen and transrectal ultrasound. J Urol 1992;147(3 pt 2): 952–955.

130. Paulson DF. Impact of radical prostatectomy in the management of clinically localized disease. J Urol 1994;152(5 pt 2):1826–1830.

131. ASTRO. Consensus Statement: Guidelines for PSA following radiation therapy. Int J Radiat Oncol Biol Phys 1997;37: 1035–1041.

132. Noble RL. Hormonal control of growth and progression in tumors of Nb rats and a theory of action. Cancer Res 1977; 37(1):82–94.

133. Schroder FH. Endocrine treatment of prostate cancer: recent developments and the future. Part 1: maximal androgen blockade, early vs. delayed endocrine treatment and side-effects. BJU Int 1999;83(2):161–170.

134. Kaisary AV, Tyrrell CJ, Peeling WB, Griffiths K. Comparison of LHRH analogue (Zoladex) with orchiectomy in patients with metastatic prostatic carcinoma. Br J Urol 1991;67(5):502–508.

135. Iversen P. Quality of life issues relating to endocrine treatment options. Eur Urol 1999;36(suppl 2):20–26.

136. Denis LJ, Carnelro de Moura JL, Bono A, et al. Goserelin acetate and flutamide versus bilateral orchiectomy: a phase III EORTC trial (30853). EORTC GU Group and EORTC Data Center. Urology 1993;42(2):119–129; discussion 129–130.

137. Crawford ED, Eisenberger MA, McLeod DG, et al. A controlled trial of leuprolide with and without flutamide in prostatic carcinoma. N Engl J Med 1989;321(7):419–424.

138. Denis L, Murphy GP. Overview of phase III trials on combined androgen treatment in patients with metastatic prostate cancer. Cancer (Phila) 1993;72(suppl 12):3888–3895.

139. Seidenfeld J, Samson DJ, Aronson N, et al. Relative effectiveness and cost-effectiveness of methods of androgen suppression in the treatment of advanced prostate cancer. Evid Rep Technol Assess (Summ) 1999(4):i–x, 1–246, I241–236, passim.

140. Bolla M, de Reijke TM, Zurlo A, Collette L. Adjuvant hormone therapy in locally advanced and localized prostate cancer: three EORTC trials. Front Radiat Ther Oncol 2002;36:81–86.

141. Messing EM, Manola J, Sarosdy M, Wilding G, Crawford ED, Trump D. Immediate hormonal therapy compared with observation after radical prostatectomy and pelvic lymphadenectomy in men with node-positive prostate cancer. N Engl J Med 1999; 341(24):1781–1788.

142. Orwoll ES, Klein RF. Osteoporosis in men. Endocr Rev 1995; 16(1):87–116.

143. Niewoehner CB. Osteoporosis in men. Is it more common than we think? Postgrad Med 1993;93(8):59–60, 63–70.

144. Townsend MF, Sanders WH, Northway RO, Graham SD Jr. Bone fractures associated with luteinizing hormone-releasing hormone agonists used in the treatment of prostate carcinoma. Cancer (Phila) 1997;79(3):545–550.

145. Hatano T, Oishi Y, Furuta A, Iwamuro S, Tashiro K. Incidence of bone fracture in patients receiving luteinizing hormone-releasing hormone agonists for prostate cancer. BJU Int 2000;86(4):449–452.

146. Melton LJ III, Alothman KI, Khosla S, Achenbach SJ, Oberg AL, Zincke H. Fracture risk following bilateral orchiectomy. J Urol 2003;169(5):1747–1750.

147. Daniell HW. Osteoporosis after orchiectomy for prostate cancer. J Urol 1997;157(2):439–444.

148. Kanis JA, Melton LJ III, Christiansen C, Johnston CC, Khaltaev N. The diagnosis of osteoporosis. J Bone Miner Res 1994;9(8): 1137–1141.

149. Finkelstein JS, Klibanski A, Neer RM, Greenspan SL, Rosenthal DI, Crowley WF Jr. Osteoporosis in men with idiopathic hypogonadotropic hypogonadism. Ann Intern Med 1987;106(3): 354–361.

150. Berruti A, Dogliotti L, Terrone C, et al. Changes in bone mineral density, lean body mass and fat content as measured by dual energy x-ray absorptiometry in patients with prostate cancer without apparent bone metastases given androgen deprivation therapy. J Urol 2002;167(6):2361–2367; discussion 2367.

151. Smith MR, McGovern FJ, Zietman AL, et al. Pamidronate to prevent bone loss during androgen-deprivation therapy for prostate cancer. N Engl J Med 2001;345(13):948–955.

152. Orwoll ES. Osteoporosis in men. Endocrinol Metab Clin N Am 1998;27(2):349–367.

153. Daniell HW. Osteoporosis due to androgen deprivation therapy in men with prostate cancer. Urology 2001;58(2 suppl 1): 101–107.

154. Higano CS. Management of bone loss in men with prostate cancer. J Urol 2003;170(6 pt 2):S59–S63; discussion S64.

155. Orwoll E, Ettinger M, Weiss S, et al. Alendronate for the treatment of osteoporosis in men. N Engl J Med 2000;343(9):604–610.

156. Diamond T, Campbell J, Bryant C, Lynch W. The effect of combined androgen blockade on bone turnover and bone mineral densities in men treated for prostate carcinoma: longitudinal evaluation and response to intermittent cyclic etidronate therapy. Cancer (Phila) 1998;83(8):1561–1566.

157. Higano CS. Bone loss and the evolving role of bisphosphonate therapy in prostate cancer. Urol Oncol 2003;21(5):392–398.

158. Smith MR, Eastham J, Gleason DM, Shasha D, Tchekmedyian S, Zinner N. Randomized controlled trial of zoledronic acid to prevent bone loss in men receiving androgen deprivation therapy for nonmetastatic prostate cancer. J Urol 2003;169(6): 2008–2012.

159. Vogelzang NJ, Breitbart W, Cella D, et al. Patient, caregiver, and oncologist perceptions of cancer-related fatigue: results of a tripart assessment survey. The Fatigue Coalition. Semin Hematol 1997;34(3 suppl 2):4–12.

160. Engelson ES, Rabkin JG, Rabkin R, Kotler DP. Effects of testosterone upon body composition. J Acquir Immune Defic Syndr Hum Retrovirol 1996;11(5):510–511.

161. Stone P, Hardy J, Huddart R, A'Hern R, Richards M. Fatigue in patients with prostate cancer receiving hormone therapy. Eur J Cancer 2000;36(9):1134–1141.

162. Krupp LB, LaRocca NG, Muir-Nash J, Steinberg AD. The fatigue severity scale. Application to patients with multiple sclerosis and systemic lupus erythematosus. Arch Neurol 1989;46(10):1121–1123.

163. Stone P, Richards M, A'Hern R, Hardy J. Fatigue in patients with cancers of the breast or prostate undergoing radical radiotherapy. J Pain Symptom Manag 2001;22(6):1007–1015.

164. Pawlikowska T, Chalder T, Hirsch SR, Wallace P, Wright DJ, Wessely SC. Population based study of fatigue and psychological distress. BMJ 1994;308(6931):763–766.

165. Strum SB, McDermed JE, Scholz MC, Johnson H, Tisman G. Anaemia associated with androgen deprivation in patients with prostate cancer receiving combined hormone blockade. Br J Urol 1997;79(6):933–941.

166. Herr HW, Kornblith AB, Ofman U. A comparison of the quality of life of patients with metastatic prostate cancer who received or did not receive hormonal therapy. Cancer (Phila) 1993;71(suppl 3):1143–1150.

167. Blanchard CG, Albrecht TL, Ruckdeschel JC. The crisis of cancer: psychological impact on family caregivers. Oncology (Williston Park) 1997;11(2):189–194; discussion 196, 201–202.

168. Valdimarsdottir U, Helgason AR, Furst CJ, Adolfsson J, Steineck G. The unrecognised cost of cancer patients' unrelieved symptoms: a nationwide follow-up of their surviving partners. Br J Cancer 2002;86(10):1540–1545.

169. Perry PJ, Yates WR, Williams RD, et al. Testosterone therapy in late-life major depression in males. J Clin Psychiatry 2002;63(12):1096–1101.

170. Pirl WF, Siegel GI, Goode MJ, Smith MR. Depression in men receiving androgen deprivation therapy for prostate cancer: a pilot study. Psycho-Oncology 2002;11(6):518–523.

171. Litwin MS, Lubeck DP, Stoddard ML, Pasta DJ, Flanders SC, Henning JM. Quality of life before death for men with prostate cancer: results from the CaPSURE database. J Urol 2001;165(3):871–875.

172. Melmed GY, Kwan L, Reid K, Litwin MS. Quality of life at the end of life: trends in patients with metastatic prostate cancer. Urology 2002;59(1):103–109.

173. Morris JN, Suissa S, Sherwood S, Wright SM, Greer D. Last days: a study of the quality of life of terminally ill cancer patients. J Chronic Dis 1986;39(1):47–62.

174. Steinhauser KE, Christakis NA, Clipp EC, McNeilly M, McIntyre L, Tulsky JA. Factors considered important at the end of life by patients, family, physicians, and other care providers. JAMA 2000;284(19):2476–2482.

175. Saunders Y, Ross JR, Riley J. Planning for a good death: responding to unexpected events. BMJ 2003;327(7408):204–206; discussion 206–207.

176. Murphy GP, Mettlin C, Menck H, Winchester DP, Davidson AM. National patterns of prostate cancer treatment by radical prostatectomy: results of a survey by the American College of Surgeons Commission on Cancer. J Urol 1994;152(5 pt 2):1817–1819.

177. Talcott JA, Rieker P, Clark JA, et al. Patient-reported symptoms after primary therapy for early prostate cancer: results of a prospective cohort study. J Clin Oncol 1998;16(1):275–283.

178. Stanford JL, Feng Z, Hamilton AS, et al. Urinary and sexual function after radical prostatectomy for clinically localized prostate cancer: the Prostate Cancer Outcomes Study. JAMA 2000;283(3):354–360.

1 3

Physical and Psychosocial Issues in Lung Cancer Survivors

Linda Sarna, Frederic W. Grannis, Jr., and Anne Coscarelli

Lung cancer emerged during the 20th century as an epidemic of enormous proportions.[1] A rare disease at the beginning of the past century, lung cancer continues to be one of the most common cancers in the world, affecting 174,470 Americans (92,700 men and 81,770 women) in 2006.[2] Mirroring changes in smoking patterns, the incidence of lung cancer among men continues to decline. Large-scale smoking among women occurred almost 20 years after men in the United States, with a subsequent delay in increased cases, peaking in the 1990s. Encouragingly, the most recent evidence demonstrates that lung cancer incidence among women is declining, as are death rates.[3] In 2000, approximately 13% of men and 17% of women (age-adjusted, 15% overall) diagnosed with lung cancer were expected to survive at least 5 years (an estimated 26,065 Americans each year).[2]

There has been minimal (albeit statistically significant) increase in the overall percentage of survivors over the past 30 years (13%, 1974–1976; 14%, 1983–1985; 15%, 1992–1999).[2] The focus of this chapter is on the emerging data describing the long-term medical and psychosocial consequences of survival from lung cancer and its treatment. In addition to length of survival, the physical, psychologic, social, and existential components of heath-related quality of life (HRQOL) data have been recognized as important outcome measures of lung cancer treatment for more than 30 years.[4,5] These measures are now a common part of clinical trials of patients with lung cancer,[6] but there is limited information about HRQOL of long-term survivors. In an extensive review of literature on HRQOL in patients with lung cancer, 151 studies were identified covering 1970–1995.[7] Almost all these studies focused on patients in treatment. Only one focused on patients with early-stage disease treated by surgery,[8] and only one study was identified with long-term survivors.[9] Since that review, there have been several additional reports[10–14] on survivors of lung cancer who were disease free and off treatment at the time of the data collection. Details of these studies and others focused on recovery after curative treatment are displayed in Table 13.1.

Lung cancer survivorship, in contrast to breast cancer survivorship, which has shaped the quantity and quality of survivorship research, is in its infancy. For the purposes of this chapter, studies published (in English) since 1980 that provide data about the physical functional status, HRQOL, symptoms, and other issues experienced by survivors after curative treatment are reviewed. Studies that only addressed cardiopulmonary function in the brief postoperative period are not included.

Survivorship and Lung Cancer

There are many survivors of lung cancer as a result of the high incidence of this disease when using the National Coalition of Cancer Survivors' definition, which is "from the point of diagnosis forward." However, with a definition that sets a defined time frame of "5-year survival" or "disease-free survival," the field of survivors is narrowed to a smaller number of patients and, thus, a more-limited opportunity for research. Survival following a diagnosis of non-small cell lung cancer depends primarily upon stage and effective treatment. Only 16% of patients are diagnosed with localized disease, 36% with regional disease, and 38% with distant metastasis.[3] Although more than 80% of patients with surgically resected stage IA disease may have 5-year disease-free survival, expectation of survival diminishes progressively through stages II and III and is rare in stage IV. If untreated, few patients, even with small peripheral stage IA tumors, survive 5 years.[15,16] The statistics for long-term survivors of limited-stage small cell lung cancer are even less optimistic. Only 6% of 144 patients with limited-stage disease treated in Canada survived longer than 5 years.[17]

Long-Term Impact of Curative Surgical Interventions

The majority of HRQOL studies including patients with lung cancer have focused on symptoms of and issues facing patients with advanced disease.[7] The quality of lung cancer survivorship and resulting physical impairment has been minimally addressed. The majority of medical issues surrounding lung cancer survivorship are related to curative surgical therapy and tend to be short term. A major consequence of the successful treatment of lung cancer arises from the

TABLE 13.1. Studies documenting symptoms, functional status, and quality of life of lung cancer survivors since 1980 (in chronologic order).

Author	Sample[a] characteristics: mean age[b], sex, ethnicity[c], education, marital status, health status	Disease characteristics/treatment/ follow-up period	Purpose/method Comparison group	Findings related to survivorship
Nou and Aberg[71]	$N = 69$ (34% of whom received surgery for cure, $n = 21$, 30% survivors) Age: 62 years Ethnicity: Swedish Health status: ND	Histology: bronchial carcinoma (1967 WHO classification) Stage: mixed Surgery: 27% pneumonectomy, 62% lobectomy, 13% nonresectional thoracotomies Follow up: 3–8 years Disease-free status not clear	Purpose: describe HRQOL and symptoms postthoracotomy, 1-month and at 3-month intervals Method: prospective evaluation of performance status by physicians Instruments: Carlens vitagram index (performance level, including working capacity, ambulation, symptoms, hospital treatment) Comparison groups: 28% nonresectional thoracotomy, 72% deceased patients	Good HRQOL among 5-year survivors: most capable of full-time work Initial preop HRQOL highest for long-term survivors Noncurative resection associated with lower HRQOL Specific information about symptoms not provided
Pelletier et al.[33]	$N = 47$ Age: 58 Sex: majority male Ethnicity: Canadian Health status: ND	Histology: ND Stage: ND Surgery: 43% pneumonectomy, 57% lobectomy Follow-up: approximately 3 months postop	Purpose: evaluate impact of lung resection on pulmonary and exercise capacity Method: prospective pre- and 3 months postop Instruments: Borg scale Spirometry, exercise testing Comparison: No	Lobectomy: 20% reduction in exercise capacity Pneumonectomy: 28% reduction in exercise capacity due to dyspnea Leg discomfort contributed to decreased exercise capacity postop; none were limited by thoracic pain Decrease in PF is a poor predictor of exercise capacity
Dajczman et al.[40]	$N = 56$ (91% with malignant disease) Age: 62 Sex: 50% male Health status: ND	Histology: ND Stage: ND Surgery: lateral thoracotomy by 1 surgeon; 13% received postoperative radiation Rx Follow-up: median 19.5 months (range 2 months–5 years), disease free at time of interview	Purpose: describe prevalence and impact of postop pain Method: cross-sectional Instrument: interview about presence, intensity, functional impact of postthoracotomy pain, and influencing factors; VAS for pain Comparison: none	Persistent pain: 55% 1 year, 45% >2 years postsurgery, 38% >3 years, 30% >4 years Pain group: 33% had constant pain, 43% numbness, 23% shoulder pain Pain interfered with daily lives (44%) Five used medication, 3 had undergone nerve block NS differences in demographic or disease/ treatment variables in groups with or without pain Patients with no pain reported functional limitations, numbness
Dales et al.[8] patients	$N = 91$ with lung cancer (of 117) Age: 65 Sex: 71% male Ethnicity: Canadian Health status: 14% had moderate/severe dyspnea preoperatively Tobacco use: 25% current smokers, 72% former smokers	Histology: ND Stage: ND Surgery: 73% Lobectomy, 20% Pneumonectomy Follow-up: up to 9 months	Purpose: compare pre and post (1, 3, 6, and 9 months) operative HRQOL Method: Prospective self-report Instruments: QL-Index, Sickness Impact Profile Clinical Dyspnea Index, Pneumoconiosis Research Unit Index Comparison: $n = 26$ who underwent thoracotomy without lung cancer	Dyspnea peaked at 3-months (34%), but continued for 10% at 6 and 9 months Patients with cancer had 2× decrease in HRQOL at 1, 3 months postop ADL returned to baseline at 6, 9 months HRQOL scores similar for all groups preop, with cancer had significantly greater deterioration postop Extent of resection and cancer dx associated with deterioration in HRQOL in SIP Older age associated with poorer scores on

Study				QL-Index
Schag et al.[9]	N = 57 Mean age: 62 Sex: 56% male Ethnicity: 93% white Education: 68% ≥ HS Marital status: 61% married Health status: 41% hypertension, 32% heart disease, 11% diabetes, 7% skin cancer, 11% alcohol use	Histology: ND Stage: disease-free Surgery: 84% had surgery (details not described) Follow-up: Mean 3.4 years since diagnosis, n=33 short-term (>2–5 years), n = 24 long-term (>5 years) survivors	Purpose: describe and compare HRQOL among lung, colon, and prostate cancer survivors Method: cross-sectional, self-report Instruments: Cancer Rehabilitation Evaluation System (CARES) HRQOL–LASA Comparison: survivors of colon (n = 117) and prostate cancer (n = 104)	Lung cancer survivors had more problems than other cancer survivors Disruptions in physical function and pain were frequent and severe problems (46% chronic pain from scars) Short-term survivors noted depression (51%) and anxiety (63%), and distress with body changes (35%), 28% report feeling overwhelmed by cancer 17%–45% report difficulties with partners (e.g., communication, expressions of affection), 79% decreased sexual contact and problems, 7%–27% difficulty in dating, 63% difficulty with memory, 25%–32% with difficulty thinking clearly Of the 1/4 working at the time of diagnosis, 96% of short-term survivors quit work due to disease and treatment
Cull et al.[48]	N=64, >2 years in remission Age: 61 (median) Sex: 51% male Ethnicity: Scottish Education: 19% > HS Health status: ND	Histology: SCLC Stage: 95% limited-stage disease Treatment: 80% PCI (50% with concurrent chemo) Follow-up: 2 to >8 years	Purpose: describe HRQOL and prevalence of neuropsychologic disturbances in long-term survivors Method: Instruments: clinical and neurologic examination, CT scan, neuropsychologic testing, HRQOL (RSC, HADS)	Abnormal neuro exams (24% of n =37), 16% with ataxia, 11% cognitive deficits; no association with abnormalities found on neuropsych testing: 81% (of 59) impaired on >1 exam, 54% ≥ 2 Most common HRQOL disruptions: fatigue (64%), lack of energy (59%), difficulty sleeping (54%), problems with concentration (54%); >1/3 had dryness of mouth, tingling hands/feet, pain/burning in eyes; psychologic distress similar to normative data for cancer survivors HADS (borderline/case level): 19% anxiety, 15% depression
Landreneau et al.[39]	N = 142 VATS, N = 97 thoracotomy (<1 year) n = 36 VAT, n = 68 thoracotomy (>1 year postoperative) Age: 60 (VATS), 59 (thoracotomy) Sex: 56% men (VATS), 42% men (thoracotomy) Health status: ND	Histology: malignant group: 66% of thoracotomy patients, 42% VATS Stage: ND Surgery: VATS, thoracotomy Follow-up: <1 year postop, >1 year postop	Purpose: compare prevalence and severity of chronic pain post-VATS vs. lateral thoracotomy Method: cross-sectional Instruments: Visual analogue scale to assess presence and intensity of discomfort, and shoulder limitations on the side of the operation Use of medication: Comparison: None	<1 year postop, VATS group had significantly less pain and shoulder dysfunction, but similar use of pain meds No significant differences >1 year postop
Hendriks et al.[23]	N = 100, N = 31 with HRQOL data (48%) response ND for HRQOL subset	ND for subset	Purpose: describe HRQOL 2.5 months postthoracotomy Methods: mailed questionnaire Instruments: EORTC QLQ = 30 Comparison: none	Good/excellent global HRQOL (56%) Poor/very poor HRQOL (26%) Higher percent of patients with pneumonectomy had lower scores Dyspnea (29%), pain (29%) no clear relationship of sx to extent of resection

(continued)

TABLE 13.1. Studies documenting symptoms, functional status, and quality of life of lung cancer survivors since 1980 (in chronologic order). (*continued*)

Author	Sample characteristics: mean age[b], sex, ethnicity[c], education, marital status, health status	Disease characteristics/treatment/ follow-up period	Purpose/method Comparison group	Findings related to survivorship
Zieren et al.[34]	N = 52 (12 months postoperative), n = 20 (pre- and postoperative data) Age: 61 years Sex: 73% male Ethnicity: German Marital status: 12% partnered Health status: ND	Histology: NSCLC Stage: ND Treatment Surgery: 81% Lobectomy, 10% pneumonectomy Adjuvant treatment: 25% radiation therapy Follow-up period: 1 year, 19% with recurrence	Purpose: describe HRQOL post surgery Method: mix of cross-sectional and prospective Instruments: EORTC HRQOL, Psychologist-rated Spitzer HRQOL Index Comparison: none	Dyspnea at exertion and pain continued at 12 months Physical dysfunction returned to preoperative level at 12 months postsurgery Emotional, social, and financial dysfunction was less severe, but continued postop Pneumonectomy was associated with more symptom distress and limitations in physical function, but not with greater emotional, social, or financial dysfunction NS differences based upon adjuvant treatment. HRQOL rated as higher by the external rater as compared to the patient. 12% employed full time Recurrence negatively impacted postop HRQOL
Bolliger et al.[30]	N = 68 Age: 61 Sex: 84% males Ethnicity: Swiss Health status: Preoperative FEV_1 = 2.38 (lobectomy), 2.50 (pneumonectomy)	Histology: ND Stage: ND Surgery: 74% lobectomy, 26% pneumonectomy Follow-up: 3 and 6 months postop	Purpose: compare effect of lobectomy and pneumonectomy on PFT, exercise capacity, and perception of symptoms Method: prospective, pre, 3, 6 months postsurgery Instruments: PFT Comparison group: none	Lobectomy: no change in exercise capacity; PFT significant decreased at 3 months and significant increased at 6 months (10% permanent loss) Exercise capacity limited by leg muscle fatigue and deconditioning Pneumonectomy: 20% reduction in exercise capacity; PFT significant lower at 3 months and did not recover at 6 months (30% permanent loss); significantly lower than lobectomy, exercise capacity limited by Dyspnea
Larsen et al.[28]	N = 57 with pre and post assessments Age: 59 (pneumonectomy); 67 (lobectomy) Sex: 72% male Ethnicity: Danish Health status: ND	Histology: NSCLC Stage: ND Surgery: 28% pneumonectomy, 72% lobectomy	Purpose: describe postop changes in cardiopulmonary function Methods Instruments: exercise testing, pulmonary function, arterial blood gas	Lobectomy: minimal change in lung function or exercise capacity Pneumonectomy: decrease in PF, but compensation due to better oxygen uptake; decrease in exercise values less than expected Change in FEV_1 was a poor predictor of change in exercise capacity Variable changes in PF and exercise capacity with some patient improving postop, some worsening, and some with little change
Mangione et al.[42]	N = 123 with lung cancer Age: 64 Sex: 54% male Ethnicity: 97% white Health status: 94% with at least 1 comorbid condition, 49% with >3	Histology: NSCLC Stage: ND Surgery: thoracotomy Follow-up: 6 and 12 months postsurgery	Purpose: examine HRQOL changes over time and compare HRQOL of patients undergoing elective surgery Method: prospective, pre- and postsurgery Instruments: SF-36, Specific Activity Scale, health transition questions and rating of general health Comparison: n = 236, with total hip arthroplasty, n = 95, repair of abdominal aortic aneurysm	Significant declines in health perceptions, physical function, role-physical, bodily pain, vitality, social function at 6 and 12 months after surgery Improvement in mental health and role-mental function over time By 12 months, physical function, bodily pain, health perceptions were lower than preop levels, but similar to population-based norms Compared to other groups, lung cancer patients continued to have the lowest health perceptions, lower role-physical and social function ratings

Study	Patient characteristics	Histology/Stage/Surgery/Follow-up	Purpose/Method/Instruments	Results
Nezu et al.[26]	N = 82 (including n = 10 undergoing lobectomy with hemodynamic data) Lobectomy: Age: 64 Sex: 84% male Ethnicity: Japanese Pneumonectomy: Age: 62 Sex: 90% male Ethnicity: Japanese Health status: FEV$_1$ % predicted: 86 (lobectomy), n = 6 hypertension, n = 2 chronic bronchitis	Histology: ND Stage: "operable" Surgery: n = 20 pneumonectomy, n = 62 lobectomy Follow-up: 3, >6 months postop	Purpose: assess effects of resection on exercise limitation Method: prospective, pre- and postop Instruments: exercise testing, spirometry, Borg scale (dyspnea) Comparison: none	Improvement in exercise capacity 3–6 months postop for lobectomy but not pneumonectomy patients Mean loss of exercise capacity (VO$_2$ max) after 6 months: 28% pneumonectomy, 13% lobectomy Changes in PF did not correlate with exercise capacity Dyspnea was a limiting factor in exercise testing for pneumonectomy (65% at 3 months, 60% after 6 months), leg discomfort continued as the limiting factor for the lobectomy group (58% at 3 months, 64% after 6 months)
Nugent et al.[36]	N = 106, n = 53 with follow-up data Age: 61–64 (by surgical procedure) Ethnicity: Irish sample Health status: Preoperative FEV$_1$ % predicted ranged from 71% to 82%	Histology: not reported Stage: ND Surgery: n = 13, pneumonectomy, n = 26, lobectomy/wedge resection, n = 13 thoracotomy (inoperable tumor) Follow-up: 3 and 6 months	Purpose: describe and compare the effects of different types of lung resections and thoracotomy alone (inoperable tumor) on exercise capacity Method: prospective, pre-, postsurgery Instruments: PF, exercise testing, Borg dyspnea scale Comparison:	Thoracotomy alone did not significantly affect exercise capacity Pneumonectomy: exercise capacity reduced by 28% Lobectomy: exercise capacity unchanged No significant difference in Borg dyspnea rating pre and post any procedures
Miyazawa et al.[27]	N = 8 Age: 67 Health status: FEV$_1$ % predicted = 67.2, VC = 3.47 Tobacco use: all had quit smoking after surgery (never smokers were excluded); smoking "piece-years" range 600–1,600	Histology: ND Stage: potentially resectable Surgery: lobectomy Follow-up: 4–6 months, 42–48 months	Purpose: to examine postop changes in cardiopulmonary function Method: prospective Instruments: PF, exercise testing, hemodynamic monitoring, Fletcher, Hugh-Jones' dyspnea index Comparison: none	None had any symptoms before surgery 63% had increased dyspnea scores at 4–6 months; at 42–48 months, all had decreased to preop levels except for 1 patient Symptoms not directly related to physiologic outcomes FEV$_1$ % predicted increased postop (77% at 4–6 months; at 72% 42–48 months); airway resistance at preop levels over time Long-term decrease in cardiopulmonary function
Sugiura et al.[41]	N = 22 VATS, N = 22 thoracotomy Age: 62 (VATS), 61 (thoracotomy) Sex: 83% men (VATS), 38% thoracotomy Health status: ND	Histology: NSCLC Stage: stage I Surgery: VATS, thoracotomy Follow-up: mean 21 months (VATS), 30 months (thoracotomy)	Purpose: describe and compare HRQOL post-VAT with thoracotomy Method: prospective; Instruments: self-report questionnaire regarding chest pain, arm/shoulder limitations, time to return to preop activity, satisfaction Comparison: none	NS differences in patient characteristics Significantly decreased in chronic pain, return to ADL, and improved satisfaction with VATS At 12 months, no patient who received the VATS reported posthoracotomy pain; 4 patients in thoracotomy group required narcotics at 12 months
Uchitomi et al.[14]	N = 223 with successful surgical resection Age: 63 years Ethnicity: Japanese Marital status: 82% married Education: 21% ≥ HS Health status: 23% < 70% predicted FEV$_1$, 6% history of depression Tobacco use: 41% current smokers, 24% former smokers	Histology: 68% adenocarcinoma, 21% squamous carcinoma Stage: 92% stage I or II Treatment: 96% lobectomy, 5% pneumonectomy Follow-up: 1 and 3 months postresection	Purpose: to describe depression at 1, 3 months post curative resection Method: prospective; Instruments: Psychiatric interview at baseline using criteria from the DSMMD, Profile of Mood States	Major or minor depressions: at 1 month (9.0%), at 2 months (9.4%), at 3 months (5.8%) Education level related to depression in the perioperative phase Depression preop was related to subsequent depression Lack of confidence in confidants (social support), pain and diminished performance status significantly associated with depression at 3 months

(continued)

TABLE 13.1. Studies documenting symptoms, functional status, and quality of life of lung cancer survivors since 1980 (in chronologic order). *(continued)*

Author	Sample characteristics: mean age,[b] sex, ethnicity, education, marital status, health status	Disease characteristics/treatment/ follow-up period	Purpose/method Comparison group	Findings related to survivorship
Uchitomi et al.[60]	N = 226 patients with curative disease Age: 62 years Sex: 61% male Ethnicity: Japanese Education: 66% > JHS Marital status: 82% married Health status: 22% < 70 & FEV₁% predicted 31% with prior history of depression, 43% with moderate/severe dyspnea	Histology: NSCLC, Stage: 76% stage I, 16% stage II Surgery: curative resection Follow-up: 3 months	Purpose: describe impact of physician support on psychologic responses post curative surgery Method: prospective; Instruments: Structured interviews 1 and 3 months after surgery using DSM-III-R, Profile of Mood States, Mental Adjustment to Cancer	Depression: 9% at 1 month, 6% at 3 months postop; 26% had hx of depression History of depression was related to psychologic distress postsurgery Dyspnea, FEV₁, and PS related to psychologic distress at 3 months 24% used the physician and 4% used nurses for social support Physician support related to decreased psychologic distress, helplessness/ hopelessness, and increased fighting spirit, not related to depression Physician support was the sole factor in a multivariate regression related to increased fighting spirit for females and patients with no hx of depression
Handy et al.[29]	N = 139, n = 103 with 6-month data Age: 62 years Sex: 59% male Health status: Respiratory function: mean predicted FEV₁ 76% Comorbid conditions: 30%, cardiac, 16% diabetes, 15% peripheral vascular disease Tobacco use: 40% smoking within 8 weeks of surgery	Histology: ND Stage: 67% had stage I or II Surgery: pneumonectomy (8%), lobectomy (78%) 58% had open thoracotomy, 1% video-assisted thoracotomy, 5% muscle-sparing thoracotomy Follow-up: 6 months (12% died within 6 months), includes 7 with metastatic disease	Purpose: compare functional status and QOL preop and 6-month post lung resection. Design: prospective Methods: prospective; Instruments: Short-Form 36, Ferrans and Powers Quality of Life Index Control: Age-matched healthy controls	Functional health status impaired Preop pain, impaired physical status, role function, social functioning, and mental health were present 6 months postsurgery Dyspnea significantly worse postop General health status, energy level unchanged Postthoracotomy/neuropathic pain was an issue for 8 subjects No age or gender differences Pre-operative DLCO (<45% predicted), not FEV₁, predicted postop HRQOL Adjuvant treatment, 6-minute walk, extent of resection, complications did not predict HRQOL 6 months after surgery
Li et al.[44]	N = 51 Age: 63 years (VATS), 67 years (thoracotomy) Sex: 74% male Ethnicity: Chinese Marital status: 71% married	Histology: 55% adenocarcinoma, 20% squamous Surgery: VATS (n = 27), thoracotomy (n = 24) Follow-up: minimum of 6-months postsurgery (range 6–75 months; for VAT (mean 34 months), for thoracotomy (mean 39 months)	Purpose: compare HRQOL and symptoms between VATS and thoracotomy Design: cross-sectional Instruments: EORTC-C30 core questionnaire, EORTC QLQ-LC13 (Chinese versions) Investigator developed additional surgery-related questions	NS differences in HRQOL or symptoms between VATS group and open thoracotomy group According to EORTC ratings: good to high level of functioning Symptoms continued, including fatigue, coughing, dyspnea, thoracotomy pain (74% VATS, thoracotomy, 75%) Most severe symptoms included coughing, fatigue, and arm/shoulder pain; 44% reported financial difficulties
Sarna et al.[10]	N = 142 (5-year minimum disease-free survivors of NSCLC) Age: 71 years Sex: 46% male Ethnicity: 83% Caucasian Marital status: 47% married Education: 28% ≥ HS Health status: 50% FEV₁ < 70% 60% had at least 1 comorbid condition, 50% reported 2 conditions (heart disease, 29% and cataracts, 55%, most	Histology: 59% adenocarcinoma, 35% squamous Stage: 80% stage I and II Surgery: 12% pneumonectomy, 74% lobectomy, 11% segmental/wedge Follow-up period: 10 years, range 5–21 years	Purpose: describe HRQOL Method: cross-sectional Instruments: HRQOL-Survivor, SF-36, CES-D, spirometry Comparison group: population-based norms	Majority reported positive attitudes: 71% described as hopeful; 50% described cancer as contributing to positive life experiences; 22% depressed (CES-D ≥ 16) Most serious issues: fatigue (27%), pain (24%), anxiety (30%), changes in self-concept (21%), changes in appearance (20%), 34% reported families experienced significant distress Lower HRQOL associated with depressed mood and being Caucasian Lower physical HRQOL linked to older age, poorer PF, living alone, longer time since diagnosis, depressed mood, more comorbid conditions

Reference	Sample characteristics	Clinical characteristics	Study design	Results
	common); 9% with second primary lung cancer, 17% with history of other cancers. Tobacco use: 76% former smokers, 13% current smokers			Most survivors had healthy lifestyles. Good/excellent health (37%), fair/poor health (30%). NS difference based upon clinical or demographic characteristics. 67% of smokers quit after diagnosis; 16% never smokers. Current smokers (13%) more likely to be male (32%) and single (60%), 28% exposed to secondhand smoke, 58% used alcohol (16% quit after diagnosis), 51% overweight (BMI ≥ 25); 16% obese (BMI ≥ 30). Current smoking, exposure to second-hand smoke, current drinking, and BMI ≥ 25 were significant predictors of poor health perceptions
Evangelista et al.[13]	As described above		Purpose: describe health perceptions and risk behaviors of survivors. Method: cross-sectional. Instruments: Perceived health status item (from Short-Form 36), self-report and biochemical verification of tobacco use, self-reported alcohol use, spirometry, BMI. Comparison group: none	
Maliski et al.[12]	I = 29 survivors within another study[10]. Age 72, 55% men. Marital status: 55% married. Ethnicity: 69% white. Education: 52% >HS. Health status: FEV1 % predicted, 59.8%. Average of 1.75 comorbid conditions. Tobacco use: 10% current smoking, 79% former smokers	Histology: 48% adenocarcinoma, 48% squamous cell. Stage: 72% stage I, 10% stage II. Surgery: 79%, lobectomy/wedge resection. Follow-up period: mean 11 years	Purpose: describe the survivorship experience in long-term survivors. Method: cross-sectional, qualitative interviews, self-report questionnaires, pulmonary function. Instruments: Interview questions about survivorship experience CES-D Spirometry. Comparison group: none	Themes related to physical and emotional well-being: (1) appreciation for life and a changed outlook, (2) taking control and appreciation of health, (3) overcoming and rationalizing changes in physical ability, (4) changed lifestyle, (5) giving and receiving support. 31% met CES-D criteria for potential depression and those in that group had more negative views of survivorship
Myrdal et al.[35]	N = 112, NSCLC. Age 67. Sex: 57% male. Ethnicity: Swedish. Health status: Preoperative pulmonary function: 33% < 60% FEV1. Tobacco use: 70% former, 11% current smokers	Histology: ND. Stage: 67% stage I, 17% stage II. Surgery: 22% pneumonectomy, 76% lobectomy. Follow-up: mean 48 months, range, 4–48 months	Purpose: describe symptoms and HRQOL postsurgery. Method: cross-sectional, mailed survey. Instruments SF-36, HADS, assessment of pulmonary symptoms. Comparison group: N = 121 post-CABG	Bodily pain was the only SF-36 subscale similar to a normative cohort. HRQOL scores comparable to patients who underwent CABG except for physical function, which was significantly lower. Social and mental health scores similar to normative standards. Dyspnea on exertion higher among those with lung cancer. 20% of patients had possible depression. Compared to never and former smokers, smokers had lower mental health (SF-36) and higher ratings of depression and anxiety
De Leyn et al.[20]	N = 77. Age: ND. Sex: ND. Ethnicity: Belgian. Health status: ND	Histology: bronchogenic ca. Stage: Surgery: sleeve-lobectomy. Follow-up: early postop recovery, 45.6% at 5 years	Purpose: to describe postop complications. Instruments: medical record. Comparison: none	Exercise tolerance and HRQOL acceptable and better than that reported for pneumonectomy. Five developed an anastomotic suture and required subsequent pneumonectomy

(continued)

TABLE 13.1. Studies documenting symptoms, functional status, and quality of life of lung cancer survivors since 1980 (in chronologic order). *(continued)*

Author	Sample[a] characteristics: mean age[b], sex, ethnicity[c], education, marital status, health status	Disease characteristics/treatment/ follow-up period	Purpose/method Comparison group	Findings related to survivorship
Welcker et al.[135]	N = 65 (n = 22 with 1-year follow-up data) Age: 65 Sex: 71% male Ethnicity: German Health status: ND	Histology: NSCLC Stage: surgery for surgical intent Surgery: variety of surgical procedures (n = 2 pneumonectomy, n = 36 lobectomy) Follow-up: 1+ year postsurgery	Purpose: to examine cost and quality of life after thoracic surgery Methods: retrospective, cross-sectional, mailed survey Instruments: SF-36, cost indicators, Qualys Comparison: none	SF-36 ratings for 2-year survivors generally lower than normative scores for those with COPD and with cancer Gain of 4.62 Qualys, with higher costs associated with resection with more-advanced stages and complexity of surgery
Nomori et al.[32]	N = 220 VATS: 28 ALT: 28 AAT: 28 PLT: 28 Age: 61–62/group Sex: 71% male	Histology Stage: 65% stage I, 10% stage II Surgery: VATS, ALT, AAT, PLT Follow-up: pre-, 1, 2, 4, 12, 24 weeks postsurgery for PF; 1	Purpose: compare differences in functional impairment by type of surgery Methods: retrospective Instruments: PFT, 6MW Comparison:	VC in all groups increased over time PLT had the greatest impairment in VC 24 weeks after surgery and in 6MW 1 week postsurgery; better functional recovery was associated with VATS and ALT procedures
Pompeo et al.[21]	N = 16 Age: 65 Ethnicity: Italian Health status: All had severe and diffuse emphysema before surgery	Histology: 9 adenocarcinoma, 5 squamous, 2 large cell Stage: 11 (T1N)M0, 5, T2N0M0 Surgery: VATS (n = 5 LVR, n = 3 wedge resections, n = 2 segmentectomy), open thoracotomy (n = 6 lobectomy) Follow-up: 46 months	Purpose: describe HRQOL in lung cancer patients with emphysema who underwent resection plus lung volume reduction Method: prospective assessments: preop, 6 (n = 16), 12 (n = 15), 24 (n = 13), 36 months (n = 9) Instruments: SF-36, Medical Research Council Dyspnea Index, 6-minute walk test, self-report postthoracotomy pain Spirometry Control: n = 16 healthy adults	Patients with end-stage emphysema and stage 1 lung cancer benefited from surgical resection Significant improvement HRQOL domains and dyspnea at 6 months, continuing through 36 months Some differences based upon type of resection No differences between lobectomy and VATS patients Pain peaked at 6 months and continued for a small subset throughout the assessment period 68% 5-year survival Analysis includes patients with recurrence and metastasis
Sarna et al.[11]	As described above[10]	As described above[10]	Purpose: describe respiratory symptoms and PF of long-term survivors Method: cross-sectional Instruments: self-report of respiratory symptoms, spirometry, SF-36 Control: none	2/3 of survivors reported respiratory symptoms: 39% dyspnea, 31% wheezing, 28% phlegm, 25% cough; 21% reported that they stayed most of the day in bed because of symptoms % predicted FEV₁ 68%; 21 % predicted <50% FEV₁ 36% moderate/severe obstructive and/or restrictive ventilatory impairment Survivors exposed to secondhand smoke 3× more likely to have respiratory symptoms Respiratory symptoms related to reduced physical function, role-limits physical, vitality, social functioning, general health, and increased bodily pain

ND, no data; NS, not significant; ADL, activities of daily living; SF-36, Short form-36; PF, pulmonary function, VAS, visual analogue scale; Qualys; quality-adjusted life years; VATS, video-assisted thoracoscopic surgery; MST, muscle-sparing thoracotomy; AAT, anteroaxillary thoracotomy; ALT, anterior limited thoracotomy; PLT, posterolateral thoracotomy; 6MW, 6-minute walk; SCLC, small cell lung cancer; PCI, prophylactic cranial irradiation; CT, computed tomography; neuropsych, neuropsychometric testing; HRQOL, health-related quality of life; RSC, Rotterdam Symptom Checklist; HADS, Hospital Anxiety Depression Scale.

[a] All available data reported.
[b] Mean age.
[c] In most cases denotes country of study

requirement for partial ablation of a vital organ. The pneumonectomy has been used successfully for lung cancer treatment since the 1930s.[18] Evidence-based strategies to enhance HRQOL, improve symptom control, and support recovery after curative surgery for lung cancer are almost nonexistent. Although the normal healthy individual can sustain the loss of one entire lung (pneumonectomy), most patients with lung cancer have comorbid illness. Many patients have sustained cardiopulmonary damage from long-term smoking and have increased risk of mortality following pneumonectomy (or in some cases even after lobectomy or limited resection). When comparing sleeve lobectomy with pneumonectomy, a meta-analysis of published studies from 1990 to 2003, using quality-adjusted life years (QALYS) as one of the outcomes, found that sleeve lobectomy resulted in better survival, and for patients who did not have recurrence, better HRQOL.[19] Other studies also support the superiority of lobectomy over pneumonectomy in terms of physical recovery.[20]

One recent advance in the treatment of early-stage lung cancer is limited resection performed by video-assisted thoracoscopic techniques (VAT) in patients with poor lung function. Patients with limited respiratory reserve are at increased risk for perioperative respiratory complications. Recent experience with the use of thoracoscopic procedures in benign lung disorders, especially emphysema, confirms that limited thoracoscopic lung resections can be performed safely in this setting, under select circumstances. Thoracoscopic pulmonary resection requires less time in hospital and reduces the duration of postoperative pain and disability. Better understanding of pulmonary function tests (PFTs) and limits of resection now allow resection of small peripheral tumors in patients with poor pulmonary function via open segmental resection, thoracoscopic wedge resection, or a combination of reduction pneumoplasty with wedge resection in carefully selected patients. The lung cancer surgery can even serve as a lung volume reduction intervention for these compromised patients. In a small study of 16 stage I non-small cell lung cancer survivors with severe emphysema who underwent a variety of surgical resections, including lung volume reduction, 68% had 5-year survival. These carefully selected patients had improved HRQOL (as measured by the SF-36), especially in physical functioning and reduction in dyspnea 2 years after surgery.[21]

As displayed in Table 13.1, a number of studies have identified lingering symptoms and issues faced by lung cancer survivors in the months and years after potentially curative treatment. Some prospective studies suggest a pattern of symptom resolution with full recovery 6 months after surgery, but others point to ongoing problems years later. Some studies have included comparison groups of patients with other forms of cancer or patients without cancer who underwent similar surgical procedures (e.g., thoracotomy). Although some studies have included mixed stage and histology of patients with lung cancer, the majority of studies address the issues of survivors of non-small cell lung cancer who underwent surgical resection with minimal attention to those with small cell lung cancer or those who have undergone adjuvant treatment. These posttreatment data, including both physical as well as emotional well-being, identify a range of issues faced by survivors of lung cancer and underscore the need to develop supportive care interventions. The perceptions of HRQOL by survivors are important, as they are linked to severity of symptom distress and have been associated with long-term survival.[22] Pneumonectomy has been more clearly associated with ongoing symptoms and reduced HRQOL.[23] Because of the lack of prospective data, few studies have reported patterns of symptom occurrence and resolution after curative treatment. A cross-sectional study of patterns of symptom distress studied 117 patients with lung cancer, enrolled within 100 days of diagnosis and receiving a variety of treatments. It found that those patients receiving surgery (n = 45) were noted to have decreased symptoms over a 6-month period.[24]

Available data describing the prevalence and patterns of lingering symptoms (dyspnea, pain, altered functional status/fatigue, emotional distress, cognitive difficulties, relationships, sexual dysfunction, and alterations in communication abilities) reported in long-term lung cancer survivors are described next.

Dyspnea and Pulmonary Impairment

The loss of functional lung tissue as a result of lung cancer surgery may result in transitory and permanent reductions in pulmonary function and, for some, physical disability. Pulmonary function can be affected by lung cancer and its treatment, by the consequences of the patient's past tobacco use, and by comorbid disease.[25] Changes in pulmonary function are variable and not a clear predictor of exercise capacity,[26] severity of dyspnea,[27] patients' perceptions of physical disruptions in day-to-day activities,[28] or even HRQOL outcomes.[10,29,30] Larsen et al.[28] note the variability of performance of lung cancer patients after resection. Based upon physiologic differences, resection of the right lung (contributing to 55% of overall lung function) might lead to more severe pulmonary consequences.[18] There are clear differences based upon the extent of resection. Bolliger et al.[31] reported reduction in PFT in the immediate postoperative period with recovery at the 6-month period for patients who underwent lobectomy. This recovery was not seen for patients who underwent pneumonectomy, similar to findings by Nezu et al.[26] Several studies support the benefit of the VATS procedure in improved functional recovery as compared to other approaches.[32]

Although dyspnea is not always a consequence of surgical treatment, the majority of studies reported ongoing problems of breathlessness in some survivors, often linked with reduction in exercise capacity.[8,21,23,26,27,29,30,33–35] Dales et al.[8] reported an increase in the prevalence of severe dyspnea in the first 3 months postthoracotomy, with reductions at 6 and 9 months, but with the continuance of severe dyspnea for 10% of the patients. Nugent et al.[36] reported long-term deficits in exercise performance in patients undergoing a pneumonectomy, with limited changes after lobectomy. The symptom dyspnea was the limiting factor in performance in exercise tests for the pneumonectomy group. Pelletier et al.[33] cited dyspnea as a factor attributing to dropout in exercise programs postthoracotomy. Zieren et al.[34] also reported continued dyspnea at exertion 1 year after surgery. However, Nugent et al.[36] reported no changes in dyspnea after surgery.

In a study comparing VATS to thoractomy, dyspnea (85% versus 75%) and cough (82% versus 75%) were continuing problems more than a year after surgery for both groups. Aging, tobacco use and comorbid conditions, in particular, may influence respiratory symptoms and level of pulmonary function. Uchitomi et al.[37] report the significant relationship of dyspnea to emotional distress in the postoperative period. This relationship was also reported by Sarna et al.[10] However, there is little research specifically looking at these issues in a systematic way. In addition to dyspnea, respiratory symptoms such as cough, phlegm, and wheezing continue to plague some long-term survivors and diminish HRQOL.[11]

Pain

In a recent review,[38] Rogers et al. reported on the incidence of chronic mild to moderate postthoracotomy pain, which was described as "under-rated" and affecting approximately 50% of patients. Chronic postthoracotomy pain along the incision line often has neuropathic features. It is less often associated with initial lung cancer surgery, but has been linked with tumor recurrence.[38] The etiology of long-term pain is not well established but may be caused by intercostal nerve damage. Several of the studies reviewed (see Table 13.1) describe persistent pain for some long-term survivors.[9,10,21,23,29,34,35,39–42] Not all studies are limited to patients with lung cancer; some included others who received a thoracotomy. Reports of lingering pain vary. Schag et al.[9] reported that 46% of survivors experience pain from scars postsurgery and 24% report aches and pains. In a study of 85 patients, 26 had moderate to severe pain 1 month after surgery. Gotoda and colleagues[43] reported that female gender and pain immediately postthoracotomy were predictive of pain 1 month and 1 year after surgery. Handy et al.[29] reported continued pain 6 months after surgery. Similarly, Pompeo et al.[21] and Zieren et al.[34] reported continued pain for some patients even 1 year after surgery. Pompeo et al.[21] also identified a subset of patients who continued to have lingering pain. However, Mangione et al.[42] and Myrdal et al.[35] reported that pain scores after surgery were similar to population norms 1 to 2 years after surgery.

Although the prevalence of chronic pain may be expected to differ by surgical procedure, especially with the emergence of the muscle- and nerve-sparing VATS procedure, reports do not consistently support significant differences. Landreneau et al.[39] reported less pain and shoulder dysfunction, but not a difference in use of pain medication.[44] Pain was reported by 71% of the thoracotomy group and 67% of the VATS group. Comparing the VATS with thoracotomy, specific type of pain included thoracotomy pain (74% versus 75%), chest pain (48% versus 29%), and arm or shoulder pain (59% versus 46%). One-third of both groups (33%) reported shoulder dysfunction. Neither Pompeo et al.[21] or Li et al.[44] report significant differences in pain when comparing lobectomy and VATS procedures. However, another study did support a beneficial difference.[41] Treatment strategies of postthoracotomy pain vary,[45] and reports for definitive treatment from clinical trials are not available.

Another painful and disabling condition is frozen shoulder, a potential postsurgical risk[46] affecting lung cancer survivors. However, there are no known studies describing the prevalence of this condition among survivors of lung cancer.

Altered Functional Status/Fatigue

Level of postoperative physical disability is an important consideration in examining the HRQOL of survivors. Although it is often related to dyspnea, decreased functional status may have other contributing factors as well, and the measurement is different. In fact, in surveying the views of a patient population at risk for lung cancer surgery ($n = 64$), many stated they would not undergo life-saving surgery if it resulted in permanent physical disability.[47] Early studies considering recovery from lung cancer surgery focused almost exclusively on pulmonary and cardiovascular function, exercise capacity, and predictors of those at risk for severe disability. Mangione et al.[42] note recovery of physical function after thoracotomy at 12 months, but never to preoperative levels. Compared to other surgical groups (hip replacement, repair of aortic aneurysm), survivors of lung cancer had lower physical function. In a small prospective study of recovery after lobectomy, Miyazawa et al.[27] reported that recovery to preoperative levels occurred approximately 1 year after surgery for most, but not all, patients. Improvement in exercise capacity also was noted by Nezu et al.,[26] but not for those who underwent pneumonectomy.

Many of these studies are limited in that a preoperative assessment was lacking and time since surgery in the postoperative assessment varied. Additionally, multiple factors, including comorbid conditions (e.g., emphysema) and impairments (e.g., arthritis), were not considered as contributors to physical function after surgery. When exercise performance is limited, deconditioning (often described as leg cramps) as well as dyspnea are factors.[33] In an older population of lung cancer survivors, comparison of physical function with other patient populations or normative standards is useful. In the 5-year survival group,[10] HRQOL scores for physical components showed a somewhat poorer status compared to norms of patients with cancer, older adults, and those with other chronic lung disease.

In addition to functional decline, fatigue has been identified as a troublesome symptom. It is unclear if these are associated with aging or comorbidity because few studies have comparison groups. In the study by Li and colleagues,[44] fatigue was the most commonly reported symptom more than 1 year postsurgery for patients who underwent a VATS (74%) or thoracotomy (92%), as was the case with long-term survivors of small cell lung cancer.[48] Fatigue also may accompany other symptoms. In a cross-sectional study assessing symptom distress in women with primary or recurrent lung cancer within the past 5 years, Sarna[49] found that when fatigue was present, 41% experienced frequent pain, 31% insomnia, 23% breathing difficulties, and 21% cough. No studies have reported fatigue after lung cancer surgery with adjuvant chemotherapy.

There appears to be a subset of survivors that reports reduction in energy and increased fatigue. In a cross-sectional study of 130 older patients with lung cancer 3 months after diagnosis (including 34 treated with surgery), risk for impaired physical functioning was strongly linked to preexisting physical impairment and symptom distress.[50] In Schag et al.'s study of lung cancer survivors,[9] almost all the shorter-term survivors reported significant decreases in their energy (84%). Fatigue also was the most common symptom reported by Sarna et al.[10] With the lack of age-matched comparison groups, it is difficult to tell how dissimilar these reports are from the population of older adults without cancer and with/or without other chronic illnesses. Schag reported on this issue comparing cancer patients to health controls using the same instrument. She notes that 84% of survivors had problems with functional health status compared to 22% of healthy controls in a previous study.[51]

Emotional Distress

Presenting evidence on the psychosocial issues and concerns of survivors of lung cancer is both a simple and complicated task. It is simple because there is a paucity of information and it is complicated by the absence of data and the clear definitions of survivor. It is important to note that positive as well as negative consequences may result from the experience of lung cancer.[52] In the qualitative study,[12] survivors described existential changes prompting them to "seeing life as a gift," "appreciating the little things in life," and "trying to live life to its fullest." However, some reflect that life after lung cancer is not a normal life, and there were multiple statements related to uncertainty. A review of available data provides support for the hypothesis that a subset of survivors experience ongoing psychologic distress such as anxiety and depression. Handy et al.[29] reported impaired mental health 6 months posttreatment, but Mangione et al.[42] noted improvement in mental health over time. Different measures were used to measure depression in the studies reviewed, and it is difficult to know whether the responses reflect a diagnosable depression (major or minor) or reflect a state of depressed feelings. Interestingly, in contrast to differences in physical function, pneumonectomy was not necessarily associated with greater emotional or social dysfunction.[34]

Depression

It may seem surprising to find reports of depression among the "fortunate few" who do survive lung cancer. The findings of disease-free survivors are surprisingly consistent with other studies that have looked at the global population of lung cancer patients which includes all stages of disease. Depression and emotional distress have been reported as higher among people with lung cancer than people with other cancers.[53] It is estimated that the incidence of depression in patients with lung cancer of all stages ranges from 15% to 44%.[7,14,54–57] Depressed mood in patients with cancer has been linked to increased reporting of symptoms.[8,57] In a study of 95 patients with newly diagnosed lung cancer of all stages, depression was linked to poorer prognosis.[58]

Interestingly, in a prospective study of survival and positive attitude (optimism) before a randomized clinical trial of chemotherapy and radiation therapy for unresectable non-small cell lung cancer,[59] mood did not influence or correlate with overall survival. According to Uchitomi's findings, depression did decrease over the year after surgery.[14,37,60] However Sarna et al.[10] reported that one of five long-term survivors required further workup for depression because of high CES-D scores and this score was also a major predictor of ratings of HRQOL. These reports underscore the importance of screening for depression as part of follow-up care. Depression is treatable, but it is unknown how many lung cancer survivors have this clinical diagnosis and are treated.

Anxiety and Fears of Recurrence

Many patients who survive a first lung cancer develop a second cancer, either a second primary lung cancer or a local recurrence. Additionally, patients with prior lung cancer are at high risk of development of second tobacco-caused cancers other than lung cancer. A few prospective studies[34] have noted significantly lower HRQOL scores for survivors who experienced recurrence compared to scores of those who remained disease free. The threat of recurrence is not unique to lung cancer survivors, and this fear has been noted in studies of disease-free survivors. In Schag et al.'s study,[9] 63% of lung cancer survivors reported anxiety, and 58% had worries about a cancer recurrence. Sarna et al.[10] reported 30% with anxiety, with 12% of survivors fearful of a second cancer, 11% fearful of a recurrence, and 11% fearful of metastatic disease.

Ongoing and quality communication with the healthcare team is essential throughout to course of treatment and during recovery. Because lung cancer has been so frequently fatal for patients, communications around survivorship issues and HRQOL may seem less important than for other patients with a better prognosis. However, it is important to recognize that there are phases of treatment, and it may be important to identify fears and issues facing survivors that lead to education, information, and interventions. For example, discussions about the potential consequences of curative treatment do not have to be limited to informing patients of potential risks.[61,62] It also can be an opportunity to prepare patients for survivorship. Resources available for rehabilitative support, including psychologic support, can be included in the plan for care.

Cognitive Difficulties

A meta-analysis of seven clinical trials demonstrated that prophylactic cranial irradiation (PCI) increased disease-free survival and decreased risk of brain metastasis for patients with small cell lung cancer.[63] Since the 1980s neurologic toxicity has emerged as a concern for some long-term survivors.[64] These problems include a range of abnormalities including problems with memory, concentration, parasthesias, and gait.[48,65–67] However, the etiology of cognitive impairment is not clear, with suggestions of abnormalities present before treatment.[17,67] Comprehensive information about the impact of cognitive impairment on HRQOL is needed in this population.

Cognitive problems also have been reported in survivors of non-small cell lung cancer. In Schag's study[9] (including patients with both small cell and non-small cell lung cancer), the majority (63%) of the short-term survivors noted that they had difficulty remembering things. Diminished ability to think clearly was associated with a diminished interest or pleasure in a recent study evaluating somatic symptoms of patients with lung cancer with major depression.[68] Sorting out cognitive difficulties from the effects of depression is an ongoing issue in cancer research but may be particularly relevant for this population.

Relationships

There are limited data describing the impact of lung cancer on marital and other relationships. In many studies information about marital status or living situations is unknown. Difficulties with relationships with families and friends were uncovered both by Schag et al.[9] and Sarna et al.,[10] but it is hard to determine if social support changed and whether there is an ongoing impact. This is clearly an area that could use additional investigation. Additionally, information about the impact of lung cancer on employment is limited.

Sexual Dysfunction

Disruptions in sexual function may be an issue for survivors of lung cancer as a result of diminished physical functional status, but data are practically nonexistent. Schag's study[9] reported on a range of activities related to intimacy among married and single individuals. In a study of 69 women with lung cancer,[69] including 38% treated with curative intent, sexual disruptions were reported by more than 20% of the sample.

Communication Ability

Complications of surgical treatment of lung cancer also could include vocal cord paralysis, although data about the prevalence of this condition among long-term survivors are lacking. Recurrent laryngeal nerve damage resulting from pneumonectomy, mediastinoscopy, or tumor invasion can result in laryngeal paralysis or paresis, causing hoarseness and soft whispery voice. This problem can have a profound impact on communication and ultimately HRQOL. In a rare study of 28 patients with vocal cord paralysis from cancer or its treatment (including 25% with lung cancer), HRQOL improved after thryoplasty.[70] Cancer patients had HRQOL and voice improvement similar to that of patients who received treatment for benign conditions. Improvements in HRQOL included physical function aspects that could be negatively affected by glottic incompetency.

Economic Impact

A few studies reviewed noted employment status and the impact of the disease on work situation, although many patients were retired at the time of diagnosis.[9,10] In some studies, return to work was viewed as a proxy for HRQOL among long-term survivors.[71,72] The impact of altered physical functional capacity after curative treatment and the long-term economic consequences on these survivors are unknown.

Support and Psychosocial Intervention

There is limited evidence as to the impact of community resources on the recovery and adaptation of lung cancer survivors. Community-based and philanthropic organizations have historically provided cancer patients and their families with essential services that have been unavailable from traditional medical sources, and reliance on these organizations is growing. A recent study[73] evaluated the resources that are available nationwide to provide support for patients with cancer and their family members, how these resources are used, and whom they serve. The primary mission of the organizations that participated in the study (32 of the 41 identi-fied) was information/referral centered. Of the 31 organizations reviewed, not 1 was devoted to patients with lung cancer, although two-thirds were specifically dedicated to patients with cancers other than lung. Problems identified for the one database of patients indicated that there is a strong need for assistance with personal adjustment to illness, financial concerns, home care, and transportation. The study also noted that the patients that are at the highest risk for developing cancer and dying of it are the least likely to utilize formal support networks. In addition, there were gaps noted in service provision. As medical environments provide less assistance for psychosocial needs, it will become incumbent upon these communities to provide assistance for patients, especially for those with lung cancer.

The Ted Mann Family Resource Center at UCLA's Jonsson Comprehensive Cancer Center has developed an approach to helping patients cope with the diagnosis of lung cancer at all phases of the disease. Funded by the surviving spouse of a patient who died of lung cancer, the Ann and John Nickoll Lung Cancer Support Program has established a variety of services for patients and family members. Patients and family members receive individual contact and psychosocial evaluation by a psychologist or social worker. Patients are offered a variety of services, including informational booklets with a library of resources, a support group for patients with lung cancer and their family members, lectures by healthcare professionals on the topic of lung cancer, individual and group programs to teach relaxation exercises and cognitive coping skills, and assistance with access to reliable web sites. Patients who are depressed receive individual counseling and are referred to psychiatry for medication evaluation if they are amenable to this type of intervention. Patients have welcomed this program of support. Some of the patients have commented, "Now we have what the breast cancer patients have," the standard by which all cancers are currently measured. The greatest difficulty that patients with lung cancer face, however, is the fact that so many cancers are found at a late stage, and patients must not only deal with the diagnosis of cancer but may have to grapple with declining function and the loss of their life in a relatively short period of time after the diagnosis. Although as yet untested, this resource may provide a model for comprehensive support for people living with lung cancer.

There is a small, but growing, network of patients and families who are participating in advocacy efforts that are primarily Internet based, as displayed in Table 13.2. Each of these organizations provides information about disease and treatment, organizes political advocacy efforts, and has a mission oriented toward better care and research for patients with lung cancer and links to other resources. These resources offer tips and suggest areas of need and intervention for survivors of lung cancer.

Although research on psychosocial interventions for a variety of types of cancer patients is not reviewed here, there is an extensive literature documenting the efficacy of a variety of interventions in diverse patient populations. These interventions are oriented toward improving the quality of life of patients with cancer through education, individual support, and groups. A recent meta-analysis of 37 published controlled studies that investigated the effectiveness of psychosocial interventions on HRQOL in adult cancer patients found that psychosocial interventions with durations of more

TABLE 13.2.   Resources for lung cancer survivors.

Organization	Web site	Purpose/mission
Alliance for Lung Cancer Advocacy, Support, and Education	www.alcase.org	National not-for-profit organization dedicated solely to helping people with lung cancer, and those who are at risk for the disease, to improve quality of life through advocacy, support, and education
American Cancer Society	www.cancer.org	Nonprofit provides general cancer educational and support services, including a Lung Cancer Resource Center that describes lung cancer, its risk factors, prevention, causes, detection, symptoms, diagnosis, staging, and treatment
American Society of Clinical Oncology	www.asco.org; www.plwc.org	Site run by the American Society of Clinical Oncology; provides up-to-date scientific information about lung cancer treatment, including links to many patient-focused resources
Cancer Care	www.lungcancer.org	Informational website sponsored CancerCare
Lung Cancer Online Foundation	www.lungcanceronline.org	Focus on improving the quality of care and quality of life for people with lung cancer by funding lung cancer research and providing information to patients and families; provides a comprehensive, annotated directory to Internet information and resources for patients and families
Lung Cancer Survivors for Change	www.lchelp.com/mambo	An organization composed of ordinary people who have survived lung cancer as well as family members of people living with lung cancer
National Coalition of Lung Cancer Survivors (NCCS)	www.canceradvocacy.org	Survivor-led advocacy organization working exclusively on behalf of this country's more than 9 million cancer survivors and the millions more touched by this disease; founded in 1986, NCCS continues to lead the cancer survivorship movement
Roy Castle Foundation	www.roycastle.org	Provides patient support and information network throughout Great Britain; every lung cancer patient and their family will have access to a comprehensive support, information, and advocacy service for all issues concerning lung cancer
Ted Mann Family Resource Center, UCLA Jonsson Comprehensive Cancer Center	www.CancerResources.mednet.ucla.edu	Provides education through streaming video as well as articles on all phases of the disease, including survivorship, and caregiver-oriented materials
Women Against Lung Cancer	www.4walc.org	Special focus on women with lung cancer, educates the public and health care professionals about women and lung cancer; provides a web listing of many lung cancer resources

than 12 weeks were more effective than interventions of shorter duration.[74]

Health Behaviors

Little is known about the health behaviors (tobacco use, alcohol use, nutrition/weight) and changes that may occur in response to the diagnosis or the perceived health status of lung cancer survivors. In an analysis of these factors, Evangelista et al.[13] reported that 70% of 5-year survivors reported their health to be good to excellent. Continued smoking, exposure to second-hand smoke, current alcohol use, and being overweight (body mass index of 25 or more) were significant predictors of poor health perceptions.

Tobacco Use and Cessation

Assessment of current and former smoking of lung cancer survivors is relevant because of the potential impact on recurrence, second primaries,[75–80] and comorbid conditions.

Smoking cessation can slow the decline in pulmonary function, and if smokers quit before extensive pulmonary damage, they may never develop clinically significant chronic obstructive pulmonary disease (COPD).[81] Approximately 90% of lung cancer cases are attributed to lifetime smoking.[82,83] Smoking continues to be the leading cause of preventable death in the United States,[84] and tobacco control is a priority for the American Society of Clinical Oncology.[85]

Rarely included in analysis of clinical trial data on survivorship are data about tobacco use. Amount of smoking (30 or more pack-years) has been shown to be an independent prognostic factor in a study of 375 patients who underwent complete surgical resection for stage I non-small cell lung cancer from 1981 to 1993.[86] Smoking is receiving special attention during clinical trials investigating efficacy of lung cancer screening.[87] At the time of surgery for lung cancer, many smokers may quit. However, some are unable to do so,[78,88–94] and others restart smoking during recovery. In Dresler et al.'s report,[93] 23% of patients who quit within the 2 weeks before surgery relapsed, and 61% who did not quit before surgery continued to smoke. She reports that 89% of smokers acknowledged receiving physician advice to stop smoking. Patients at highest risk for return to smoking were those with the briefest quit time before surgery. In a study of long-term survivors,[13] 13% continued to smoke after curative surgery. There have been several attempts to provide targeted smoking cessation interventions for survivors of cancer, including lung cancer.[79,95,96] However, it is important to note that former smokers continue to be at lifelong increased risk for lung cancer.[78,97] Minimal attention has been given to the risks of exposure to second-hand smoke, also a risk factor for lung cancer. This exposure was reported among 28% of disease-free survivors.[13]

Patients with lung cancer, including long-term survivors, may receive more attributions of blame and responsibility for their disease because of their smoking behavior. Clinically, patients have noted that they feel a judgment that comes from others (healthcare providers, family members, and friends) that they are responsible for their disease if they smoked. Additionally, patients who never smoked or who quit long before their diagnosis may feel unfairly judged. In a qualitative study of 45 patients with lung cancer, patients reported feeling stigmatized because of their smoking. Regardless of current smoking status, patients believed that that past or current smoking affected their quality of care, and for this reason, some concealed their diagnosis.[98] The individual smoker is blamed for his or her illness; even though he or she may have become addicted as a youth, little blame is aimed at the tobacco industry that misled the public about health risks. Only a few studies have explored causal attributions that might affect a patient's response to the diagnosis of lung cancer, especially in the case of a smoking history. There are data to suggest that medical staff's attitudes toward patients may be influenced by these factors as well.[99] In a study that looked at lung cancer patients' own attributions for the cause of their illness, it was found that while smoking cigarettes was the most frequently suggested causal factor, patients also tried to minimize the impact.[100] Eighty-one percent of patients put forward at least one statement that served to qualify or argue the relevance of smoking as the cause. For example, 41% of the patients indicated that "they didn't really know where the disease came from," others argued "they had always led a normal/healthy life, that non-smokers also got lung cancer, that there must be other causes for lung cancer, and that they had always been healthy." Patients are able to reduce their sense of guilt by diluting the cause of the disease; this allows the person to feel some responsibility without shouldering the full sense of blame. Despite the potential causes and responsibilities, there is a need to understand more about these processes and their impact on coping; however, understanding what patients must cope with is a significant concern.

Alcohol Use and Substance Abuse

Although tobacco use is associated with increased risk of alcohol use, few studies have reported on alcohol use or substance abuse among people with cancer, including lung cancer survivors. Among 5-year survivors,[13] 58% were reported to have had a drink in the previous month, with 3% reporting more than 8 drinks in one sitting. As described previously, alcohol use among survivors was associated with poorer perceptions of health.

Nutrition and Weight

There are limited data about weight, nutritional intake, and physical activity that can be used to recommend lifestyle changes for lung cancer survivors. Evangelista et al.[13] reported that 51% of survivors were overweight, including 23% with a body mass index of 30 or more. Recently, a panel of experts convened by the American Cancer Society reviewed the available scientific evidence regarding the benefit of nutritional and activity interventions to decrease recurrence, improve overall survival, and increase HRQOL. They concluded (with an indication of the strength of the evidence as "probable" or "possible" benefit) that lung cancer survivors should strive for a healthy weight during treatment and recovery, and increase fruit, vegetable, and omega 3 fatty acids uptake (especially in the face of weight loss).[101] Additionally, increased activity after treatment was recommended to increase overall survival and HRQOL. There was insufficient evidence for recommendations regarding total fat intake or intake of fiber or soy. The negative impact of tobacco use on decreasing nutrition was noted. Limited information is available about nutritional supplements and the lung cancer survivor, although two previous trials of beta-carotene pills demonstrated an increased risk of lung cancer in smokers.[102,103] A current clinical trial is investigating the potential benefit of selenium supplements in reducing risk of lung cancer recurrence.[104]

Factors Associated with Increased Problems

Although prognostic variables associated with survival have been well studied, factors associated with increased morbidity and diminished HRQOL among disease-free survivors have received limited attention. Age, sex, race/ethnicity, socioeconomic status, and comorbidity have been suggested to contribute to differences.

Age

Older age at diagnosis may influence recovery needs as well as occurrence of long-term sequelae. With the growing number of older Americans, many of whom have had a lifetime of tobacco use and exposure, lung cancer incidence among the elderly can be expected to climb along with the burden of other tobacco-related comorbidities.[84] In a study of patients with limited small cell lung cancer, older patients were more likely to have poorer performance status, more likely to experience poorer survival, and less likely to receive the full extent of optimal treatment.[105] However, older age and comorbidity were not directly related to survival. In Sarna's study,[10] older age was associated with poorer physical function. In a study of physical functioning among older cancer patients, patients who were 3 to 6 weeks post lung cancer surgery ($n = 32$) had significantly lower physical function and more limitations than older patients who had undergone surgery for breast, colon, or prostate surgery.[106] In a cross-sectional study of 133 older patients with lung cancer (over 65 years of age) with various stages of disease and treatment ($n = 26$, including 11 with adjuvant treatment), prior physical function, symptom severity, and older age were predictors of diminished physical functioning.[107]

Sex Differences

As reviewed by Patel et al.,[108] there are important sex differences in lung cancer that may affect survivorship, including the generally female advantage for long-term survival, and differential response to treatment. However, women may be at increased susceptibility to the carcinogens of tobacco[109] and are more likely to be diagnosed with adenocarcinoma.[108,110] Additionally, younger female nonsmokers appear to be at increased risk for lung cancer.[111] However, sex differences in physical and psychologic dimensions of HRQOL are less clear among long-term survivors. None of the studies reviewed supported sex differences in pulmonary function of exercise capacity, although many had only a small subset of women. Sarna et al.[10] reported that women survivors were more likely to live alone and had significantly higher ratings in the existential/spiritual domain of HRQOL as compared to men. In the study by Uchitomi et al.,[60] findings indicate that female patients, but not male patients, did benefit from physicians' social support.

Race/Ethnicity and Socioeconomic Status

Lung cancer incidence varies by race/ethnicity and social status, and these differences have been attributed to differences in lung cancer survivorship.[112] Over 45 million Americans continue to smoke. The gap between smoking among the higher and lower socioeconomic classes is widening, with 32.9% of those below the poverty line smoking as compared to 22.2% at or above the poverty level.[113] Lung cancer is fast becoming a cancer of the impoverished, poorly educated, and ethnic minorities,[114,115] but it is not clear how these factors influence survivorship. Tobacco use has been suggested as a cause of the large differential in male black cancer deaths over the past several decades.[116] African-Americans are less likely to be diagnosed with localized disease as compared to whites (14% versus 16%), and there has been minimal change in survivorship over time (1974–1976, 11%; 1983–1985, 11%; 1992–1999, 12%).[2] A variety of factors have been suggested to account for this disturbing difference, including differences in access to care. Using Surveillance, Epidemiology, and End Results (SEER) data between 1985 and 1993 for black (n = 860) and white (n = 10,124) patients with resectable non-small cell lung cancer, 12.7% fewer black patients in comparison with white patients received potentially curative resection.[117] This unequal treatment resulted in racial differences in survival, as has been reported by others.[118]

Long-term survivors of lung cancer are more likely to come from higher socioeconomic groups.[112] Socioeconomic status has been related to stage at diagnosis and, thus, survivorship.[118,119] Using SEER data for all races from 1995–1999, for those below the poverty rate, 25.3% and 59% of lung cancer patients were diagnosed with regional and distant disease, respectively. Additionally, in a prospective cross-sectional study of 129 newly diagnosed patients with non-small cell lung cancer (including 6 who received surgery), those with lower socioeconomic status, regardless of clinical status, had more health problems and poorer quality of life than those who were affluent.[120]

Comorbidity

In evaluating the HRQOL and health status of survivors, the presence of comorbid conditions, especially those associated with tobacco-related illnesses, may more directly affect HRQOL ratings than the cancer or its treatment. However, there has been limited investigation in this area. Few studies reviewed have adequately documented comorbid conditions among patients who have undergone surgery for lung cancer.[121] In a survey (including preoperative patient history) of 2,189 patients who underwent surgery for lung cancer in Spain, 73% reported at least one comorbid condition, including 50% COPD, 16.5% hypertension, 13.5% heart disease, 10% peripheral vascular disease, and 9% diabetes. Comorbidity was higher in older age groups, but smoking status was not reported. These findings of comorbidity were similar to findings of Sarna et al.[10] among 142 disease-free survivors, in which 70% reported one or more conditions: 28.9% heart disease, 17.6% COPD, 16.9% peptic ulcer disease, 13.4% diabetes, and 16% with reports of other cancers. Fewer comorbid conditions were significantly related to higher physical HRQOL scores, especially for survivors with known heart disease, and contributed to the statistical model for overall HRQOL. Schag et al.[9] found similar results: 32% cardiovascular disease, 41% hypertension, 11% diabetes, and 28% other illnesses; however, a comorbidity index was not predictive of HRQOL for the lung cancer survivors. The Karnofsky performance status was significant, which may be in part a surrogate for the combined effect of comorbid illnesses.

Long-term tobacco use can complicate recovery from lung cancer and its treatment[122] and increase the potential for other and tobacco-related comorbid conditions. Because smoking is a major risk for cardiovascular disease and increases the risk of disease in the presence of other risk factors (e.g., untreated hypertension),[123] the assessment of the impact of tobacco-related comorbidity is essential to survivorship concerns. Additionally, chronic obstructive pulmonary disease (COPD), now the fourth leading cause of death in the United States, continues to increase, especially among women.[123] Similar to lung cancer, more than 90% of cases of COPD are due to smoking; 15% of smokers develop significant COPD.[81] Additionally, COPD has been postulated as a risk factor for lung cancer.[124] Lung function declines more rapidly in smokers as compared to nonsmokers and is associated with progressive disability.[125] Twenty-five percent of patients with small cell lung cancer were noted to have COPD at diagnosis, and 15% had heart disease; however, the prevalence among the 60 long-term survivors is not reported.[72] In a cross-sectional study of 129 older patients with lung cancer at various stages of disease, an average of 3.1 comorbid conditions was reported.[107]

Limits to Current Studies of Lung Cancer Survivors

There are numerous limitations to the current studies describing issues facing lung cancer survivors. A variety of instruments have been used, limiting comparisons across studies. Several have used standardized instruments such as the Center for Epidemiology Status-Depression (CES-D) to assess depression that allow score comparison with normal populations. Other studies have allowed comparison of scores across cancer survivors. Comparing survivors of lung cancer to other populations of survivors of cancer and to populations without major illness is essential in evaluating generalizability of research among survivors. However, further qualitative studies also are needed that provide details about the survivors' lives, identifying positive and negative outcomes.

To determine if these findings are different from or similar to those in others with chronic illness or others with cancer, comparison groups are important. This differences are beyond the extent of surgery alone, as long-term survivors were noted to have higher preoperative HRQOL, when compared to those who suffered recurrence.[71] A health utility score, a global indicator of health reflecting HRQOL, allows for comparisons across studies. This strategy was used in a study using population-based cross-sectional data from the National Health Interview Survey (1998 cohort) of 692 long-term survivors recovering from surgical cancer treatment: breast (*n* = 377), colon (*n* = 169), melanoma (*n* = 92), and lung cancer (*n* = 54, 50% females). In the acute less than 1-year time period, the scores for the lung cancer survivors (0.42, with 1.0 indicating perfect health), were significantly lower than for the other survivor groups.[126] However, the scores in the longer term cohort (more than 5 years) increased by 47% to 0.62. The presence of pain and angina contributed to poorer scores in long-term survivors. In Schag's study,[9] there was a greater frequency of psychologic distress in patients with lung cancer than the survivors of colon and prostate cancer.

Recommendations to Support Recovery of Lung Cancer Survivors

Based on the available evidence, several interventions are essential to decrease morbidity and promote HRQOL among lung cancer survivors. As a diagnosis of any life-threatening illness such as lung cancer offers clinicians a "teachable moment", recovery can be the impetus for important life changes and behavioral interventions. (1) All lung cancer survivors who smoke must be offered/referred to support and resources to promote tobacco cessation. (2) Because a significant number of survivors experience serious emotional distress in the face of curative treatment, vigilant attention is needed in the ongoing assessment to detect psychosocial problems and to ensure referral for subsequent treatment of those with clinical symptomatology. (3) There should be ongoing assessment and treatment of postthoracotomy pain. (4) Physical rehabilitation must be promoted, especially among those with evidence of disability before curative treatment. (5) Interventions to provide interventions to support relief of dyspnea should be offered to those with this symptom. (6) Changes in lifestyle including healthy diet and activity to promote HRQOL and reduce disability should be supported. (7) There should be identification of and intervention with high-risk patients with known risk factors for morbidity after curative treatment.

A comprehensive wellness approach to survivorship requires that clinicians challenge existing nihilistic views of the curability of lung cancer in general, including negative attitudes toward investing in efforts to support HRQOL regardless of the length of survival. Many of these interventions may be synergistic, such as the decrease in depression associated with exercise. Additionally, those with stable disease may live for many years with lung cancer. Although they may not be "disease free," they should not be neglected in the efforts to improve coping and living with uncertainty while reducing physical and emotional distress.

Future Research

The excellent survival of individuals treated with adequate surgical resection in stage 1 non-small cell lung cancer suggests that increasing survivorship is linked with early detection. Henschke and her colleagues at Cornell University conducted a prospective single-arm trial of low-dose noncontrast spiral computerized tomography (CT) in high-risk patients and demonstrated that CT is three times as sensitive in the detection of small pulmonary nodules as chest roentgenogram and that 80% of lung cancer is detected by this methodology in stage IA.[127]

The National Lung Screening Trial is underway to evaluate current and former smokers aged 55 to 74 at risk for cancer.[128] Findings from standard chest X-rays will be compared with spiral computed tomography (CT) scans to see if early detection of small potentially curable lesions will result in reduced deaths from lung cancer. Thus, an increased number of disease-free survivors might be anticipated, making information about the issues associated with survivorship all the more important. Regardless of efforts to prevent tobacco use and to support cessation, former smokers will continue at higher risk. Hundreds of thousands of Americans will be at risk for lung cancer in the next decades. It is also important to acknowledge the lack of information about long-term survivors with advanced-stage disease. For example, in a few selected cases of patients with isolated brain metastasis, long term survival (more than 10 years) occurred after surgical removal of tumor.[129]

Much more evidence is needed to provide a clear understanding and support for interventions to prevent or reduce physical and psychosocial sequelae of lung cancer and its treatment.[130] Further research is needed to monitor the course of symptoms post treatment and to evaluate strategies for reducing overall symptom burden and improving HRQOL. The studies reviewed are limited primarily because of small sample size and the cross-sectional nature of the design. There are almost no prospective studies documenting the course of survivors who have received adjuvant treatment. Although Schumacher et al. reported that preoperative chemoradiation did not significantly reduce HRQOL in 54 patients in the immediate posttreatment time frame, data for long-term survivors were not available.[131] There is almost no information available about the issues of survivors of small cell lung cancer. Although smoking cessation is included in recommendations for follow-up and surveillance,[132] it is clear from this review of the literature that there is strong evidence to support monitoring physical and emotional well-being after treatment as well.

There are minimal reports of efforts to promote wellness after curative treatment or to examine the efficacy of rehabilitation programs for lung cancer survivors. Future research needs to address the wide range of problems with an eye toward developing a body of literature in which one study can be compared with another. Further research is needed to evaluate available instruments and determine how to get the most information, to provide opportunities for comparison and generalizations across studies, and to not overburden respondents. The work to date represents a start in the understanding of the needs of lung cancer survivors, but it raises more questions than it answers. Some have expressed concerns that if the perception of the physician is that surgery would result in substantial reduction in HRQOL, curative treatment would not be offered, regardless of the patient's view.[133] There are subsets of patients who have significant difficulties in a range of areas. More research is needed in non-white samples, from a variety of socioeconomic strata, and the inclusion of family members will provide a more complete view of the impact and needs of survivors.

Intervention studies such as targeting depressed patients might involve both psychologic interventions oriented toward cognitive coping as well as medication trials. The role of multidisciplinary care teams involved in the coaching, support, and physical reconditioning posttreatment need to be explored. The interaction between beliefs and behaviors on the part of the medical team with the patients' belief systems may lead to ways to create greater support and interaction. Additionally, the involvement of survivor participants in the development and monitoring of this research would be useful.

Limiting research for survivors of lung cancer to the disease-free period after 5 years is far too narrow. There is limited knowledge about the period after treatment is completed and before recurrence or second primaries. Newer therapies for advanced non-small cell lung cancer have resulted in improved HRQOL and symptom relief.[134] These needs and issues faced by these survivors with stable disease also need attention.

The evidence base for frequency and type of screening test is important. This information is important in exploring the need for rehabilitation and support. According to findings from available research, lung cancer survivors are diverse, with different profiles of comorbidity, and different vulnerabilities and needs for rehabilitation. Future studies are needed to explore the need to test tailored assessments and interventions so that those at highest risk are appropriately treated to prevent unnecessary short- and long-term morbidity. Because of the relatively small number of lung cancer survivors, the development of a database through a clinical trial mechanism would be useful. Additionally, the quality and the impact of the explosion of web-based sources for cancer survivors, including lung cancer survivors, on HRQOL has not been evaluated.

References

1. Centers for Disease Control. Ten great public health achievements—United States, 1900–1999. MMWR (Morb Mortal Wkly Rep) 1999;48:241–243.
2. Jemal A, Siegel R, Ward E, Murray T, Xu J, Smigal C, Thun MJ. Cancer statistics, 2006. CA Cancer J Clin 2006;56:106–130.
3. Jemal A, Clegg LX, Ward E, et al. Annual report to the nation on the status of cancer, 1975–2001, with a special feature regarding survival. Cancer (Phila) 2004;101:3–27.
4. Carlens EDG, Nou E. Comparative measurements of quality of survival of lung cancer patients after diagnosis. Scand J Respir Dis 1970;51:268–275.
5. Carlens EDG, Nou E. An attempt to include "quality of life" in evaluation of survival in bronchial cancer therapy. Bronches 1971;21:215–219.
6. Sarna L, Reidinger MS. Assessment of quality of life and symptom improvement in lung cancer clinical trials. Semin Oncol 2004;31(suppl 9):1–10.
7. Montazeri A, Gillis CR, McEwen J. Quality of life in patients with lung cancer: a review of literature from 1970 to 1995. Chest 1998;113:467–481.
8. Dales RE, Belanger R, Shamiji FM, et al. Quality of life following thoracotomy for lung cancer. J Clin Epidemiol 1994;47: 1443–1449.
9. Schag CAC, Ganz PA, Wing DS, et al. Quality of life in adult survivors of lung, colon and prostate cancer. Qual Life Res 1994;3:127–141.
10. Sarna L, Padilla G, Holmes C, et al. Quality of life of long-term survivors of non-small cell lung cancer. J Clin Oncol 2002;20: 2920–2929.
11. Sarna L, Evangelista L, Tashkin D, et al. Impact of respiratory symptoms and pulmonary function on quality of life of long-term survivors of non-small cell lung cancer. Chest 2004;125: 439–445.
12. Maliski SL, Sarna L, Evangelista L, et al. The aftermath of lung cancer: balancing the good and bad. Cancer Nurs 2003;26: 237–244.
13. Evangelista LS, Sarna L, Brecht ML, et al. Health perceptions and risk behaviors of lung cancer survivors. Heart Lung 2003;32: 131–139.
14. Uchitomi Y, Mikami I, Kugaya A, et al. Depression after successful treatment for nonsmall cell lung carcinoma. A 3-month follow-up study. Cancer (Phila) 2000;89:1172–1179.
15. Motohiro A, Ueda H, Komatsu H, et al. Prognosis of non-surgically treated, clinical stage I lung cancer patients in Japan. Lung Cancer 2002;36:65–69.
16. McGarry RC, Song G, des Rosiers P, et al. Observation-only management of early stage, medically inoperable lung cancer: poor outcome. Chest 2002;2002:1155–1158.
17. Tai THP, Yu E, Dickof P, et al. Prophylactic cranial irradiation revisited: cost-effectiveness and quality of life in small-cell lung cancer. Int J Radiat Oncol Biol Phys 2002;52:68–74.
18. Fuentes PA. Pneumonectomy: historical perspective and prospective insight. Eur J Cardiothorac Surg 2003;23:439–445.
19. Ferguson MK, Lehman AG. Sleeve lobectomy or pneumonectomy: optimal management strategy using decision analysis techniques. Ann Thorac Surg 2003;76:1782–1788.
20. De Leyn P, Rots W, Deneffe G, et al. Sleeve lobectomy for non-small cell lung cancer. Acta Chir Belg 2003;103:570–576.
21. Pompeo E, De Dominicis E, Ambrogi V, et al. Quality of life after tailored combined surgery for stage 1 non-small-cell lung cancer and severe emphysema. Ann Thorac Surg 2003;76:1821–1827.
22. Montazeri A, Milroy R, Hole D, et al. Anxiety and depression in patients with lung cancer before and after diagnosis: findings from a population in Glasgow, Scotland. J Epidemiol Community Health 1998;52(3):203–204.
23. Hendriks J, Van Schil P, Van Meerbeeck J, et al. Short-term survival after major pulmonary resections for bronchogenic carcinoma. Acta Chir Belg 1996;96:273–279.
24. Cooley M. Patterns of symptom distress in adults receiving treatment for lung cancer. J Palliat Care 2002;18:150–159.
25. Pelkonen M, Notkola I-L, Tukianinen H, et al. Smoking cessation, decline in pulmonary function and total mortality: a 30 year follow up study among the Finnish cohorts of the Seven Counties Study. Thorax 2001;56:703–707.
26. Nezu K, Kushibe K, Tojo T, et al. Recovery and limitation of exercise capacity after lung resection for lung cancer. Chest 1998;113:1511–1516.

27. Miyazawa M, Haniuda M, Nishimura H, et al. Long-term effects of pulmonary resection on cardiopulmonary function. J Am Coll Surg 1999;189:26–33.

28. Larsen KR, Svendsen UG, Milman N, et al. Cardiopulmonary function at rest and during exercise for bronchial resection for bronchial carcinoma. Ann Thorac Surg 1997;64:960–964.

29. Handy JR, Asaph JW, Skokan L, et al. What happens to patients undergoing lung cancer surgery? Outcomes and quality of life before and after surgery. Chest 2002;122:21–30.

30. Bolliger CT, Jordan P, Soler M, et al. Pulmonary function and exercise capacity after lung resection. Eur Respir J 1996;9:415–421.

31. Bolliger CT, Zellweger JJP, Danielsson T, et al. Influence of long-term smoking reduction on health risk markers and quality of life. Nicotine Tobacco Res 2002;4:433–439.

32. Nomori H, Ohtsuka T, Horio H, et al. Difference in the impairment of vital capacity and 6-minute walking after a lobectomy performed by thoracoscopic surgery, an anterior limited thoracotomy, an anteroaxillary thoracotomy, and a posterolateral thoracotomy. Surg Today 2003;33:7–12.

33. Pelletier C, Lapointe L, LeBlanc P. Effects of lung resection on pulmonary function and exercise capacity. Thorax 1990;1990:497–502.

34. Zieren HU, Muller JM, Hamberger U, et al. Quality of life after surgical therapy of bronchogenic carcinoma. Eur J Cardiothorac Surg 1996;10:233–237.

35. Myrdal G, Valtysdottir S, Lambe M, et al. Quality of life following lung cancer surgery. Thorax 2003;58:194–197.

36. Nugent AM, Steele IC, Carragher AM, et al. Effect of thoracotomy and lung resection on exercise capacity in patients with lung cancer. Thorax 1999;54:334–338.

37. Uchitomi Y, Mikami I, Nagai K, et al. Depression and psychological distress in patients during the year after curative resection of non-small cell lung cancer. J Clin Oncol 2003;21:69–77.

38. Rogers ML, Duffy JP. Surgical aspects of chronic post-thoracotomy pain. Eur J Cardiothorac Surg 2000;19:711–716.

39. Landreneau RJ, Mack MJ, Hazelrigg SR, et al. Prevalence of chronic pain after pulmonary resection by thoracotomy or video-assisted thoracic surgery. J Cardiovasc Surg 1995;109:1085–1086.

40. Dajczman E, Gordon A, Kreisman H, et al. Long-term postthoracotomy pain. Chest 1991;99:270–274.

41. Sugiura H, Morikawa T, Kaji M, et al. Long-term benefits for the quality of life after video-assisted thoracoscopic lobectomy in patients with lung cancer. Surg Laparosc Endosc Percutan Tech 1999;9:403–408.

42. Mangione CM, Goldman L, Orav J, et al. Health-related quality of life after elective surgery. J Gen Intern Med 1997;12:686–697.

43. Gotoda Y, Kambara N, Sakai T, et al. The morbidity, time course and predictive factors for persistent post-thoracotomy pain. Eur J Pain 2001;5:89–96.

44. Li WW, Lee TW, Lam SS, et al. Quality of life following lung cancer resection: video-assisted thoracic surgery versus thoracotomy. Chest 2002;122:584–589.

45. d'Amours RH, Riegler FX, Little AG. Pathogenesis and management of persistent postthoracotomy pain. Chest Surg Clin N Am 1998;8:703–722.

46. Goldberg BA, Scarlat MM, Harryman DT. Management of the stiff shoulder. J Orthop Sci 1999;4:462–471.

47. Cykert S, Kissling G, Hansen CJ. Patient preferences regarding possible outcomes of lung resection. Chest 2000;117:1551–1559.

48. Cull A, Gregor A, Hopwood P, et al. Neurological and cognitive impairment in long-term survivors of small cell lung cancer. Eur J Cancer 1994;30A:1067–1074.

49. Sarna L. Correlates of symptom distress in women with lung cancer. Cancer Pract 1993;1:21–28.

50. Kurz ME, Kurtz JC, Stommel M, et al. Predictors of physical functioning among geriatric patients small cell or non-small cell lung cancer 3 months after diagnosis. Support Care Cancer 1999;7:328–331.

51. Schag CC, Heinrich RL. The impact of cancer on daily living. A comparison with cardiac patients and health controls. Rehabil Psychol 1986;31:157–167.

52. Zebrack BJ. Cancer survivor identity and quality of life. Cancer Pract 2000;8:238–242.

53. Zabora J, Brintzenhofeszoc K, Curbow B, et al. The prevalence of psychological distress by cancer site. Psycho-Oncology 2001;10:19–28.

54. Ginsberg ML, Quirt C, Ginsberg AD, et al. Psychiatric illnesses and psychosocial concerns of patients with newly diagnosed lung cancer. Can Med Assoc J 1995;152:1961–1963.

55. Hopwood PS. Depression in patients with lung cancer: prevalence and risk factors. J Clin Oncol 2000;18:893–903.

56. Hughes JE. Depressive illness and lung cancer. II. Follow-up of inoperable patients. Eur J Surg Oncol 1985;11:21–24.

57. Kurtz ME, Kurtz JC, Stommel M, et al. Predictors of depressive symptomatology of geriatric patients with lung cancer: a longitudinal analysis. Psycho-Oncology 2002;11:12–22.

58. Buccheri G. Depressive reactions to lung cancer are common and often followed by poor outcome. Eur Respir J 1998;11:173–178.

59. Schofield P, Ball D, Smith JG, et al. Optimism and survival in lung carcinoma patients. Cancer (Phila) 2004;100:1276–1282.

60. Uchitomi Y, Mikami I, Kugaya A, et al. Physician support and patient psychologic responses after surgery for non-small cell lung carcinoma: a prospective observational study. Cancer (Phila) 2001;92:1926–1935.

61. Dowie J, Wildman M. Choosing the surgical mortality threshold for high risk patients with stage Ia non-small cell lung cancer: insights from decision analysis. Thorax 2002;57:7–10.

62. Treasure T. Whose lung is it anyway? Thorax 2002;57:3–4.

63. Auperin A, Arriagada R, Pignon JP, et al. Prophylactic cranial irradiation for patients with small-cell lung cancer in complete remission. Prophylactic cranial irradiation overview collaborative group. N Engl J Med 1999;12:476–484.

64. Turrisi AT, Sherman CA. The treatment of limited small cell lung cancer: a report of the progress made and future prospects. Eur J Cancer 2002;38:279–291.

65. Johnson BE, Becker B, Goff WB, et al. Neurologic, neuropsychologic, computed cranial tomography scan abnormalities in 2- to 10-year survivors of small-cell lung cancer. J Clin Oncol 1985;3:1659–1667.

66. Albain KS, Crowley JJ, Livingston RB. Long-term survival and toxicity in small cell lung cancer. Chest 1991;99:1425–1432.

67. van Oosterhout AGM, Ganzevles PGJ, Wilmink JT, et al. Sequelae in long-term survivors of small cell lung cancer. Int J Radiat Oncol Biol Phys 1996;34:1037–1044.

68. Akechi T, Akizuke N, Sakuma K, et al. Somatic symptoms for diagnosing major depression in cancer patients. Psychosomatics 2003;44:244–248.

69. Sarna L. Women with lung cancer: impact on quality of life. Qual Life Res 1993;2:13–22.

70. Billante CR, Specto B, Hudson M, et al. Voice outcome following thyroplasty in patients with cancer-related vocal fold paralysis. Auris Nasus Larynx 2001;28:315–321.

71. Nou E, Aberg T. Quality of survival in patients with surgically treated bronchial carcinoma. Thorax 1980;35:255–263.

72. Lassen U, Osterlind K, Hansen M, et al. Long-term survival in small-cell lung cancer: posttreatment characteristics in patients surviving 5 to 18+ years. An analysis of 1,714 consecutive patients. J Clin Oncol 1995;13:1215–1220.

73. Shelby RA, Taylor KL, Kerner JF, et al. The role of community-based and philanthropic organizations in meeting cancer patient and caregiver needs. CA Cancer J Clin 2002;52:229–246.

74. Pukrop R, Rehse B. Effects of psychosocial interventions on quality of life in adult cancer patients: meta analysis of 37 published controlled outcome studies. Patient Educ Counsel 2003;50:179–186.

75. Johnson BE. Second lung cancers in patients after treatment for an initial lung cancer. JNCI 1998;90:1335–1345.

76. Johnson-Early A, Cohen MH, Minna JD, et al. Smoking abstinence and small cell lung cancer survival: an association. JAMA 1980;244:2175–2179.

77. Kawahara M, Ushijima S, Kamimori T, et al. Second primary tumours in more than 2-year disease-free survivors of small-cell lung cancer in Japan: the role of smoking cessation. Br J Cancer 1998;78:409–412.

78. Richardson GE, Tucker MA, Venzon DJ. Smoking cessation after successful treatment of small-cell lung cancer is associated with fewer smoking-related second primary cancers. Ann Intern Med 1993;119:383–390.

79. Gritz E, Vidrine DJ, Lazev AB. Smoking cessation in cancer patients: never too late to quit. In: Given B, Given CW, Champion V, et al. (eds). Evidence-Based Interventions in Oncology. New York: Springer, 2004.

80. Videtic GMM, Stitt LW, Dar R, et al. Continued cigarette smoking by patients receiving concurrent chemoradiotherapy for limited-stage small-cell lung cancer is associated with decreased survival. J Clin Oncol 2003;21:1544–1549.

81. Anthonisen N, Connett JE, Kiley JP, et al. Effects of smoking intervention and the use of an inhaled anticholinergic bronchodilator on the rate of decline of FEV1. The Lung Health Study. JAMA 1994;272:1497–1505.

82. Peto R, Darby S, Deo H, et al. Smoking, smoking cessation, and lung cancer in the UK since 1950: combination of national statistics with two case control studies. BMJ 2000;321:323–329.

83. Doll R, Peto R, Boreham J, et al. Mortality in relation to smoking: 50 years' observation on male British doctors. BMJ 2004. doi: 10.1136/bmj.38142.554479.AE, retrieved July 15, 2004.

84. Mokdad AH, Marks JS, Stroup DF, et al. Actual causes of death in the United States, 2000. JAMA 2004;291:1238–1245.

85. American Society of Clinical Oncology. American Society of Clinical Oncology Policy Statement Update: Tobacco control—reducing cancer incidence and saving lives. J Clin Oncol 2003; 21:2777–2786.

86. Fujisawa T, Iizasa T, Saitoh Y, et al. Smoking before surgery predicts poor long-term survival in patients with stage I non-small cell lung carcinomas. J Clin Oncol 1999;17:2086–2091.

87. Clarke MM, Cox LS, Jett JR, et al. Effectiveness of smoking cessation self-help materials in a lung cancer screening population. Lung Cancer 2004;44:13–21.

88. Cox L, Africano N, Tercyak K, et al. Nicotine dependence treatment for patients with cancer: review and recommendations. Cancer (Phila) 2003;98:632–644.

89. Cox LS, Sloan JA, Patten CA, et al. Smoking behavior of 226 patients with diagnosis of stage IIIA/IIIB non-small cell lung cancer. Psycho-Oncology 2002;11:472–478.

90. Davison G, Duffy M. Smoking habits of long-term survivors of surgery for lung cancer. Thorax 1982;37:331–333.

91. Gritz ER, Nisenbaum R, Elashoff RE, et al. Smoking behavior following diagnosis in patients with stage I non-small cell lung cancer. Cancer Causes Control 1991;2:105–112.

92. Sridhar KS, Raub WA Jr. Present and past smoking history and other predisposing factors in 100 lung cancer patients. Chest 1992;101:19–25.

93. Dresler CM, Bailey M, Roper CR, et al. Smoking cessation and lung cancer resection. Chest 1996;110:1199–1202.

94. Grannis FW. The lung cancer and cigarette smoking web page: a pilot study in telehealth promotion on the World Wide Web. Can Respir J 2001;8:333–337.

95. Browning KK, Ahijevych KA, Ross P, et al. Implementing the Agency for Health Care Policy and Research's Smoking Cessation Guideline in a Lung Cancer Surgery Clinic. Oncol Nurs Forum 2000;27:1248–1254.

96. Wewers ME, Jenkins L, Mignery T. A nurse-managed smoking cessation during diagnostic testing for lung cancer. Oncol Nurs Forum 1997;24:1419–1422.

97. Ebbert JO, Yang P, Vachon CM, et al. Lung cancer risk reduction after smoking cessation: observations from a prospective cohort of women. J Clin Oncol 2003;21:921–926.

98. Chapple A, Ziebland S, McPherson A. Stigma, shame, and blame experienced by patients with lung cancer: a qualitative study. BMJ 2004. doi: 10.1136/bmj.38111.639734.7c (published June 11), retrieved July 15, 2004.

99. Marteu T, Riordan DC. Staff attitudes towards patients: the influence of causal attributions for illness. Br J Clin Psychol 1992;31:107–110.

100. Faller H, Schilling S, Lang H. Causal attribution and adaptation among lung cancer patients. J Psychosom Res 1995;39:619–627.

101. Brown JK, Byers T, Doyle C, et al. Nutrition and physical activity during and after cancer treatment: an American Cancer Society guide for informed choices. CA A Cancer J Clin 2003;53:268–291.

102. The Alpha Tocopherol Betacarotene Prevention Study Group. The effect of vitamin E and betacarotene on the incidence of lung cancer and other cancers in male smokers. N Engl J Med 1994;330:1029–1035.

103. Omenn G, Goodman G, Thornquist M, et al. Effects of a combination of betacarotene and vitamin A on lung cancer and cardiovascular disease. N Engl J Med 1996;334:1150–1155.

104. Phase III randomized chemoprevention study of selenium in participants with previously resected stage I non-small cell lung cancer (Protocol ID E-5597). http://www.cancer.gov/ClinicalTrials/, retrieved July 15, 2004.

105. Ludbrook JJ, Truong PT, MacNeil MV, et al. Do age and comorbidity impact treatment allocation and outcomes in limited stage small-cell lung cancer? A community-based population analysis. Int J Radiat Oncol Biol Phys 2003;55:1321–1330.

106. Kurz ME, Kurtz JC, Stommel M, et al. Loss of physical functioning among geriatric cancer patients: relationships to cancer site, treatment, comorbidity and age. Eur J Cancer 1997;33: 2352–2358.

107. Kurtz ME, Kurtz JC, Stommel M, et al. Symptomatology and loss of physical functioning among geriatric patients with lung cancer. J Pain Symptom Manag 2000;19:249–256.

108. Patel JD, Bach PB, Kris MG. Lung cancer in US women: a contemporary epidemic. JAMA 2004;291:1763–1768.

109. Henschke CI, Miettinen OS. Women's susceptibility to tobacco carcinogens. Lung Cancer 2004;43:1–5.

110. Thun M, Lally C, Flannery J, et al. Cigarette smoking and changes in histopathology of lung cancer. JNCI 1997;89: 1580–1586.

111. Lienert T, Serke N, Schofeld N, et al. Lung cancer in young females. Eur Respir J 2000;16:986–990.

112. Singh GK, Miller BA, Hankey BF. Changing area socioeconomic patterns in U.S. cancer mortality, 1950–1998. Part II: Lung and colorectal cancers. JNCI 2002;94:916–925.

113. Centers for Disease Control and Prevention. Cigarette smoking among adults: United States, 2002. MMWR 2004;53:427–431.

114. Barbeau EM, Krieger N, Soobader MJ. Working class matters: socioeconomic disadvantage, race/ethnicity, gender, and smoking in NHIS 2000. Am J Public Health 2003;94:269–278.

115. Centers for Disease Control and Prevention. Prevalence of cigarette use among 14 racial/ethnic populations—United States, 1999–2001. MMWR (Morbid Mort Wkly Rep) 2004;53: 49–52.

116. Leisktikow B. Lung cancer rates as an index of tobacco smoke exposures: validation against black male–non-lung cancer death rates, 1969–2000. Prev Med 2004;38:511–515.

117. Bach PB, Cramer LD, Warren JL, et al. Racial differences in the treatment of early-stage lung cancer. N Engl J Med 1999;341: 1198–1205.

118. Greenwald HP, Polissar NH, Borgatta EF, et al. Social factors, treatment, and survival in early-stage non-small cell lung cancer. Am J Public Health 1998;88:1681–1684.

119. Ward E, Jemal A, Cokkinides V, et al. Cancer disparities by race/ethnicity and socioeconomic status. CA A Cancer J Clin 2004;54:78–93.

120. Montazeri A, Hole DJ, Milroy R, et al. Quality of life in lung cancer patients: does socioeconomic status matter? Health Qual Life Outcomes 2003;1:19–24.

121. Lopez-Encuentra A. Bronchogenic Carcinoma Co-Operative Group: comorbidity inoperable lung cancer. A multicenter descriptive study on 2992 patients. Lung Cancer 2002;35:263–269.

122. Gritz E. Facilitating smoking cessation in cancer patients. Tobacco Control 2000;i50(suppl 1):50.

123. U.S. Department of Health and Human Services. The health consequences of tobacco use: a report of the Surgeon General. Atlanta, GA: U.S. Department of Health and Human Services, Public Health Service, Centers for Disease Control and Prevention, National Center for Chronic Disease Prevention and Health Promotion, Office on Smoking and Health, 2003.

124. Nakayma M, Satoh H, Sekizawa K. Risk of cancers in COPD patients. Chest 2003;123:1775.

125. Beck GJ, Doyle CA, Schachter EN. Smoking and lung function. Am Rev Respir Dis 1981;123:149–155.

126. Ko CY, Maggard M, Livingston EH. Evaluating health utility in patients with melanoma, breast cancer, colon cancer, and lung cancer. A nationwide, population-based assessment. J Surg Res 2003;114:1–5.

127. Henschke CI, McCauley DI, Yankelevitz DF, et al. Early lung cancer action project: overall design and findings from baseline screening. Lancet 1999;354:99–105.

128. Patz EF, Swensen SJ, Herndon RE. Estimate of lung cancer mortality from low-dose spiral computed tomography screening trials: implications for current mass screening recommendations. J Clin Oncol 2004;22:2202–2206.

129. Shahidi H, Kvale PA. Long-term survival following surgical treatment of solitary brain metastasis in non-small cell lung cancer. Chest 1996;109:271–276.

130. Dow KH. Challenges and opportunities in cancer survivorship research. Oncol Nurs Forum 2003;30:455–469.

131. Schumacher A, Riesenbeck D, Braunheim M, et al. Combined modality treatment for locally advanced non-small cell lung cancer: preoperative chemoradiation does not result in poorer quality of life. Lung Cancer 2004;44:89–97.

132. Colice GL, Rubins J, Unger M. Follow-up and surveillance of the lung cancer patient following curative-intent therapy. Chest 2003;123:272S–283S.

133. McManus K. Concerns of poor quality of life should not deprive patients of the opportunity for curative surgery. Thorax 2003;58:189.

134. Natale RB. Effects of ZD 1839 (Iressa, Gefitinib) treatment on symptoms and quality of life in patients with advanced non-small cell lung cancer. Semin Oncol 2004;31:23–30.

135. Welcker K, Marian P, Thetter O, et al. Cost and quality of life in thoracic surgery. Thorac Cardiovasc Surg 2003;51:260–266.

14

Cancer Survivorship Issues in Colorectal Cancer

Clifford Y. Ko and Patricia A. Ganz

Epidemiologic Trends That Will Influence the Number of Colon and Rectal Cancer Survivors

Colon and rectal cancers (CRC) are among the most common adult malignancies worldwide, and for a variety of reasons, the numbers of survivors of colorectal cancer are likely to increase in coming years. The incidence of these cancers doubles with each successive decade of life beyond 50 years, and with the expansion of the older population in the coming years, the absolute numbers of CRC patients in the United States will grow substantially.[1] It is estimated that by the year 2030 the number of persons over the age of 65 years will have doubled and the number of persons over the age of 85 years will have quadrupled (see Chapter 16).[2] Given this expanding and aging population, projections suggest that the numbers of CRC patients may increase by as much as 30%.[3] Thus, with these profound demographic changes, it will be imperative to have a better understanding of the late effects and health care needs of long-term CRC survivors.

In addition to the increased incidence of colorectal cancer, advances in the detection and treatment are contributing to improved survival outcomes for patients with this disease. Earlier detection of CRC leads to better survival through downstaging of the disease. Several large population-based studies have demonstrated that increasingly more colon and rectal cancers are being detected at an earlier stage through screening.[4–9] Data from the Surveillance, Epidemiology, and End Results (SEER) program[10] demonstrate an increasing proportion of localized colon cancers for the population 65 years and older: in the 1970s, 36% of tumors were localized; in the 1980s, 39% were localized; and in the 1990s, this increased to 42%. Similarly, the proportion of localized rectal cancers has increased from 46% to 49% from the 1970s to the 1990s.

In addition, there is an anticipated growth for the number of CRC survivors secondary to secular trends in screening for this disease. As CRC screening becomes more widespread through current health promotion campaigns, there will be an accelerated shift to earlier-stage disease, contributing further to a stage-related increase in the numbers of long-term survivors. The benefits of earlier stage on survival are demonstrated by looking at data on survival by stage (1992–1998):

the 5-year survival for regional tumors (i.e., AJCC stage III) is 65.2%, while for localized colon and rectal cancers (i.e., AJCC stage I and II) the survival rate is 90.1%.[10] Overall, we can be optimistic about better outcomes and long-term survival for CRC patients in the decades ahead.

Finally, there are increasing numbers of CRC survivors because of advances in medical treatments. For example, the surgical technique of total mesorectal excision for rectal cancers has significantly decreased the likelihood of local recurrence,[11] and the use of radiation therapy in the disease both decreases local recurrence and improves overall survival.[12,13] Studies have also demonstrated the efficacy of various adjuvant chemotherapy regimens for improving survival in colon cancer patients.[14–16] The benefits of these improvements in detection and treatment are also reflected in population-based survival rates for CRC. In reviewing the latest data from the SEER program database, the overall 5-year survival rate for colon and rectal cancer for all races and both sexes is 61.9%.[10] This rate is significantly better than 1974–1976, which was 49.8% (P less than 0.05). Furthermore, the survival for patients under 65 years of age versus over 65 years is not dramatically different (63% versus 61.3%), which shows that the elderly with colorectal cancer achieve long-term survival as well. Data for survival beyond 5 years are also available through SEER and have shown similar improvements. For example, the 10-year survival for colon and rectal cancer patients improved from 44.7% in 1975 to 55.3% in 1989. For all these cited reasons, there will be a growing number of CRC survivors in the decades ahead.

Given that the number of CRC survivors is increasing, there are a number of important issues pertinent solely to this cancer site—some that are related to the CRC treatments, and others that are related to specific characteristics of the population that survives colorectal cancer (e.g., the level of comorbidity in this elderly population). The following sections address these survivorship issues. First, the treatment-related issues are discussed, including prevalence, symptomology, and quality of life. The subsequent sections examine issues related to the comorbidity and use of medical services for the CRC survivors population as a whole. The last part of this chapter discusses strategies that may help to improve survivorship outcomes now and in the future.

Treatment-Specific Survivorship Issues

Treatment of colorectal cancer is often multidisciplinary, depending on the stage of disease and whether or not the cancer arises in the colon or the rectum. More specifically, the treatment modalities can include surgical resection and chemotherapy for colon cancer and surgical resection, chemotherapy, and radiation therapy for rectal cancer. Although the current first-line chemotherapeutics do not have appreciable long-term effects on survivors, surgery and radiation therapy can have associated lasting morbidities that affect the function and quality of life of survivors long after the cancer is treated. A description of the pertinent effects related to surgical resection and radiation therapy is presented next.

Survivorship Issues Related to Surgery

Surgical resection is the mainstay of curative treatment for colon and rectal cancers.[17] The surgical procedure requires removal of a segment of colon and/or rectum where the tumor is located, as well as the associated blood vessels and draining lymph nodes.[11,18] In addition, if there is evidence of metastatic disease, this tissue (e.g., liver, omentum) is also removed or biopsied at the time of initial surgery.[19] Currently, most operations are performed through an open vertical incision up to 30 to 40 cm in length through the abdominal wall. This open approach has associated risks of complications that may be important for colorectal cancer survivors in relation to function status and quality of life. Of note, trials have been reported regarding laparoscopic colon cancer resections. This latter issue is discussed at the end of the chapter.

Long-Term Complications of Abdominal Surgery

Several possible surgery-associated problems can occur in the short and long term that will affect colorectal cancer survivors. In the acute period, clinical complications may include wound infections (3%–26%), intraabdominal infections (2%–5%), and anastomotic leaks (2%–10%), all of which may require rehospitalization and possible additional invasive (e.g., surgical) procedures.[20–22] However, more important for longer-term survivors of CRC are the issues that occur beyond the acute period: three important issues are bowel obstructions, abdominal wall hernias, and functional problems. Complications from bowel obstruction can occur any time after surgery (e.g., weeks to years), and the presentation can range from imminent bowel necrosis that requires immediate surgery to chronic cyclic episodes of debilitating pain that may require hospitalization, intravenous hydration, and gastrointestinal decompression with use of nasogastric drainage. In one study of 472 consecutive patients operated on for colorectal cancer who were followed for a median period greater than 5 years, small bowel obstruction necessitating an operation occurred in 10% after resection with curative intent and in 4% after a palliative operation.[23] Obstruction is particularly relevant to survivors of CRC because it always has the potential of being a sign of tumor recurrence. In this same study, although benign adhesions accounted for 51% of the obstructions, local tumor recurrence and carcinomatosis accounted for 49%.

Another potential surgical complication for colorectal cancer survivors is an *abdominal wall hernia*. Abdominal wall hernias can potentially lead to pain, limitation of activities, and the need for emergent surgery for possible bowel strangulation. It has been estimated that hernias at the incision site (i.e., incisional hernias) occur in approximately 4% to 10% of patients after open surgical procedures.[24,25] However, the rate increases to as high as 20% for patients whose wounds are infected. As only 50% of incisional hernias become evident within 6 months after an operation, many will continue to have this problem much beyond the acute recovery of their surgery. Overall, more than 100,000 incisional hernia repairs are performed each year in the United States, and the rate of reoperation for such repairs is high (the 5-year reoperative rate was 24% after an initial operation).[26,27]

Although intestinal obstruction and incision hernias are two of the most common (and generic) potentially chronic problems associated with open colon or open rectal cancer surgery, there are some unique factors that are specifically pertinent to survivors of rectal cancer who have undergone complete or partial proctectomy, especially if radiation therapy is also used. These issues include functional problems in three areas: fecal dysfunction and incontinence, sexual dysfunction, and urinary bladder dysfunction. These areas, which may substantially affect survivors, are discussed next.

Bowel Changes/Dysfunction

One role of the rectum is storage of fecal material. When the rectum is resected for cancer, the storage capacity of the rectum's replacement, the colon (e.g., usually the descending or sigmoid colon), is substantially less, and therefore frequent, clustered, and/or incomplete bowel movements can ensue.[28] Also, because of possible nerve damage from surgery or radiation therapy, anal sphincter function may be further affected, and the degree of incontinence may be worsened.[29]

Many providers and patients alike strongly prefer a sphincter-sparing procedure; however, it is necessary for the patient/survivor to understand that bowel dysfunction may occur even in the presence of sphincter preservation. In part, the level of the anastomosis is extremely relevant to subsequent function. A low colorectal or a coloanal anastomosis (i.e., an anastomosis performed immediately adjacent to the sphincter muscles) is associated with a higher frequency of defecation and more fecal leakage and incontinence than a high colorectal anastomosis. In addition, defecatory problems can occur as a result of surgical trauma or the effects of radiation therapy to the anal sphincter and its innervation, even when sphincter preservation is performed.

Overall, the most common bowel-related symptoms following rectal resection are increased frequency of bowel motion, urgency, fecal leakage, and incontinence. However, also reported by patients to some degree are diarrhea, constipation, and excessive flatus. These are clearly important issues for rectal cancer survivors because even though their cancer may be cured, their function and quality of life may be severely diminished as a result of bowel-related symptoms, even if the anal sphincter is spared.

A short-term single-institution series recently reported that 56% of patients who underwent sphincter preservation for rectal cancer reported unfavorable function and were all

TABLE 14.1. Bowel dysfunction in rectal cancer survivors.

Bowel dysfunction (overall)	56%–60%
Fecal leakage	44%–64%
Pad usage	18%–39%
Four or more bowel movements/day	16%–22%
Urgency	22%–24%
Unable to defer defecation 15 min	73%
Unable to defer defecation 5 min	27%
Bowel dysfunction requiring ostomy	5%

Source: References 28–30.

TABLE 14.3. Sexual dysfunction in rectal cancer survivors.

Sexual dysfunction (overall)	14%–95%
Male	33%–95%
Female	14%–67%
Low anterior resection	42%–45%
Abdominal perineal resection	25%–90%
Sexual dysfunction following autonomic nerve preservation surgery	4%–14%

Source: References 36–40.

dissatisfied with their quality of life.[30] Although few long-term data are available, small case series have shown that bowel dysfunction and incontinence is often a chronic issue for many rectal cancer survivors who undergo sphincter preservation. Table 14.1 highlights some of the functional outcomes in rectal cancer survivors.

OSTOMY ISSUES

In patients who undergo abdominoperineal resection, not only do pelvic dissection and rectal resection influence survivorship issues, but the presence of a permanent colostomy also has strong influence on survivors. First, stoma-related problems are common. In a series of 203 patients with end sigmoid colostomies, the 13-year actuarial risk of paracolostomy complications was 58%. Paracolostomy hernia was the most common complication (36% at 10 years).[31] Other stoma-related complications may occur in survivors, including stomal prolapse (12%), skin-related problems (e.g., excoriation) (12%), and stenosis of the stomal opening (7%).[31,32] In a survey study of almost 400 ostomates, 51% had skin problems (e.g., rashes) and 36% had leakage; 80% reported some change in lifestyle[33] (Table 14.2).

In addition to complications, several studies have compared postoperative psychosocial adjustment and quality of life in ostomy and nonostomy patients, including concerns regarding sexuality, limitations of activity, and bowel function. These quality of life issues related to ostomy are discussed later in this chapter. It is important that clinicians make use of referral of patients to enterostomal therapists who are able to address both the physical and psychosocial sequelae of having a stoma. Their consultation is valuable throughout the course of survivorship from preoperative to short- and long-term periods. Stoma support groups exist in many communities and are another resource.[34,35]

SEXUAL DYSFUNCTION

Sexual problems are associated with surgical and radiation therapies that affect the tissues/organs of the pelvis and the

TABLE 14.2. Colostomy problems in rectal cancer survivors.

Colostomy problems (overall)	21%–76%
Parastomal hernia	37%
Leakage	36%
Prolapse	12%
Skin problems	12%
Stomal stenosis	7%

Source: References 31, 33.

nerves that innervate them (Table 14.3). The potential sexual dysfunctions for males include erectile dysfunction and ejaculatory difficulties (inability to ejaculate or retrograde ejaculation).[36] Disruption of the parasympathetic nerve network interferes with penile erection, and sympathetic nerve disruption impairs normal ejaculation. The incidence of sexual dysfunction increases with advancing patient age and is higher after abdominoperineal resection (i.e., removal of the rectum and placement of a permanent colostomy) than after anterior resection. A conventional rectal cancer resection in men is associated with postoperative impotence and retrograde ejaculation or both in 25% to 100% of cases.[37–39]

In females, the most common postoperative sexual complaint is dyspareunia, which may include loss of vaginal lubrication and inability to achieve orgasm. Although somewhat difficult to objectively assess, sexual activity has been used as a surrogate measure. Of those women who are sexually active before surgery, 47% to 86% remain sexually active after surgery. Other studies have demonstrated that while 55% to 58% of women remain sexually active after sphincter preservation surgery, only 10% to 39% remain sexually active after an abdominoperineal resection.[37,38,40] In some women who have undergone a posterior vaginectomy in addition to an abdominoperineal dissection, sexual intercourse may be impossible because of a stenotic vaginal introitus.

Havenga et al.[38] surveyed 54 women after total mesorectal excision (i.e., a surgical technique that removes the rectal mesentery and is associated with lower cancer recurrence rates) with autonomic nerve preservation for carcinoma of the rectum (44 low anterior resection, 10 abdominoperineal resection) and found that 95% of women remained interested in sex, 86% remained sexually active, 85% continued to experience vaginal lubrication during arousal, and 91% maintained their ability to achieve orgasm postoperatively. Although the most common postoperative sexual complaint was dyspareunia, the incidence was not significantly changed from the preoperative to postoperative periods.[38] Just as with men, the best possible outcome is achieved by careful sharp dissection with preservation of the pelvic autonomic nerves. Additional data regarding nerve-preserving surgery are presented at the end of the chapter.

UROLOGIC DYSFUNCTION

Bladder dysfunction has been reported to occur in 7% to 68% of patients after low rectal cancer resection; however, the incidence is generally quoted to be around 30% in most series.[41] Urologic dysfunction includes problems such as incomplete emptying, urgency, overflow or stress incontinence, loss of bladder sensation, dysuria, and chronic urinary tract infections. Similar to sexual dysfunction, the majority of voiding difficulties have been shown to be neurogenic in origin. Parasympathetic denervation is specific to urologic dysfunction in this setting. Although a neurogenic bladder may occur in as many as 50% of men after abdominoperineal resection, voiding difficulties resolve in the majority within 3 to 6 months after surgery.[41,42] In addition to neurogenic problems, mechanical and physiologic issues plays a role as bladder neck angulation following surgery, and the presence of benign prostatic hypertrophy (particularly in this age group) also contributes to urologic dysfunction.

As with sexuality, urinary difficulties are more often associated with abdominoperineal resection than with anterior resection. Balslev and Harling[43] identified urologic symptoms such as dysuria and incontinence in 29 of 31 patients who underwent abdominoperineal resection. As with sexual dysfunction, favorable outcomes may be achieved by careful sharp dissection with preservation of pelvic anastomotic nerves.

Survivorship Issues Regarding Radiation Therapy

According to National Cancer Institute (NCI)-developed guidelines, stage II and III rectal cancer patients should receive radiation therapy.[44] Studies have subsequently shown that radiation therapy decreases local recurrence as well as increases survival.[12] However, radiation therapy can have potentially serious late effects for the rectal cancer survivor. While short-term (acute) complications of radiotherapy may include lethargy, nausea, diarrhea, and skin changes (i.e., erythema and/or desquamation), and also develop to some degree in the majority of patients during treatment, they are generally self-limiting.[45]

For the long-term rectal cancer survivor who underwent radiation therapy, it is important to evaluate the morbidity, pelvic floor function, and quality of life. In this regard, delayed radiation toxicities have been reported and include radiation enteritis (4%), small bowel obstruction (5%), and rectal stricture (5%); this is in addition to the bowel, sexual, and urinary dysfunction discussed earlier that may be compounded by radiation-induced pelvic nerve injuries.[46] Regarding the latter two issues, although sexual and urologic function is poorly studied, data suggest that radiation has a negative impact in both men and women.[47]

Bowel function after radiation therapy is an important issue. There are several studies that are generally consistent and show that bowel function, as measured by frequency, urgency, evacuation, sensation, and/or continence, is impaired after radiation therapy when compared with patients not treated with radiation.[47]

The Swedish Rectal Cancer randomized controlled trial[12] has shown that preoperative high-dose radiotherapy improves survival and decreases local recurrence; they have also studied the long-term bowel function following radiation therapy (XRT) and anterior resection. The authors found that the median frequency of bowel movements was higher in the XRT plus surgery group versus the surgery-only group (20 versus 10 bowel movements per week; P less than 0.0001).[12,48] Additionally, urgency, emptying difficulties, and incontinence for loose stools were more common in the XRT plus surgery group (all P less than 0.0001). In terms of quality of life, 30% of the XRT plus surgery group stated that their

TABLE 14.4. Bowel issues in rectal cancer patients following radiation.

Diarrhea	39%
Nocturnal defecation	36%
Use of pad/diaper	32%
Number of bowel movements per day	0.5–3.5

Source: References 45–50, 84.

social life was impaired because of bowel dysfunction compared to 10% of the surgery-only group (P less than 0.01).[48]

Another study of rectal cancer patients undergoing surgical resection with or without radiation therapy found similar results that the irradiated group had more diarrhea (39% versus 13%; $P = 0.005$) and more nocturnal defecation (36% versus 15%; $P = 0.03$) compared with the nonirradiated group.[49]

Looking at slightly longer outcomes, a recent study examined rectal cancer patients between 2 and 8 years following surgical resection with no radiation, preoperative radiation, or postoperative radiation.[50] They found that the postoperative radiation group had more episodes of clustered bowel movements (P less than 0.02) than either the preoperative radiation group or the no-radiation group. The authors attributed the adverse effects of postoperative radiation therapy to irradiation of the neorectum, which is spared when radiation is given preoperatively (Table 14.4).

Along these same lines, manometric studies of low anterior resection patients with and without chemoradiation shows that resting pressure, resting volume, and maximal tolerable volume of the neorectum was significantly worsened in the irradiated group after radiation compared with before radiation. These same parameters did not change in the nonirradiated group.[51]

Quality of Life in Colorectal Cancer Survivors

Some of the earliest studies of quality of life (QOL) in cancer patients were done by Ganz and colleagues using a newly developed instrument called the Cancer Inventory of Problem Situations (CIPS), which was later renamed the Cancer Rehabilitation Evaluation System (CARES).[52–56] These studies were conducted with heterogeneous samples of cancer patients and survivors, with several common cancers being represented, including 277 CRC patients and survivors.[55] In one of the first published studies to examine quality of life in adult cancer survivors, Schag et al.[53] reported on a sample of lung, colon, and prostate cancer disease-free survivors that compared QOL outcomes across disease sites as well as by length of survivorship (short-term, less than 2 years after diagnosis; intermediate-term, 2–5 years after diagnosis; long-term, more than 5 years after diagnosis). This particular study included a total of 117 CRC survivors, with 27 of them being long-term survivors. In comparing the CRC survivors across the three time periods of survivorship, the long-term survivors reported significantly better QOL on a global single-item rating of QOL, as well as better psychosocial functioning on the CARES, compared with the short- and intermediate-term survivors. Specific problems that were frequent and severe in CRC survivors were difficulty in doing physical activities, reduction

TABLE 14.5. Proportion of colon cancer survivors with issues rated as frequent/severe.

Difficulty with bending or lifting	42%
Difficulty with walking/moving around	26%
Difficulty doing physical activities	50%
Difficulty driving	5%
Not engaged in recreational activities	33%
Has frequent pain	30%
Difficulty thinking clearly	45%

Source: Reference 53.

in energy, difficulty doing recreational activities, having trouble gaining weight, worry about whether treatments worked, body image problems, problems with sexual interest and functioning, and at-work concerns such as difficulty talking to others about the cancer, difficulty asking for time off from work for treatment, and worrying about being fired (Table 14.5). Across all the CRC survivors, significant predictors of QOL were the Karnofsky Performance Status score, type of hospital setting in which treatment was received (higher QOL in a private hospital in comparison to a VA, teaching hospital, public hospital, or HMO), gender (males better QOL than females), and work status (nonworking survivors reported better QOL). In this model, comorbid conditions nearly reached significance, with better QOL associated with fewer comorbid conditions.[53] These findings suggest that a variety of factors influence QOL in CRC survivors and that they are important to address in treatment planning (Table 14.6).

A more-recent study of 227 colorectal cancer survivors by Ramsey et al. examined the quality of life after more than 5 years of survivorship. They found that survivors report a relatively uniform and high QOL. In addition, the presence and severity of comorbid conditions and low income status were more predictive of overall QOL than the stage of cancer. Interestingly, compared to age-matched controls, long term survivors reported higher overall QOL, although problems remained such as frequent bowel movements (16%), diarrhea (49%), and depression.[57]

With the advent of new surgical techniques that allow for the performance of lower-level anastomoses for rectal cancer resection, there has been a strong push for sphincter-sparing procedures. In a review of quality of life articles regarding the presence of an ostomy, Sprangers[58] identified studies that addressed at least one of four aspects (i.e., physical, psychologic, social, and sexual) for stoma versus nonstoma patients. The authors found that both patient cohorts were troubled by

TABLE 14.6. Treatment strategies for improving survivorship quality of life, function, and outcomes.

1. Informed discussion of expectations following treatment
2. Address coexistent disease throughout care and survivorship
3. Consider laparoscopic approach if appropriate
4. If colostomy will be performed, consider marking the site preoperatively.
5. Consider ostomy support group.
6. Consider transanal excision if appropriate
7. Consider neoadjuvant radiation (vs. adjuvant)
8. Autonomic nerve preservation techniques
9. Create neorectum with coloplasty or colonic J pouch

frequent or irregular bowel movements and diarrhea. Also, although both patient groups reported restrictions in their social functioning, colostomy patients reported a higher prevalence of these problems. Finally, stoma patients reported higher levels of psychologic distress as well as more impaired sexual dysfunction. Overall, this review shows that although both stoma and nonstoma survivors have impaired function and quality of life, nonstoma patients might fare better than do stoma patients.

Increasingly more sphincter-preserving procedures are being performed, but other recent studies show that it remains unclear whether quality of life has definitively improved.[59] It should be noted that these studies comparing sphincter-sparing resection with abdominoperineal resection/permanent colostomy are nonrandomized and therefore may be biased with regard to patient selection. The results are nonetheless interesting, particularly because a randomized controlled trial will likely never be performed.

A study by Grumann et al.[60] examined 73 rectal cancer patients and compared quality of life in patients undergoing anterior resection (AR; e.g., sphincter preservation) or abdominoperineal resection (APR). All patients were treated for cure and were disease free throughout the study. QOL was evaluated before surgery and at two time points following surgery (6–9 months, and 14–15 months). The findings revealed that on most scales the rectal cancer survivors who had an APR had superior, although not significantly better, scores than the AR patients. Of note, APR patients had significantly less constipation and diarrhea than AR patients, and also had significantly less sleeplessness; for example, the AR patients reported significantly more sleep disturbances than APR patients. On further comparison of low anterior resection versus high anterior resection, low anterior resection patients had significantly lower total QOL, role function, social function, body image, and future perspective, and more gastrointestinal- and defecation-related symptoms, than patients undergoing high anterior resection.

In another quality of life study of ostomates versus nonostomate rectal cancer survivors, a 4-year prospective study by Engel et al. examined 329 rectal cancer patients in Germany and demonstrated somewhat different findings.[61] Overall, survivors who underwent anterior resection had better QOL scores than APR patients (i.e., stoma patients had significantly worse QOL scores than nonstoma patients). High anterior resection patients had significantly better scores than both low anterior resection patients and APR patients. Interestingly, APR patients' QOL scores did not improve over time.

The somewhat inconsistent findings of these studies highlight the likely selection bias that is inherent in nonrandomized observational studies. These studies do illustrate, however, the importance of having informed discussions between the patient and provider regarding options, benefits, risks, and overall expectations.

Role of Comorbid Conditions in CRC Survivors

With the earlier detection of colorectal cancer due to improved screening, there will be increasing numbers of older survivors who have a greater likelihood of comorbid conditions. Healthcare providers for these survivors will have to address the disease of colorectal cancer (including the follow-up surveillance) as well as issues related to comorbid diseases. Coordinating the efforts of disease prevention, disease surveillance, and addressing the active issues of comorbidities is a complex task that requires good coordination among healthcare providers.

Few studies are available that have specifically characterized the burden of comorbid conditions in colorectal cancer survivors, partly because of the difficulty of obtaining this type of data. One study of colorectal cancer survivors (5+ years following diagnosis) using a mailed survey found the most common comorbid conditions were arthritis/rheumatism (20%), congestive heart failure (6%), hypertension (5%), angina (5%), and myocardial infarction (4%).[57]

In another study using a large population-based, nationwide, patient interview, comorbidities and use of services were characterized in colon cancer patients who were 1 to 3 years past diagnosis.[62] The study showed that 75% of survivors had reported having a major comorbid disease. The most common comorbid condition was cardiovascular related (55%), followed by hypertension (46%), arthritis (44%), coronary heart disease (13%), and pulmonary-related comorbidity (11%). Of note, almost 1 of 10 survivors reported having a history of a myocardial infarction. Also prevalent was diabetes, which was present in 14% of survivors, of which 57% were insulin dependent.

The potential significance of having diabetes is seen in a study by Meyerhardt et al.,[63] which showed that at 5 years, colon cancer patients with diabetes mellitus, compared with colon cancer patients without diabetes, had a significantly worse disease-free survival, overall survival, and recurrence-free survival. Median survival was 6 years and 11.3 years for diabetics and nondiabetics, respectively. Although cause of death was not explicitly studied in detail, compared with patients without a history of diabetes, those with diabetes had a 42% increased risk of death from any cause (P less than 0.0001). Further studies are needed to determine if better management of a comorbid condition such as diabetes will influence survival after a diagnosis of colon cancer.

While the available evidence in this regard is sparse, these studies highlight the potential issues related to the prevalence, detection, and need for treatment of comorbid conditions in a colorectal cancer survivor cohort. This is especially relevant as survival times increase from colorectal cancer; it is likely that the comorbidity prevalence and severity will increase as well.

Healthcare Utilization in CRC Survivors

There have been relatively few studies that have characterized the colorectal cancer patient's use of healthcare services following treatment of the cancer. One important study has examined the use of surveillance related to colorectal cancer survivors. A study by Lafata et al. examined the use of CRC surveillance tests in more than 250 colorectal cancer survivors enrolled in a large managed care organization.[64] The specific surveillance tests included colonic examinations, carcinoembryonic antigen (CEA) testing, and metastatic disease testing. The study demonstrated that within 18 months of treatment, 55% of the cohort received a colon examination,

71% received CEA testing, and 59% received metastatic disease screening tests. While it may be difficult to evaluate these findings without the breakdown of cancer stage, it is noteworthy that race/ethnicity disparities were demonstrated. Whites were more likely than minorities to receive CEA testing ($P = 0.04$) and also tended to be more likely to receive a colon examination ($P = 0.09$). Moreover, socioeconomic disparities were apparent. As the median household income increased, so too did the likelihood of colon examination and metastatic disease testing ($P = 0.03$, $P = 0.01$, respectively). The presence of disparate care is an important issue for colorectal cancer survivors.

One other study provides limited characterization of the use of services of colon cancer patients 1 to 3 years after diagnosis.[62] In this survey-based study, the report showed that 95% of the cohort had a usual source of care and that 66% saw a primary care provider in the past 12 months. Of note, 84% saw a specialist in the past 12 months, and 68% were in the emergency room at least once during that same time period. Eighteen percent reported having had home care in the prior year. It is evident that these survivors need and obtain medical care, both for cancer surveillance as well as the comorbid conditions. It appears, however, that there may be room for improvements. Using the receipt of preventive care measures as a rough proxy for appropriate receipt of health care, the study found that only 53% of the survivors received a flu shot in the past year. Moreover, further pulmonary and/or new cancer concerns arise because the study shows that 33% still smoked tobacco, with 27% overall reported to smoke daily.

Ongoing Issues: Changes in Treatments to Minimize Treatment Morbidity

From the discussions presented here, one can see that there are considerable short- and long-term problems associated with CRC treatment. As such, there is great interest in using efficacious treatments with less morbidity. Treatment modifications that are continually being clinically defined and used include laparoscopic-assisted surgery, the use of local excision of rectal cancers, the use of nerve-sparing surgical techniques, possibly using radiation therapy less frequently, and the use of chemoprevention. The following section briefly summarizes the current issues that surround these treatments.

Laparoscopic Surgery

Although an open approach has been the traditional method of performing colorectal cancer surgery, recently there have been studies that have demonstrated the advantages of laparoscopic resection. In brief, the advantages are smaller incisions, less pain, decreased length of stay, a decrease in the incisional hernia rate, and possible less adhesion formation. A recent randomized controlled trial (RCT) compared the efficacy of laparoscopic-assisted colectomy with open colectomy and found that patients having the former approach recovered faster, had lower blood loss, and had lower morbidity (P less than 0.001). Finally, the authors report that the probability of cancer-related survival was higher in the laparoscopic-assisted group ($P = 0.02$), as the Cox model showed that laparoscopic-assisted approach was independently associated with reduced risk of tumor relapse, death from any cause, and death from a cancer-related cause compared to open colectomy.[65]

A trial of the laparoscopic versus open approach for colon cancer treatment has also been performed in North America. Regarding quality of life issues, Weeks et al. demonstrated that the global quality of life was significantly higher at 2 weeks following the laparoscopic approach.[66] Additionally, the laparoscopic patients required significantly fewer days of parenteral and oral narcotics. Of note, however, is that no differences in QOL were demonstrated at 2 months following surgery. Importantly, the survival and recurrence results of this trial were not statistically different, which thus suggests that in appropriately performed operations, laparoscopic colon cancer resections can be performed safely.[67]

In the future, it is likely that increasingly more laparoscopically assisted surgical resections of colon and rectal cancers will be performed; however, it remains a priority that, with the laparoscopic approach, appropriately indicated and safe cancer resections are performed.

Local Excision for Rectal Cancer

Several researchers have reported that local excision with or without chemoradiation therapy is an alternative approach for sphincter preservation in patients with locally invasive rectal carcinoma.[68–71] While local excision has been performed in the past for early-stage rectal cancers, complete indications, appropriateness, and long-term results have not been finalized at this point. Local excision is performed transanally and is fundamentally a wide excisional biopsy. The rationale for this procedure is that for those patients with favorable prognosis rectal tumors confined to the bowel wall where removal of the draining lymphatic tissue would not add any oncologic benefit, local excision would be adequate and appropriate.

The technique can be relatively simple or very difficult, depending on such things as body habitus and the location and size of the tumor. In brief, using retractors or an operating proctoscope, the lesion is excised transanally with an adequate margin of normal tissue. Currently, local excision of T1 lesions with good prognostic factors (e.g., well differentiated) yields good results, and the use of adjuvant therapy in T2 lesions and lesions with high-risk factors has also been associated with favorable results. This literature is discussed in further detail in other chapters. Regarding survivors, however, meticulous follow-up is essential for early detection of local recurrences, which possibly allows for good results from salvage surgery.

In terms of function and quality of life, what is clearly advantageous regarding a transanal excision of a rectal cancer is that the potential morbidity associated with either a low anterior resection, coloanal, or an abdominoperineal resection (e.g., fecal incontinence, sexual and urologic dysfunction) is virtually eliminated (unless adjuvant radiation therapy is also performed).

Surgical Creation of a Neorectum to Improve Bowel-Related Function

One of the functions of the rectum is storage, and in this regard the rectum is a capacitance organ. When the rectum is resected for rectal cancer and the colon is put in its place, it is understandable that bowel function is worsened. In this regard, to overcome the functional deficiencies attributed to the loss of rectal capacity and decrease in compliance, studies have demonstrated how the creation of a neorectum improves bowel function. The two most common techniques to create a neorectum are the colonic J pouch and the coloplasty.

Creation of a J pouch involves folding over the lower 6 to 8 cm of the colon to make a "J" configuration. This J pouch basically doubles the lumen diameter over the straight colon. The J pouch has been compared to straight colon anastomoses in several RCTs and has been shown to result in better function. Bowel movement frequency, continence to liquids and gas, and cancer-specific quality of life are better with the J pouch.[28,72,73]

Another option is the coloplasty, which has been described and primarily developed in the past 5 years. Creation of a coloplasty involves making a 6- to 8-cm longitudinal incision in the lower colon and then suturing the incision closed in a transverse direction. This technique creates a larger pouch toward the lower end of the colon, just above the site of the anastomosis. RCTs of coloplasty versus J pouch have basically demonstrated an equivalent outcome in terms of bowel function (stool frequency, clustering of bowel movements, and urgency), continence, and quality of life.[73,74] What may be advantageous for the coloplasty is the maintenance of bowel length for performance of an anastomosis and a less bulky neorectum for patients with an especially narrow pelvis. In an unpublished review, the use of neorectal pouches in rectal cancer patients is below 25%.

Necessity of Radiation Therapy: When Not to Use It

The excellent results reported by Heald[11,75] and others utilizing "optimal surgery" (i.e., total mesorectal excision) without routine adjuvant therapy, the results of the NSABP R-02 trial, and other work bring to the forefront the controversy of omitting radiation therapy in the face of optimal surgery. Because the main purpose of radiation therapy is to improve local control, can optimally performed surgery in appropriately selected patients obviate the need for radiation therapy?

Heald examined this issue performing total mesorectal excisions for his patients with rectal cancer.[11,75] Total mesorectal excision involves complete removal of all the rectal mesentery, which includes the lymph nodes adjacent to the rectum. In a series of 419 consecutive rectal cancer patients, cancer-specific survival of all surgically treated patients was 68% at 5 years and 66% at 10 years. The local recurrence rate was 6% at 5 years and 8% at 10 years. In 405 "curative" resections, the local recurrence rate was 3% at 5 years and 4% at 10 years. Disease-free survival in this group was 80% at 5 years and 78% at 10 years. In his series overall, Heald found that rectal cancer can be cured by surgical therapy alone in 2 of 3 patients undergoing surgical excision in all stages and in 4 of 5 patients having curative resections [it should be noted that a small percentage of the series did receive chemotherapy (6%) and preoperative radiation (9%)].

A similar case series study of a specific tumor stage (i.e., T3N0M0) has demonstrated that adequate surgery will result in superb oncological outcomes, without use of adjuvant radiation therapy. In a single institutional series, Merchant et al.

showed that sharp mesorectal excision for T3N0M0 rectal cancers results in a local recurrence rate of less than 10% without the use of adjuvant therapy.[76]

Although not specifically tested, the National Surgical Adjuvant Bowel Program's R-02 trial is consistent with the nonuse of adjuvant radiation therapy. In this RCT, eligible patients ($n = 694$) with Dukes' B or C carcinoma of the rectum were randomly assigned to receive either postoperative adjuvant chemotherapy alone ($n = 348$) or chemotherapy with postoperative radiotherapy ($n = 346$).[77] The results showed that postoperative radiotherapy resulted in no beneficial effect on disease-free survival ($P = 0.90$) or overall survival ($P = 0.89$), regardless of chemotherapy. It should be noted, however, that radiation therapy did reduce the cumulative incidence of locoregional relapse from 13% to 8% at 5-year follow-up ($P = 0.02$).

In a review of the literature, Meagher et al.[78] reported that radiotherapy has only been demonstrated to significantly improve survival in one individual study and one recent meta-analysis. Although the local recurrence rates in the no-radiotherapy arm of these studies were 27% and 21% to 36.5%, respectively, in more-recent studies, with lower local recurrence rates reflecting modern surgical standards, no survival advantage has been found. While it is currently unknown whether radiotherapy improves patients' quality of life, studies have demonstrated that radiotherapy does bring about both acute and long-term detrimental effects on quality of life. Finally, these authors report that 17 to 20 patients need to undergo adjuvant radiotherapy to prevent 1 local recurrence,[78] questioning the appropriateness of radiation therapy as a general rule.

Data are available that supports the opposite sentiment. In contrast to the foregoing views, an important and recently published interim report from the Dutch Colorectal Cancer Group compared preoperative radiotherapy (20Gy over 5 days) followed by total mesorectal resection (924 patients) with total mesorectal excision alone (937 patients), that is, no radiation therapy.[13] At 2 years, no difference in overall survival was demonstrated; however, the rate of local recurrence at 2 years was significantly lower in the radiation group (2.4% versus 8.2%; P less than 0.0001). This study demonstrates that local recurrence is lessened with adjuvant radiation therapy, even with the use of "optimal surgery."

Overall, several issues remain regarding the use of radiation therapy in rectal cancer. First, will differences in local recurrence rates affect survival rates when examined in the long term? Second, is the toxicity of radiation therapy warranted with a decrease in local recurrence? Finally, can we select patients based on preoperative stage or tumor grade who should (and should not) receive radiation therapy?

Surgical Nerve-Sparing Techniques

Nerve preservation is important when performing rectal cancer surgery. Havenga et al.[37] evaluated sexual and urinary function after total mesorectal excision with autonomic nerve preservation was performed in patients with tumors situated within 12 cm of the anal verge. The ability to engage in intercourse was maintained by 86% of the male patients under 60 years of age and 67% of those age over 60 or undergoing APR, with a mean of 80% of preoperative penile rigidity. The ability to achieve orgasm was retained in 87%

of men and 91% of women, with arousal and lubrication present in 85% of the women. There were no severe urinary dysfunctions.

Masui et al.[79] evaluated sexual function in 134 men who had histologically curative resections with varying degrees of autonomic nerve preservation. All were under 65 years of age and all were sexually active preoperatively; 49% had tumors above the peritoneal reflection and 52% below. These patients were interviewed at least 1 year after surgery. Erection was maintained in 93% of those with complete nerve preservation, 82% when there was a hemilateral nerve preservation, and 61% with only pelvic plexus preservation. The respective proportions with erectile rigidity and duration sufficient for vaginal insertion were 90%, 53%, and 26%. Ejaculation potencies were 82%, 47%, and 0%. Although 96% of patients reported orgasm preoperatively, 94% of men with complete preservation, 65% with hemilateral preservation, and 22% with plexus preservation reported orgasm postoperatively. The combining of total mesorectal incision with autonomic nerve preservation is essential to reducing the long-term genitourinary morbidity of rectal cancer resection. These results suggest that preservation of sexual function is dependent on careful operative technique with preservation of the pelvic autonomic nerves. The low incidence of injury after curative total mesorectal incision also stands in contradiction to earlier admonitions that if erection and ejaculation were maintained then the operation was not curative.

Chemoprevention for Survivors

An important area of cancer research that may potentially impact the mecial treatment for colorectal cancer survivors is chemoprevention. Chemoprevention is the use of specific agents to prevent, inhibit, or reverse tumorigenic progression to invasive cancer. It is not intended to treat invasive carcinomas and therefore should be clearly distinguished from chemotherapy. The main goals of chemoprevention are to block the original initiation of the carcinogenic process, to arrest or reverse further progression of premalignant cells into becoming invasive or metastatic. Agents that have been investigated for chemopreventative activity in CRC include NSAIDs, calcium, antioxidant vitamins, and selenium.

Most of the work in chemoprevention of CRC has been performed in NSAIDs because of biologic evidence of the role of the cyclooxygenase pathway in CRC pathogenesis. More specifically, animal studies have demonstrated that NSAIDs function to stop colorectal carcinogenesis by blocking prostaglandin synthesis. Of the various available NSAIDs, sulindac is the most extensively studied. One study by Waddell et al. demonstrated that at doses ranging from 150 to 400 mg per day, colorectal polyps in FAP were eliminated. Importantly, the polyps regrew after sulindac was stopped, but then the polyps disappeared again after sulindac was reinstituted.[80]

Other studies have shown contrary results. A more recent RCT of 41 young (age 8 to 25 years) familial adenomatous polyposis (FAP) patients who were phenotypically unaffected received either 75 or 150 mg sulindac orally twice a day or identical-appearing placebo tablets for 48 months. This study found that after 4 years of treatment, adenomas developed in 9 of 21 subjects (43%) in the sulindac group and 11 of 20 subjects in the placebo group (55%) ($P = 0.54$). There were no significant differences in the mean number ($P = 0.69$) or size ($P = 0.17$) of polyps between the groups. While this study was performed in FAP patients and not in survivors, it did demonstrate that standard doses of sulindac did not prevent the development of adenomas.[81]

The role and effect of NSAIDs are still to be determined. Important to their use of NSAIDs for chemoprevention is the level of associated toxicity. A recent Japanese study of sulindac 300 mg per day showed that five of six patients had drug related complications, which ranged from severe nausea and vomiting to multiple ulcers of the small bowel and stomach.[82]

Recently, aspirin, which irreversibly affects the cyclooxygenase pathway, has been reported to decrease adenoma formation. In a randomized controlled study, 1,121 patients with a history of biopsy-proven adenomas were randomized to receive placebo (372 patients), 81 mg aspirin (377 patients), or 325 mg aspirin (372 patients) daily. Follow-up colonoscopy demonstrated that the incidence of one or more adenomas was 47% in the placebo group, 38% in the group given 81 mg aspirin per day, and 45% in the group given 325 mg aspirin per day (global $P = 0.04$). Unadjusted relative risks of any adenoma (as compared with the placebo group) were 0.81 in the 81-mg group (95% confidence interval, 0.69–0.96) and 0.96 in the 325-mg group (95% confidence interval, 0.81–1.13). For advanced neoplasms (adenomas measuring at least 1 cm in diameter or with tubulovillous or villous features, severe dysplasia, or invasive cancer), the respective relative risks were 0.59 (95%, 0.38–0.92) and 0.83 (95% confidence interval, 0.55–1.23).[83]

A separate randomized controlled trial of 635 colorectal cancer survivors who were randomized to receive either 325 mg aspirin per day or placebo corroborates these findings. The mean (±SD) number of adenomas was lower in the aspirin group than the placebo group (0.30 ± 0.87 versus 0.49 ± 0.99; $P = 0.003$ by the Wilcoxon test). The adjusted relative risk of any recurrent adenoma in the aspirin group, as compared with the placebo group, was 0.65 (95% confidence interval, 0.46–0.91). The time to the detection of a first adenoma was longer in the aspirin group than in the placebo group (hazard ratio for the detection of a new polyp, 0.64; 95% confidence interval, 0.43–0.94; $P = 0.022$).[84]

For colorectal cancer survivors in the future, chemoprevention appears to be a promising modality. There are ongoing large randomized controlled trials to address these issues and define the optimal prevention strategy.

Future Work

It is clear that there is a paucity of good evidence regarding colorectal cancer survivorship issues. Because the number of survivors will be increasing, this will be an important topic of study in the future. Specific issues include addressing the morbidities associated with the different treatment modalities, identifying and focusing on the presence of comorbidities in this elderly patient population, and improving the performance of CRC surveillance (without disparities).

References

1. Jemal A, Siegel R, Ward E, Murray T, Xu J, Smigal C, Thun MJ. Cancer statistics, 2006. CA Cancer J Clin 2006;56:106–130.

2. Hutchins LF, Unger JM, Crowley JJ, Coltman CA Jr, Albain KS. Underrepresentation of patients 65 years of age or older in cancer-treatment trials. N Engl J Med 1999;341:2061–2067.

3. Etzioni DA, Liu JH, Maggard MA, Ko CY. The aging population and its impact on the surgery workforce. Ann Surg 2003;238:170–177.

4. Mandel JS, Bond JH, Church TR, et al. Reducing mortality from colorectal cancer by screening for fecal occult blood. Minnesota Colon Cancer Control Study. N Engl J Med 1993;328:1365–1371.

5. Mandel JS, Church TR, Bond JH, et al. The effect of fecal occult-blood screening on the incidence of colorectal cancer. N Engl J Med 2000;343:1603–1607.

6. Kronborg O, Fenger C, Olsen J, Jorgensen OD, Sondergaard O. Randomised study of screening for colorectal cancer with faecal-occult-blood test. Lancet 1996;348:1467–1471.

7. Hardcastle JD, Chamberlain JO, Robinson MH, et al. Randomised controlled trial of faecal-occult-blood screening for colorectal cancer. Lancet 1996;348:1472–1477.

8. Ransohoff DF, Sandler RS. Clinical practice. Screening for colorectal cancer. N Engl J Med 2002;346:40–44.

9. Troisi RJ, Freedman AN, Devesa SS. Incidence of colorectal carcinoma in the U.S.: an update of trends by gender, race, age, subsite, and stage, 1975–1994. Cancer (Phila) 1999;85:1670–1676.

10. SEER. www.seer.cancer.gov 2004.

11. Heald RJ, Moran BJ, Ryall RD, Sexton R, MacFarlane JK. Rectal cancer: the Basingstoke experience of total mesorectal excision, 1978–1997. Arch Surg 1998;133:894–899.

12. Improved survival with preoperative radiotherapy in resectable rectal cancer. Swedish Rectal Cancer Trial. N Engl J Med 1997;336:980–987.

13. Kapiteijn E, Marijnen CA, Nagtegaal ID, et al. Preoperative radiotherapy combined with total mesorectal excision for resectable rectal cancer. N Engl J Med 2001;345:638–646.

14. Rao S, Cunningham D. Adjuvant therapy for colon cancer in the new millennium. Scand J Surg 2003;92:57–64.

15. O'Connell MJ, Laurie JA, Kahn M, et al. Prospectively randomized trial of postoperative adjuvant chemotherapy in patients with high-risk colon cancer. J Clin Oncol 1998;16:295–300.

16. Arkenau HT, Bermann A, Rettig K, Strohmeyer G, Porschen R. 5-Fluorouracil plus leucovorin is an effective adjuvant chemotherapy in curatively resected stage III colon cancer: long-term follow-up results of the adjCCA-01 trial. Ann Oncol 2003;14:395–399.

17. Schwartz SI, Shires GT, Spencer FC, Daly JM, Fischer JE, Galloway AC (eds). Principles of Surgery, 7th ed. New York: McGraw Hill, 1999.

18. Joseph NE, Sigurdson ER, Hanlon AL, et al. Accuracy of determining nodal negativity in colorectal cancer on the basis of the number of nodes retrieved on resection. Ann Surg Oncol 2003;10:213–218.

19. Kemeny N, Huang Y, Cohen AM, et al. Hepatic arterial infusion of chemotherapy after resection of hepatic metastases from colorectal cancer. N Engl J Med 1999;341:2039–2048.

20. Gordon PH, Nivatvongs S. Surgery of the Colon, Rectum, and Anus. London: Saunders, 2001.

21. Corman MC. Surgery of the Colon and Rectum. Philadelphia: Lippincott Williams & Wilkins. 2001.

22. Smith R, Bohl J, McElearney S, et al. Wound infection after elective colorectal resection. Ann Surg 2004;239:599–605.

23. Edna TH, Bjerkeset T, Loe B. Small bowel obstruction in patients previously operated on for colorectal cancer. Eur J Surg 1998;164:587–592.

24. Cameron J (ed). Current Surgical Therapy, 7th ed. St. Louis: Mosby, 2001.

25. Cahalane MJ, Shapiro ME, Silen W, et al. Abdominal incision: decision or indecision? Lancet 1989;1:146–148.

26. Millikan KW. Incisional hernia repair. Surg Clin N Am 2003;83:1223–1234.

27. Flum DR, Horvath K, Koepsell T. Have outcomes of incisional hernia repair improved with time? A population-based analysis. Ann Surg 2003;237:129–135.

28. Sailer M, Fuchs KH, Fein M, Thiede A. Randomized clinical trial comparing quality of life after straight and pouch coloanal reconstruction. Br J Surg 2002;89:1108–1117.

29. Mancini R, Cosimelli M, Filippini A, et al. Nerve-sparing surgery in rectal cancer: feasibility and functional results. J Exp Clin Cancer Res 2000;19:35–40.

30. Chatwin NA, Ribordy M, Givel JC. Clinical outcomes and quality of life after low anterior resection for rectal cancer. Eur J Surg 2002;168:297–301.

31. Londono-Schimmer EE, Leong AP, Phillips RK. Life table analysis of stomal complications following colostomy. Dis Colon Rectum 1994;37:916–920.

32. Makela J, Turku P, Laitinen S. Analysis of late stomal complications following ostomy surgery. Ann Chir Gynaecol 1997; 86:305–310.

33. Nugent KP, Daniels P, Stewart B, Patankar R, Johnson CD. Quality of life in stoma patients. Dis Colon Rectum 1999;42: 1569–1574.

34. Bass EM, Del Pino A, Tan A, Pearl RK, Orsay CP, Abcarian H. Does preoperative stoma marking and education by the enterostomal therapist affect outcome? Dis Colon Rectum 1997;40: 440–442.

35. Sprangers MA, Taal BG, Aaronson NK, te Velde A. Quality of life in colorectal cancer. Stoma vs. nonstoma patients. Dis Colon Rectum 1995;38:361–369.

36. Beck D, Wexner SD eds) Fundamentals of Anorectal Surgery. London: Saunders, 1998.

37. Havenga K, DeRuiter MC, Enker WE, Welvaart K. Anatomical basis of autonomic nerve-preserving total mesorectal excision for rectal cancer. Br J Surg 1996;83:384–388.

38. Havenga K, Enker WE, McDermott K, Cohen AM, Minsky BD, Guillem J. Male and female sexual and urinary function after total mesorectal excision with autonomic nerve preservation for carcinoma of the rectum. J Am Coll Surg 1996;182:495–502.

39. Enker WE, Havenga K, Polyak T, Thaler H, Cranor M. Abdominoperineal resection via total mesorectal excision and autonomic nerve preservation for low rectal cancer. World J Surg 1997;21:715–720.

40. van Driel MF, Weymar Schultz WC, van de Wiel HB, Hahn DE, Mensink HJ. Female sexual functioning after radical surgical treatment of rectal and bladder cancer. Eur J Surg Oncol 1993; 19:183–187.

41. Rothenberger DA, Wong WD. Abdominoperineal resection for adenocarcinoma of the low rectum. World J Surg 1992;16: 478–485.

42. Havenga K, Enker WE, Norstein J, et al. Improved survival and local control after total mesorectal excision or D3 lymphadenectomy in the treatment of primary rectal cancer: an international analysis of 1411 patients. Eur J Surg Oncol 1999; 25:368–374.

43. Balslev I, Harling H. Sexual dysfunction following operation for carcinoma of the rectum. Dis Colon Rectum 1983;26:785–788.

44. NIH CC. Adjuvant therapy for patients with colon and rectal cancer. JAMA 1990;264:1444–1450.

45. Guren MG, Dueland S, Skovlund E, Fossa SD, Poulsen JP, Tveit KM. Quality of life during radiotherapy for rectal cancer. Eur J Cancer 2003;39:587–594.

46. Ooi BS, Tjandra JJ, Green MD. Morbidities of adjuvant chemotherapy and radiotherapy for resectable rectal cancer: an overview. Dis Colon Rectum 1999;42:403–418.

47. Temple LK, Wong WD, Minsky B. The impact of radiation on functional outcomes in patients with rectal cancer and sphincter preservation. Semin Radiat Oncol 2003;13:469–477.

48. Dahlberg M, Glimelius B, Graf W, Pahlman L. Preoperative irradiation affects functional results after surgery for rectal cancer: results from a randomized study. Dis Colon Rectum 1998;41: 543–549; discussion 549–551.

49. Dehni N, McNamara DA, Schlegel RD, Guiguet M, Tiret E, Parc R. Clinical effects of preoperative radiation therapy on anorectal function after proctectomy and colonic J-pouch-anal anastomosis. Dis Colon Rectum 2002;45:1635–1640.

50. Nathanson DR, Espat NJ, Nash GM, et al. Evaluation of preoperative and postoperative radiotherapy on long-term functional results of straight coloanal anastomosis. Dis Colon Rectum 2003;46:888–894.

51. Ammann K, Kirchmayr W, Klaus A, et al. Impact of neoadjuvant chemoradiation on anal sphincter function in patients with carcinoma of the midrectum and low rectum. Arch Surg 2003; 138:257–261.

52. Schag CA, Ganz PA, Heinrich RL. Cancer Rehabilitation Evaluation System–short form (CARES-SF). A cancer specific rehabilitation and quality of life instrument. Cancer (Phila) 1991;68:1406–1413.

53. Schag CA, Ganz PA, Wing DS, Sim MS, Lee JJ. Quality of life in adult survivors of lung, colon and prostate cancer. Qual Life Res 1994;3:127–141.

54. Schag CA, Heinrich RL, Aadland RL, Ganz PA. Assessing problems of cancer patients: psychometric properties of the cancer inventory of problem situations. Health Psychol 1990; 9:83–102.

55. Ganz PA, Schag CA, Lee JJ, Sim MS. The CARES: a generic measure of health-related quality of life for patients with cancer. Qual Life Res 1992;1:19–29.

56. Heinrich RL, Schag CC, Ganz PA. Living with cancer: the Cancer Inventory of Problem Situations. J Clin Psychol 1984; 40:972–980.

57. Ramsey SD, Berry K, Moinpour C, Giedzinska A, Andersen MR. Quality of life in long term survivors of colorectal cancer. Am J Gastroenterol 2002;97:1228–1234.

58. Sprangers MA. Quality-of-life assessment in colorectal cancer patients: evaluation of cancer therapies. Semin Oncol 1999;26: 691–696.

59. Allal A, Bieri S, Pelloni A, et al. Sphincter-sparing surgery after preoperative radiotherapy for low rectal cancers: feasibility, oncologic results and quality of life outcomes. Br J Cancer 2000; 82:1131–1137.

60. Grumann MM, Noack EM, Hoffmann IA, Schlag PM. Comparison of quality of life in patients undergoing abdominoperineal extirpation or anterior resection for rectal cancer. Ann Surg 2001;233:149–156.

61. Engel J, Kerr J, Schlesinger-Raab A, Eckel R, Sauer H, Holzel D. Quality of life in rectal cancer patients: a four-year prospective study. Ann Surg 2003;238:203–213.

62. Ko C, Chaudhry S. The need for a multidisciplinary approach to cancer care. J Surg Res 2002;105:53–57.

63. Meyerhardt JA, Catalano PJ, Haller DG, et al. Impact of diabetes mellitus on outcomes in patients with colon cancer. J Clin Oncol 2003;21:433–440.

64. Lafata JE, Johnson CC, Ben-Menachem T, Morlock RJ. Sociodemographic differences in the receipt of colorectal cancer surveillance care following treatment with curative intent. Med Care 2001;39:361–372.

65. Lacy AM, Garcia-Valdecasas JC, Delgado S, et al. Laparoscopy-assisted colectomy versus open colectomy for treatment of nonmetastatic colon cancer: a randomised trial. Lancet 2002;359: 2224–2229.

66. Weeks JC, Nelson H, Gelber S, Sargent D, Schroeder G. Short-term quality-of-life outcomes following laparoscopic-assisted colectomy vs. open colectomy for colon cancer: a randomized trial. JAMA 2002;287:321–328.

67. Group COoSTS. A comparison of laparoscopically assisted and open colectomy for colon cancer. N Engl J Med 2004;350: 2050–2059.

68. Paty PB, Nash GM, Baron P, et al. Long-term results of local excision for rectal cancer. Ann Surg 2002;236:522–529; discussion 529–530.

69. Saclarides TJ. Transanal endoscopic microsurgery: a single surgeon's experience. Arch Surg 1998;133:598–599.

70. Rothenberger DA, Garcia-Aguilar J. Role of local excision in the treatment of rectal cancer. Semin Surg Oncol 2000;19: 367–375.

71. Blair S, Ellenhorn JD. Transanal excision for low rectal cancers is curative in early-stage disease with favorable histology. Am Surg 2000;66:817–820.

72. Furst A, Burghofer K, Hutzel L, Jauch KW. Neorectal reservoir is not the functional principle of the colonic J-pouch: the volume of a short colonic J-pouch does not differ from a straight coloanal anastomosis. Dis Colon Rectum 2002;45:660–667.

73. Furst A, Suttner S, Agha A, Beham A, Jauch KW. Colonic J-pouch vs. coloplasty following resection of distal rectal cancer: early results of a prospective, randomized, pilot study. Dis Colon Rectum 2003;46:1161–1166.

74. Ho YH, Brown S, Heah SM, et al. Comparison of J-pouch and coloplasty pouch for low rectal cancers: a randomized, controlled trial investigating functional results and comparative anastomotic leak rates. Ann Surg 2002;236:49–55.

75. Heald RJ. Total mesorectal exsicion (TME). Acta Chir Iugosl 2000;47:17–18.

76. Merchant NB, Guillem JG, Paty PB, et al. T3N0 rectal cancer: results following sharp mesorectal excision and no adjuvant therapy. J Gastrointest Surg 1999;3:642–647.

77. Wolmark N, Wieand HS, Hyams DM, et al. Randomized trial of postoperative adjuvant chemotherapy with or without radiotherapy for carcinoma of the rectum: National Surgical Adjuvant Breast and Bowel Project Protocol R-02. J Natl Cancer Inst 2000; 92:388–396.

78. Meagher AP, Ward RL. Current evidence does not support routine adjuvant radiotherapy for rectal cancer. ANZ J Surg 2002;72:835–840.

79. Masui H, Ike H, Yamaguchi S, Oki S, Shimada H. Male sexual function after autonomic nerve-preserving operation for rectal cancer. Dis Colon Rectum 1996;39:1140–1145.

80. Waddell WR, Ganser GF, Cerise EJ, Loughry RW. Sulindac for polyposis of the colon. Am J Surg 1989;157:175–179.

81. Giardiello FM, Yang VW, Hylind LM, et al. Primary chemoprevention of familial adenomatous polyposis with sulindac. N Engl J Med 2002;346:1054–1059.

82. Ishikawa H, Akedo I, Suzuki T, Narahara H, Otani T. Adverse effects of sulindac used for prevention of colorectal cancer. J Natl Cancer Inst 1997;89:1381.

83. Baron JA, Cole BF, Sandler RS, et al. A randomized trial of aspirin to prevent colorectal adenomas. N Engl J Med 2003;348(10): 891–899.

84. Sandler RS, Halabi S, Baron JA, et al. A randomized trial of aspirin to prevent colorectal adenomas in patients with previous colorectal cancer. N Engl J Med 2003;348:883–890.

Medical and Psychosocial Issues in Transplant Survivors

Karen L. Syrjala, Paul Martin, Joachim Deeg, and Michael Boeckh

Survival rates for hematopoietic cell transplantation (HCT) have improved with advances in supportive care that have reduced acute, transplant-related mortality. More than 40,000 transplants were performed worldwide in 2002, mostly for the treatment of leukemia, lymphoma, or multiple myeloma.[1] The probability of successful transplantation is generally greater for patients transplanted early in their disease course, for younger patients, and for patients who receive stem cells from donors whose human leukocyte antigens (HLA) match the patient's. For survivors who receive HCT for acute leukemia or chronic myeloid leukemia and who remain free of disease after 2 years, the probability of living 5 or more years is 89%.[2]

HCT survivors experience short and long-term problems similar to those of many other cancer survivors who receive systemic high-dose therapy. In addition, patients receiving stem cells from a related or unrelated donor (allogeneic) rather than receiving their own stem cells (autologous) experience complications related to the immunologic reaction of donor cells against the patient's cells and tissues. Chronic graft-versus-host disease (GVHD) occurs in about 60% of patients who survive the acute transplant-related toxicities and can persist for years. It is generally treated with immunosuppressive medications, often including high-dose glucocorticoids. Extended immunosuppression leads to several other vulnerabilities in allogeneic HCT recipients beyond that which is seen in other cancer survivors. Some of these effects result from GVHD itself; others are a consequence of the treatments used for GVHD.

Although evidence-based conclusions from HCT clinical trials are plentiful, research on survivor medical and quality of life issues is limited and largely descriptive. Randomized controlled trials are few, in part because they are difficult to accomplish with widely dispersed patients who, until recently, represented a small percentage of the cancer survivor population. Effective treatment of chronic GVHD without dependence on high-dose glucocorticoids is a primary need for improving both survival and quality of life for allogeneic transplant survivors. Evidence is needed regarding the risks and effective treatments for fungal and pulmonary complications as well as bone- and joint-related problems such as osteoporosis and avascular necrosis.

Chronic Graft-Versus-Host Disease

Chronic GVHD is a pleiotropic syndrome with onset generally occurring between 3 and 24 months after HCT from an allogeneic donor.[3–5] Clinical manifestations of chronic GVHD are highly variable and resemble an overlap of several collagen vascular diseases, with frequent involvement of the skin, liver, eyes, mouth, sinuses, and esophagus, and less-frequent involvement of serosal surfaces, lungs, lower gastrointestinal tract, female genitalia, and fascia. Major causes of morbidity include scleroderma, contractures, ulceration, keratoconjunctivitis, esophageal and vaginal strictures, obstructive pulmonary disease, and weight loss with or without malabsorption. Uncontrolled chronic GVHD interferes with immune reconstitution and is strongly associated with increased risks of opportunistic infections and death.

Studies have provided a good understanding of risk factors for development of chronic GVHD and risk factors for mortality among patients with newly diagnosed GVHD. Five-year survival rates for patients with newly diagnosed *standard-risk* chronic GVHD have remained at approximately 70%, and 5-year survival rates for those with "high-risk" chronic GVHD have remained at 40% to 50%. In aggregate, only 50% of patients with chronic GVHD are able to discontinue immunosuppressive treatment within 5 years after the diagnosis, and 10% require continued treatment beyond 5 years. The remaining 40% die or develop recurrent malignancy before chronic GVHD resolves. Prolonged treatment with high-dose glucocorticoids causes considerable morbidity, leading to a desperate need for agents that can decrease the dependence on steroids for controlling the disease.

Prevention of Chronic GVHD

Results of retrospective analyses and Phase 3 clinical trials have identified a variety of risk factors for the development of chronic GVHD after allogeneic HCT (Table 15.1). Risk factors that cannot be controlled as part of medical management include older age of the patient, the use of a female donor, and the use of an unrelated donor or HLA-mismatched related donor as opposed to an HLA-identical sibling.[3,5] Risk factors that can be controlled as part of medical management are related to the use of marrow versus growth factor-mobilized blood as the source of hematopoietic cells, the numbers of T cells and CD34-positive cells in the graft, the use of prednisone for prevention of GVHD after the transplant, and the duration of cyclosporine administration.

The use of growth factor-mobilized peripheral blood as opposed to marrow as a source of stem cells clearly increases the risk of chronic GVHD[6] and may prolong the duration of immunosuppression needed to control chronic GVHD.[7] These results are consistent with findings that the risk of chronic GVHD increases after administration of nonmobilized buffy coat cells to prevent rejection after marrow transplantation for treatment of aplastic anemia.[8] Despite these observations, the choice between mobilized blood cells and marrow depends primarily on the evaluation of other endpoints, such as survival or relapse-free survival, which are more important than the risk of chronic GVHD per se.

The increased risk of chronic GVHD after transplantation with mobilized blood could reflect the 10-fold-higher number of T cells in the graft as compared to marrow. However, results of retrospective studies that correlated the cellular composition of mobilized apheresis products with a variety of outcomes after transplant did not support this interpretation. Instead, chronic GVHD was associated with high numbers of CD34-positive cells in the graft.[9,10] Mechanisms to explain this unexpected association remain to be defined.

Results of an early randomized trial[11] and many Phase 2 studies have suggested that depletion of T cells from the graft decreases the risk of chronic GVHD, and this suggestion was initially confirmed by results from a large retrospective review of data from the International Bone Marrow Transplant Registry (IBMTR).[12] A subsequent review of data in the IBMTR, however, unexpectedly showed a higher risk of chronic GVHD among patients who received HLA-mismatched marrow treated with "narrow specificity" antibodies compared to those who received marrow that was treated by other methods or that was not treated.[13] Preliminary results of a recent randomized controlled trial showed that T-cell depletion did not decrease the risk of chronic GVHD.[14] Recent evidence has suggested that depletion of donor T cells by in vivo administration of rabbit antithymocyte globulin (ATG) may reduce the risk of chronic GVHD.[15]

Taken together, the T-cell depletion trials and ATG trials have produced inconsistent results regarding the relationship between the T-cell content of the graft and risk of chronic GVHD, making it difficult to reach a general conclusion. The possible association between the number of CD34 cells in the graft and risk of chronic GVHD needs confirmation from additional studies.

Four randomized clinical trials have evaluated the effects of prophylactic glucocorticoid administration after allogeneic marrow transplantation.[16–19] In each of these studies, the primary endpoint was the development of acute GVHD, and chronic GVHD was a secondary endpoint. Results with respect to chronic GVHD were inconsistent, despite enrollment of 108 to 186 patients in each study. The weight of the evidence suggests that prophylactic administration of glucocorticoids after marrow transplantation is likely to increase rather than decrease the risk of chronic GVHD.

Two randomized trials[20,21] and one sequential cohort study[22] have evaluated the risk of chronic GVHD as related to the duration of cyclosporine administration. Taken together, the consistent results of these trials suggest that prolonged administration of cyclosporine might yield a modest reduction in the risk of chronic GVHD, but the effect was too small to reach statistical significance in the two randomized trials.

Results from Phase 2 studies suggested that thalidomide might be effective for treatment of chronic GVHD, but results from a Phase 3 study showed that mortality was increased when thalidomide was administered before the onset of chronic GVHD.[23]

Treatment of Chronic GVHD

Anecdotal experience and retrospective reviews during the 1970s and early 1980s demonstrated that untreated clinical extensive chronic GVHD generally causes severe disability related to scleroderma, contractures, strictures, pulmonary disease, and keratoconjunctivitis (Table 15.2).[3–5] Administration of prednisone late in the natural history of the disease provided little benefit. Early administration of prednisone appeared to prevent disability but did not greatly affect survival. Retrospective reviews have identified a variety of factors associated with an increased risk of mortality from causes other than recurrent malignancy among patients with chronic GVHD.[3,5] The most consistently reported findings indicate an increased risk of transplant-related mortality among patients who have direct progression from acute to chronic GVHD or a platelet count less than $100,000/\mu L$ at the diagnosis of GVHD. The term high-risk chronic GVHD has been used to describe cases with either of these characteristics, whereas standard-risk chronic GVHD excludes cases with either of these characteristics.

An early double-blind randomized trial was carried out to determine whether administration of azathioprine together with prednisone might be more effective than prednisone alone for treatment of newly diagnosed chronic GVHD.[24] The results unexpectedly showed inferior outcomes for patients in the azathioprine arm. The difference in survival was attributed to an increased incidence of infections in the azathioprine arm.

Results of sequential Phase 2 studies suggested that survival among patients with high-risk chronic GVHD might be improved by combined treatment with cyclosporine and prednisone.[24,25] In a subsequent randomized prospective trial, however, cyclosporine did not provide a survival benefit, although the incidence of avascular necrosis was decreased in the cyclosporine arm, suggesting a steroid-sparing effect.[26]

Results of several Phase 2 studies suggested that thalidomide might be effective for treatment of steroid-refractory chronic GVHD, but subsequent randomized trials showed no benefit with the use of thalidomide.[27,28]

TABLE 15.1. Clinical trials of prevention of chronic graft-versus-host disease.

Author	Reference	Year	Number of patients	Randomized (Y/N)	Diagnosis/ stage of disease	Intervention/design	Follow-up	Relative risk/outcomes	Survival statistics	Conclusions/ comments
Mitsuyasu et al.	11	1986	40	Y	Leukemia	T-cell-depleted marrow compared with unmodified marrow; methotrexate or cyclosporine also given to prevent GVHD; RCT	1–2 years	Decreased incidence of chronic GVHD with T-cell-depleted marrow (5% versus 25%)	No significant difference between arms	T-cell depletion increased the risk of recurrent malignancy after the transplant
Marmont et al.	12	1991	3,211	N	Leukemia	T-cell-depleted marrow compared with unmodified marrow; retrospective multicenter cohort study	3–8 years	Relative risk of chronic GVHD = 0.56 with T-cell depletion compared to unmodified marrow ($P < 0.0001$)	Decreased leukemia-free survival with T-cell depletion	T-cell depletion increased the risk of recurrent malignancy after the transplant
Champlin et al.	13	2000	1,868	N	Leukemia	T-cell-depleted marrow compared with unmodified marrow; depletion with "narrow specificity" antibodies compared to other methods; retrospective multicenter cohort study	4 months to 11 years	Relative risk of chronic GVHD = 1.5 for marrow treated with "narrow specificity" antibodies compared to untreated marrow ($P < 0.0003$)	Leukemia-free survival better after T-cell depletion with "narrow specificity" antibodies compared to other methods; no significant difference in leukemia-free survival with "narrow specificity" antibodies compared to unmodified marrow	The use of "broad specificity" methods that deplete natural killer cells and T cells from HLA-mismatched donor marrow appeared to have detrimental effects on outcome
Wagner et al.	14	2002	410	Y	Mostly leukemia	T-cell-depleted marrow and immunosuppression with cyclosporine compared with unmodified marrow and immunosuppression with methotrexate and cyclosporine; multicenter RCT	2–6 years	Incidence of chronic GVHD = 24% with T-cell depletion and 29% with unmodified marrow	T-cell depletion was associated with an increased risk of recurrent malignancy among patients with chronic myeloid leukemia; leukemia-free survival was similar in the two arms for patients with other diseases	T-cell depletion decreased the risk of severe acute GVHD but did not improve survival
Bacigalupo et al.	15	2001	109	Y	Hematologic malignancies	Conventional pretransplant conditioning with or without rabbit antithymocyte globulin administered at two different doses; two consecutive RCT		Incidence of chronic GVHD = 39% with ATG and 62% without ($P = 0.04$)	No difference in survival between arms	Use of ATG at the higher dose was associated with an increased risk of infections
Storb et al.	16	1990	147	Y	Mostly leukemia	Posttransplant immunosuppression using methotrexate plus cyclosporine, with or without prednisone administered throughout the first 35 days after transplant; two studies, one RCT and the other a prospective cohort study	1.5–3 years	Incidence of chronic GVHD = 62% with prednisone and 40% without ($P = 0.01$)	No difference in survival between arms	Use of prednisone increased the risk of chronic GVHD

Study	Ref	Year	N	RCT	Population	Intervention	Follow-up	Chronic GVHD outcome	Survival outcome	Acute GVHD/conclusion
Deeg et al.	180	1997	122	Y	Hematologic malignancy	Posttransplant immunosuppression with cyclosporine with or without methylprednisolone administered between days 7 and 72 after transplant; RCT	0.5–3.5 years	Incidence of chronic GVHD = 44% with methylprednisolone and 21% without ($P = 0.02$)	No difference in survival between arms	Incidence of acute GVHD was 60% with methylprednisolone and 73% without ($P = 0.01$)
Chao et al.	18	2000	193	Y	Leukemia	Posttransplant immunosuppression plus methotrexate plus cyclosporine with or without prednisone administered between days 7 and 180 after transplant; RCT	1–6 years	Incidence of chronic GVHD = 46% with prednisone and 52% without ($P = 0.38$)	No difference in survival between arms	Incidence of acute GVHD was 18% with prednisone and 20% without ($P = 0.6$)
Ruutu et al.	181	2000	108	Y	Hematologic malignancy	Posttransplant immunosuppression using methotrexate plus cyclosporine with or without methylprednisolone administered between days 14 and 110 after transplant; RCT	4–9 years	Incidence of chronic GVHD = 35% with methylprednisolone and 48% without ($P = 0.17$)	No difference in survival between arms	Incidence of acute GVHD was 19% with methylprednisolone and 56% without ($P = 0.0001$)
Storb et al.	20	1997	103	Y	Mostly leukemia	Posttransplant immunosuppression using methotrexate plus cyclosporine administered to day 60 or day 180 among patients who did not have GVHD on day 60; RCT	1–10 years	Incidence of chronic GVHD = 54% in the day 60 arm and 43% in the day 180 arm ($P = 0.26$)	Possible increase in transplant-related mortality in day 60 arm among patients with GVHD before day 60	No benefit from prolonged administration of cyclosporine among patients who did not have acute GVHD
Kansu et al.	21	2001	162	Y	Mostly leukemia	Patients eligible if they had a prior history of acute GVHD or if skin biopsy showed histologic evidence of GVHD on day 80; RCT comparing administration of cyclosporine for 6 or 24 months	2–9 years	Incidence of chronic GVHD = 39% in the 24-month arm and 51% in the 6-month arm ($P = 0.24$); hazard ratio = 0.76 ($P = 0.25$)	No difference in survival	Prolonged administration of cyclosporine did not greatly decrease the incidence of chronic GVHD
Mengarelli et al.	22	2003	57	N	Hematologic malignancy	Patients received peripheral blood cells from an HLA-identical sibling, and cyclosporine was administered for either 6 or 12 months in two consecutive retrospective cohorts	1–4 years	Incidence of chronic GVHD = 25% in the 12-month group and 69% in the 6-month group; hazard ratio = 0.2 (adjusted $P = 0.008$)	No difference in survival	Prolonged administration of cyclosporine appeared to decrease the incidence of chronic GVHD
Chao et al.	23	1996	59	Y	Hematologic malignancy	Administration of thalidomide or placebo beginning at day 80 after transplant; double-blind RCT	6 months to 3 years	Incidence of chronic GVHD = 64% with thalidomide and 38% with placebo ($P = 0.06$)	Increased mortality in the thalidomide arm ($P = 0.006$)	Administration of thalidomide was unexpectedly found to be harmful

GVHD, graft-versus-host disease; RCT, randomized controlled trial; ATG, antithymocyte globulin.

TABLE 15.2. Clinical trials of chronic graft-versus-host disease.

Author	Reference	Year	Number of patients	Randomized (Y/N)	Diagnosis/stage of disease	Intervention/design	Follow-up	Relative risk/ outcomes	Survival statistics	Conclusions/comments
Sullivan et al.	25	1988	126	Y	Newly diagnosed chronic GVHD and platelet count >100,000/µL	Prednisone with or without azathioprine; double-blind RCT	Minimum of 3.8 years	Not stated	47% survival at 5 years with prednisone plus azathioprine, 61% with prednisone plus placebo ($P = 0.03$)	Results demonstrate inferior outcomes when azathioprine was used to treat chronic GVHD
Koc et al.	26	2002	287	Y	Newly diagnosed chronic GVHD and platelet count >100,000/µL	Prednisone with or without continued administration of cyclosporine; RCT	4–14 years	Incidence of nonrelapse mortality at 5 years = 17% with prednisone plus cyclosporine, 13% with prednisone; hazard ratio = 1.55 ($P = 0.11$)	67% survival at 5 years with prednisone plus cyclosporine, 72% with prednisone; hazard ratio = 1.35 ($P = 0.13$) 61% survival without recurrent malignancy at 5 years with prednisone plus cyclosporine, 71% with prednisone; hazard ratio = 1.51 ($P = 0.03$)	Subset analysis suggested increased mortality among patients with chronic GVHD that evolved directly from acute GVHD Incidence of avascular necrosis was lower with prednisone plus cyclosporine than with prednisone alone
Arora et al.	27	2001	54	Y	Newly diagnosed chronic GVHD	Prednisone and cyclosporine with or without thalidomide (200–800 mg/day); double-blind RCT	0.5–4.8 years	Incidence of partial or complete response at 2, 6, and 12 months = 83%, 88% and 85% with thalidomide, 89%, 84%, and 73% without thalidomide	66% at 2 years with thalidomide, 54% without thalidomide ($P = 0.85$)	High response rate was observed in both groups; study was terminated early due to low accrual rate
Koc et al.	28	2000	52	Y	Newly diagnosed chronic GVHD with platelet count <100,000/µL or progressive onset from acute GVHD as high-risk features	Prednisone and cyclosporine or tacrolimus with or without thalidomide (200–800 mg/day); double-blind RCT	Not reported	No statistically significant difference in transplant-related mortality	49% survival at 4 years with thalidomide, 47% without thalidomide ($P = 0.87$)	Thalidomide caused intolerable side effects, leading to premature discontinuation of administration in 92% of patients; the duration of thalidomide administration was not sufficient to allow assessment of efficacy

Phase 2 studies have been carried out to evaluate the use of many immunosuppressive agents for treatment of steroid-refractory chronic GVHD. The small number of enrolled patients, the widely divergent enrollment criteria and poorly defined efficacy criteria, and the lack of controls hamper the interpretation of these studies. Efficacy is generally reported as improvement in symptoms or signs of chronic GVHD at any time after introduction of the additional immunosuppressive treatment. The duration of clinical improvement is typically not taken into account, and survival data are difficult to interpret because of variable follow-up and possible selection biases in enrollment. In the absence of pharmacokinetic evaluation, studies of this type typically do not add useful information to the available safety profile of approved immunosuppressive agents. Trial designs with prior specification of criteria for judging efficacy according to robust and meaningful endpoints would help to make the results of Phase 2 studies more informative.

Emerging Challenges in Chronic GVHD

Advances in supportive care have reduced morbidity, but survival for patients with newly diagnosed chronic GVHD has not changed since the mid-1980s.[3,5] In the past, investigators have taken the highly empirical approach of testing virtually any available immunosuppressive agent for treatment of chronic GVHD, because the pathophysiology of chronic GVHD is complex and poorly understood. Development of a more-direct approach will require an improved understanding of the pathophysiologic mechanisms leading to chronic GVHD.

Infections

A susceptibility to late infectious complications persists because of residual immunodeficiency that is observed in all HCT recipients, not only those with allogeneic donors,[29] although infection risk is increased with the additional immunosuppression associated with chronic GVHD and its treatment (Table 15.3).

Bacterial

There is a significant risk for severe infection with encapsulating bacteria (*Streptococcus pneumoniae, Haemophilus influenzae*) after HCT in the setting of chronic GVHD.[30] Patients may develop rapidly progressive disease, which is often fatal. The presumed explanation for bacteremic pneumococcal infections is that HCT patients lose and do not subsequently make opsonizing antibody to encapsulated gram-positive organisms, even after recovery from infection.[30] Patients also respond poorly to immunization with prototype pneumococcal vaccines for the first 1 to 2 years after transplant, although response again improves with time.[31,32] Immunization with the available pneumococcal vaccines provides incomplete protection for those most in need, that is, patients with chronic GVHD.[33]

Antibacterial prophylaxis is recommended in patients with chronic GVHD to prevent both bacteremic pneumococcal and other infection, although no randomized placebo-controlled trials have been performed.[34] The 23-valent pneumococcal polysaccharide vaccine (12 and 24 months after transplantation) and the *Haemophilus influenzae* B conjugate vaccine (12, 14, and 24 months after transplantation) are recommended in standard guidelines.[34] However, these vaccinations are not 100% protective; the 7-valent conjugated pneumococcal vaccine has not been evaluated in transplant recipients.

Althouogh penicillin appears to work for this indication, the recent emergence of penicillin-resistant pneumococci make it a less preferable choice.[35] Rather, trimethoprim-sulfamethoxazole (TMP-SMX) given once daily (80 mg TMP component) provides protection both against *Pneumocystis jiroveci* pneumonia (PCP), encapsulated bacteria, and possibly also against toxoplasmosis. Controlled trial data are not available to evaluate the efficacy of such prophylaxis, but retrospective study of nonrandomized treatment groups indicates that patients with chronic GVHD who receive TMP-SMX prophylaxis have a significantly lower incidence of infection.[29] Oral penicillins should be reserved for patients who are unable to tolerate daily TMP-SMX. No reports exist about new quinolones or macrolides for this indication.

Because infection with other organisms including both *Staphylococcus* species and gram-negative aerobic bacteria also occurs, empirical antibiotic treatment of HCT patients admitted with clinical sepsis should include broad-spectrum coverage until the identity of the infecting organisms is known.

Viral

Varicella-zoster virus (VZV) disease is the most common viral infection late after HCT.[36-40] Median time of onset is 5 months after transplant, and most cases occur within the first year. However, VZV disease can occur up to several years after transplantation, especially in the setting of chronic GVHD. A subgroup at particularly high risk for VZV infection is VZV-seropositive allogeneic transplant recipients of age greater than 10 years who received total-body irradiation (TBI). In one study, the risk of VZV disease was 44% during the first 3 years after transplant among these patients.[41] Abdominal infections without skin manifestations are observed occasionally. These manifestations carry a high mortality, and the clinical hallmark is rapidly rising transaminases. In an unpublished randomized double-blind trial, oral acyclovir at a dose of 800 mg twice daily for 1 year prevented VZV infection after HCT without rebound disease after discontinuation of prophylaxis. This treatment may be particularly useful in patients with continued chronic GVHD.[37] Strategies that used lower doses for a shorter duration resulted in a high number of infections after discontinuation of prophylaxis.[42]

Cytomegalovirus (CMV) seropositive transplant recipients and recipients of stem cell products from a seropositive donor continue to be at risk for late CMV disease if they have chronic GVHD and/or have reactivated CMV during the first 100 days after transplantation.[43-46] The majority of late disease occurs during the first year after transplantation, but there may be cases until 3 years after transplant if immunosuppression continues. Clinical manifestation of late CMV disease may differ from the typical pneumonia and gastrointestinal disease seen earlier. Cases of retinitis, late marrow failure, and encephalitis have been described.[47] Outcome of late CMV disease is poor, with pneumonia having the highest

TABLE 15.3. Infections after hematopoietic cell transplantation (HCT).

Author	Reference	Year	Number of patients	Randomized (Y/N)	Diagnosis/ stage of disease	Intervention/design	Median follow-up 12 months	Relative risk/hazard ratio	Conclusions/results
Ljungman et al.	42	1986	42	Y	Various	RCT	Not reported	Not reported	Acyclovir prophylaxis given for 6 months leads to prevention of HSV and VZV infection during prophylaxis but frequent recurrence of VZV after discontinuation
Locksley et al.	36	1985	1,394	N	Various	Cohort study	NR	3.6 (allogeneic transplantation) 1.6 (chronic GVHD) 1.5 (ATG)	Risk factors for dissemination of VZV or death: GVHD (all deaths within 9 months after transplantation)
Han et al.	37	1994	1,186	N	Various	Cohort study	NR	Not reported	VZV seropositive + age > 10 years + radiation pretransplant: 44% VZV infection
Boeckh et al.	46	2003	146	N	Allogeneic, CMV seropositive	Cohort study	NR	3.3 (CMV reactivation <day 100 for late CMV disease)	Late CMV disease common Late viremia associated with poor survival
Peggs et al.	48	2000	81	N	Allogeneic, CMV seropositive	Prospective cohort study	13.5 months	Not reported	No late CMV disease with PCR-based surveillance and preemptive therapy for 6 months
Marr et al.	49	2002	1,682	N	All types of transplants	Retrospective cohort study	NR	6.7 (GVHD) 6.6 (CMV disease)	Late aspergillosis common GVHD, CMV disease increase risk of aspergillosis >6 months
Fukuda et al.	50	2003	163	N	Nonmyeloablative conditioning	Cohort study	23 months	2.8 (acute GVHD) 3.7 (chronic GVHD) 13.3 (CMV disease)	15% invasive mold infection 5% invasive candidiasis Steroids associated with poor outcome of disease

HSV, herpes simplex virus; VZV, varicella-zoster virus; CMV, cytomegalovirus; PCR, polymerase chain reaction; NR, not reported.

mortality.[46] About one-third of patients who survive the first episode of late disease will suffer a relapse after a median of 3 months.[46] Continued monitoring [pp65 antigenemia, polymerase chain reaction (PCR) for CMV DNA] and use of preemptive therapy in high-risk patients is useful in the management of patients at risk for late CMV disease.[46,48]

HCT recipients with chronic GVHD continue to be at risk for acquisition of respiratory virus infections such as respiratory syncytial virus, influenza viruses, and parainfluenza viruses. Seasonal vaccination of close contacts with the inactivated vaccine is recommended.[34] Recipient vaccination starting at 6 months after transplantation is also recommended.[34] Less commonly, late impaired graft function has been described in association with human herpes virus (HHV)-6 and human parvovirus B 19.

Fungal

Late invasive aspergillosis is an increasingly frequent event in allogeneic graft recipients with chronic GVHD and preceding viral infections (i.e., CMV, respiratory viruses), possibly due to an immunosuppressive effect of these viruses.[49] Recipients of lower-dose conditioning regimens who have GVHD are also at risk for late mold infections.[50] In contrast, invasive candidiasis occurs infrequently after day 100.[50,51] The outcomes of both mold and candidal infections in this setting remain poor. Mold-active drugs are now available (itraconazole, voriconazole). However, the efficacy and toxicity of long-term prophylaxis have not been tested in randomized fashion in this setting. Sensitive diagnostic tests (aspergillus galactomannan assay, PCR) can be used for early diagnosis of disease.

Pneumocystis jiroveci Pneumonia (PCP)

With the availability of effective prophylaxis, early cases of *Pneumocystis jiroveci* pneumonia (PCP) are only rarely seen late after transplant.[52] Most cases occur in a setting of poor adherence or in patients who are unable to tolerate TMP-SMX because of side effects or allergy, or who received ineffective alternative prophylaxis regimens.[53] Standard guidelines following allogeneic transplantation recommend prophylaxis for the duration of drug-induced immunosuppression.[34] However, the optimal duration of prophylaxis after autologous transplant is currently poorly defined, as recent data suggest that there is late PCP in autologous graft recipients as well.[54] Approximately 15% to 30% of HCT recipients require alternative prophylaxis regimens at some time after transplantation.[55] Reasons for requiring alternative prophylaxis include allergy to TMP-SMX, gastrointestinal intolerance, increased transaminases, and neutropenia. Very few data exist on the efficacy and toxicity of alternative prophylaxis regimens. Daily dapsone appears to be superior to inhaled pentamidine.[55] As it has overall superior results, TMP-SMX should be given whenever possible. Desensitization should be attempted in all patients with allergy to TMP-SMX.[52] Only limited data exist on atovaquone.[56]

The clinical syndrome of PCP is indistinguishable both clinically and radiologically from other nonbacterial pneumonias. The diagnosis is established either by bronchoalveolar lavage (BAL), induced sputum, or thoracoscopic or open lung biopsy. The treatment of choice is high-dose intravenous TMP-SMX in combination with a short course of corticosteroids based on results in human immunodeficiency virus (HIV)-infected patients.[57] Of the alternative agents used in the HIV setting (intravenous pentamidine, atovaquone, clindamycin/primaquine, dapsone/trimethoprim, and trimetrexate), clindamycin/primaquine appears to be most effective for treatment of disease.[58]

Distinctions in Adult and Pediatric Presentation, Course, and Treatment

Virtually no data exist on differences in infection risk and outcome among survivors of HCT. Whether immune reconstitution is faster in younger individuals has not been studied. However, if chronic GVHD is present, all available data suggest that children have the same infectious risk as adults. The exposure to respiratory viruses may even be higher if children are exposed to group settings. Certain contraindications for use of antimicrobials (e.g., quinolones) should be considered in the management of children.

Emerging Challenges in Infection

The major challenge is to design infection prevention strategies for survivors of HCT with persistent severe immunosuppression. These patients are not only at risk for VZV, PCP, and encapsulated bacteria but also for CMV and invasive mold infections. Strategies need to be easy to administer, effective, and well tolerated. With increasing long-term use of antimicrobials, resistance may become a challenge in the future.

Other Medical Complications

Pulmonary

Chronic pulmonary complications affect at least 15% to 20% of patients after HCT, and pulmonary dysfunction is an important risk factor for delayed mortality. However, current knowledge is based exclusively on retrospective analyses (Table 15.4).

LATE-ONSET PNEUMONITIS

Late-onset interstitial pneumonitis usually occurs in patients with chronic GVHD.[59] Most require therapy with immunosuppressive agents; treatment with bronchodilators is usually ineffective. However, late pneumonias occur also in the absence of GVHD, and even after autologous transplantation in patients who have not previously had pulmonary disease, with an incidence of 31% at 4 years. The prognosis is generally good with bacterial etiology, but mortality reaches 80% with fungal or polymicrobial pneumonia.[54]

RESTRICTIVE PULMONARY DISEASE

Pretransplant and posttransplant abnormal pulmonary function tests (PFTs), in particular decreased diffusing capacity (DLCO) and increased oxygen gradient [P(A-a) O_2], are associated with higher posttransplant mortality than seen in

TABLE 15.4. Pulmonary complications after HCT.

Author	Reference	Year	Number of patients	Randomized (Y/N)	Diagnosis/stage of disease	Intervention/design	Follow-up	Relative risk/outcomes/predictors	Disease-free survival (or survival statistics)	Conclusions/results
Chien et al.	63	2003	1,131	N	Various	Retrospective cohort study	1–11 years	AFO associated with decrease in FEV_1 >5%/year, decreased pretransplant FEV_1/FVC, acute and chronic GVHD, respiratory virus infection Among patients with chronic GVHD, those with AFO have a higher risk of mortality (HR 2.3, 95% CI 1.63.3) than patients without AFO Risk increases with increasing age (RR 1.7–2.5) for patients more than 20 to more than 60 years of age and patients with quiescent (RR 1.6) or progressive onset (RR 1.9) of chronic GVHD	AFO attribution to mortality, all patients (those with chronic GVHD): 9% (22%) 12% (27), 18% (40) at 3, 5, and 10 years, respectively	75% of AFO occurred in patients with chronic GVHD AFO is more frequent than previously reported and has a major negative impact on long-term survival, particularly in patients with chronic GVHD
Chen et al.	54	2003	1,359	N	Various	Retrospective cohort study	0.01–5 years	Risk factors include: patient age, HLA non-identity, and chronic GVHD among allogeneic recipients (none identified for autologous)	Cumulative incidence of first pneumonia at 4 years was 31% (18% for autologous, 34% for HLA-identical allogeneic, 39% for other allogeneic/unrelated) Survival rates were best with bacterial (71%), and worst with multimicrobial pneumonias (8%)	Pneumonia is frequent, even late after transplantation and poses a significant risk, particularly among patients more than 40 years of age, and in patients with chronic GVHD

Reference		Year	N			Study type		Results		Conclusions
Crawford et al.	60	1995	906	N	Various	Retrospective cohort study	1–9 years	Restrictive lung defect at 3 months after transplant or ≥15% decline in total lung capacity from baseline was associated with a twofold increase in risk of nonrelapse mortality (respiratory failure)	Death from respiratory failure occurred in 1.9% of patients with normal or unchanging total lung capacity, compared to 5.3% in patients with restrictive ventilatory defects; chronic GVHD did not appear to influence the rate of death with respiratory failure	Impaired total lung capacity, impaired airflow, and decreased diffusing capacity all had a negative impact on survival
Sullivan et al.	68	1996	250	Y	Various	IV immunoglobulin (500 mg/kg/month) between days 90 and days xvs. none; RCT		No difference in systemic infections; localized infections marginally more frequent in controls ($P = 0.07$); after 2 years total infections less common in controls ($P = 0.03$)	No difference	Prophylactic administration of IV immunoglobulin, in the absence of hypogammaglobulinemia, has no demonstrable benefit, and in fact may delay endogenous immune recovery
Freudenberger et al.	69	2003	49 patients 161 controls	N	Various	Case-control study	Sequentially	Risk factors for bronchiolitis obliterans organizing pneumonia (BOOP): acute ($P = 0.002$) and chronic ($P = 0.02$) GVHD; progressive onset chronic GVHD ($P = 0.001$); skin involvement with acute (HR 4.6), and oral (HR 5.9) and gut involvement (HR 6.6)	5-year survival 31% in patients with BOOP vs. 45% in controls ($P = 0.05$)	BOOP is more frequent in patients with acute or chronic GVHD Steroid treatment has no recognizable therapeutic effect

AFO, air flow obstruction.

patients with normal tests.[60] Restrictive defects, defined as a decrease in total lung capacity to less than 80% of predicted values, are present in one-third of all patients studied. Changes are not correlated with the type of conditioning regimen or with chronic GVHD and generally do not produce severe symptoms. However, becuase they are associated with an increase in late mortality, routine evaluation of lung function after HCT is warranted.[61] Aggressive therapy of any infection of the respiratory tract is indicated.

OBSTRUCTIVE PULMONARY DISEASE

Air flow obstruction (AFO), defined as decreased expiratory airflow, in particular, a decrease in the proportion of air that can be exhaled over the first second of expiration, may represent sequelae to extensive restrictive changes in the small airways or may be related to small airway destruction.[62] Both acute and chronic GVHD are important risk factors for AFO, and thereby affect long-term survival, with 75% of AFO cases occurring among patients with chronic GVHD, particularly those with quiescent or progressive onset (see Table 15.4).[63] There is generally no response to bronchodilator treatment; 30% to 40% of patients improve on glucocorticoids. Few patients with end-stage disease have been treated successfully with cadaveric lung transplants.[64,65]

BRONCHIOLITIS OBLITERANS

Progressive bronchiolitis obliterans has been reported in 10% of patients with chronic GVHD.[66,67] Chest radiographs may show hyperinflation of the lungs and flattening of the diaphragm, but abnormalities are best identified by high-resolution computed tomography (CT) scans (inspiratory and expiratory cuts). PFTs show a reduction in forced midexpiratory flow to 10% or 20% of predicted values and moderate to severe reduction in forced vital capacity. The diffusion capacity is usually normal. Pulmonary ventilation scans show decreased activity patterns corresponding to areas of obliteration of bronchiolar walls along with atelectatic areas. Histologic changes are thought to be due to a graft-versus-host reaction, possibly aggravated by infections.

The clinical course of bronchiolitis varies from mild, with slow deterioration, to diffuse necrotizing fatal bronchiolitis. Severe disease may not respond to glucocorticoids, but corticosteroids in combination with calcineurin inhibitors or possibly azathioprine can stabilize PFTs and improve outcome. It is of note that a randomized trial examining the effect of intravenous immunoglobulin on chronic GVHD and bronchiolitis showed a marked decrease in the incidence of obliterative bronchiolitis in all patients such that an effect of intravenous Ig was not apparent.[68]

Bronchiolitis obliterans organizing pneumonia (BOOP) histologically shows polypoid masses of granulation tissue in the bronchioles and alveolar sacs as well as infiltration of alveolar septa by mononuclear cells. A recent analysis of results in 6,523 patients transplanted at the Fred Hutchinson Cancer Research Center revealed 51 cases of BOOP, all but 2 after allogeneic transplants.[69,70] BOOP was diagnosed at 5 to 2,819 (median, 108) days after HCT. The chest radiograph was abnormal in 47 patients. Most patients presented with fever, dyspnea, or cough, but 23% were asymptomatic. Most patients respond to glucocorticosteroids (1–2 mg/kg), which often must be continued for 6 months or longer.

Osteoporosis

Dual-energy X-ray absorptiometry (DEXA), a semiquantitative method to assess bone mineral density (BMD), is a validated method commonly used to detect osteoporosis [as defined by a Z-score of less than or equal to 2.5 standard deviations (SD) below sex- and age-related mean bone mineral density (BMD)] and osteopenia (defined by a Z-score of 1.0 to 2.4 SD below sex- and age-related mean BMD). Reduction of bone mass using DEXA has been reported in approximately 40% of men and women at 1 year after allogeneic HCT, with nontraumatic fractures in 11% by 3 years.[71] Risk factors include number of days and dose of glucocorticoids and number of days of cyclosporine or tacrolimus used for treating chronic GVHD.

In women, supplementation with estrogens and medroxyprogesterone can increase bone mass after HCT.[72] However, there may be increased risks of cardiovascular diseases (venous thrombosis, strokes, pulmonary emboli) and breast cancer in postmenopausal women given conjugated equine estrogen (0.625 mg) with medroxyprogesterone (2.5 mg).[73] This possibility is of concern because HCT recipients are at risk for secondary malignancies even without hormone therapy. Thus, the overall risks and benefits of hormone replacement in this situation remain to be determined. Lower doses of estrogen alone (after hysterectomy) or combined with progestin (in women with uterus intact) have been used for the management of bone loss in other patient populations.[74] Alternative regimens of bisphosphonates or hormone therapy have not been tested in clinical trials for efficacy or safety in women after HCT either for osteoporosis prevention or for postmenopausal symptoms.

Aseptic Necrosis

Avascular necrosis, especially in weight-bearing joints, is a classic side effect of glucocorticoid therapy and has been reported in 4% to 10% of allogeneic HCT survivors as early as 2 months and as late as 10 years posttransplant.[75–77] The hip is the joint most frequently affected (two-thirds of all cases). In most patients more than one joint is affected. One-third of patients with this disease required joint replacement at 2 to 42 months.[76] A case-control study of 87 patients with avascular necrosis found that posttransplant glucocorticoid use and TBI given in preparation for HCT were significant risk factors.[78] In addition to glucocorticoid therapy, male gender (relative risk, 4.2) and age greater than 15 years (relative risk, 3.8) were risk factors.

Endocrinology

THYROID

Overt or compensated hypothyroidism and the "euthyroid sick syndrome" [ETS; low free triiodothyronine, free thyroxine, or both, along with normal or low thyroid-stimulating hormone (TSH)] are the most frequent thyroid abnormalities following transplantation (Table 15.5).[79] In one study ETS was associated with a significantly lower survival than observed in patients not affected by ETS (34.5% versus 96.2%; P less than 0.0001).[80,81] The risk of hypothyroidism is increased in patients who received pretransplant cranial

TABLE 15.5. Endocrine function, and growth and development.

Author	Reference	Year	Number of patients	Randomized (Y/N)	Diagnosis/stage of disease	Intervention/design	Follow-up	Relative risk/outcomes/predictors	Conclusions/results
Leung et al.	182	2000	43	N	Various with chemotherapy alone vs. chemo + cranial irradiation vs. chemo +TBI HCT	Retrospective cohort study	Median 13 years	Decreased height by 0.21 SD with chemo vs. 1.2 with chemo + cranial vs.1.33 with HCT	Importance of irradiation; growth hormone deficiency only with HCT
Thomas et al.	183	1993	49	N	Various	Retrospective cohort study	1–3 years	TBI 1,000 cGy single vs. 1,200–1,440 cGy fractionated dose; decrease in height of 0.2–0.9 SD vs. 0.09–0.2 SD; accentuated by cranial irradiation	Irradiation impairs growth; more so as single dose, and even further with cranial irradiation; growth hormone is helpful; should be instituted early (before the growth lag is >1.5 SD); dose should be adjusted for puberty
Sanders	184	1991	63 (55) (154)	N	Various	Retrospective cohort study	>12 years	Cyclophosphamide alone leads to little delay; TBI, single dose (71%; 83%) more than fractionated (49%; 58%) delays development	Cyclophosphamide by itself is well tolerated; little if any delay and normal rates of pregnancy Busulfan has intermediate effect TBI results in marked impairment
Sanders	83	2004	145/93 128/98	N	Various	Retrospective cohort study	1–12 years	Cyclophosphamide alone, 54% of women recover normal function; among men, 95% normal Sertoli cellfunction, 61% normal FSH, with busulfan/cyclophosphamide, only 2 of 93 women recovered ovarian function. Among men 65% showed azoospermia	Significant impairment of gonadal function with busulfan-containing regimens; less so with cyclophosphamide
Sanders	83	2004	562 498	N	Various	Retrospective cohort study	1–14 years	1,000 cGy single or 1,200–1,575 fractionated TBI, 83 women recovered ovarian function at 3–7 years; in men Leydig cell function was generally preserved, but Sertoli cell function was impaired in the majority	TBI has major impact; high frequency of sexual dysfunction, decrease in libido (associated with decreased testosterone in men) Chronic GVHD further impairs function. In women, systemic and topical vaginal hormone application is indicated

TBI, total-body irradiation; FSH, follicle-stimulating hormone.

irradiation or irradiation to the neck (e.g., for Hodgkin's disease).[82] All patients who have received irradiation to the thyroid should be followed for life with annual physical evaluation and thyroid function studies as indicated.[82]

ADRENAL GLANDS

Many HCT patients receive glucocorticoid therapy. Endogenous cortisol production is suppressed, and any superimposed stress may cause a relative adrenal insufficiency. However, lasting adrenal dysfunction appears to be uncommon. One study in 78 patients showed 24% to have subnormal 11-deoxycortisol levels following discontinuation of glucocorticoid therapy at 1 to 8 years posttransplant. No patient was symptomatic, and the proportion of patients affected did not increase with time posttransplant.[83,84]

HYPOTHALAMIC–PITUITARY AXIS

Cranial irradiation, with or without TBI, affects the pituitary gland.[85–87] Thyrotropin-releasing hormone (TRH) may be low early posttransplant, and TRH-induced TSH responses may be subnormal and delayed.[85] Release of gonadotropin in response to luteinizing hormone-releasing hormone (LHRH) may be elevated.[85] Prolactin secretion and the pituitary–adrenal axis are usually intact. Growth hormone levels are decreased after cranial irradiation, and deficiency becomes apparent earlier with younger age at transplant.[83,86]

GONADAL FUNCTION, PUBERTY, AND FERTILITY

Chemotherapy and TBI regimens used before hematopoietic transplantation for malignancies usually cause gonadal failure. Puberty and menarche are markedly delayed or may not occur, and fertility is infrequently regained in either men or women.

In men, testosterone levels usually decline as a result of transplant conditioning, but recover by 1 year posttransplant. Decreased libido, reduced bone mineral density, and low testosterone levels after transplant are indications for testosterone replacement unless contraindicated for other reasons. Risk for short stature is increased in males and those who are younger if they also receive TBI.[88]

Permanent ovarian failure invariably occurs in women who receive busulfan and cyclophosphamide pretransplant, whereas recovery of ovarian function has been observed after transplant in 54% of younger patients less than 26 years conditioned with cyclophosphamide only, and in 10% of younger patients who received more than 1,000 cGy TBI with cyclophosphamide. Pregnancy, although not common, has occurred following high-dose HCT, with increased risk for spontaneous abortion after TBI and preterm delivery of low birth weight babies. However, no increased risk of congenital abnormalities has been observed.[89,90] Lack of hormone therapy by 1 year after HCT for women with ovarian failure is a risk factor for sexual dissatisfaction at 3 years after HCT.[91] Vasomotor and sexual complaints 6 months after HCT improve after the start of hormone therapy, based on results from a nonrandomized pre–post cohort study.[92]

Safety of hormone therapy after transplantation has not been reported; thus, hormone replacement for survivors must be individualized. Males treated with testosterone may be at increased risk for prostate hypertrophy and prostate carcinoma. A nonrandomized cohort study has reported that hormone therapy in women does not influence chronic GVHD activity between 3 and 24 months after starting the hormone therapy (most of whom were also receiving cyclosporine) after allogeneic HCT.[93] Unfortunately, combined estrogen and progestin was recently found to increase the risk of cardiovascular disease and to increase the risk of invasive breast cancer after 3 years of therapy in naturally postmenopausal older women who had not had transplants, but no effect on survival was observed.[73] Human pituitary growth hormone replacement has been associated with increased risk of mortality from colorectal and Hodgkin's disease in a cohort study, a study not conducted in survivors of HCT.[94] These relative risks versus the consequences of delayed pubertal development, extremely short stature, attainment of peak bone mass, osteoporosis, and other quality of life factors need to be weighed along with hormone alternatives. If hormone therapy is elected, duration of treatment and a monitoring plan for complications should be part of the treatment plan.

Emerging Challenges in Medical Complications

Most treatment strategies for pulmonary, bone, and endocrine complications in transplant survivors are empirical rather than evidence based. Safety and toxicity of hormone therapies and efficacy of treatments for all medical complications need to be examined further, but in general are those that apply to the population at large.

Late Medical Complications

As large numbers of survivors live longer, late complications are being recognized. With fractionated TBI, 30% to 47% of HCT recipients have cataracts by 5 to 7 years; without TBI, 10% to 16% have cataracts, most often those who received corticosteroids for longer than 3 months.[95,96] Keratoconjunctivitis sicca syndrome is seen in up to 40% of patients with chronic GVHD. Other risk factors include female gender, older age, and methotrexate for GVHD prophylaxis.[97] Other than hepatitis, iron overload is the primary identified hepatic late effect; 22% of survivors showed fibrosis at a median follow-up of 5 years.[98] After mean follow-up of 7 years for four randomized trials comparing busulfan plus cyclophosphamide regimens with cyclophosphamide plus TBI in 488 survivors, late complications have not been noted to differ, with the exceptions of cataracts (more common after busulfan) and alopecia (more common after TBI).[96] Of greatest concern because of their potential lethality are second cancers and cardiovascular effects of transplantation.

Second Cancers

Lymphoproliferative disorders after HCT [posttransplant lymphoproliferative disorder (PTLD)], generally of B-cell lineage, occur mostly in allogeneic transplant recipients.[99,100] T-cell PTLD, non-Hodgkin's lymphoma and Hodgkin's disease have also been reported (Table 15.6). More than 80% of cases of PTLD are diagnosed within 1 year of transplantation, with peak occurrence (120 cases/10,000 patients/year) at 2 to 5 months.[101] The incidence is highest in patients

TABLE 15.6. Malignancies after HCT.

Author	Reference	Year	Number of patients	Randomized (Y/N)	Diagnosis/ stage of disease	Intervention/ design	Duration of follow-up	Relative risk/outcomes/ predictors	Conclusions/results
Metayer et al.	109	2003	56 patients, 168 controls	N	Hodgkin's disease; non-Hodgkin's lymphoma	Multicenter retrospective case-control study	Not reported	Pretransplant use of mechlorethamine ($P = 0.04$) or chlorambucil ($P = 0.009$) significantly increased the risk of MDS/AML after autologous transplantation; conditioning with TBI $\geq 1{,}320$ cGy increased risk ($P = 0.03$)	The risk of MDS/AML after autologous transplants for Hodgkin's disease or non-Hodgkin's lymphoma is significantly increased with pretransplant use of alkylating agents and high-dose TBI in preparation for transplantation
Curtis et al.	110	1997	19,229	N	Various	Retrospective multicenter cohort study	Median 3.5 years	Ratio of observed/ expected cases was 2.7. The risk was 8.3 fold increased in patients surviving >10 years. Younger age, higher doses of TBI, chronic GVHD, and male sex were risk factors	Solid tumors, in particular malignant melanoma, cancers of the buccal cavity, liver, brain, thyroid, bone, and connective tissue were increased. Cancers of the buccal cavity were prominent among male patients and patients with chronic GVHD. Lifelong surveillance is indicated
Curtis et al.	101	1999	18,014	N	Various	Retrospective multicenter cohort study	<1 month to >10 years	Cumulative incidence 1% at 10 years. Unrelated or HLA non-identical transplants, T-cell depletion of donor marrow, use of ATG or anti-CD3 monoclonal antibody, acute GVHD, and conditioning with TBI were risk factors	Most lymphopro-liferative disorders occurred within 5 months of transplantation; late cases are rare. Risk factors are cumulative. The use of broadly reactive monoclonal antibodies was associated with a lower risk than narrowly reactive anti-T-cell antibodies

DS, myelodysplasias; AML, acute myeloid leukemia.

transplanted for immunodeficiency disorders. Risk factors include the use of ATG or anti-CD3 monoclonal antibody (MAB) for acute GVHD prophylaxis or in the preparative regimen, use of TBI in the conditioning regimen, T-cell depletion of donor marrow, unrelated donor or HLA nonidentical-related donor, and primary immunodeficiency disease. The impact of risk factors is additive (or synergistic). Increasing intensity of posttransplant immunosuppression in patients who are otherwise at low risk significantly increases the incidence of PTLD.[100] The best approach to prevent Epstein–Barr virus (EBV)-related PTLD currently is close monitoring and preemptive therapy with anti-CD20 monoclonal antibody (325 mg) in patients with rising EBV titers. Additional doses of anti-CD20 antibody can be given if high EBV titers persist.

Rare T-cell proliferative disorders with or without EBV association have been reported.[102] None was associated with HTLV1, HIV, or HHV-6 infection. Several cases of late-occurring lymphomas have been reported,[103–105] some linked to EBV infection (just as early-onset PTLD), and others associated with T-cell depletion of the graft.

"Secondary" myelodysplasias (MDS) and acute myeloid leukemia (AML) occur after conventional chemotherapy with or without radiotherapy for Hodgkin's disease, non-Hodgkin's lymphoma, and solid tumors,[106] as well as after autologous HCT.[103,107,108] After autologous HCT, incidence rates of 4% to 18% have been reported.

A case-control study analyzed data on 56 patients who developed MDS/leukemia and 168 controls within a cohort of 2,739 patients with Hodgkin's disease or non-Hodgkin's lymphoma transplanted at 12 institutions.[109] MDS/AML was significantly correlated with the intensity of pretransplant chemotherapy, specifically mechlorethamine [relative risk (RR), 2.0 and 4.3 for doses of less than 50 or 50 mg/m^2 or more, respectively], and chlorambucil (RR, 3.8 and 8.4 for duration of less than 10 or 10 months or more; $P = 0.0009$) compared to cyclophosphamide. Also, higher doses of TBI (more than 1,200 cGy) used for transplant conditioning tended to carry a higher risk (RR, 4.7).

A spectrum of tumors including glioblastoma, melanoma, squamous cell carcinoma, adenocarcinoma, hepatoma, and basal cell carcinoma has been reported. A recent study analyzed results in 19,220 patients (97.2% allogeneic, 2.8% syngeneic recipients) transplanted between 1964 and 1992.[110] There were 80 solid tumors for an observed/expected (O:E) ratio of 2.7 (P less than 0.001). In 10-year survivors, the risk increased eightfold. The tumor incidence was 2.2% at 10 years and 6.7% at 15 years. The risk increased significantly for melanoma (O:E, 5.0), cancers of the oral cavity (11.1), liver (7.5), central nervous system (CNS) (7.6), thyroid (6.6), bone (13.4), and connective tissue (8.0). The risk was highest for the youngest patients and declined with age. Preliminary data from an ongoing nested case-control study in a cohort of 29,737 patients suggest that duration of chronic GVHD for more than 2 years and prolonged therapy are risk factors, in particular for the development of squamous cell carcinoma.

Cardiovascular Effects

Cardiac insufficiency and coronary artery disease are known complications of intensive cytotoxic therapy, in particular, high-dose anthracycline and mediastinal irradiation. Cardiac insufficiency may also be seen in patients conditioned with cyclophosphamide 200 mg/kg, usually early, sometimes

before conditioning is completed, although the overall incidence is low and approximately 0.7% are life threatening or fatal.[111] Late cardiomyopathy has occasionally been observed and treated successfully by orthotopic cardiac transplantation.[112]

Coronary artery disease and thrombotic events have been reported at various time intervals after HCT.[113,114] Hyperlipidemia and hyperglycemia are common in patients treated with calcineurin inhibitors, rapamycin, and glucocorticosteroids. Although data are lacking, potential risk factors for the development of coronary disease in long-term survivors of HCT include treatment with estrogen/progesterone and inactivity due to fatigue or other causes.

Functional and Quality of Life Outcomes

Many cross-sectional cohort studies, and a smaller number of prospective longitudinal cohort or case-control studies, have defined functional and psychosocial outcomes after HCT. These investigations consistently find that 85% to 90% of survivors of HCT do well in their return to "normal" life in the domains of physical, psychologic, social, existential, and overall subjective quality of life, although specific residual problems remain for many.[2,115,116] Physical recovery returns to pretransplant levels by 1 year for most survivors. However, return to work and emotional recovery may take longer.[117–119] Although physical recovery is more rapid for autologous transplant recipients, results are inconsistent as to whether function continues better for autologous survivors after 1 year.[118,120] Risk factors for poorer quality of life include older age, being female, and chronic GVHD.[118,121–124] Specifically, females have a more difficult time in the areas of sexuality, fatigue, emotional adaptation, and return to work.[116,123–126] After resolution of chronic GVHD, survivor function seems to be equal to those patients who did not have chronic GVHD.[118,127] Cross-sectional studies of survivors 5 to 18 years after HCT do not suggest deterioration over time in quality of life.[124,128,129] Residual symptoms that are most common and remain after 5 years in at least a third of survivors, based on a survey of 125 adults, include sexual dysfunction, emotional reactivity and fears, fatigue, joint and muscle pains, eye problems, sleep disruption, financial and insurance worries, cognitive concerns, and social roles and relationships.[128] Only 7% of this cohort was disabled and 74% was employed; the number who considered homemaking their job was not reported, but only 3 survivors were seeking employment.

Rates of return to work continue to rise until 5 years after HCT. By 3 or more years after HCT, between 72% and 89% of patients have returned to full-time work or school.[96,119,124,127] Survivors who are older, female, have had chronic myeloid leukemia, or have had extensive chronic GVHD are at risk for incomplete resumption of work or school activity after 5 years.[124,127] A nonrandomized cohort-controlled trial found that HCT survivors who received a 3- to 4-week inpatient rehabilitation program demonstrated no difference in employment when compared with a group of patients who did not receive this rehabilitation.[130]

Pediatric survivor quality of life is similar to adults. A cohort study compared 120 survivors who had HCT as children 5 or more years previously, with 114 survivors of childhood leukemia who had received chemotherapy without transplant, and 149 age- and gender-matched nontransplanted comparison subjects.[131] The HCT survivors reported more major illness, physician visits, diabetes, second malignancies, and poorer physical health than participants in either of the other two cohorts. Both survivor groups reported more health or life insurance refusals (25% and 33% versus 3% for comparison subjects). Marital status and mental health did not differ between cohorts, and other psychosocial factors also did not differ.[131] Other researchers have found comparable results. Investigators who compared adolescents and young adults 2 to 13 years after HCT or bone cancer found that[132] the groups did not differ in adjustment or perceived quality of life, with the exception that HCT survivors reported higher anxiety and feelings of sensitivity and vulnerability. Other researchers have reported that pediatric survivors do better than their peers in psychosocial domains.[133] The rate of successful return to school (85% to 95%) is similar to rates of return to work in adult survivors.[134]

Fatigue

Fatigue is the one of the most persistent symptoms beyond the first year after HCT. A multicenter longitudinal cohort study of fatigue and sleep disturbance in 172 adult survivors more than 12 months after HCT, followed again 18 months after the first assessment, found that a majority reported at least mild problems at both time points, with 15% to 20% reporting moderate to severe problems.[135] Risk factors for sleep but not fatigue included older age, receipt of TBI, and female sex. Problems did not resolve over time, and no specific risk factors for fatigue were identified. Other studies have reported age to be a risk factor for fatigue.[128] A cohort study of breast cancer 20-month survivors after autologous HCT found significantly higher levels of fatigue than in a matched noncancer cohort of women,[136] and another longitudinal cohort study reported that more than 80% of survivors at both 100 days and 1 year reported "I tire easily".[137] Many biologic mechanisms have been postulated to explain fatigue following HCT or other cancer treatments. Considered among potential causes are effects of interleukins and interferons, anemia, metabolic abnormalities, infection, immunosuppression, gonadal insufficiency, TBI, sleep disruption, lack of physical activity, depression, systemic medications such as corticosteroids, and other medications. However, evidence does not clearly support any of these causes over others in HCT survivors.[138] Treatments for fatigue and physical strength have been tested in randomized or nonrandomized trials using exercise, erythropoietin, or coping skills that included relaxation training. Results show improved fatigue and reduced medical complications.[139–141] However, these studies have focused on the acute phase of treatment, not fatigue in survivors.

Neurologic and Cognitive Deficits

Neurologic complications are numerous during acute treatment and as a consequence of chronic GVHD treatment. Neuroradiologic studies have determined that changes such as cortical atrophy and ventricular enlargement occur in some patients after HCT conditioning chemotherapy or total body irradiation.[142] Chronic GVHD-related CNS neurotoxicities

seem to resolve with discontinuation of the drug causing the problems unless stroke or other permanent brain events occur.[143–146] An adult cohort study[146] tested 66 patients with neurologic examination, magnetic resonance imaging, and neuropsychologic exams from 8 months to 5 years after transplant. Neuropsychologic deficits did not correlate with pathology seen in neurologic or imaging tests. Pathology on neuroradiologic examination was greater for patients with progressive-onset chronic GVHD or corticosteroid or cyclosporine use. Meanwhile, long-term cyclosporine use and age increased the risk for neuropsychologic impairment.

Twenty percent to 56% of patients enter transplant with cognitive deficits that could interfere with function.[147–149] Thus, without knowing the pretransplant function of a patient, it is not possible to determine whether long-term problems are a consequence of transplantation, or of treatment predating HCT, or instead are outcomes of depression, anxiety, or fatigue. Patient complaints about cognitive difficulties following transplantation are prevalent. However, complaints do not always match objective neuropsychologic test results[150,151] and more likely correlate with subjective anxiety, depression, and fatigue.

Mechanisms underlying cognitive impairment related to chemotherapy remain uncertain but include (1) direct neurotoxic injury, (2) secondary inflammatory response, (3) microvascular injury leading to obstruction, and (4) altered neurotransmitter levels.[152] Data indicate that TBI has significant diffuse effects on neuropsychologic function in the short term, but toxicities resolve with time if doses are 12 Gy or less.[153–156] A study of patients tested pretransplant and at 80 days and 1 year after transplantation found major decrements at 80 days, but recovery of function to pretransplant levels by 1 year, in most neuropsychologic areas tested.[149] A cross-sectional study reported impairment in 25% of allogeneic transplant recipients 2 or more years posttransplant.[151]

Among survivors of pediatric transplantation, a prospective longitudinal cohort study of 102 pediatric survivors found no declines at 1- or 3-year follow-up testing of patients over the age of 5 at the time of transplant.[157] However, younger patients, particularly those under 3 years of age, do have some risk of IQ decline over time posttransplant.[157–159] Testing of children before and at 1 year and 3 years after transplant indicates no difference in performance based on whether the child received TBI.[159,160]

To date, there is no indication that adult cognitive abilities decline more rapidly after HCT when compared with nontransplanted adults.[155] By 1 or 2 years posttransplant, approximately 55% to 60% of adult allogeneic HCT survivors and 32% of autologous breast cancer survivors have some evidence of neuropsychologic impairment on objective tests versus 17% of standard-dose chemotherapy recipients.[149–151] Surprisingly, few risk factors specific to HCT have been identified as predictors of long-term deficits. Rather, accumulated difficulties in overall health, fatigue, mood, and physical function predict deficits (Table 15.7).

Sexual Function

Both men and women report lower rates of sexual activity and satisfaction after HCT than before transplantation and in comparison with either the general population or patients who receive chemotherapy without transplantation (Table 15.8). This result is consistent across time points after

TABLE 15.7. Neuropsychologic function after HCT.

Author	Reference	Year	Number of patients	Disease/stage	Intervention/design	Follow-up	Relative risk/outcomes	Conclusions/results
Arvidson et al.	158	1999	26	Pediatric hematologic malignancies with autologous HCT	Cohort study	8–10 years post-HCT	Risk for impairment increased with younger age, longer follow-up time	Children treated with auto HCT had average IQ; however, deficits in memory and attention were seen
Harder et al.	151	2002	40	Progression-free adult survivors of allogeneic HCT including TBI	Cohort study	22–82 months after HCT	Predictors of poor performance included fatigue, global health, educational level, subjective cognitive complaints, physical functioning, social functioning, mood, employment status	Mild to moderate cognitive impairment found in 60% Compared with healthy population norms, areas most likely to be affected were selective attention and executive function, information processing speed, verbal learning, and verbal and visual memory HCT may lead to cognitive complaints and late cognitive deficits in long-term adult survivors
Kramer et al.	159	1997	67: 1 year after HCT 26: 3 years after HCT	Pediatric HCT	Prospective cohort study	1 year or 3 years	Not reported	Significant decline in IQ was seen between baseline and 1 year Although IQ was lower at 1 year, no further changes were evident at 3-year follow-up
Padovan et al.	146	1998	66	Various adults	Cohort study	Mean 34 months post-HCT	Risk factors for neuropsychologic impairment were age, long time post-HCT, intrathecal methotrexate, long-term cyclosporine, progressive chronic GVHD	Mild cognitive deficit, especially impaired memory, seen in more than 1/3 of allogeneic-HCT patients; lower risk of pathologic neurologic exam after auto-HCT
Peper et al.	154	2000	14: before TBI and HCT, 20: after TBI and autologous HCT 11: controls with renal insufficiency	Adult acute leukemias, lymphoma	Cohort and case-control study	32 months and 8.8 years	Brain atrophy increase was associated primarily with pretransplant irradiation or methotrexate No medical factors were associated with cognitive deficits	Neurologic deficits seen in one new case after HCT All brain atrophy measures were within normal range, but were slightly increased after TBI Cognitive deficit levels were not significant Power may have been inadequate to detect clinically meaningful differences Some tests were associated with ventricle index results No decline in cognitive function seen long term

Author	Ref	Year	N	Population	Study design	Follow-up	Risk factors	Results
Phipps et al.	157	2000	102 survivors to 1 year with 54 followed to 3 years	Pediatric HCT	Prospective cohort study	3 years	Younger age showed more decline over time; <3 years particularly vulnerable	No significant changes on global measures of VC intelligence or academic achievement at either 1 or 3 years after an HCT HCT with or without TBI entails minimal risk of late neurocognitive sequelae in patients who are 6 years of age or older
Simms et al.	160	1998	122	Pediatric HCT recipients with no previous cranial irradiation	Prospective cohort study	1 year	None identified	No statistically significant differences between the two groups Regression analysis failed to identify treatment, age, or gender effects Suggests that neuropsychologic functioning 1 year after HCT was not detrimentally affected by chemotherapy or TBI
Syrjala et al.	149	2004	142	Adults with malignancy receiving first allogeneic HCT	Prospective cohort study	80 days and 1 year	2.76 RR (CI = 1.01–7.55) for impaired motor dexterity in patients actively receiving cyclosporine, tacrolimus or my cophenolate mofetil vs. not 2.99 RR (CI = 1.08–8.30) for impairment on any test pretransplant in patients with no previous chemotherapy, or only hydroxyurea before HCT	Performance on all tests declined from pretransplant to 80 days and improved by 1 year to pretransplant levels on all tests except strength and dexterity Verbal fluency and memory recovered by 1 year but remained below norms suggesting that these long term cognitive decrements were not a result of HCT treatment in most patients
van Dam et al.	150	1998	34: autologous HCT 36: standard dose 34: controls, stage I, no chemotherapy	Adult breast cancer	Case-control and cohort study	Mean 2 years, minimum 6 months	8.2 RR (CI = 1.8–37.7) for HCT vs. control 3.5 RR (CI = 1.1–12.8) for HCT vs. standard chemotherapy	Patients with high-dose chemo have a greater risk of cognitive impairment than patients with standard dose
Wenz et al.	155	2000	58	Adult hyperfractionated TBI with autologous HCT	Prospective cohort study	Median 27 months	None found	No measurable radiation damage found

TABLE 15.8. Sexual function after HCT.

Author	Reference	Year	Number of patients	Randomized (Y/N)	Diagnosis/stage of disease	Intervention/design	Follow-up	Relative risk/outcomes	Conclusions/results
Balleari et al.	93	2002	39 received hormone therapy; 32 controls	N	Premenopausal women treated with autologous transplant for hematologic malignancies	Case-control study	24 months	No increased risk of chronic GVHD activity with hormone therapy	No differences observed in chronic GVHD activity score between HRT and controls after 3, 6, 12, and 24 months
Chatterjee et al.	169	2002	8	N	Males after HCT for lymphoma, with hypogonadism, erectile dysfunction, diminished libido and ejaculatory disorders; all had Leydig cell insufficiency with or without frank serum testosterone insufficiency; all but one had cavernosal arterial insufficiency	Case series Patients received intramuscular testosterone cypionate (250 mg 4× weekly) and 50–100 mg of sildenafil orally one to two times per week for 6 months	6 months	Not reported	All patients responded favorably; results suggest therapy is a safe and effective approach in recipients of high-dose therapy with erectile dysfunction after HCT
Chatterjee et al.	185	2000	24 HCT survivors 10 healthy controls	N	Males after HCT with hypogonadism and erectile dysfunction	Case-control study	Mean 34 months	TBI increases risk for Leydig cell insufficiency; cavernosal vascular insufficiency increased risk of erectile dysfunction	Testosterone levels were lower than controls but within normal range Cavernosal arterial insufficiency found in 11/14 of TBI-treated and 3/10 chemotherapy treated patients Testosterone therapy improved libido but not erectile dysfunction
Molassiotis et al.	164	1995	29 HCT survivors 30 non-HCT cancer survivors 119 controls	N	Males after autologous and allogeneic HCT	Case-control study	Mean 35.6 months	Risk increased with TBI	FSH and LH increased throughout years after HCT Hyperprolactinemia observed only in the second year after HCT; testosterone levels were normal Long-term HCT survivors had similar psychosexual adjustment to non-HCT cancer survivors Major problems were erectile difficulties (37.9%), low sexual desire (37.9%), altered body image (20.7%)

	Author	Year	N		Disease	Design	Duration	Results
186	Mumma et al.	1992	26 HCT survivors 33 non-HCT survivors	N	Acute leukemia	Cohort study	Mean 47 months for HCT; 64 months for non-HCT	No differences between HCT and conventional chemotherapy. Compared with controls, women had decreased sexual frequency and satisfaction; both men and women had poorer body image. Longer time since cancer treatment predicted greater frequency of sexual activity in women but poorer body image for both men and women
91	Syrjala et al.	1998	407	N	Various	Prospective cohort study	1 and 3 years	Pretransplant men and women did not differ in sexual satisfaction. After 1 and 3 years women were more dissatisfied and had more problems. No pretransplant factors predicted 3-year outcomes for women. At 3 years, 80% of women and 29% of men had at least one sexual problem. Male sexual dissatisfaction at 3 years was predicted by older age, not being married, pretransplant sexual dissatisfaction, and poorer psychologic function. Females were more dissatisfied at 3 years if they did not receive hormone therapy by 1 year and if they were less satisfied at 1 year
166	Syrjala et al.	2000	185 HCT survivors 94 non-HCT survivors 121 controls	N	Various	Cohort study	1–10 years	Hormone therapy was not associated with sexual function. HCT survivors and females have high levels of sexual dysfunction. Risk of poorer sexual function for: HCT survivors vs. controls, females, shorter time since HCT for females, postmenopausal status for females, extensive chronic GVHD for males
165	Watson et al.	1999	168 HCT, 311 non-HCT	N	AML	Cohort study	Median 14 months	Sexual function correlated with fatigue and emotional function. Sexual function worse in HCT, females, older
163	Wingard et al.	1992	126	N	Various HCT survivors	Cohort study	Mean 47 months	22% were dissatisfied with sexual function. 24% of men had erectile difficulty; 13% had ejaculation difficulty. For women, hormone therapy was not associated with satisfaction. Sexual satisfaction correlated with serum estrogen or testosterone levels though levels were within normal range. Satisfaction increased with younger age and satisfaction with appearance, life, and partner relationship

HCT, and across ages at time of transplantation, in both prospective longitudinal and cohort comparison studies.[91,115,120,123,161–165] Before HCT, 42% of females and 14% of males report one or more sexual problems, compared with 17% to 35% of the general population of females and up to 19% of males.[91] By 3 years after HCT, the prevalence of problems increases to 80% of females and 29% of males. Risk factors include, for women, initiation of hormone therapy after 1 year posttransplantation and chronic GVHD, and, for men, older age, chronic GVHD, and psychologic function before HCT.[91,165,166]

Long-term problems for females are presumably caused by ovarian failure and consequent endocrine changes or by chronic GVHD-related vaginal introital stenosis and mucosal changes.[167] Prospective cohort studies indicate that hormone therapy with oral estrogen improves or prevents more serious decline in sexual function in women after HCT but does not eliminate problems.[91,93] Because hormone replacement has been widely prescribed after HCT, vasomotor symptoms and other menopausal syndromes have been less commonly reported than sexual dysfunction. However, with new concerns about the long-term risks of hormone therapy, menopausal symptoms and hormone alternatives need to be reconsidered. We have found no clinical trials comparing treatments for female sexual dysfunction after HCT despite the well-recognized prevalence of problems. Descriptions of clinical interventions for women recommend vaginal lubricants to improve comfort as well as counseling with sexual partners. Some couples do well after brief counseling that provides education, facilitates communication, and encourages gradually increasing intimacy behaviors and relearning pleasurable sexual strategies rather than avoiding sexual activity.[168]

Male sexual problems have been attributed to gonadal and cavernosal arterial insufficiency, with resulting libido and erectile dysfunction.[169] Results from a small case-series of eight patients 6 months after HCT suggested that testosterone injections and sildenafil one to two times per week improved sexual performance for men with erectile dysfunction, low libido, and ejaculatory disorders.[169] However, other data indicate that most males recover testosterone levels and sexual function between 6 months and 1 year after transplantation.[170] Thus, without controlled clinical trials, it is unclear whether sexual function in the treated men would have recovered without treatment.

Psychologic Adaptation

Rates of depression and anxiety among HCT recipients are higher than population norms. Prospective studies have reported depressive symptoms in 43% to 53% of survivors at some time during or after HCT.[127,137] Rates of both general anxiety and depression decline from pretransplant to 1 year and then stabilize.[117,127] Depression is of particular concern because studies have found it to be a risk factor for mortality and poorer long-term physical and psychologic functioning after HCT.[117,127,171,172] More prevalent than clinical syndromes of depression or anxiety are subclinical elevations in emotions that continue long term.[128] Worries and concerns related to health and survival decline gradually between discharge and 3 years.[127,173] However, other concerns increase after the first year, including work, relationships, finances,

and social and family issues.[137] Children, similar to adults, appear to be distressed during treatment but then to recover psychologically.[174]

Emerging Challenges in Functional and Quality of Life Outcomes

Evidence related to functional and quality of life outcomes indicate that physical capability improves within 1 year whereas treatment-related distress and return to work resolve by 2 to 3 years. Other problems do not resolve without treatment; for instance, sexual dysfunction, fatigue, and reduced social activities persist past 5 years. Long-term impact of HCT on cognitive function remains undefined for adults. The clearest challenge is to increase testing of treatments to improve outcomes for those problems that persist.

Emerging Issues

Nonmyeloablative Transplants

Both the pretransplant conditioning regimen and posttransplant donor immune-mediated mechanisms account for elimination of malignant cells in the recipient. Conventional high-dose, myeloablative pretransplant conditioning regimens have been designed to prevent graft rejection and to eliminate as many malignant cells as possible, but these regimens are not well tolerated in older patients or in those who are not in good medical condition at the time of the transplant. During the past 5 years, improvements have been made in posttransplant immunosuppressive regimens so that low-dose, nonmyeloablative pretransplant conditioning regimens are sufficient to prevent graft rejection. This treatment strategy relies heavily on immune-mediated mechanisms to eliminate malignant cells when immunosuppressive medications are gradually withdrawn after the transplant.

Results from many Phase 2 studies have suggested that low-dose, nonmyeloablative pretransplant conditioning regimens cause much less posttransplant morbidity than conventional, high-dose myeloablative conditioning regimens during the first month after the transplant. This impression has been confirmed by comparing skin, liver, and gastrointestinal morbidity between two cohorts of patients who had either a myeloablative or nonmyeloablative conditioning regimen.[175] Morbidity after the first month, however, was similar in the two groups. The proportion of patients who needed treatment for either acute or chronic GVHD was lower among patients who received a nonmyeloablative conditioning regimen, and the time to onset of GVHD was delayed. Randomized trials have not yet been carried out to compare results with the two types of conditioning regimens.

Caregiver and Family Needs

Caregiving by a spouse, parent, or other family member or friend is vital to recovery after HCT. Longitudinal studies find that emotional distress in caregivers peaks during the first 2 weeks of treatment[176] while fatigue peaks at 3 months.[177] Mothers of pediatric HCT patients seem to suffer the greatest emotional strain in the course of their child's treatment.[178] In a case-matched, longitudinal, prospective cohort study that also included nontransplant controls, spouse caregivers reported greater depression and anxiety than patients throughout the first year after HCT.[179] Female caregivers also were at higher risk of marital dissatisfaction than male caregivers. Little else has been published about the financial or family costs of HCT. Particularly lacking is information on family responses after an HCT recipient dies.

Conclusions

Medical and quality of life issues facing survivors of HCT have been well described, as have risk factors for major medical complications. In contrast, few randomized controlled trials have tested efficacy of treatments for chronic GVHD or infectious, pulmonary, endocrine, or functional problems. For most medical complications, treatment choices are based on Phase 2 data or historical case-control studies. Evidence for treatment of functional or quality of life problems such as fatigue, sexual dysfunction, or cognitive deficits must be extrapolated either from studies during the acute phase of treatment, as for fatigue, or from research with other populations of patients, as with sexual dysfunction, cognitive deficits, or psychosocial adaptation.

The foremost risk factors for mortality and morbidity in survivors are chronic GVHD and its treatment, infection, or malignancy recurrence. However, if transplant recipients survive without malignancy recurrence, their physical and psychosocial quality of life is excellent for more than 80%, whether they have autologous or allogeneic transplant, whether or not they have clinical extensive chronic GVHD, and regardless of age. Although males have higher rates of mortality, female survivors are at greater risk for functional and psychosocial complications. Recent descriptive studies indicate that most survivors perceive long-term benefits as well as losses as a consequence of their disease and HCT. Although second cancers are more prevalent in survivors and problems with insurance and cataracts have been documented, few other late effects of HCT have been detected thus far.

Acknowledgments. This work was supported by grants from the National Cancer Institute CA63030, CA79880, CA102542, and CA18029. We thank Ashley Walter, Bonnie Larson, and Helen Crawford for assistance with the research review and manuscript preparation.

References

1. Loberiza F. Report on state of the art in blood and marrow transplantation: part I of the IBMTR/ABMTR summary slides with guide. IBMTR/ABMTR Newsl 2003;10:7–10.
2. Socie G, Stone JV, Wingard JR, et al. Long-term survival and late deaths after allogeneic bone marrow transplantation: late effects working committee of the International Bone Marrow Transplant Registry. N Engl J Med 1999;341:14–21.
3. Sullivan KM. Graft-versus-host disease. In: Thomas ED, Blume KG, Forman SJ (eds). Hematopoietic Cell Transplantation, 2nd ed. Boston: Blackwell Science, 1999:515–536.
4. Vogelsang GB. How I treat chronic graft-versus-host disease. Blood 2001;97:1196–1201.
5. Lee SJ, Vogelsang G, Flowers MED. Chronic graft-versus-host disease. Biol Blood Marrow Transplant 2003;9:215–233.
6. Cutler C, Giri S, Jeyapalan S, et al. Acute and chronic graft-versus-host disease after allogeneic peripheral-blood stem-cell and bone marrow transplantation: a meta-analysis. J Clin Oncol 2001;19:3685–3691.
7. Flowers MED, Parker PM, Johnston LJ, et al. Comparison of chronic graft-versus-host disease after transplantation of peripheral blood stem cells versus bone marrow in allogeneic recipients: long-term follow-up of a randomized trial. Blood 2002;100: 415–419.
8. Storb R, Doney KC, Thomas ED, et al. Marrow transplantation with or without donor buffy coat cells for 65 transfused aplastic anemia patients. Blood 1982;59:236–246.
9. Zaucha JM, Gooley T, Bensinger WI, et al. CD34 cell dose in granulocyte colony-stimulating factor-mobilized peripheral blood mononuclear cell grafts affects engraftment kinetics and development of extensive chronic graft-versus-host disease after human leukocyte antigen-identical sibling transplantation. Blood 2001;98:3221–3227.
10. Przepiorka D, Anderlini P, Saliba R, et al. Chronic graft-versus-host disease after allogeneic blood stem cell transplantation. Blood 2001;98:1695–1700.
11. Mitsuyasu RT, Champlin RE, Gale RP, et al. Treatment of donor bone marrow with monoclonal anti-T-cell antibody and complement for the prevention of graft-versus-host disease. Ann Intern Med 1986;105:20–26.
12. Marmont AM, Horowitz MM, Gale RP, et al. T-cell depletion of HLA-identical transplants in leukemia. Blood 1991;78: 2120–2130.
13. Champlin RE, Passweg JR, Zhang MJ, et al. T-cell depletion of bone marrow transplants for leukemia from donors other than HLA-identical siblings: advantage of T-cell antibodies with narrow specificities. Blood 2000;95:3996–4003.
14. Wagner JE, Thompson JS, Carter S, et al. Impact of graft-versus-host disease (GVHD) prophylaxis on 3-year disease-free survival (DFS): results of a multi-center, randomized phase II–III trial comparing T cell depletion/cyclosporine (TCD) and methotrexate/cyclosporine (M/C) in 410 recipients of unrelated donor bone marrow (BM). Blood 2002;100:75a–76a.
15. Bacigalupo A, Lamparelli T, Bruzzi P, et al. Antithymocyte globulin for graft-versus-host disease prophylaxis in transplants from unrelated donors: 2 randomized studies from Gruppo Italiano Trapianti Midollo Osseo (GITMO). Blood 2001;98:2942–2947.
16. Storb R, Pepe M, Anasetti C, et al. What role for prednisone in prevention of acute graft-versus-host disease in patients undergoing marrow transplants? Blood 1990;76:1037–1045.
17. Deeg HJ, Lin D, Leisenring W, et al. Cyclosporine or cyclosporine plus methylprednisolone for prophylaxis of graft-versus-host disease: a prospective, randomized trial. Blood 1997;89: 3880–3887.
18. Chao NJ, Snyder DS, Jain M, et al. Equivalence of 2 effective graft-versus-host disease prophylaxis regimens: results of a prospective double-blind randomized trial. Biol Blood Marrow Transplant 2000;6:254–261.
19. Ruutu T, Volin L, Parkkali T, et al. Cyclosporine, methotrexate, and methylprednisolone compared with cyclosporine and methotrexate for the prevention of graft-versus-host disease in bone marrow transplantation from HLA-identical sibling donor: a prospective randomized study. Blood 2000;96:2391–2398.
20. Storb R, Leisenring W, Anasetti C, et al. Methotrexate and cyclosporine for graft-vs.-host disease prevention: what length of therapy with cyclosporine? Biol Blood Marrow Transplant 1997; 3:194–201.
21. Kansu E, Gooley T, Flowers MED, et al. Administration of cyclosporine for 24 months compared with 6 months for prevention of chronic graft-versus-host disease: a prospective randomized clinical trial [brief report]. Blood 2001;98:3868–3870.

22. Mengarelli A, Iori AP, Romano A, et al. One-year cyclosporine prophylaxis reduces the risk of developing extensive chronic graft-versus-host disease after allogeneic peripheral blood stem cell transplantation. Haematologica 2003;88:315–323.

23. Chao NJ, Parker PM, Niland JC, et al. Paradoxical effect of thalidomide prophylaxis on chronic graft-vs.-host disease. Biol Blood Marrow Transplant 1996;2:86–92.

24. Sullivan KM, Witherspoon RP, Storb R, et al. Prednisone and azathioprine compared with prednisone and placebo for treatment of chronic graft-versus-host disease: prognostic influence of prolonged thrombocytopenia after allogeneic marrow transplantation. Blood 1988;72:546–554.

25. Sullivan KM, Witherspoon RP, Storb R, et al. Alternating-day cyclosporine and prednisone for treatment of high-risk chronic graft-versus-host disease. Blood 1988;72:555–561.

26. Koc S, Leisenring W, Flowers MED, et al. Therapy for chronic graft-versus-host disease: a randomized trial comparing cyclosporine plus prednisone versus prednisone alone. Blood 2002; 100:48–51.

27. Arora M, Wagner JE, Davies SM, et al. Randomized clinical trial of thalidomide, cyclosporine, and prednisone versus cyclosporine and prednisone as initial therapy for chronic graft-versus-host disease. Biol Blood Marrow Transplant 2001;7: 265–273.

28. Koc S, Leisenring W, Flowers MED, et al. Thalidomide for treatment of patients with chronic graft-versus-host disease. Blood 2000;96:3995–3996.

29. Storek J, Dawson MA, Storer B, et al. Immune reconstitution after allogeneic marrow transplantation compared with blood stem cell transplantation. Blood 2001;97:3380–3389.

30. Winston DJ, Schiffman G, Wang DC, et al. Pneumococcal infections after human bone marrow transplantation. Ann Intern Med 1979;91:835–841.

31. Witherspoon RP, Storb R, Ochs HD, et al. Recovery of antibody production in human allogeneic marrow graft recipients: influence of time posttransplantation, the presence or absence of chronic graft-versus-host disease, and antithymocyte globulin treatment. Blood 1981;58:360–368.

32. Storek J, Viganego F, Dawson MA, et al. Factors affecting antibody levels after allogeneic hematopoietic cell transplantation. Blood 2003;101:3319–3324.

33. Singhal S, Mehta J. Reimmunization after blood or marrow stem cell transplantation. Bone Marrow Transplant 1999;23:637–646.

34. Centers for Disease Control and Prevention, Infectious Disease Society of America, American Society of Blood and Marrow Transplantation. Guidelines for preventing opportunistic infections among hematopoietic stem cell transplant recipients. MMWR (Morbid Mort Wkly Rep) 2000;49:1–125.

35. D'Antonio D, Di Bartolomeo P, Iacone A, et al. Meningitis due to penicillin-resistant *Streptococcus pneumoniae* in patients with chronic graft-versus-host disease. Bone Marrow Transplant 1992;9:299–300.

36. Locksley RM, Flournoy N, Sullivan KM, et al. Infection with varicella-zoster virus infection after marrow transplantation. J Infect Dis 1985;152:1172–1181.

37. Han CS, Miller W, Haake R, et al. Varicella zoster infection after bone marrow transplantation: incidence, risk factors and complications. Bone Marrow Transplant 1994;13:277–283.

38. Koc Y, Miller KB, Schenkein DP, et al. Varicella zoster virus infections following allogeneic bone marrow transplantation: frequency, risk factors, and clinical outcome. Biol Blood Marrow Transplant 2000;6:44–49.

39. Bilgrami S, Chakraborty NG, Rodriguez-Pinero F, et al. Varicella zoster virus infection associated with high-dose chemotherapy and autologous stem-cell rescue. Bone Marrow Transplant 1999; 23:469–474.

40. Schuchter LM, Wingard JR, Piantadosi S, et al. Herpes zoster infection after autologous bone marrow transplantation. Blood 1989;74:1424–1427.

41. Bowden RA, Roger KS, Meyers JD. Oral acyclovir for the long-term suppression of varicella zoster virus infection after marrow transplantation. In: 29th Interscience Conference on Antimicrobial Agents and Chemotherapy 1989, p 62.

42. Ljungman P, Wilczek H, Gahrton G, et al. Long-term acyclovir prophylaxis in bone marrow transplant recipients and lymphocyte proliferation responses to herpes virus antigens *in vitro*. Bone Marrow Transplant 1986;1:185–192.

43. Boeckh M, Gooley TA, Myerson D, et al. Cytomegalovirus pp65 antigenemia-guided early treatment with ganciclovir versus ganciclovir at engraftment after allogeneic marrow transplantation: a randomized double-blind study. Blood 1996;88:4063–4071.

44. Krause H, Hebart H, Jahn G, et al. Screening for CMV-specific T cell proliferation to identify patients at risk of developing late onset CMV disease. Bone Marrow Transplant 1997;19: 1111–1116.

45. Zaia JA, Gallez-Hawkins GM, Tegtmeier BR, et al. Late cytomegalovirus disease in marrow transplantation is predicted by virus load in plasma. J Infect Dis 1997;176:782–785.

46. Boeckh M, Leisenring W, Riddell SR, et al. Late cytomegalovirus disease and mortality in recipients of allogeneic hematopoietic stem cell transplants: importance of viral load and T-cell immunity. Blood 2003;101:407–414.

47. Crippa F, Corey L, Chuang EL, et al. Virological, clinical, and ophthalmologic features of cytomegalovirus retinitis after hematopoietic stem cell transplantation. Clin Infect Dis 2001; 32:214–219.

48. Peggs KS, Preiser W, Kottaridis PD, et al. Extended routine polymerase chain reaction surveillance and pre-emptive antiviral therapy for cytomegalovirus after allogeneic transplantation. Br J Haematol 2000;111:782–790.

49. Marr KA, Carter RA, Boeckh M, et al. Invasive aspergillosis in allogeneic stem cell transplant recipients: changes in epidemiology and risk factors. Blood 2002;100:4358–4366.

50. Fukuda T, Boeckh M, Carter RA, et al. Risks and outcomes of invasive fungal infections in recipients of allogeneic hematopoietic stem cell transplants after nonmyeloablative conditioning. Blood 2003;102:827–833.

51. Marr KA, Seidel K, Slavin M, et al. Prolonged fluconazole prophylaxis is associated with persistent protection against candidiasis-related death in allogeneic marrow transplant recipients: long-term follow-up of a randomized, placebo-controlled trial. Blood 2000;96:2055–2061.

52. Souza JP, Boeckh M, Gooley TA, et al. High rates of *Pneumocystis carinii* pneumonia in allogeneic blood and marrow transplant recipients receiving dapsone prophylaxis. Clin Infect Dis 1999;29:1467–1471.

53. Tuan I-Z, Dennison D, Weisdorf DJ. *Pneumocystis carinii* pneumonitis following bone marrow transplantation. Bone Marrow Transplant 1992;10:267–272.

54. Chen C-S, Boeckh M, Seidel K, et al. Incidence, risk factors and mortality from pneumonia developing late after hematopoietic stem cell transplantation. Bone Marrow Transplant 2003;32: 515–522.

55. Vasconcelles MJ, Bernardo MV, King C, et al. Aerosolized pentamidine as pneumocystis prophylaxis after bone marrow transplantation is inferior to other regimens and is associated with decreased survival and an increased risk of other infections. Biol Blood Marrow Transplant 2000;6:35–43.

56. Colby C, McAfee S, Sackstein R, et al. A prospective randomized trial comparing the toxicity and safety of atovaquone with trimethoprim/sulfamethoxazole as *Pneumocystis carinii* pneumonia prophylaxis following autologous peripheral blood stem cell transplantation. Bone Marrow Transplant 1999;24: 897–902.

57. Gagnon S, Boota AM, Fischl MA, et al. Corticosteroids as adjunctive therapy for severe Pneumocystis carinii pneumonia in the acquired immunodeficiency syndrome. A double-blind, placebo-controlled trial. N Engl J Med 1990;323:1444–1450.

58. Smego RA Jr, Nagar S, Maloba B, et al. A meta-analysis of salvage therapy for *Pneumocystis carinii* pneumonia. Arch Intern Med 2001;161:1529–1533.

59. Kantrow SP, Hackman RC, Boeckh M, et al. Idiopathic pneumonia syndrome: changing spectrum of lung injury after marrow transplantation. Transplantation 1997;63:1079–1086.

60. Crawford SW, Pepe M, Lin D, et al. Abnormalities of pulmonary function tests after marrow transplantation predict nonrelapse mortality. Am J Respir Crit Care Med 1995;152:690–695.

61. Crawford SW. Respiratory infections following organ transplantation. Curr Opin Pulmonary Med 1995;1:209–215.

62. Clark JG, Schwartz DA, Flournoy N, et al. Risk factors for airflow obstruction in recipients of bone marrow transplants. Ann Intern Med 1987;107:648–656.

63. Chien JW, Martin PJ, Gooley TA, et al. Airflow obstruction after myeloablative allogeneic hematopoietic stem cell transplantation. Am J Respir Crit Care Med 2003;168:208–214.

64. Boas SR, Noyes BE, Kurland G, et al. Pediatric lung transplantation for graft-versus-host disease following bone marrow transplantation. Chest 1994;105:1584–1586.

65. Spray TL, Mallory GB, Canter CB, Huddleston CB. Pediatric lung transplantation. Indications, techniques, and early results. J Thorac Cardiovasc Surg 1994;107:990–999; discussion 999–1000.

66. Sullivan KM, Mori M, Witherspoon R, et al. Alternating-day cyclosporine and prednisone (CSP/PRED) treatment of chronic graft-vs.-host disease (GVHD): Predictors of survival. Blood 1990;76(suppl 1):568a.

67. Philit F, Wiesendanger T, Archimbaud E, et al. Post-transplant obstructive lung disease ("bronchiolitis obliterans"): a clinical comparative study of bone marrow and lung transplant patients. Eur Resp J 1995;8:551–558.

68. Sullivan KM, Storek J, Kopecky KJ, et al. A controlled trial of long-term administration of intravenous immunoglobulin to prevent late infection and chronic graft-vs.-host disease after marrow transplantation: clinical outcome and effect on subsequent immune recovery. Biol Blood and Marrow Transplant 1996;2:44–53.

69. Freudenberger TD, Madtes DK, Curtis JR, et al. Association between acute and chronic graft-versus-host disease and bronchiolitis obliterans organizing pneumonia in recipients of hematopoietic stem cell transplants. Blood 2003;102:3822–3828.

70. Palmas A, Tefferi A, Myers JL, et al. Late-onset noninfectious pulmonary complications after allogeneic bone marrow transplantation. Br J Haematol 1998;100:680–687.

71. Stern JM, Sullivan KM, Ott SM, et al. Bone density loss after allogeneic hematopoietic stem cell transplantation: a prospective study. Biol Blood Marrow Transplant 2001;7:257–264.

72. Castelo-Branco C, Rovira M, Pons F, et al. The effect of hormone replacement therapy on bone mass in patients with ovarian failure due to bone marrow transplantation. Maturitas 1996;23:307–312.

73. Rossouw JE, Anderson GL, Prentice RL, et al. Risks and benefits of estrogen plus progestin in healthy postmenopausal women. JAMA 2002;288:321–333.

74. Lindsay R, Gallagher JC, Kleerekoper M, et al. Effect of lower doses of conjugated equine estrogens with and without medroxyprogesterone acetate on bone in early postmenopausal women. JAMA 2002;287:2668–2676.

75. Fink JC, Leisenring WM, Sullivan KM, et al. Avascular necrosis following bone marrow transplantation: a case-control study. Bone (NY) 1998;22:67–71.

76. Socié G, Cahn JY, Carmelo J, et al. Avascular necrosis of bone after allogeneic bone marrow transplantation: analysis of risk factors for 4,388 patients by the Societe Francaise de Greffe de Moelle (SFGM). Br J Haematol 1997;97:865–870.

77. Fletcher BD, Crom DB, Krance RA, et al. Radiation-induced bone abnormalities after bone marrow transplantation for childhood leukemia. Radiology 1994;191:231–235.

78. Fink JC, Leisenring WM, Sullivan KM, et al. Avascular necrosis following bone marrow transplantation: a case-control study. Bone (NY) 1998;22:67–71.

79. Toubert ME, Socié G, Gluckman E, et al. Short- and long-term follow-up of thyroid dysfunction after allogeneic bone marrow transplantation without the use of preparative total body irradiation. Br J Haematol 1997;98:453–457.

80. Thomas BC, Stanhope R, Plowman PN, et al. Endocrine function following single fraction and fractionated total body irradiation for bone marrow transplantation in childhood. Acta Endocrinol 1993;128:508–512.

81. Boulad F, Bromley M, Black P, et al. Thyroid dysfunction following bone marrow transplantation using hyperfractionated radiation. Bone Marrow Transplant 1995;15:71–76.

82. Neglia JP, Nesbit ME, Jr. Care and treatment of long-term survivors of childhood cancer [review]. Cancer (Phila) 1993;71:3386–3391.

83. Sanders JE. Growth and development after hematopoietic cell transplantation. In: Blume KG, Forman SJ, Appelbaum FR (eds). Thomas' Hematopoietic Cell Transplantation, 3rd ed. Oxford: Blackwell, 2004:929–943.

84. Sierra J, Bjerke J, Hansen J, et al. Marrow transplants from unrelated donors as treatment for acute leukemia. Leuk Lymphoma 2000;39:495–507.

85. Kubota C, Shinohara O, Hinohara T, et al. Changes in hypothalamic-pituitary function following bone marrow transplantation in children. Acta Paediatr Jpn 1994;36:37–43.

86. Brauner R, Adan L, Souberbielle JC, et al. Contribution of growth hormone deficiency to the growth failure that follows bone marrow transplantation. J Pediatr 1997;130:785–792.

87. Clement-De Boers A, Oostdijk W, Van Weel-Sipman MH, et al. Final height and hormonal function after bone marrow transplantation in children. J Pediatr 1996;129:544–550.

88. Cohen A, Rovelli A, Bakker B, et al. Final height of patients who underwent bone marrow transplantation for hematological disorders during childhood: a study by the Working Party for Late Effects–EBMT. Blood 1999;93:4109–4115.

89. Sanders JE, Hawley J, Levy W, et al. Pregnancies following high-dose cyclophosphamide with or without high-dose busulfan or total-body irradiation and bone marrow transplantation. Blood 1996;87:3045–3052.

90. Salooja N, Szydlo RM, Socie G, et al. Pregnancy outcomes after peripheral blood or bone marrow transplantation: a retrospective survey. Lancet 2001;358:271–276.

91. Syrjala KL, Roth-Roemer SL, Abrams JR, et al. Prevalence and predictors of sexual dysfunction in long-term survivors of marrow transplantation. J Clin Oncol 1998;16:3148–3157.

92. Spinelli S, Chiodi S, Bacigalupo A, et al. Ovarian recovery after total body irradiation and allogeneic bone marrow transplantation: long-term follow up of 79 females. Bone Marrow Transplant 1994;14:373–380.

93. Balleari E, Garre S, van Lint MT, et al. Hormone replacement therapy and chronic graft-versus-host disease activity in women treated with bone marrow transplantation for hematologic malignancies. Ann NY Acad Sciences 2002;966:187–192.

94. Swerdlow AJ, Higgins CD, Adlard P, et al. Risk of cancer in patients treated with human pituitary growth hormone in the UK, 1959–85: a cohort study. Lancet 2002;360:273–277.

95. Benyunes MC, Sullivan KM, Deeg HJ, et al. Cataracts after bone marrow transplantation: long-term follow-up of adults treated with fractionated total body irradiation. Int J Radiat Oncol Biol Phys 1995;32:661–670.

96. Socie G, Clift RA, Blaise D, et al. Busulfan plus cyclophosphamide compared with total-body irradiation plus cyclophosphamide before marrow transplantation for myeloid leukemia: long-term follow-up of 4 randomized studies. Blood 2001;98:3569–3574.

97. Tichelli A, Duell T, Weiss M, et al. Late-onset keratoconjunctivitis sicca syndrome after bone marrow transplantation: incidence and risk factors. European Group on Blood and Marrow Transplantation (EBMT) Working Party on Late Effects. Bone Marrow Transplant 1996;17:1105–1111.

98. Strasser SI, Sullivan KM, Myerson D, et al. Cirrhosis of the liver in long-term marrow transplant survivors. Blood 1999;93: 3259–3266.

99. Shepherd JD, Gascoyne RD, Barnett MJ, et al. Polyclonal Epstein–Barr virus-associated lymphoproliferative disorder following autografting for chronic myeloid leukemia. Bone Marrow Transplant 1995;15:639–641.

100. O'Reilly RJ, Lacerda JF, Lucas KG, et al. Adoptive cell therapy with donor lymphocytes for EBV-associated lymphomas developing after allogeneic marrow transplants. In: DeVita VT, Jr., Hellman S, Rosenberg SA (eds). Important Advances in Oncology. Philadelphia: Lippincott, 1996:149–166.

101. Curtis RE, Travis LB, Rowlings PA, et al. Risk of lymphoproliferative disorders after bone marrow transplantation: a multi-institutional study. Blood 1999;94:2208–2216.

102. Hanson MN, Morrison VA, Peterson BA, et al. Posttransplant T-cell lymphoproliferative disorders–an aggressive, late complication of solid-organ transplantation. Blood 1996;88:3626–3633.

103. Deeg HJ, Socié G. Malignancies after hematopoietic stem cell transplantation: many questions, some answers. Blood 1998; 91:1833–1844.

104. Meignin V, Devergie A, Brice P, et al. Hodgkin's disease of donor origin after allogeneic bone marrow transplantation for myelogenous chronic luekiemia [review]. Transplantation 1998; 65:595–597.

105. Schouten HC, Hopman AH, Haesevoets AM, et al. Large-cell anaplastic non-Hodgkin's lymphoma originating in donor cells after allogeneic bone marrow transplantation. Br J Haematol 1995;91:162–166.

106. Travis LB, Curtis RE, Stovall M, et al. Risk of leukemia following treatment for non-Hodgkin's lymphoma. J Natl Cancer Inst 1994;86:1450–1457.

107. Chao NJ, Nademanee AP, Long GD, et al. Importance of bone marrow cytogenetic evaluation before autologous bone marrow transplantation for Hodgkin's disease. J Clin Oncol 1991; 9:1575–1579.

108. Stone RM. Myelodysplastic syndrome after autologous transplantation for lymphoma: the price of progress? Blood 1994;83:3437–3440.

109. Metayer C, Curtis RE, Vose J, et al. Myelodysplastic syndrome and acute myeloid leukemia after autotransplantation for lymphoma: a multicenter case-control study. Blood 2003;101: 2015–2023.

110. Curtis RE, Rowlings PA, Deeg HJ, et al. Solid cancers after bone marrow transplantation. N Engl J Med 1997;336:897–904.

111. Murdych T, Weisdorf DJ. Serious cardiac complications during bone marrow transplantation at the University of Minnesota, 1977–1997. Bone Marrow Transplant 2001;28:283–287.

112. Ramrakha PS, Marks DI, O'Brien SG, et al. Orthotopic cardiac transplantation for dilated cardiomyopathy after allogeneic bone marrow transplantation. Clin Transplant 1994;8:23–26.

113. Kakavas PW, Ghalie R, Parrillo JE, et al. Angiotensin converting enzyme inhibitors in bone marrow transplant recipients with depressed left ventricular function. Bone Marrow Transplant 1995;15:859–861.

114. Hochster H, Wasserheit C, Speyer J. Cardiotoxicity and cardioprotection during chemotherapy [review]. Curr Opin Oncol 1995;7:304–309.

115. Bush NE, Donaldson GW, Haberman MH, et al. Conditional and unconditional estimation of multidimensional quality of life after hematopoietic stem cell transplantation: a longitudinal follow-up of 415 patients. Biol Blood Marrow Transplant 2000; 6:576–591.

116. Wingard JR, Curbow B, Baker F, et al. Health, functional status, and employment of adult survivors of bone marrow transplantation. Ann Intern Med 1991;114:113–118.

117. Broers S, Kaptein AA, Cessie SL, et al. Psychological functioning and quality of life following bone marrow transplantation: a 3-year follow-up study. J Psychosom Res 2000;48:11–21.

118. Lee SJ, Fairclough D, Parsons SK, et al. Recovery after stem-cell transplantation for hematologic diseases. J Clin Oncol 2001;19: 242–252.

119. Syrjala KL, Chapko MK, Vitaliano PP, et al. Recovery after allogeneic marrow transplantation: prospective study of predictors of long-term physical and psychosocial functioning. Bone Marrow Transplant 1993:11:319–327.

120. Zittoun R, Suciu S, Watson M, et al. Quality of life in patients with acute myelogenous leukemia in prolonged first complete remission after bone marrow transplantation [allogeneic or autologous] or chemotherapy: a cross-sectional study of the EORTC-GIMEMA AML 8 A trial. Bone Marrow Transplant 1997;20:307–315.

121. Andrykowski MA, Bruehl S, Brady MJ, et al. Physical and psychosocial status of adults one year after bone marrow transplantation: a prospective study. Bone Marrow Transplant 1995;15:837–844.

122. Brezden CB, Phillips KA, Abdolell M, et al. Cognitive function in breast cancer patients receiving adjuvant chemotherapy. J Clin Oncol 2000;18:2695–2701.

123. Chiodi S, Spinelli S, Ravera G, et al. Quality of life in 244 recipients of allogeneic bone marrow transplantation. Br J Haematol 2000;110:614–619.

124. Duell T, van Lint MT, Ljungman P, et al. Health and functional status of long-term survivors of bone marrow transplantation. Ann Intern Med 1997;126:184–192.

125. Heinonen H, Volin L, Uutela A, et al. Quality of life and factors related to perceived satisfaction with quality of life after allogeneic bone marrow transplantation. Ann Hematol 2001;80: 137–143.

126. Prieto JM, Saez R, Carreras E, et al. Physical and psychosocial functioning of 117 survivors of bone marrow transplantation. Bone Marrow Transplant 1996;17:1133–1142.

127. Syrjala KL, Langer SL, Abrams JR, et al. Recovery and long-term function after hematopoietic cell transplantation for leukemia or lymphoma. JAMA 2004;291(19):2335–2343.

128. Bush NE, Haberman M, Donaldson G, et al. Quality of life of 125 adults surviving 6–18 years after bone marrow transplantation. Soc Sci Med 1995;40:479–490.

129. Kiss TL, Abdolell M, Jamal N, et al. Long-term medical outcomes and quality of life assessment of patients with chronic myeloid leukemia followed at least 10 years after allogeneic bone marrow transplantation. J Clin Oncol 2002;20:2334–2343.

130. Hensel M, Egerer G, Schneeweiss A, et al. Quality of life and rehabilitation in social and professional life after autologous stem cell transplantation. Ann Oncol 2002;13:209–217.

131. Sanders JE, Syrjala KL, Hoffmeister PA, et al. Quality of life (QOL) of adult survivors of childhood leukemia treated with chemotherapy (CT) or bone marrow transplant (BMT). Blood 2001;98:741a.

132. Felder-Puig R, Peters C, Matthes-Martin S, et al. Psychosocial adjustment of pediatric patients after allogeneic stem cell transplantation. Bone Marrow Transplant 1999;24:75–80.

133. Badell I, Igual L, Gomez P, et al. Quality of life in young adults having received a BMT during childhood: a GETMON study. Bone Marrow Transplant 1998;21(suppl 2):S68–S71

134. Schmidt GM, Niland JC, Forman SJ, et al. Extended follow-up in 212 long-term allogeneic bone marrow transplant survivors. Transplantation 1993;55:551–557.

135. Andrykowski MA, Carpenter JS, Greiner CB, et al. Energy level and sleep quality following bone marrow transplantation. Bone Marrow Transplant 1997;20:669–679.

136. Hann DM, Jacobsen PB, Martin SC, et al. Fatigue in women treated with bone marrow transplantation for breast cancer: a comparison with women with no history of cancer. Support Care Cancer 1997;5:44–52.

137. McQuellon RP, Russell GB, Rambo TD, et al. Quality of life and psychological distress of bone marrow transplant recipients: the "time trajectory" to recovery over the first year. Bone Marrow Transplant 1998;21:477–486.

138. Knobel H, Loge JH, Nordøy T, et al. High level of fatigue in lymphoma patients treated with high dose therapy. J Pain Symptom Manag 2000;19:446–456.

139. Baron F, Sautois B, Baudoux E, et al. Optimization of recombinant human erythropoietin therapy after allogeneic hematopoietic stem cell transplantation. Exp Hematol 2002;30:546–554.

140. Dimeo FC, Stieglitz RD, Novelli-Fischer U, et al. Effects of physical activity on the fatigue and psychologic status of cancer patients during chemotherapy. Cancer (Phila) 1999;85:2273–2277.

141. Gaston-Johansson F, Fall-Dickson JM, Nanda J, et al. The effectiveness of the comprehensive coping strategy program on clinical outcomes in breast cancer autologous bone marrow transplantation. Cancer Nurs 2000;23:277–285.

142. Jager HR, Williams EJ, Savage DG, et al. Assessment of brain changes with registered MR before and after bone marrow transplantation for chronic myeloid leukemia. Am J Neurorad 1996;17:1275–1282.

143. Provenzale JM, Graham ML. Reversible leukoencephalopathy associated with graft-versus-host disease: MR findings. Am J Neurorad 1996;17:1290–1294.

144. Openshaw H, Slatkin NE, Smith E. Eye movement disorders in bone marrow transplant patients on cyclosporin and ganciclovir. Bone Marrow Transplant 1997;19:503–505.

145. Shah AK. Cyclosporine A neurotoxicity among bone marrow transplant recipients [review]. Clin Neuropharmacol 1999;22:67–73.

146. Padovan CS, Yousry TA, Schleuning M, et al. Neurological and neuroradiological findings in long-term survivors of allogeneic bone marrow transplantation. Ann Neurol 1998;43:627–633.

147. Andrykowski MA, Schmitt FA, Gregg ME, et al. Neuropsychologic impairment in adult bone marrow transplant candidates. Cancer (Phila) 1992;70:2288–2297.

148. Meyers CA, Weitzner M, Byrne K, et al. Evaluation of the neurobehavioral functioning of patients before, during, and after bone marrow transplantation. J Clin Oncol 1994;12:820–826.

149. Syrjala KL, Dikmen S, Roth-Roemer S. Neuropsychological changes from pretransplant to one year in patients receiving myeloablative allogeneic hematopoietic cell transplant. Blood 2004;104:3386–3392.

150. van Dam FS, Schagen SB, Muller MJ, et al. Impairment of cognitive function in women receiving adjuvant treatment for high-risk breast cancer: high-dose versus standard-dose chemotherapy. J Natl Cancer Inst 1998;90:210–218.

151. Harder H, Cornelissen JJ, Van Gool AR, et al. Cognitive functioning and quality of life in long-term adult survivors of bone marrow transplantation. Cancer (Phila) 2002;95:183–192.

152. Saykin A, Ahles T, McDonald BC. Mechanisms of chemotherapy-induced cognitive disorders: neuropsychological, pathophysiological, and neuroimaging perspectives. Semin Clin Neuropsychol 2003;8:201–216.

153. Andrykowski MA, Altmaier EM, Barnett RL, et al. Cognitive dysfunction in adult survivors of allogeneic marrow transplantation: relationship to dose of total body irradiation. Bone Marrow Transplant 1990;6:269–276.

154. Peper M, Steinvorth S, Schraube P, et al. Neurobehavioral toxicity of total body irradiation: a follow-up in long-term survivors. Int J Radiat Oncol Biol Phys 2000;46:303–311.

155. Wenz F, Steinvorth S, Lohr F, et al. Prospective evaluation of delayed central nervous system [CNS] toxicity of hyperfraction-ated total body irradiation [TBI]. Int J Radiat Oncol Biol Phys 2000;48:1497–1501.

156. Fann JR, Roth-Roemer S, Burington BE, et al. Delirium in patients undergoing hematopoietic stem cell transplantation. Cancer (Phila) 2002;95:1971–1981.

157. Phipps S, Dunavant M, Srivastava DK, et al. Cognitive and academic functioning in survivors of pediatric bone marrow transplantation. J Clin Oncol 2000;18:1004–1011.

158. Arvidson J, Kihlgren M, Hall C, et al. Neuropsychological functioning after treatment for hematological malignancies in childhood, including autologous bone marrow transplantation. Pediatr Hematol Oncol 1999;16:9–21.

159. Kramer JH, Crittenden MR, DeSantes K, et al. Cognitive and adaptive behavior 1 and 3 years following bone marrow transplantation. Bone Marrow Transplant 1997;19:607–613.

160. Simms S, Kazak AE, Gannon T, et al. Neuropsychological outcome of children undergoing bone marrow transplantation. Bone Marrow Transplant 1998;22:181–184.

161. Howell SJ, Radford JA, Smets EM, et al. Fatigue, sexual function and mood following treatment for haematological malignancy: the impact of mild Leydig cell dysfunction. Br J Can 2000;82:789–793.

162. Schimmer AD, Ali V, Stewart AK, et al. Male sexual function after autologous blood or marrow transplantation. Biol Blood Marrow Transplant 2001;7:279–283.

163. Wingard JR, Curbow B, Baker F, et al. Sexual satisfaction in survivors of bone marrow transplantation. Bone Marrow Transplant 1992;9:185–190.

164. Molassiotis A, van den Akker OB, Milligan DW, et al. Gonadal function and psychosexual adjustment in male long-term survivors of bone marrow transplantation. Bone Marrow Transplant 1995;16:253–259.

165. Watson M, Wheatley K, Harrison GA, et al. Severe adverse impact on sexual functioning and fertility of bone marrow transplantation, either allogeneic or autologous, compared with consolidation chemotherapy alone: analysis of the MRC AML 10 trial. Cancer (Phila) 1999;86:1231–1239.

166. Syrjala KL, Schroeder TC, Abrams JR, et al. Sexual function measurement and outcomes in cancer survivors and matched controls. J Sex Res 2000;37:213–225.

167. Schubert MA, Sullivan KM, Schubert MM, et al. Gynecological abnormalities following allogeneic bone marrow transplantation. Bone Marrow Transplant 1990;5:425–430.

168. Syrjala KL, Powell-Emsbo S, Garrett K, et al. Focus Forward: Recovery Tips and Tools for Transplant Recipients and Caregivers. Seattle: Fred Hutchinson Cancer Research Center, 2002.

169. Chatterjee R, Kottaridis PD, McGarrigle HH, et al. Management of erectile dysfunction by combination therapy with testosterone and sildenafil in recipients of high-dose therapy for haematological malignances. Bone Marrow Transplant 2002;29:607–610.

170. Kauppila M, Viikari J, Irjala K, et al. The hypothalamus-pituitary-gonad axis and testicular function in male patients after treatment for haematological malignancies. J Intern Med 1998;244:411–416.

171. Loberiza FR Jr, Rizzo JD, Bredeson CN, et al. Association of depressive syndrome and early deaths among patients after stem-cell transplantation for malignant disease. J Clin Oncol 2002;20:2118–2126.

172. Molassiotis A, van den Akker OB, Milligan DW, et al. Symptom distress, coping style and biological variables as predictors of survival after bone marrow transplantation. J Psychosom Res 1997;42:275–285.

173. Fife BL, Huster GA, Cornetta KG, et al. Longitudinal study of adaptation to the stress of bone marrow transplantation. J Clin Oncol 2000;18:1539–1549.

174. Phipps S, Dunavant M, Garvie PA, et al. Acute health-related quality of life in children undergoing stem cell transplant: I.

Descriptive outcomes. Bone Marrow Transplant 2002;29: 425–434.

175. Mielcarek M, Martin PJ, Leisenring W, et al. Graft-versus-host disease after nonmyeloablative versus conventional hematopoietic stem cell transplantation. Blood 2002;100:175a.

176. Foxall M, Gaston-Johansson F. Burden and health outcomes of family caregivers of hospitalized bone marrow transplant patients. J Adv Nurs 1996;24:915–923.

177. Zabora JR, Smith ED, Baker F, et al. The family: the other side of bone marrow transplantation. J Psychosoc Oncol 1992;10: 35–46.

178. Manne S, DuHamel K, Nereo N, et al. Predictors of PTSD in mothers of children undergoing bone marrow transplantation: the role of cognitive and social processes. J Pediatr Psychol 2002;27:607–617.

179. Langer SL, Abrams JR, Syrjala KL. Caregiver and patient marital satisfaction and affect following hematopoietic stem cell transplantation: a prospective, longitudinal investigation. Psycho-Oncology 2003;12:239–253.

180. Deeg HJ, Lin D, Leisenring W, et al. Cyclosporine or cyclosporine plus methylprednisolone for prophylaxis of graft-versus-host disease: a prospective, randomized trial. Blood 1997;89: 3880–3887.

181. Ruutu T, Volin L, Parkkali T, et al. Cyclosporine, methotrexate, and methylprednisolone compared with cyclosporine and methotrexate for the prevention of graft-versus-host disease in bone marrow transplantation from HLA-identical sibling donor: a prospective randomized study. Blood 2000;96:2391–2398.

182. Leung W, Hudson M, Zhu Y, et al. Late effects in survivors of infant leukemia. Leukemia 2000;14:1185–1190.

183. Thomas BC, Stanhope R, Plowman PN, et al. Growth following single fraction and fractionated total body irradiation for bone marrow transplantation. Eur J Pediatr 1993;152:888–892.

184. Sanders JE, and the Seattle Marrow Transplant Team. The impact of marrow transplant preparative regimens on subsequent growth and development. Semin Hematol 1991;28: 244–249.

185. Chatterjee R, Andrews HO, McGarrigle HH, et al. Cavernosal arterial insufficiency is a major component of erectile dysfunction in some recipients of high-dose chemotherapy/chemoradiotherapy for haematological malignancies. Bone Marrow Transplant 2000;25:1185–1189.

186. Mumma GH, Mashberg D, Lesko LM. Long-term psychosexual adjustment of acute leukemia survivors: impact of marrow transplantation versus conventional chemotherapy. Gen Hosp Psychiatry 1992;14(1):43–55.

16

Cancer Survivorship Issues in Older Adults

Karim S. Malek and Rebecca A. Silliman

Epidemiology

Cancer Burden in Older Adults

Advancing age comes bundled with increased cancer incidence and mortality.[1,2] Indeed, the median age at diagnosis of all cancers combined is 69 years for men and 67 years for women.[3] Age-adjusted cancer incidence is ten times higher in the 65+ population compared to their younger counterparts (2,151.2 versus 208.8/100,000 persons).[2] Similarly, age-adjusted cancer mortality is 15-fold higher in the 65+ population (1,068.2 versus 67.3/100,000 persons).[2] Figures 16.1 and 16.2 illustrate the proportions of the commonest cancers incidence and mortality in the 65+ population.[2] As a result, while the total US population is expected to grow by 9% between 1990 and 2010, the incidence of cancer is expected to increase by a disproportionate 32% in the same timeframe.[4,5] These trends are mirrored in countries across the globe.[6,7]

These figures have pressed many private and public institutions to sponsor the development of geriatric oncology as a separate subspecialty. Recent literature has seen a surge in the number of seminal publications specifically devoted to the management of older patients with cancer.[8–11] Geriatric oncology is a rapidly growing field and, while not exhaustive, this chapter will outline the challenges that are unique to this new discipline and briefly explore future research directions.

How Old Is Old?

Physiologically, there are no data to favor one particular age cutoff over the other. Although chronological aging and organ function decline with advancing age are undeniable realities, individual organ functions decline at different rates in different persons. This makes the older population a heterogeneous group when it comes to life expectancy, functional status and secondarily for geriatric oncologists, cancer treatment benefits and tolerance.

A Practical Approach to Geriatric Oncology

Geriatric oncologists are faced with a two-sided challenge: on the one hand, they have to carefully select evidence-based data that are applicable to older cancer patients from an ever-expanding oncology literature addressed to a wider audience. This is a difficult task given the limited representation of older individuals in cancer clinical trials.[12] Indeed, even after removing age as an exclusion criterion from collaborative group trials, only 13% of all participants in the Southwest Oncology Group (SWOG) and 8% of all participants in the European Organization for Research and Treatment of Cancer (EORTC) clinical trials are older than 70,[13,14] compared to 47% of the total US population with cancer in the same age group.[13] A retrospective review of National Cancer Institute (NCI) sponsored clinical trials active between 1997 and 2000 yielded similar conclusions.[15] On the other hand, treating cancer in older patients requires that four unique points be addressed.

ESTIMATING THE PATIENT'S LIFE EXPECTANCY

While the *average* life expectancy of the general population has doubled in the last century,[16] it is important to note that those who live close to or beyond the *average* expectancy are not condemned to imminent death, but contrarily, have the highest odds of surviving even longer.[17] The average life expectancy at ages 65, 75, and 85 years is, respectively, 17.5, 11.2, and 6 years.[18] This concept is key in avoiding the temptation of under-treating older patients based solely on their advanced age.[18,19]

EVALUATING THE PATIENT'S COMORBIDITIES AND FUNCTIONAL STATUS

Eighty percent of individuals who are 65 years of age or older have at least one comorbidity.[20] Advancing age is associated with an increased vulnerability to multiple comorbidities—such as diabetes, hypertension, arthritis and heart diseases—as well as other age-related conditions, including dementia, incontinence, and balance disorders. The interaction of comorbidity and cancer is a very complex one and is the subject of a detailed discussion below (see **Comorbidity and Cancer**). Comorbidities are independent predictors of survival in cancer patients.[21,22] Accounting for them is an essential step in the management of older patients with cancer.

There are many tools to assess comorbidity with variable content and different goals,[23–26] but there is no consensus on which one to use in routine Geriatric Oncology. Additionally, these tools often require lengthy administration, rendering them less practical for regular use in a busy oncology practice. For example, the Multi-dimensional Assessment of Cancer in the Elderly (MACE), although specifically developed to evaluate comorbidity in older cancer patients, requires 27+/−7 minutes for scoring.[27] We and others have implemented shorter screening questionnaires as a practical substitute to exhaustive geriatric assessment scales (Table 16.1).[28,29] This screening questionnaire can often be

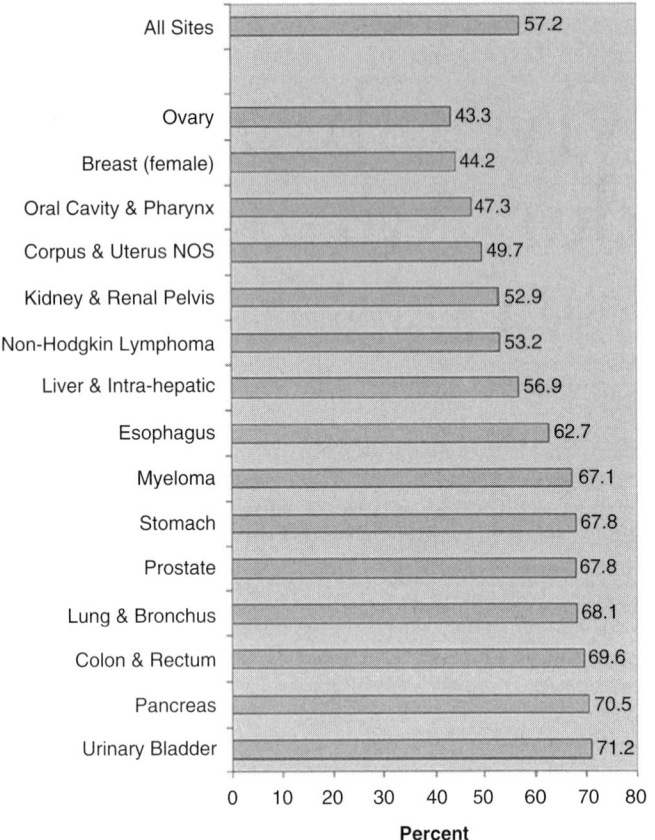

FIGURE 16.1. Age-adjusted cancer incidence in the 65+ population.   **FIGURE 16.2.** Age-adjusted cancer mortality in the 65+ population.

TABLE 16.1.   Geriatric Screening Questionnaire.*

To be filled by the patient (Yes/No)

1. Have you lost 10 pounds or more in the last 6 months without trying to do so?

2. How are you able to walk?
   Independent _____
   Assist _____ Cane _____ Walker _____
   Dependent _____

3. A) In the past year, have you ever lost your urine and gotten wet?
   B) If you have answered "Yes" to the above question, have you lost urine on at least 6 separate days?

4. Are you able to:
   • Do strenuous activities, like fast walking or biking?
   • Do heavy work around the house like washing windows, walls or floors?
   • Go shopping for groceries or clothes?
   • Get to places out of walking distances?
   • Bathe (either a sponge bath or tub bath) or shave?
   • Dress, like putting on a shirt, buttoning or zipping, or putting on shoes?

5. Do you feel that your needs at home are not being met?

To be filled by healthcare professional

6. Do you feel unsafe or threatened by someone around you?

7. Do you often feel sad or depressed?

8. I am going to give you the names of 3 objects. Please repeat them after me: "Apple, penny, table".
   Recall at one minute: _____ (of 3)

*Adapted from Reuben and Moore et al.[28,30]

self-administered by the patient with minimal help from family members. The sensitivity, specificity, positive, and negative predictive values of the questionnaire items are well established.[30] Results of the screening test are reported as part of the initial geriatric oncology evaluation and the test subsequently can be repeated at the physician's discretion. Patients who perform poorly in the initial screening test are candidates for referral to a geriatrician who would then perform a comprehensive geriatric assessment.

INCREASED SUSCEPTIBILITY TO TREATMENT TOXICITY IN OLDER PATIENTS

This is the subject of ongoing research and is one of the main barriers to extrapolating clinical trial data obtained from younger trial participants to older cancer patients. Older patients are more susceptible to the side effects of chemotherapeutic agents.[31] Additionally, cancer treatment modalities may impact older patients in a unique fashion. For example, a chemotherapeutic agent that causes peripheral neuropathy may worsen imbalance in an older individual and increase his/her risks of falling and the subsequent morbidity that ensues. Increased treatment toxicity may also negatively affect an often-compromised quality of life. The common problem of polypharmacy in older age increases the likelihood of drug to drug and/or drug to food interactions.[32–34] The impact of treatment modalities on older cancer patients is detailed in "Specific Cancer Management Issues in the Older Population" (p. 219).

PUTTING TREATMENT BENEFITS IN PERSPECTIVE: ABSOLUTE VERSUS RELATIVE GAINS

Barring untoward side effects, a treatment that offers a 25% relative reduction of mortality at ten years may be an attractive modality for a 65-year-old patient, whose average life expectancy is otherwise 17.5 years. The same relative risk reduction may not, however, represent a significant survival gain in an 85-year-old with the same disease stage, and whose life expectancy is limited to 6 years. Treatment gains and side effects should be carefully weighed against the individual's life expectancy *and* quality of life. How comorbidities impact life expectancy is also an integral part of the equation.[21,22]

Comorbidity and Cancer

Importance of Integrating Comorbidity and Cancer

Comorbidity is defined as the presence of more than one concomitant chronic health condition in an individual. Conditions such as diabetes, hypertension, and/or other age-related conditions—such as limited self-reliance, dementia, malnutrition or incontinence—represent a problem of significant magnitude while managing older patients. Eighty percent of individuals who are 65 and older have at least one comorbidity; 30% have 3–4 while 15% have seven or more such conditions.[19,21] The routine incorporation of comorbidity assessment in the practice of geriatric oncology is easily justifiable since clinicians must make cancer treatment decisions in the context of preexisting morbidities.[35,36] Moreover,

comorbidity and cancer interact intimately. They impact stage at diagnosis,[37] as well as survival, independent of a patient's age and/or tumor stage.[22,38] They also compete with cancer as a cause of death and increase the risks of disability among cancer patients.[21,39] Their presence is often associated with the receipt of less definitive cancer therapy,[40] which in turn leads to poorer treatment outcomes.[17] On the other hand, cancer and its treatment modalities—even the adjunct ones—may impact preexisting morbidities. For example, steroids are potent antiemetics but they can wreck havoc on diabetic control. Similarly, erythropoietin is an effective treatment for cancer-related anemia, but it can worsen hypertension. This is especially true given that older patients are generally more susceptible to developing treatment-related side effects.[31] The concomitant management of comorbidities and cancer presents its own challenges since primary and specialty care may not always be well-coordinated. Patients themselves may not think that the continued management of other conditions is as important after a cancer diagnosis is established.

Sources of Comorbidity Data

Multiple sources could be exploited to collect comorbidity data and they should ideally be used in a complementary fashion:

(1) *Medical records* are widely considered to be the most comprehensive source of information. They are easily accessible to multiple providers with the spreading computerization of clinical care. Limitations include the inconsistent access between hospitals and patients,[41] as well as the introduction of a bias resulting from varying health care utilization among patients.

(2) *In medical interviews*, patients are often a good source of data if they were made aware of their comorbidities in prior medical encounters. Some studies have demonstrated that patients are as reliable as medical records as a source of their comorbidity,[42] although reliability obviously decreases with dementia and recall problems. Medical interviews are good means to assess the *severity* of comorbidities, since their impact on functional status can be directly appreciated.

(3) *In administrative datasets*, the computerization of billing information has resulted in large databases that are often coded using ICD-9-CM nomenclatures. These, however, are seldom complete as conditions could be addressed by clinicians but not adequately translated onto billing records. Other limitations include the inconsistent translation between some comorbidity indices and ICD-9-CM coding[43–45] and the lack of data on severity of comorbidity.

Note that some comorbidities are often overlooked and therefore underrecorded in routine clinical practice. Depression and anxiety are classic examples of underrecognized morbidities.[46,47] Others include cognitive impairment, malnutrition, and anemia.

Comorbidity Indices

There are multiple tools to evaluate and score morbidities, each with different goals and outcomes.[22,25,27,48–52] Their descriptions are outlined in Table 16.2. As stated earlier, there is no consensus on which tool is best adapted to routine clinical practice.[24,26]

TABLE 16.2. Commonly used comorbidity indices.

	Description	Advantages	Disadvantages
Charlson Index[25]	Provides an overall score based on a composite of values assigned to 19 comorbidity conditions; estimates risk of death from comorbid conditions	• Shorter administration time than ICED • Validated in evaluation breast cancer patients • Derived from medical records	• No measure of severity of comorbidity • No functional • Dichotomous
Satariano and Ragland[22]	Modified Charlson index providing survival estimates in breast cancer	• Validated in breast cancer patients	• No measure of severity of comorbidity • No functional evaluation
Index of Co-Existing Diseases (ICED)[51–52]	Integrates measures of ten functional areas, each divided into three levels of severity; chart-based review	• Provides functional evaluation • Provides and estimate of severity of disease	• Average overall reliability (kappa 0.5–0.6) and Index of Disease Severity subindex (kappa 0.4–0.5)
Kaplan and Feinstein[50]	Assigns scores from 1 to 3 to comorbidity in various organ systems	• Provides an estimate of severity of disease • Validated in several cancers, including breast, prostate and head and neck	• No functional evaluation
Multidimensional Assessment of Cancer in the Elderly (MACE)[27]	Integrates measures of comorbidity, functional status, depression, balance, physical function and disability	• Validated in cancer patients • Provides a structured evaluation of functional status	• Lengthy administration (27 +/− 7 min)
Multiple Informants Analysis[48]	Combined scoring of the Charlson, ICED, PS and American Society of Anesthesiologists Index	• Superior in estimating the overall effect of comorbidity than separate models that included only one index	• Lengthy administration (average: 30 minutes*)

*T Lash, personal communication.

Quantification of the Impact of Comorbidities on Cancer

This area has largely benefited from the work of Yancik et al., using a cohort of male and female colon cancer patients who were 55 years and older as a model.[21] High and moderate-impact comorbidities were identified (Table 16.3). The rela-tionship between the number of comorbidities and overall survival was reported: Patients with 5 or more comorbidities had lower survival rates than those who have 4 or less (Mor-tality risk ratio = 1.44 in patients with 5 to 6 comorbidities and 1.85 in those with 7 or more). Comorbidities with the highest association with increased mortality were also iden-tified (Table 16.4).

Cancer Screening in Older Individuals

Cancer screening in older individuals comes with its own sets of problems and characteristics:[53]

TABLE 16.3. High- and moderate-impact comorbidities.

High-impact comorbidities

History	Current
Cardiac	Cardiac
Arrest	Angina
Congestive heart failure	Arrhythmias
Lung	Myocardial infarction
Emphysema	Valvular disease
Renal failure	Type 1 diabetes
	Cancer

Moderate-impact comorbidities

Current
  Alcohol Abuse
  Anemia
  Asthma
  Deep vein thrombosis
  Depression
  Gastrointestinal diseases
  Hypertension
  Lipid abnormalities
  Liver diseases
  Mental diseases
  Stroke/Transient ischemic attack
  Tobacco abuse

Source: Adapted from Yancik et al.[21]

TABLE 16.4. Specific comorbidities and mortality risk ratio in patients with colon cancer.

Comorbidity	Mortality risk ratio
Liver disease	3.04
Other serious comorbidity	2.33
Alcohol abuse	2.20
Deep vein thrombosis	2.06
Renal failure	1.99
Emphysema	1.67
Depression	1.63
Thyroid/glandular disease	1.49
Severe heart disease (high-impact)	1.48
Diabetes mellitus	1.37
Anemia	1.25

Source: Adapted from Yancik et al.[21]

(1) The characteristics of a given screening test may change with age. For example, the sensitivity and specificity of mammography gradually increases with advancing age.[54] Similarly, the specificity of PSA screening for prostate cancer decreases with age because of the increased prevalence of benign prostatic hyperplasia.

(2) Tumors may have a different biology in older patients (e.g., slower growth rate).[55] This leads to an increased detection of slowly growing tumors, known as length-time bias.

(3) Older individuals have a shorter life expectancy compared to younger counterparts, by virtue of their advanced age or associated comorbidities. The detection of an asymptomatic tumor may not translate into a longer survival in the older individual, therefore questioning the rationale of screening at extremes of age. In general terms, the impact of screening is evident 3 to 5 years later and the value of screening may be therefore limited in individuals with shorter life expectancy.[56,57]

(4) This over-detection of clinically nonsignificant tumors may lead to treatments that adversely affect the quality of life of the older individual and may represent an unjustified healthcare cost to the community.[56]

Specific Cancer Management Issues in the Older Population: Treatment Modalities

Older cancer patients benefit from the same treatment modalities widely used in the management of cancer, including surgery, radiation therapy and chemotherapy. The following section highlights how these modalities are applied to older cancer patients. However, treatment choices in older patients go beyond the mere age-associated physiological and/or pathological changes. Older patients often have a different outlook on life, caring more about their quality of life rather than longevity; how they opt for one therapeutic modality over the other has not been fully studied. Additionally, social and/or financial considerations may ultimately affect their choice. For example, lumpectomy followed by radiation therapy for breast cancer has yielded similar survival results as a more extensive mastectomy, however older patients may still opt for mastectomy since it obviates the need for postoperative radiation therapy, which requires additional logistic arrangements over several weeks.

Cancer Surgery in Older Patients

Surgery is an integral part of a multimodality approach to the treatment of most cancers; its use is very frequently a prerequisite for treatment plans with a curative intent. Geriatric surgery has been the subject of excellent reviews elsewhere.[58–60] The following section highlights some of its most salient aspects.

INCREASED OPERATIVE RISKS IN OLDER AGE

Surgery has advanced by giant leaps in the latter part of the twentieth century. It has benefited from innovative technology, safer anesthetics agents, the advent of a large array of antibiotics, enhanced intra-operative monitoring, and post-operative intensive care. Surgical risks have been proportionally withered. Age-related physiologic changes and accumulating comorbidities continue, however, to expose older patients to specific risks.[61–64] These changes involve all major organ systems (see Table 16.5).

PREOPERATIVE RISK ASSESSMENT

Careful preoperative evaluation of older patients is a crucial step in estimating operative risk and plan interventions to reduce them to a minimum.[65] Controversy persists over how extensive preoperative risk assessments should be.[66–69] Of interest, several preoperative risk assessment scales consider age per se as a factor that increases the risks of an adverse cardiac event in noncardiac surgical interventions. For example, age >70 years contributes 5 points to the Goldman index of cardiac risk in noncardiac surgical procedures.[70,71] Similarly, being 80 years of age or older automatically puts a patient in class II (out of possible V) in the American Society of Anesthesia (ASA) scale.[72] However, these scales remain heavily weighted by the presence or absence of comorbid conditions, rather than by age alone. For example, clinical evidence of congestive heart failure and a history of recent myocardial infarction contribute 11 and 10 points respectively to the Goldman index,[70] overshadowing the more limited contribution of age to the final score.

REDUCTION OF OPERATIVE RISKS

Multiple interventions have been advocated to reduce operative risks in older patients. These include (1) correction of

TABLE 16.5. Age-related changes and increased surgical risks.

Organ system	Physiologic and pathologic age-related changes	Surgical risks
Cardiovascular	• Increased atherosclerosis • Increased risk of arrhythmias • Decreased ventricular distensibility • Increased dependence on preload	• Increased sensitivity to fluid shifts • Increased risk of cardiac ischemia • Increased risk of congestive heart failure
Kidney	• Decreased renal mass • Decreased renal blood flow • Decreased GFR	• Risks of acid-base balance disturbances • Risk of electrolytes imbalance • Increased sensitivity to renally cleared drugs • Increased risk of renal ischemia
Liver	• Decreased hepatic mass • Decreased hepatic blood flow	• Increased sensitivity to hepatically cleared drugs
Pulmonary	• Decreased pulmonary volumes • Decreased compliance • Decreased ciliary function	• Risk of postoperative atelectasis • Risk of postoperative pneumonia
Central Nervous System	• Decreased cerebral mass • Decreased cerebral blood flow • Dementia	• Difficulty obtaining informed consent • Risk of postoperative delirium • Slow postoperative recovery and prolonged hospitalization

reversible metabolic parameters,[73] (2) use of beta-blockers to reduce perioperative mortality from cardiac events,[65] (3) adequate blood pressure control,[65] (4) close monitoring of volume status using invasive pulmonary artery catheters,[74] although their benefit is contested,[75] and (5) most importantly, avoid the delay in surgery which exposes the patient to higher risks of needing an emergent intervention,[59] or a more extensive surgery secondary to tumor progression.

In conclusion, surgical risks related to aging are mostly related to coexisting morbidities, rather than to age by itself. Therefore, older patients should not be denied a chance at curative treatment based on their age alone.

Radiation Therapy in Older Cancer Patients

Like surgery, radiation therapy plays a central role in the treatment of older cancer patients, both as part of a multi-modality approach and/or with a palliative intent.[76] There are no convincing data that tissue tolerance to radiation therapy is different in older than in younger patients. Most laboratory data were obtained in rapidly growing tissue cultures and apply only to acute radiation toxicity.[77] Tolerance of radiation therapy in older patients is modulated by existing comorbidities. Specifics of radiation treatment in older patients with breast, lung, gastrointestinal and genitourinary cancers are beyond the scope of this chapter and have been extensively reviewed elsewhere.[78,79] Radiation therapy improves the quality of life in older patients and it has proven especially efficacious in controlling tumor-induced pain.[80–82] Social issues such as transportation continue to pose a significant logistic and financial burden on those who lost their physical and/or financial independence.

Chemotherapy in Older Cancer Patients

Chemotherapy is a mainstay treatment for many types of cancer. Two retrospective trials showed that chemotherapy toxicity does not differ between older and younger patients.[83,84] Results of these trials, however, should be carefully interpreted, since stringent exclusion criteria may preclude their generalization to the average older patient. The pharmacology of individual antineoplastic agents in older patients is extensively reviewed elsewhere.[85]

Every aspect of drug pharmacokinetics is potentially affected in older patients and this explains in part why they have an increased rate of chemotherapy toxicity.

Absorption

Mucosal atrophy, decreased gastrointestinal motility, and splanchnic blood flow are all documented changes in older patients and can account for decreased absorption of drugs in the older population.[86] This is especially important given that an increasing number of new chemotherapeutic agents, such as capecitabine and imatinib, are orally administered.

Distribution

Several factors affect drug distribution in older patients: (1) Decreased body water by about 20% in older patients leads to decreased volume of distribution of polar drugs, such as methotrexate and mitomycin-C. (2) Plasma albumin decreases by an average of 15% to 20% in older patients, leading to an increased unbound fraction of protein-bound drugs such as etoposide, anthracyclins, and taxanes.[87] (3) Increased body fat leads to increased half-life and lower clearance of fat-soluble agents. (4) Changes in the shape of the area under the curve (AUC), with water soluble drugs show higher plasma concentrations and shorter half-lives, while fat-soluble drugs show lower plasma concentrations and prolonged half-lives. These changes affect both drug efficacy and toxicity profile. (5) Anemia can significantly increase the toxicity of red-blood-cell-bound drugs such as taxanes and anthracyclines.

Hepatic Clearance

Decreased liver size and reduced hepatic blood flow both contribute to reduced clearance of hepatically cleared chemotherapeutic agents.[88] Several of the Cytochrome P450 enzyme activity decline with age, leaving the patient at risk for increased toxicity from delayed clearance.[89,90] Moreover, older patients are commonly subject to polypharmacy. CYP3A4 is inhibited by a large number of commonly prescribed drugs, leaving patients at risk for increased of toxicity from CYP3A4-dependant chemotherapy agents, such as cyclophosphamide, ifosfamide, taxanes, tamoxifen, and vinca alkaloids.

Renal Clearance

Glomerular filtration rate (GFR) steadily decreases at the rate of 1 ml/year in individuals who are 40 years or older.[91] This decrease is not proportionally translated into an increased serum creatinine value because of the parallel reduction in muscle mass. Serum creatinine and estimates of creatinine clearance such as the Cockroft-Gault formula may therefore overestimate the renal GFR.[92] This in turn may result in increased serum levels and toxicity of any of the renally excreted agents. Drugs such as carboplatinum and bleomycin should have their doses reduced by 25% to 30% in moderate renal insufficiency (creatinine clearance of 10 to 30 ml/min), whereas the use of other agents such as cisplatinum, methotrexate and nitrosoureas should be completely avoided.

Prevention of Chemotherapy-Induced Toxicity in Older Patients

Neutropenia

Older patients are at a higher risk of hematopoietic toxicity because of limited hematopoietic reserves and decreased response to hematopoietic growth factors.[93] Older patients are more liable to develop clinically significant neutropenia, although this finding was contested by other studies.[84,94] Several trials have demonstrated the value of adding a granulocyte colony-stimulating factor (G-CSF) to moderately myelosuppressive chemotherapy regimens.[95–97] These trials provide the bases for the regular use of G-CSF in older patients receiving such chemotherapy. Although G-CSF use is associated with reduced neutropenia and risk of sepsis, complete remissions and overall survival remain generally unchanged.[98]

Anemia

Anemia of chronic disease is a common complication of cancer and its various treatment modalities. Several studies have shown that anemia is an independent predictor of survival in older individuals.[99-101] Anemia significantly impacts quality of life, with increased fatigue,[102] difficulty in concentrating, impaired memory,[103] and increased susceptibility to complications from red blood cell-bound chemotherapy agents.[104] Synthetic erythropoietin use has been associated with relief of anemia of chronic disease and improved quality of life.[105] Newer agents, such as glycosylated erythropoietin, have a very long half-life that allows their administration on a bimonthly basis. Interestingly, concomitant G-CSF administration may augment erythropoietin efficacy in treating anemia in diseases such as myelodysplastic syndromes.[106]

MUCOSITIS AND DIARRHEA

Two reports have yielded contrasting results regarding the incidence of mucositis in older cancer patients. One argues for an increased incidence, while the other states that there were no age-associated differences in the incidence of gastrointestinal toxicities.[107,108] Interventions to reduce oral mucositis include oral cryotherapy, careful oral hygiene. The use of G-CSF is associated with reduced mucosal ulcerations, presumably through its effect in increasing salivary neutrophils.

Cancer Survivorship in Older Adults

Recent and anticipated demographic changes in the United States have magnified the concentration of cancer survivors among persons ≥65 years of age. At present 61% of the estimated 10.1 million cancer survivors are ≥65 years of age[109] and the number of incident cases in this age group is expected to double over the next 30 years.[110] Furthermore, recent gains in life expectancy have occurred at the end of life. For example, the average life expectancy of a 75 year old woman is nearly 12 years (17 years if healthy), and that of an 85 year old woman is 5.9 years (9.6 years if healthy).[111] These gains mean that older persons have, on average, longer periods of time when they are at risk for recurrences and of dying of their cancers than was true in the past, and this magnifies the importance of cancer survivorship in this population.

Yet very little is known about long-term cancer survivorship in older adults. Recent investigators have taken advantage of national probability surveys, including the National Health Interview Survey[112] and the Medicare Current Beneficiary Survey[113] to compare the health and functional status of older cancer survivors to that of older persons without cancer. Both have documented poorer health and functional status among cancer survivors, compared to persons without cancer. Although these surveys reflect large representative samples, study limitations include reliance on self-report of cancer, comorbidities, and functional status; unknown and presumably varying lengths of survivorship; and cross-sectional study designs. Furthermore, they include no detail about stage at diagnosis and treatment.

In spite of the lack of systematic data, attention to three key considerations will serve to enhance the quality of life of these older cancer survivors: (1) surveillance for recurrence and attention to attendant fears, (2) management of persisting side effects related to cancer therapies, and (3) management of comorbid conditions and attention to appropriate preventive strategies. Using the example of breast cancer, we address each of these in turn.

Guidelines for breast cancer survivors' care recommend annual history, physical examination and mammography, but no surveillance with blood chemistry tests or X-rays for distant metastases unless symptoms warrant.[114-116] This is because clinical trials of intensive follow-up (physical examination, mammography, blood tests, and X-rays) of breast cancer patients have demonstrated that recurrences can be detected slightly earlier using this approach, but that there is no difference in survival.[117,118] The lack of a survival benefit is because asymptomatic recurrences represent only a minority of recurrences (about 15% to 25%).[119] Published studies suggest that older women are at risk for receipt of less than guideline surveillance.[120-121] However, the consequences of this undersurveillance have not been well studied. Indeed, a recent systematic review of surveillance mammography after treatment of primary breast cancer highlights surveillance in older women as a key area for further study.[122]

Side effects of therapy also can be problematic for older persons and interact with coexisting conditions. In the context of breast cancer, these include, for example, radiation and chronic obstructive pulmonary disease; chemotherapy-induced peripheral neuropathy and hip or knee osteoarthritis or gait disorders; and radiation/axillary dissection and shoulder problems, including rotator cuff injuries, tendonitis, and bursitis. A recent observational study of older women with early stage breast cancer documented that over half reported a decline in upper body function over a four-year period, compared to 10% in a similarly aged sample of older women without breast cancer.[123]

As noted earlier, comorbidity is a major risk factor for mortality and this is also true for older breast cancer patients, particularly the oldest old (≥85 years of age) where 82% of women die of conditions other than breast cancer.[40] Furthermore, there is evidence suggesting that a breast cancer diagnosis interacts with comorbidity to increase the risk of death from causes other than breast cancer.[22,124] Putative explanations include tumor-host interactions, long-term adverse affects of therapy, and/or lack of quality care and management of other conditions. Although recent analyses of the SEER-Medicare database suggest that older breast cancer survivors receive high quality preventive services, disparities related to older age, being African American, being of lower socioeconomic status, living in rural areas, and not receiving care in a teaching hospital have been observed.[125] Whether a diagnosis of breast cancer is associated with an increased burden of disease or modifies the quality of care for prevalent conditions when compared to similar women is unknown. It is likely that both are true. Thus, careful attention to preventive interventions such as influenza vaccination, assessment of bone health, and colorectal cancer screening, as well as management of existing conditions and the early identification and management of new ones is critical. In the setting of multiple physician providers, as occurs commonly in cancer care for older adults, this requires meticulous communication among them so that responsibilities for management are clear.

Summary

Cancer care for older adults is challenging—from diagnosis and initial care through long-term survivorship. The evidence on which to base sound clinical decisions is modest, but growing. As the epidemic of cancer in old age gains momentum, it behooves providers and researchers to focus attention on this important group of patients.

References

1. Ries L, Eisner M, Kosary C, et al. Surveillance, Epidemiology and End Results (SEER) Cancer Statistics Review 1975–2000. Vol. 2003; National Cancer Institute, 2003.

2. Ries L, Kosary C, Hankey B. SEER Cancer Statistics Review, 1973–1996. Bethesda, MD: National Cancer Institute, 1999.

3. Miller B, Ries L, Hankey B, Kosary C, Edwards B. Cancer Statistics Review 1973–1989: National Cancer Institute, 1992.

4. Kennedy B, Bushhouse S, Benber A. Minnesota population cancer risks. Cancer 1994;73:724–729.

5. Mettlin C. New evidence of progress in the National Cancer Program. Cancer 1996;78:2043–2044.

6. Levi F, Vecchia CL, Lucchini F, et al. Worldwide trends in cancer mortality in the elderly, 1955–1992. Eur J Cancer 1996;32A:652–672.

7. Vecchia CL, Levi F, Lucchini F, et al. International perspectives of cancer and aging. In: Balducci L, Lyman G, Ershler W (eds). Comprehensive Geriatric Oncology. Amsterdam, The Netherlands: Harwood Academic Publishers, 1998:19–93.

8. Sargent D, Goldberg R, Jacobson S, et al. A pooled analysis of adjuvant chemotherapy for resected colon cancer in elderly patients. N Engl J Med 2001;345:1091–1097.

9. Schild S, Stella P, Geyer S, et al. The outcome of combined-modality therapy for stage III non-small cell lung cancer in the elderly. J Clin Oncol 2003;21:3201–3206.

10. Silliman RA. What constitutes optimal care for older women with breast cancer? J Clin Oncol 2003;21:3554–3556.

11. Bouchardy C, Rapiti E, Fioretta G, et al. Undertreatment strongly decreases prognosis of breast cancer in elderly women. J Clin Oncol 2003;21:3580–3587.

12. Yee K, Pater J, Pho L, et al. Enrollment of older patients in cancer treatment trials in Canada: why is age a barrier? J Clin Oncol 2003;21:1618–1623.

13. Hutchins L, Unger J, Crowley J, Coltman C, Albain K. Underrepresentation of patients 65 years of age or older in cancer-treatment trials. N Eng J Med 1999;341:2061–2067.

14. Monfardini S, Sorio R, Boes G, et al. Entry and evaluation of elderly patients in European Organization for Research and Treatment of Cancer (EORTC) new drug development studies. Cancer 1995;76:333–338.

15. Lewis JH, Kilgore ML, Goldman DP, et al. Participation of patients 65 years of age or older in cancer clinical trials. J Clin Oncol 2003;21:1383–1389.

16. Current population reports, special studies: 65+ in the United States. Washington, DC: US Bureau of the Census, 1996:2–8.

17. United States life tables, 2000. Natl Vital Stat Rep 2002;51:1–38.

18. Record high life expectancy. Stat Bull Metrop Insur Co 1993;74:28–35.

19. Moroff S, Pauker S. What to do when the patient outlives the literature, or DEALE-ing with a full deck. Medical Decision Making 1983;3:313–338.

20. Fried L, Wallace R. The complexity of chronic illness in the elderly: From clinic to community. In: Wallace R, Woolson R (eds). The Epidemiologic Study of the Elderly. New York: Oxford University Press, Inc, 1992:10–19.

21. Yancik R, Wesley M, Ries L. Comorbidity and age as predictors of risk for early mortality in male and female colon cancer patients: a population-based study. Cancer 1998;82:2123–2134.

22. Satariano W, Ragland D. The effect of comorbidity on 3-year survival of women with primary breast cancer. Ann Intern Med 1994;120:104–110.

23. Satariano W. Comorbidities and cancer. In: Hunter C, Johnson K, Muss H (eds). Cancer in the Elderly. New York: Dekker, 2000:477–499.

24. Mandeblatt J, Bierman A, Gold K, Silliman R. Constructs of burden of illness in older patients with breast cancer: a comparison of measurement methods. Health Serv Res 2001;36:1085–1107.

25. Charlson M, Pompei P, Ales K, MacKenzie C. A new method of classifying prognostic comorbidity in longitudinal studies: development and validation. J Chronic Dis 1987;40:373–383.

26. Wang P, Walker A, Tsuang M, Orav E, Levin R, Avron J. Strategies for improving comorbidity measures based on Medicare and Medicaid claims data. J Clin Epidemiol 2000;53:571–578.

27. Monfardini S, Ferrucci L, Fratino L, Lungo ID, Serraino D, Zagonel V. Validation of a multidimensional evaluation scale for use in elderly cancer patients. Cancer 1996;77:395–401.

28. Reuben D. Principles of geriatric assessment. In: Hazzard W, Blass J, Ouslander J, Tinetti M (eds). Principles of Geriatric Medicine and Gerontology. New York: McGraw-Hill, 2003:99–110.

29. Balducci L, Yates J. General guidelines for the management of older patients with cancer. Oncology (Huntingt) 2000;14:221–227.

30. Moore AA, Siu AL. Screening for common problems in ambulatory elderly: clinical confirmation of a screening instrument [see comment]. Am J Med 1996;100:438–443.

31. Chen H, Cantor A, Meyer J, et al. Can older cancer patients tolerate chemotherapy? A prospective pilot study. Cancer 2003;97:1107–1114.

32. Greenblatt D, Sellers E, Shader R. Drug therapy: drug disposition in old age. New Engl J Med 1982;306:1018–1028.

33. Shaw P. Common pitfalls in geriatric drug prescribing. Drugs 1982;23:324–328.

34. Beers M, Ouslander J. Risk factors in geriatric drug prescribing: a practical guide to avoid problems. Drugs 1989;37:105–112.

35. Yancik R, Havlik R, Wesley M. Cancer and comorbidity in older patients: A descriptive profile. Ann Epidemiol 1996;5:399–412.

36. Newschaffer C, Penberthy M, Lynne M, Desch C, Retchin S, Whittemore M. The effect of age and comorbidity in the treatment of elderly women with non-metastatic breast cancer. Arch Intern Med 1996;156:85–90.

37. Fleming S, Pursley H, Newman B, Pavlov D, Chen K. Comorbidity as a predictor of stage of illness for patients with breast cancer. Med Care 2005;43:132–140.

38. West D, Satariano W, Ragland D. Comorbidity and breast cancer survival: a comparison between black and white women. Ann Intern Med 1996;413–419.

39. Fleming S, Rastogi A, Dmitrienko A, Johnson K. A comprehensive index to predict survival based on multiple comorbidities: a focus on breast cancer. Med Care 1999;37:601–614.

40. Yancik R, Wesley M, Ries M, et al. Effect of age and comorbidity in postmenopausal breast cancer patients aged 55 years and older. JAMA 2001;285:885–892.

41. Havlick R, Yancik R, Long S, et al. The National Institute on Aging and the National Cancer Institute SEER collaborative study on comorbidity and early diagnosis of cancer in the elderly. Cancer 1994;74(suppl):2101–2106.

42. Silliman R, Lash T. Comparison of interview-based and medical record-based indices of comorbidity among breast cancer patients. Med Care 1999;37:339–349.

43. Deyo R, Cherkin D, Clol M. Adapting a clinical comorbidity index for use with ICD-9 CM-administrative databases. J Clin Epidemiol 1992;45:613–619.

44. Romano P, Roos L, Jollis J. Adapting a clinical comorbidity index for use with ICD-9-CM administrative data: differing perspectives. J Clin Epidemiol 1993;46:1075–1079.

45. Romano P, Roos L, Jollis J. Further evidence concerning the use of clinical comorbidity index with ICD-9-CM administrative data. J Clin Epidemiol 1993;46:1085–1090.

46. Small GW. Recognizing and treating anxiety in the elderly. J Clin Psychiatry. 1997;58:41–47; discussions 48–50.

47. Osborn DP, Fletcher AE, Smeeth L, et al. Factors associated with depression in a representative sample of 14 217 people aged 75 and over in the United Kingdom: results from the MRC trial of assessment and management of older people in the community. Int J Geriatr Psychiatry. 2003;18:623–630.

48. Feinstein A. The pre-therapeutic classification of comorbidity in chronic diseases. J Chron Dis 1970;23:455–469.

49. Lash T, Thwin S, Horton N, Guadagnoli E, Silliman R. Multiple informants: a new method to assess comorbidity in breast cancer patients. Am J Epidemiol 2003;157:249–257.

50. Kaplan M, Feinstein A. The importance of classifying initial comorbidity in evaluating the outcome of diabetes mellitus. J Chronic Dis 1974;27:387–404.

51. Greenfield S, Blanco D, Elashoff R, Ganz P. Patterns of care related to age of breast cancer patients. JAMA 1987;257:2766–2770.

52. Bennett C, Greenfield S, Aronow H, Ganz P, Vogelzang N, Elashoff R. Patterns of care related to age of men with prostate cancer. Cancer 1991;67:2633–2441.

53. Lyman G. Decision analysis: a way of thinking about health care in the elderly. In: Balducci L, Lyman G, Ershler W (eds). Geriatric Oncology. Philadelphia: JB Lippincott, 1992:5–14.

54. Carney P, Miglioretti D, Yankaskas B, et al. Individual and combined effects of age, breast density, and hormone replacement therapy use on the accuracy of screening mammography. Ann Intern Med 2003;138:168–175.

55. Diab S, Elledge R, Clark G. Tumor characteristics and clinical outcome of elderly women with breast cancer. J Natl Cancer Inst 2000;92:550–556.

56. Walter L, Covinsky K. Cancer screening in elderly patients. A framework for individualized decision making. JAMA 2001;285:2750–2756.

57. Law M. Screening without evidence of efficacy [see comment]. BMJ 2004;328:301–302.

58. Rosenthal RA, Zenilman ME, Katlic MR (eds). Principles and Practice of Geriatric Surgery. New York: Springer-Verlag, 2001.

59. Pofahl WE, Pories WJ. Current status and future directions of geriatric general surgery. J Am Geriatr Soc 2003;51:S351–S354.

60. Devereaux E, Kemeny M. Surgery in the elderly oncology patient. In: Hunter C, Johnson K, Muss H (eds). Cancer in the Elderly. New York: Dekker, 2000:153–186.

61. Evans B, Townsend C, Thompson J. Organ physiology of aging. Surg Clin North Am 1994;74:23–29.

62. Wynne H, Cope L, Mutch E, et al. The effect of aging upon liver volume and apparent liver blood flow in healthy man. Hepatology 1989;1989:297–301.

63. Mooney H, Roberts R, Cooksley W, et al. Alterations in the liver with ageing. Clin Gastroenterol 1985;14:757–771.

64. Rocca R. Psychosocial aspects of surgical care in the elderly patient. Surg Clin North Am 1994;74:223–243.

65. Fleisher L, Eagle K. Lowering cardiac risk in non-cardiac surgery. N Engl J Med 2001;345:1677–1682.

66. Marcello P, Roberts P. "Routine" preoperative studies: which studies in which patients? Surg Clin North Am 1996;76:11–23.

67. Velanovich V. Preoperative laboratory evaluation. J Am Coll Surg 1996;183:79–87.

68. Kaplan E, Sheiner L, Boeckmann A, et al. The usefulness of preoperative laboratory screening. JAMA 1985;253:3576–3581.

69. Roizen M, Kaplan E, Schreider B, et al. The relative roles of the history and physical examination, and laboratory testing in preoperative evaluation for outpatient surgery: the "Starling" curve of preoperative laboratory testing. Anesthesiol Clin North Am 1987;5:15.

70. Goldman L, Caldera D, Nussbaum S. Multifactorial index of cardiac risk in noncardiac surgical procedures. N Engl J Med 1977;297:845–850.

71. Goldman L. Cardiac risks and complications of noncardiac surgery. Ann Intern Med 1983;98:504–513.

72. Owens W, Felts J, Jr. ES. ASA physical status classifications: a study of consistency of ratings. Anesthesiology 1978;49:239–243.

73. Evans T. Hemodynamic and metabolic therapy in critically ill patients. N Engl J Med 2001;345:1417–1418.

74. Cooper A, Doig G, Sibbald W. Pulmonary artery catheters in the critically ill: an overview using the methodology of evidence-based medicine. Crit Care Clin 1996;12:777–794.

75. Sandman J, Hull R, Brant R, et al. A randomized, controlled trial of the use of pulmonary-artery catheters in high-risk surgical patients. N Engl J Med 2003;348:5–14.

76. Tobias J. Clinical practice of radiotherapy. Lancet 1992;339:159–163.

77. Sargent E, Burns F. Repair of radiation-induced DNA damage in rat epidermis as function of age. Rad Res 1985;102:176–181.

78. Scalliet P, Pignon T. Radiotherapy in the elderly. In: Balducci L, Lyman G, Ershler W (eds). Comprehensive Geriatric Oncology. Amsterdam, The Netherlands: Harwood Academic Publishers, 2000;421–427.

79. Mundt A. Radiation therapy and the elderly. In: Hunter C, Johnson K, Muss H (eds). Cancer in the Elderly. New York: Dekker, 2000:187–216.

80. Isenring E, Bauer J, Capra S. The scored Patient-generated Subjective Global Assessment (PG-SGA) and its association with quality of life in ambulatory patients receiving radiotherapy. Eur J Clin Nutr 2003;57:305–309.

81. Nag S, Ellis RJ, Merrick GS, et al. American Brachytherapy Society recommendations for reporting morbidity after prostate brachytherapy. Int J Radiat Oncol Biol Phys 2002;54:462–470.

82. Janda M, Johnson D, Woelfl H, et al. Measurement of quality of life in head and neck cancer patients utilizing the quality of life radiation therapy questionnaire. Strahlenther Onkol 2002;178:153–158.

83. Berg C, Carbone P. Clinical trials and drug toxicity in the elderly: the experience of the Eastern Cooperative Oncology Group. Cancer 1983;52:1986–1992.

84. Christman K, Muss H, Case L, et al. Chemotherapy of metastatic breast cancer in the elderly: the Piedmont Oncology Association experience. JAMA 1992;268:57–62.

85. Lichtman S, Skirvin J, Vemulapalli S. Pharmacology of antineoplastic agents in older cancer patients. Clin Rev Oncol Hematol 2003;46:101–114.

86. Yuen G. Altered pharmacokinetics in the elderly. Clin Geriatr Med 1990;6:257–267.

87. Wallace S, Whiting B. Factors affecting drug binding in plasma of elderly patients. Br J Clin Pharmacol 1976;3:327–330.

88. Woodhouse K, Wynne H. Age-related changes in liver size and hepatic blood flow: the influence on drug metabolism in the elderly. Clin Pharmacokinet 1998;15:287–294.

89. Soteniemi E, Arranto A, Pelkonen O, et al. Age and cytochrome P450-linked drug metabolism in humans: an analysis of 226 subjects with equal histopathologic conditions. Clin Pharmacol Ther 1997;61:331–339.

90. Vestal R. Aging and pharmacology. Cancer 1997;80:1302–1310.

91. Lindeman R, Tobin J, Shock N, et al. Longitudinal studies on the rate of decline in renal function with age. J Am Geriatr Soc 1985;33:278–285.

92. Cockroft D, Gault M. Prediction of creatinine clearance from serum creatinine. Nephron 1976;16:31–42.

93. Lipschitz D. Age-related declines in hematopoietic reserve capacity. Semin Oncol 1995;22(suppl):3–5.

94. Ibrahim N, Frye D, Buzdar A, et al. Docorubicin-based chemotherapy in elderly patients with metastatic breast cancer: tolerance and outcome. Arch Intern Med 1996;156:882–888.

95. Fisher R, Graynor E, Dahlberg S, et al. Comparison of a standard regimen (CHOP) with three intensive chemotherapy regimens

for advanced non-Hodgkin's lymphoma. N Engl J Med 1993;328:1002–1006.

96. Lyman G, Kuderer D, Djulbegovic B. Prophylactic granulocyte colony-stimulating factors in patients receiving dose-intensive cancer chemotherapy: a meta-analysis. Am J Med 2002;112: 406–411.

97. Balducci L, Lyman G. Patients aged ≥70 are at high risk for neutropenic infection and should receive hemopoietic growth factors when treated with moderately toxic chemotherapy. J Clin Oncol 2001;19:1583–1585.

98. Ozer H, Armitage J, Bennett C, et al. 2000 Update of recommendations for the use of Hematopoietic Colony-Stimulating Factors: evidence-based, clinical practice guidelines. J Clin Oncol 2000;18:3558–3585.

99. Chavez P, Volpato S, Fried L. Challenging the World Health Organization criteria for anemia in older women. J Am Geriatr Soc 2001;49 (suppl 3):10.

100. Izaks G, Westendorp R, Knoot D. The definition of anemia in older persons. JAMA 1999;281:1714–1717.

101. Kikuchi M, Inagaki T, Shinagawa N. Five-year survival of older people with anemia: variation with hemoglobin concentration. J Am Geriatr Soc 2001;49:1226–1228.

102. Gutstein H. The biologic basis of fatigue. Cancer 2001;92 (suppl):1678–1683.

103. Nissenson A. Epoetin and cognitive function. Am J Kidney Dis 1992;20 (suppl):21–24.

104. Shrijvers D, Highley M, Bruyn ED, et al. Role of red blood cells in pharmacokinetics of chemotherapeutic agents. Anticancer Drugs 1999;10:147–153.

105. Rizzo J, Lichtin A, Woolf S, et al. Use of Epoetin in patients with cancer: evidence-based clinical practice guidelines of the American Society of Clinical Oncology and the American Society of Hematology. J Clin Oncol 2002;19:4083–4107.

106. Hellstrom-Lindberg E, Ahlgren T, Begguin Y, et al. Treatment of the anemia of myelodysplastic syndromes with G-CSF plus erythropoietin: Results of a randomized phase II study and long term follow-up of 71 patients. Blood 1998;92:68–75.

107. Popescu R, Norman A, Ross P, et al. Adjuvant or palliative chemotherapy for colorectal cancer in patients 70 years or older. J Clin Oncol 1999;17:2412–2418.

108. Sargent D, Goldberg R, MacDonald J, et al. Adjuvant chemotherapy for colon cancer (CC) is beneficial without significant incrased toxicity in elderly patients (Pts): results from 3351 Pt meta-analysis [Abstract 933]. Proc Am Soc Clin Oncol 2000;19: 241a.

109. Cancer control and population sciences: research findings. http://dccps.nci.nih.gov/ocs/prevalence. Accessed August 1, 2005.

110. Edwards BK, Howe HL, Ries LA, Thun MJ, Rosenberg HM, Yancik R, et al. Annual report to the nation on the status of cancer, 1973–1999, featuring implication of age and aging on US cancer burden. Cancer 2002;94:2766–2792.

111. National Center for Health Statistics. Life Tables of the United States, 1997.

112. Hewitt M, Rowland JH, Yancik R. Cancer survivors in the United States: age, health, and disability. J Gerontol 2003;58: 82–91.

113. Stafford RS, Cyr PL. The impact of cancer on the physical function of the elderly and their utilization of health care. Cancer 1997;80:1973–1980.

114. Smith TJ, David NE, Schapira DV, et al: American Society of Clinical Oncology 1998 update of recommended breast cancer surveillance guidelines. J Clin Oncol 1999;47:1080–1082.

115. The Steering Committee on Clinical Practice Guidelines for the Care and Treatment of Breast Cancer: follow-up after treatment for breast cancer. Can Med Assoc J 1998;158(S3):S65–S70.

116. Report from the National Breast Cancer Consensus Conference. Management of newly diagnosed early breast cancer: A national approach to breast cancer control. Med J Aust 1994;161(S7): S10–S16.

117. The GIVIO Investigators. Impact of follow-up testing on survival and health-related quality of life in breast cancer patients: a multicenter randomized controlled trial. JAMA 1994;271:1587–1592.

118. Roselli Del Turco M, Palli D, Criddi A, Ciatto S, Pacini P, Distante V. Intensive diagnostic follow-up after treatment of primary breast cancer: A randomized trial. JAMA 1994;271: 1593–1597.

119. Shapira DV, Urban N. A minimalist policy for breast cancer surveillance. JAMA 1991;265:380–382.

120. Schapira MM, McAulliffe TL, Nattinger AB. Underutilization of mammography in older breast cancer survivors. Med Care 2000;38:281–289.

121. Lash TL, Silliman RA. Medical surveillance after breast cancer diagnosis. Med Care 2001;39:945–955.

122. Grunfeld E, Noorani H, McGahan L, Paszat L, Coyle D, van Walraven C, et al. Surveillance mammography after treatment of primary breast cancer. A systematic review. Breast 2002;11: 228–235.

123. Westrup JL, Lash TL, Thwin SS, Silliman RA. Risk of decline in upper-body function and symptoms among older breast cancer patients. J Gen Intern Med; under review.

124. Newschaffer CJ, Bush TL, Penberthy LE, Bellantoni M, Helzlsour K, Diener-West M. Does comorbid disease interact with cancer? An epidemiologic analysis of mortality in a cohort of elderly breast cancer patients. J Gerontol 1998;53A:M372–M378.

125. Earle CC, Burstein HJ, Winer EP, Weeks JC. Quality of non-breast cancer health maintenance among elderly breast cancer survivors. J Clin Oncol 2003;21:1447–1451.

17

Second Malignancies After Radiation Treatment and Chemotherapy for Primary Cancers

Lydia B. Zablotska, Matthew J. Matasar, and Alfred I. Neugut

Cancer survivors have been shown to have an increased risk for second malignant neoplasms (SMN). These increased risks result from genetic predisposition, harmful environmental exposures, or cancer treatment therapies. Regardless of their cause, SMNs now comprise the sixth most common group of malignancies after skin, prostate, breast, lung, and colorectal cancers.[1] It is important to emphasize that the fear of SMN related to the treatment of the first cancer diagnosis should not outweigh the positive effects of curative therapy for the first cancer. Both physicians and patients should, however, be aware of the consequences of the cancer treatment regimens, specifically radiation therapy (RT) and chemotherapy, and consider them while devising follow-up plans.

Radiation Therapy

The following are general criteria for attributing a malignancy to the effects of radiation, defined by Goolden in 1951: (a) a history of prior irradiation; (b) malignancy occurring within the prior irradiation field; (c) gross or microscopic pathologic evidence of radiation damage to the surrounding tissues; and (d) a long, latent interval between the prior irradiation and the development of the malignancy.[2–5] Only the first two criteria are considered essential.

External-beam radiation therapy has the potential for the induction of mutations in normal cells because of the harmful effects of the radiation used to kill cancer cells. Years or decades later, such mutated cells may give rise to new primary cancers.

Although ionizing radiation has been shown to cause most types of cancer, some organs and tissues appear to be more susceptible than others. Based on radiation epidemiologic studies, the most radiation-sensitive solid tissues and organs are the bone marrow, thyroid, and female breast. Bone and soft tissue sarcomas also can occur following radiation therapy.[6] In addition, cancers of the lung, stomach, colon, bladder, and esophagus have been conclusively associated with ionizing radiation exposure. Possible links have been described for cancers of the kidney, ovary, brain, and central nervous system (CNS). Cancers of other sites have not been correlated with radiation exposure.[7]

In addition to individual susceptibility, the risk of second cancers after radiation therapy depends on the total dose of radiation delivered during the course of treatment, as well as on the type and energy of the radiation. Megavoltage treatments currently in use deliver concentrated high energy to tumors, with low scatter of the radiation to areas outside of the treatment field (low peripheral doses). Orthovoltage treatments, which were used in previous decades, on the other hand, frequently injured the skin and delivered higher doses of radiation to the bone than to the surrounding tissues, and in the process produced substantial peripheral doses.

The type of dose delivery (protracted or instantaneous) also plays a role in the carcinogenesis of second malignancies. It is generally recognized that, as the exposure time for a given total dose is extended, the biologic effect is reduced. Protracted delivery of a dose over hours or days, in general, will result in less severe consequences because of reduced tumorigenic effectiveness as compared to the instantaneous delivery of the total dose.

Finally, the risks of second cancers depend on the volume of irradiated tissues and organs. Current treatment guidelines recommend that smaller fractions should be used when larger volumes need to be irradiated to decrease the acute side effects of radiation treatment. The late effects of radiotherapy could be lessened by "hyperfractionation" of radiation therapy (smaller doses twice per day over the same treatment period).[6]

Recent technologic advances (shielding, collimation of the radiation beam, use of multivoltage beams, more precise localization of tumors) have significantly reduced the irradiation of normal tissues and the risk of posttherapy new cancers. However, because radiation-associated cancers tend to appear at the same age as spontaneous cancers, patients who were exposed many years ago at young ages may, potentially, be at risk of developing SMN cancers due to radiation exposure.

Individual risks for patients are modified by such factors as their age at the time of exposure, time since exposure/survival time, gender, exposure to other carcinogens (including chemotherapy), as well as by immune and hormonal status. Although the risks associated with radiation exposure are substantially less than the risks posed by the initial tumor, it is important to know them before the start of the radiation therapy to make informed decisions about treatment regimens that might minimize the side effects of radiation therapy. This information is also important for counseling patients who are at increased risk of developing second malignancies due to other risk factors, as well as for continuing surveillance of those treated. Our knowledge of the possible adverse effects associated with radiation therapy should be used for the development of surveillance programs aimed at the early detection of cancers and campaigns to decrease negative behaviors and exposures that have been shown to promote the development of second cancers after radiation therapy.

Individual Cancers

In our review, we look at the subjects who received irradiation for treatment of nine specific primary malignant diseases and summarize the evidence from the descriptive (case reports and case series) and analytical (case-control, cohort, and randomized controlled trials) epidemiologic studies to show the current state of knowledge on the consequences of the treatment for each of the nine diseases.

After reviewing epidemiologic studies for the nine primary cancers, we compare and contrast their findings. We show that they add to our knowledge of the effects of high-dose exposures and can be used for risk estimation purposes as well as to provide both physicians and patients with the necessary information to make informed decisions regarding radiation therapy for primary cancer.

Pediatric Cancers

Various epidemiologic studies have shown that the incidence of the majority of cancers increases with age. Based on data from the Japanese survivors of the atomic bombings of Hiroshima and Nagasaki, the effect of radiation exposure is to multiply age-specific solid cancer rates by a constant radiation dose-dependent factor through lifetime. Thus, those with absorbed dose of 0.20 Sv experience a 10% increase in the risk of solid cancer above background rates. Estimates of risk also depend on age at exposure (increase by 10 years decreases relative risk for solid cancers by 130%).[8] Based on the same data, most organizations have adopted a multiplicative risk model for most solid cancers, which states that after a specified latency period, "the excess cancer risk is given by a constant factor applied to the age-dependent incidence of natural cancers in the population"[9] (p. 108) (in other words, the relative risk remains constant as subjects are followed over time).

The majority of cancers that are associated with radiation exposure, thus, will appear at the same time when spontaneous cancers of the same organ appear. The difference between exposed and unexposed populations, then, will be in the number of new incident cases. Researchers, therefore, have combined subjects with specific types of first childhood cancers and studied them as a group named "pediatric cancers."

The significance of the problem of second malignancies after pediatric cancers is underscored by the fact that survival following childhood cancer has improved markedly and now approaches 70%.[1] Thus, it is important to compare the carcinogenic potential of different treatments for primary pediatric cancers. Some pediatric cancers are more likely to be treated with radiation than others and, as a consequence, they are associated with second malignancies within the radiation field. First reports about second cancers following primary pediatric cancers started appearing in the late 1970s with the advent of new radiation treatment regimens. A large study of pediatric patients who were followed for at least 2 years after initial treatment of the primary tumor showed no association between RT and the subsequent development of leukemia.[10] Although large, this study had a very small proportion of subjects who received only RT; the majority of subjects also received chemotherapy. Thus, the effects of RT could have been obscured by the effects of treatment by various alkylating agents. In a more-recent study of childhood cancer survivors, the risk of second leukemia after RT was significantly increased eightfold.[11] The difference between the two studies could be explained by the size of the irradiation field. Patients with HD usually receive more targeted radiation treatment, whereas the cumulative doses for radiotherapy for NHL are usually smaller than the doses delivered for treatment of HD. Nevertheless, in the process of treatment, larger areas of radiosensitive tissues, such as bone marrow, are exposed to radiation.

Other second cancers that have been associated with RT for primary childhood cancers include cancers of the bone,[12] skin,[13] nervous system,[14] and thyroid gland.[15] As one would expect with solid cancer, in these studies the incidence increased with time since treatment. For example, in The Late Effects Study Group, which followed 9,000 survivors of childhood cancer, a lifetime risk of thyroid gland cancer after RT for primary childhood cancer was almost 4% after 26 years of follow-up.[15] To avoid problems associated with low power of individual studies, Ron et al. pooled data from seven individual studies to evaluate the risk of thyroid cancer following exposure to external radiation. Individual estimates of increased risk of thyroid cancer varied from 1.4 to 33.5 per Gy[16]; that is, those who were exposed to 1 Gy of radiation during RT for primary cancer had a much higher risk of developing second primary thyroid cancer compared to those who did not receive RT. This study provided strong evidence that, along with the breast and bone marrow, the thyroid gland is one of the most radiosensitive organs.

Population-based study of the occurrence of second cancers following primary childhood cancer in the five Nordic countries showed that childhood cancer survivors have a fourfold-higher risk of second cancers compared to the general population.[17] The largest increase was observed during the first 10 years following RT; however, risks remained increased throughout their lifetimes and the absolute excess of second cancers increased with time. This result probably reflects the promotional effect of radiation on the carcinogenic effects of environmental exposures.

Several publications from the large Childhood Cancer Survivor Study cohort show an increased risk of second malignant neoplasms more than 20 years after RT for primary childhood cancer. In comparison with the general population, their risk of bone second cancers, in particular bone sarcomas and breast cancer, was increased sixfold.[18]

In summary, the effects of radiation treatment for childhood cancers start to increase in early adolescence and early adulthood and continue to be increased later in life. Bone marrow, bone and soft tissues, and breast and thyroid gland appear to be the most radiosensitive. Risk of second tumors depends on the age at exposure (the risk is greatest among those exposed at the youngest ages) and on the time since exposure. Current knowledge of the effects of ionizing radiation had an important influence on RT practices. Specifically, lead aprons and shields are currently being used to protect the most radiation-sensitive organs and tissues. In addition, advances in technology, such as utilization of wedge compensators or half-beam blocks, minimize scattering of radiation to adjacent tissues. Finally, because of the greater awareness of the effects of radiation, survivors of childhood cancers are being constantly monitored and screened for second cancers during follow-up.

Bone Marrow Transplantation

High-dose total-body irradiation (TBI) is part of the conditioning regimen for bone marrow transplantation used for treatment of leukemia and other diseases (see also Chapter 15). One of the mechanisms of development of second cancers following TBI is thought to be due to radiation-induced immunosuppression.[19] In addition to radiation-associated effects, it is also necessary to consider the effects of immunosuppressive drugs that are used concomitantly with radiation. Curtis et al. showed that patients who received TBI had an increased risk of subsequent new solid cancers compared to those who did not receive radiation treatment.[20] High doses of TBI were associated with increased risks of melanoma and cancers of the brain and thyroid. The risk was higher for recipients who were younger at the time of transplantation than for those who were older (P for trend less than 0.001).

Another registry-based study found that high-dose TBI increased the risk of subsequent solid tumors threefold [95% confidence interval (CI), 1.1, 10.3].[21] Younger age at the time of treatment increased the risk of brain and thyroid tumors. In addition, cancers of the salivary gland, bone, and connective tissues were also increased.

In summary, various studies show the trend toward an increased risk over time after transplantation and the greater risk among younger patients. Second cancers could be related to both transplant therapy and to chemotherapy treatments given before it. All these factors indicate the need for lifelong surveillance of the patients who received irradiation as part of the bone marrow transplantation.

Hodgkin's Disease

Introduction of intensive radiotherapy and chemotherapy to treat Hodgkin's disease (HD) three decades ago dramatically changed survival times and prognosis for patients with this disorder (see also Chapter 8). Long-term sequelae of treatment have become increasingly important as patients now survive for several decades. HD is a systemic cancer and radiation treatment frequently consists of irradiation of mantle fields, including all lymph node regions ('total lymphoid irradiation' with cumulative doses 20–40 Gy) or only some regions ('subtotal lymphoid irradiation' with doses less than 20 Gy), by external-radiation beams.[22] Dose–response analysis of the effects of radiation is frequently confounded by the concurrent chemotherapy in the majority of patients.

Several studies looked at breast cancer incidence and mortality, the most frequently seen second malignancy following treatment for HD. Table 17.1 summarizes the results of the most influential studies. In general, risk of breast cancer was increased and ranged from 2 to 75 times compared to the risk in the general population. Most cancers appeared within or at the margin of the radiation field, and the risk increased with dose. Investigators from the Late Effects Study Group estimated that the cumulative probability of breast cancer at age 40 following radiation exposure for HD in childhood is close to 35% (following a median dose of radiotherapy of 40 Gy).[23]

Clemons et al.[22] reviewed 18 epidemiologic studies on the risk of breast cancer in patients treated with radiation for HD. They concluded that women between the ages of puberty and 30 years are at the highest risk. Data on the use of exogenous estrogen hormones, age at first pregnancy, and prevalence of early menopause were not available to control for possible

TABLE 17.1. Studies of breast cancer risk among patients treated for primary Hodgkin's disease.

Reference	Year	RT and follow-up	Age at the time of first treatment	SIR and 95% CI
Hancock et al.[114]	1993	1961–1989	Mean age 25 years	SIR = 4.1 (2.5, 5.7)
Bhatia et al.[23]	1996	1955–1986, follow-up till 1996	Younger than 16 years old	SIR = 75.3 (44.9, 118.4)
Tinger et al.[115]	1997	1966–1974 treatment era	Mean age 30 years	4.7
Tinger et al.[115]	1997	1974–1985 treatment era	Mean age 28 years	2.2
Hudson et al.[116]	1998	1968–1990	—	SIR = 1.33 (1.12, 1.72)
Wolden et al.[117]	1998	1960–1995	Younger than 21 years	SIR = 1.26 (1.15, 1.42)
Swerdlow et al.[27]	2000	1963–1993	60% younger than 35 years old	SIR = 2.5 (1.4, 4.0)
Van Leeuwen et al.[70]	2000	1966–1986	Younger than 40 years old	SIR = 7.7 (4.3, 12.7)

RT, radiotherapy; SIR, standardized incidence ratio; CI, confidence interval.

confounding effects of these variables. Breast cancers due to irradiation tend to appear after a 15-year latency period at the age from 30 to 40. Breast cancer risk is highly dependent on age at irradiation, time since irradiation, dose, and concurrent chemotherapy. These findings, along with the finding that no cases of breast cancer after radiation therapy for HD have been reported in men, suggest that the actively growing and differentiating cells of female breast tissue are particularly vulnerable to radiation exposure.

A nested case-control study of lung cancer among patients previously treated for HD found that radiation doses greater than 5 Gy increased the risk sixfold (95% CI, 2.7, 13.5).[24] Smoking acted in a multiplicative way with radiation exposure [relative risk (RR) comparing moderate-heavy smokers to nonsmokers and light smokers among those without radiation treatment was 6.0; RR comparing those with radiation treatment to those without among nonsmokers and light smokers was 7.2; RR comparing those with radiation treatment to those without among all subjects adjusting for smoking was 20.2]. Treatment with alkylating agents, on the other hand, acted additively with radiation therapy (individual risks added up to perfect additivity). Similar to other studies, increased age at diagnosis of HD was associated with an increased risk of lung cancer.

Birdwell et al.[25] noticed that high doses to the abdomen from radiation for HD cause multiple gastrointestinal (GI) cancers, including stomach, pancreas, and small intestine (RR for all GI cancers, 2.0, 95% CI, 1.0, 3.4). Risks started to increase after a latency period of 10 years and were highest among younger patients. GI cancers were similarly increased in the large study based on the International Database on HD (more than 12,000 cases)[25] and in the study of atomic bomb survivors (53% of all incident cancers in the atomic bomb study were due to cancers of the digestive system).[26]

Findings of increased risk of second cancers are further supported by the largest current study of 5,519 British patients with HD who were followed for more than 30 years.[27] Irradiated patients had a 1.7 fold (95% CI, 1.0, 2.5) higher incidence of GI cancers, 2.5 fold (95% CI, 1.4, 4.0) higher incidence of breast cancer, and 2.9 fold (95% CI, 1.9, 4.1) higher incidence of lung cancer than the general population. Risk of leukemia was increased in patients who received combined modality treatment (chemotherapy with radiotherapy) or chemotherapy alone compared to those who received RT alone. Similar to previous studies, relative risks tended to increase 5 to 10 years after treatment and decreased with increasing age at first treatment. Women older than 25 years were not at risk of increased breast cancer [RR$_{<25 \text{ years}}$, 14.4 (95% CI, 5.7, 29.3) and RR$_{25-44 \text{ years}}$, 1.6 (95% CI, 0.5, 3.7)]. A combined study of 16 population-based cancer registries in Europe and North America, which included HD patients diagnosed before the age of 21 years, also found that the risk of second malignancy decreased with increasing age at HD diagnosis and treatment on a relative scale.[28] High estimates of relative risks of second cancers in this cohort were due to low background rates in the relatively young cohort.

In summary, it appears that radiation treatment for HD increases the risk of second malignancies. Long-term risks depend on age at exposure and time since exposure. Latency periods differ from study to study, but a major increase in risks appears at 10 to 14 years of follow-up. Second cancers sometimes appear at a much younger age than similar

cancers. Radiation treatment for HD is linked to cancers of the GI tract, breast, lung, bone, and soft tissue, melanoma, and thyroid gland (Table 17.2).

Breast Cancer

Standard treatment for invasive breast cancer includes high, concentrated doses of radiation to the chest and to the lymph nodes (about 40–60 Gy total).[29] Initially, localized radiotherapy was combined with radical mastectomy, but since the mid-1980s treatment consists of breast-conserving surgery and radiotherapy. Women irradiated before the mid-1980s received higher doses of radiation to the lungs, contralateral breast, thoracic bone, and bone marrow. A small increase in risk of leukemia was shown in a cohort of women from the Connecticut Tumor Registry irradiated between 1935 and 1972.[29] Following an average dose of 5.3 Gy to the bone marrow, the risk was 16% higher in irradiated women than in nonirradiated women (90% CI, 0.6, 2.1). A larger study based on five population-based cancer registries in the United States (1973–1985)[30] found a 2.4 times increased risk (95% CI, 1.0, 5.8) of acute nonlymphocytic leukemia after radiation treatment with an average dose of 7.5 Gy over the total active bone marrow. They observed a positive dose–response relation in the data (those exposed to doses higher than 9 Gy had a 7-fold-higher risk). Increase in risk was first seen 2 years after initial treatment, and it persisted, albeit at a much lower level, 7 years after treatment. The authors described a statistical multiplicative interaction effect of radiotherapy and treatment with alkylating agents on the development of ANLL (RR for radiotherapy alone, 2.4; RR for alkylating agents therapy, 10.0; RR for combined therapy, 17.4).

Boice et al.[31] described an increase in the risk of cancer in the contralateral breast in patients from the Connecticut Tumor Registry diagnosed between 1935 and 1982. An average dose of 2.8 Gy was associated with a twofold increase in risk in 10-year survivors. Risk was significantly higher among women who were younger than 45 years at the time of radiation treatment. The investigators estimated that the absolute excess risk of contralateral breast cancer was 4.4 cases per 10,000 person-years per Gy (compared to 6.7 cases per 10,000 person-years per Gy for atomic bomb survivors).[26]

Several studies have shown a significantly increased risk of lung cancer following radiation therapy (RT) after total mastectomy. Ten-year survivors from the Connecticut Tumor Registry who were diagnosed with histologically confirmed primary invasive breast cancer between 1935 and 1971 had an 80% higher risk (95% CI, 0.8, 3.8) of developing lung cancer if they received radiotherapy as part of their initial treatment regimen compared to those not receiving initial RT (mean dose to both lungs, 9.8 Gy).[32] Risk continued to increase with time and after 15 years reached 2.8 (95% CI, 1.0, 8.2). The excess relative rate was 0.20 per Gy (95% CI, −0.62, 1.03) compared to an estimate of 0.95 per Gy (95% CI, 0.60, 1.4) for trachea, bronchus, and lung in the atomic bomb study.[26] In a case-control study from this cohort, Neugut et al.[33] assessed risk of lung cancer in relation to radiation treatment and smoking in 10-year survivors. They observed a multiplicative interaction effect if both exposures were present (OR for RT alone, 3.2; OR for smoking and no RT, 17.7; OR for both RT and smoking, 32.7).

TABLE 17.2. Studies of risks of second malignant neoplasms (SMNs) among patients treated for primary Hodgkin's disease.

Reference	Year	Design	Median follow-up, years	Site(s) of SMN	Primary treatment modalities	Estimates of risk and 95% CI
Swerdlow et al.[27]	2000	Cohort	8.5	Gastrointestinal	ChT	SIR = 1.5 (0.8, 2.5; P > 0.05)*
					ChT + RT	SIR = 3.3 (2.1, 4.8; P < 0.001)
				Lung	ChT	SIR = 3.3 (2.2, 4.7; P < 0.001)
					ChT + RT	SIR = 4.3 (2.9, 6.2; P < 0.001)
				NHL	ChT	SIR = 14.8 (8.7, 23.3; P < 0.001)
Swerdlow et al.[71]	2001	Nested case-control	8.5	Lung	MOPP + RT (vs. RT)	OR = 2.41 (1.33, 4.51; P = 0.004)
Dores et al.[18]	2002	Cohort	25	Cumulative solid tumor	ChT	RR = 2.1 (n/a; P < 0.05)
					ChT + RT	RR = 2.0 (1.9, 2.0; P < 0.05)
				Acute nonlymphcytic leukemia	ChT	RR = 36.1 (25.6, 49.3; P < 0.05)
van Leeuwen et al.[70]	2000	Cohort	14.1	Breast	RT	RR = 7.7 (4.3, 12.7)
					ChT + RT	RR = 7.5 (2.7, 16.3)
					ChT + RT + salvage	RR = 1.4 (0.2, 5.1)
				Nonbreast solid tumor	RT	RR = 4.9 (3.0, 7.4)
					ChT + RT	RR = 4.4 (2.0, 8.3)
					ChT + RT + salvage	RR = 10.0 (6.8, 14.3)
				Gastrointestinal	RT	RR = 3.7 (1.0, 9.5)
					ChT + RT	RR = 7.8 (2.1, 20.0)
					ChT + RT + salvage	RR = 13 (6.2, 23.9)
Neglia et al.[18]	2001	Cohort	5	Cumulative SMN	Not specified	RR = 2.34 (1.44, 3.81)
				Breast		RR = 4.89 (0.95, 25.24)
				Leukemia		RR = 3.99 (0.84, 18.88)
				Soft tissue sarcoma		RR = 10.32 (1.18, 90.18)
				Thyroid		RR = 1.74 (0.50, 6.01)
Bhatia et al.[23]	1996	Cohort	11.4	Cumulative SMN	Not specified	SIR 18.1 (14.3, 22.3)
				Breast		SIR 75.3 (44.9, 118.4)
				Leukemia		SIR 78.8 (56.6, 123.2)
				Leukemia	ChT	RR = 1,091 (344, 2256)
					ChT + RT	RR = 439 (270, 645)
				Non-Hodgkin's lymphoma	ChT	RR = 60 (0.02, 235)
					ChT + RT	RR = 23 (6, 50)
Metayer et al.[28]	2000	Cohort	10.5	Cumulative SMN	Not specified	RR = 7.7 (6.6, 8.8)
				Breast		RR = 14.1 (P < 0.05)
				Thyroid		RR = 13.7 (8.6, 20.7)
				Leukemia		RR = 20.9 (13.9, 30.3)
				Non-Hodgkin's lymphoma		RR = 27.4 (17.9, 40.2)
Green et al.[69]	2000	Cohort	17.1	*Cumulative SMN (male)	Not specified	RR = 9.39 (4.05, 18.49, P < 0.00001)
					RT	RR = 12.32 (2.54, 36.01, P < 0.005)
					ChT + RT	RR = 8.64 (2.81, 20.16, P < 0.001)
				Cumulative SMN (female)	Not specified	RR = 10.16 (5.56, 17.05, P < 0.00001)
					RT	RR = 4.46 (0.92, 13.02, P = 0.062)
					ChT + RT	RR = 15.93 (7.95, 28.51, P < 0.00001)

OR, odds ratio; NHL, non-Hodgkin's lymphoma; RR, relative risk; ChT, chemotherapy; RT, radiation therapy; SMN, second malignant neoplasm.
*P value of significance.

As was noted earlier, radiation treatment regimens have changed over the past two decades, lowering radiation doses to the lungs.[34] In a large population-based study from the SEER (Surveillance, Epidemiology, and End Results) database of subjects diagnosed and followed up from 1973 till the end of 1998, the risk of cancer in the ipsilateral lung 10 to 14 years after RT and radical mastectomy was increased by 2.06 (95% CI, 1.53, 2.78), whereas the risk of ipsilateral lung cancer 10 to 14 years after conservative surgery (lumpectomy) and adjuvant RT was not increased (RR, 0.80; 95% CI, 0.23, 2.84).[35] Studies of other cohorts also showed increased risk of second cancers following breast cancer.[36] Another SEER-based study showed that the standardized incidence ratio (SIR) of esophageal cancer after RT for primary breast cancer was 54% higher than in the general population (95% CI, 1.27, 1.84).[37] Risk increased with time, reaching 5.42 (95% CI, 2.33, 10.68) for esophageal squamous cell carcinoma 10 years after radiotherapy. No information on smoking or alcohol consumption was available.

Gynecologic Cancers

Hormones, in general, in these cancers could play an important role in the timing of late effects of radiation treatment, their dependence on the age at exposure, and time since exposure. Some studies do not have data on the use of exogenous estrogen hormones, age at first pregnancy, time of menopause, and other factors related to hormonal status. Therefore, possible confounding effects of these variables could not be evaluated.

CANCER OF THE UTERUS

Curtis et al. examined the relationship of leukemia risk to radiation dose following radiotherapy of the uterine corpus in a nested case-control study based on a cohort of women drawn from nine population-based registries in the United States and Europe.[38] After external-beam therapy (mean dose, 9.88 Gy), cases were two times more likely to develop leukemia (excluding chronic lymphocytic leukemia) than matched controls (ERR, 0.13 per Gy; 95% CI, 0.04, 0.27).

Based primarily on data from the cohort of atomic bomb survivors, the association between radiation exposure and development of leukemia appears to depend on total dose to the bone marrow, total percent of the person's bone marrow exposed to radiation, and the dose rate at which radiation was delivered. As was mentioned earlier, the dose response for atomic bomb survivors is linear-quadratic for doses below 4 Gy (ERR, 4.8 per Sv).[39] The difference between the estimates from the Curtis et al. study and the estimate from the LSS cohort can be partly explained by the killing of stem cells of the bone marrow at high doses. Treatment regimens with low-dose-rate radiation (e.g., brachytherapy) were more leukemogenic per unit dose than external-beam therapy, perhaps due to the repair of radiation damage in protracted exposure regimens.

As a result of a wide field of radiation encompassed by the partial-body radiation treatment (only parts of the body are irradiated as opposed to the total-body irradiation as in bone marrow transplantation) of cancer of the corpus uteri, patients are also at risk of developing second solid cancers. Subjects with primary cancer of the uterine cervix from a Swedish cancer registry had a 20% higher risk of developing a second malignancy compared to the population rates.[40] Organs situated in the immediate proximity to the radiation field had the highest risk of second cancer (colon, vulva, and bladder) 9 years after initial treatment. A fourfold increase in leukemia was observed 3 to 9 years after exposure, but it was based on a small number of cases (95% CI, 1.68, 8.59).

OVARIAN CANCER

A SEER-based study of long-term survivors of ovarian cancer found a twofold-increased risk of leukemia 5 to 9 years after radiotherapy,[41] although several case-control studies did not.[42,43] A twofold increase in risk was also observed for all solid cancers 10 to 14 years after exposure (P less than 0.05).[41] Significant associations were seen for cancers of connective tissue, bladder, and pancreas. A case-control study of ovarian cancer survivors who later developed bladder tumor showed that those treated with radiotherapy alone had a twofold-higher risk (95% CI, 0.77, 4.9).[44]

In summary, RT for gynecologic cancers has been linked to the development of various second primary malignancies. They mainly experience increased risks of second malignan-cies of the organs situated in immediate proximity to the radiation field as well as leukemia.

Testicular Cancer

Testicular cancer is the most common cancer in men in the age group 20 to 44 years.[1] Early reports showed that these patients are at increased risk of second cancers following 10 to 15 years after radiotherapy.[45] Significant increases were observed for all solid cancers (RR, 1.6; 95% CI, 1.3, 2.1), gastrointestinal cancers (RR, 2.6; 95% CI, 1.7, 3.9), and leukemia (RR, 5.1; 95% CI, 1.4, 13.0).

A large population-based study of testicular cancer survivors in 1997 confirmed an increased risk of stomach, bladder, and pancreatic cancers by twofold. Overall risk was similar after seminomas (SIR, 1.42) or nonseminomatous tumors (SIR, 1.50). The largest investigation to date of leukemia following testicular cancer was done in the follow-up of the same cohort.[46] Those treated with radiotherapy had a three times higher risk of developing leukemia (95% CI, 0.7, 22.0). This risk is similar to the risks estimated after radiation therapy for cancers of the cervix,[47] breast,[30] or Hodgkin's disease.[48] Although atomic bomb survivors received lower doses of radiation, they experienced higher risks than medically irradiated subjects mainly because the dose was delivered to the entire body without dose fractionation.[49]

In summary, because testicular cancer is a disease of men under the age of 40 years, they are at increased risk of developing second malignancies later in life. In particular, both physicians and patients should be aware of increased risks of second cancers located in the bladder, lungs, connective tissue, and stomach. These patients should be under continuous surveillance for possible second cancer. In addition, because of the high risks of lung cancer, patients should be advised to quit smoking.

Prostate Cancer

In a large population-based retrospective cohort study of survivors of first primary prostate cancer in the Detroit metropolitan area who were diagnosed between 1973 and 1982, the overall risk of second malignancies was similar to the rates of cancer in the general population.[50] Subanalyses, however, showed that prostate cancer survivors were at increased risk of bladder cancer (SIR, 1.49; 95% CI, 1.07–2.02) when compared to the Detroit-area male population. Researchers concluded that the magnitude of relative and absolute risks did not suggest the presence of large risks associated with radiation treatment. In another large population-based study from the database of the Connecticut Tumor Registry, comparison of the risk of developing a SMN cancer following prostate irradiation compared to the underlying risk in patients with prostate cancer showed that the risks were not significantly different, at any time period and in all age groups, between the two groups of patients.[51] Short follow-up (mean follow-up under 4 years) could have contributed to these negative findings. However, more careful investigation of the cases who survived more than 10 years again showed no significantly increased risk of second malignancy following radiation therapy for primary prostate cancer.[52]

In the largest to date epidemiologic study of second cancers after prostate cancer based on the SEER database, a cohort of patients who received radiation treatment sometime between 1973 and 1990 showed a significant 50% increase in risk of second primary bladder cancer.[53] Risk remained increased for at least 8 years after initial radiation treatment. There was no increased risk of rectal carcinoma or leukemia after this type of radiation exposure.

In summary, prostate cancer is the most common male cancer in the United States, with nearly 200,000 men diagnosed annually.[1] Findings regarding the effect of RT for prostate cancer have been conflicting. If present, risks are probably significantly lower than risks described for other first cancers. This fact could be explained by smaller doses and less-aggressive treatments.

Lung Cancer

In a large retrospective cohort study of 2-year survivors of primary small cell lung cancer, patients who received RT experienced a 13-fold increase in the risk of second primaries among those who received chest irradiation, whereas non-irradiated patients experienced only a 7-fold increase compared to that of the general population.[54] The highest risk was observed among those who continued smoking, with evidence of an interaction between chest irradiation and continued smoking (RR, 21). Risks continued to increase with time after radiation treatment.

In a large population-based study based on the Finnish Tumor Registry lung cancer patients treated with RT between 1953 and 1989, there was a significant increase in the risk of esophageal cancer and leukemia among lung cancer patients subject to radiotherapy.[55] The risk of a second cancer among lung cancer patients increased with the length of follow-up.

Colorectal Cancer

In the past, radiotherapy was not widely used to treat colorectal cancer. There are, consequently, only a few epidemiologic studies of the effects of radiation in colorectal cancers. These studies have shown that patients with primary cancers of the colon and rectum have small increases in risks of SMN cancers as a result of radiation therapies. In particular, irradiation increases the risk of second primaries of the breast, uterus, ovaries, and other pelvic organs in the radiation field.[1,56]

Chemotherapy

That only a small percentage of individuals receiving a given chemotherapeutic regimen will go on to develop a SMN suggests that individual variations play a role in this process. Indeed, it has become apparent that a number of individual factors contribute in part to this risk. Germ-line mutations have long been recognized to predispose to primary malignancies; indeed, more than 40 genes have been cloned that, when mutated from the wild-type, are known to increase the susceptibility to malignancy.[57] Although the mechanisms of this increased susceptibility are variable, it has become apparent that many individuals with these germ-line mutations are at heightened risk of SMN and, specifically, treatment-associated malignancies.

Next we explore the various factors that contribute to the risk of SMN among patients treated with systemic chemotherapy, including the organ affected by the primary cancer, the chemotherapeutic agents employed, and host factors such as environmental exposures and immune status.

Individual Cancers

Although the use of chemotherapeutic alkylating agents imparts a risk of secondary malignancy, particularly secondary leukemia, the concern regarding SMNs is not restricted to their use alone. Indeed, for many of the hematologic and solid malignancies, there are concerns about the potential for patients to experience treatment-related neoplasms. Evidence for such an association is stronger for some malignancies, weaker for others; in some malignancies, there are as yet no convincing data regarding an elevated risk of SMN as a result of treatment. Whether this lack of effect is due to an inability of cancer chemotherapy to significantly prolong life, or whether it reflects a truly low oncogenic potential of the agents employed, is difficult to determine; what is clear, however, is that as chemotherapeutic regimens continue to become both more complex and more effective, the challenge of treatment-related SMN will require ongoing vigilance.

Pediatric Cancers

Acute Lymphocytic Leukemia

A number of reports have been published regarding the risk of treatment-associated malignancies following treatment of childhood acute lymphocytic leukemia (ALL). Children treated with all the most common protocols in ALL therapy, including the Berlin–Frankfurt–Munster (BFM) protocol, Children's Cancer Group protocol, and the Dana–Farber protocol, experience an estimated risk of SMN within 15 years of treatment ranging from 2.5% to 3.3%, although children receiving weekly or twice-weekly epipodophyllotoxin have been found to have a 12% cumulative incidence of secondary myelogenous leukemia.[14,58–60] Despite these concerning statistics, the BFM study failed to find an association between a specific chemotherapeutic agent and subsequent acute myeloid leukemia (AML); 12 of the 16 cases of secondary AML they report had not received epipodophyllotoxin.[60] Patients in these groups who also received craniospinal radiation were found to be at an increased risk of a number of radiation-induced SMNs, including primary CNS malignancy, thyroid cancer, and skin cancers; more-recent ALL protocols have rejected craniospinal radiotherapy in favor of intrathecal chemotherapy for younger patients without evidence of CNS involvement at initiation of therapy.

An additional risk of SMN among patients treated during childhood for ALL is that of malignant melanoma. It had been reported that patients receiving monthly maintenance therapy of vincristine and prednisone, weekly methotrexate, and daily 6-mercaptopurine (6-MP) were found to have an increased number of melanocytic nevi and dysplastic nevi; on this basis, concern was raised that these patients may be at higher risk of subsequent malignant melanoma than the general population.[61] Whether such an effect will be seen with more modern maintenance regimens has not yet been determined.

SARCOMA

In contrast to the specific case of RB-associated sarcoma, the treatment and sequelae from therapy of primary pediatric sarcoma have been well studied. Among these patients, a consistent and long-lasting rate of SMN following intensive chemotherapy of sarcoma has been identified. The reported cumulative incidence of solid SMN among patients treated for Ewing's sarcoma ranges from 5% at 15 years of follow-up to more than 20% at 20 years, whereas the risk of leukemia has been estimated in the range of 2%.[62–64] These patients went on to develop a variety of hematologic complications, including myelodysplasia (MDS) as well as AML and ALL, between 1 and 8 years after therapy for Ewing's sarcoma. Secondary sarcomas within the field of radiotherapy have been described as well; no clear association with systemic chemotherapy has yet been established for these SMNs.

Treatment of pediatric rhabdomyosarcoma has also been associated with the development of SMNs. The latency period for these patients appears to be slightly longer, with a median time to diagnosis of between 5 and 11 years following initial treatment.[65,66] The cumulative incidence of SMN following rhabdomyosarcoma appears to be similar to that found in Ewing's sarcoma, but unlike the case of Ewing's sarcoma, this risk seems to be at least in part attributable to a potentiating effect of systemic chemotherapy.[62,67] Although solid tumor SMNs appear to be salvageable with multimodal therapy, hematologic SMNs following treatment for pediatric sarcoma appear to share the generally poor prognosis of secondary leukemias more commonly seen with epipodophyllotoxins and alkylating agents.[64,66]

WILM'S TUMOR

Long-term follow-up data gathered by the National Wilms Tumor Study Group (NWTSG) demonstrated that, between 1969 and 1991, patients treated in childhood for Wilm's tumor went on to develop an eightfold-greater risk of SMN.[68] These malignancies consisted of both solid tumors, largely within the field of irradiation, and hematologic malignancies, including both lymphomas and leukemias. The NWTSG reported that their cohort had developed carcinomas of the breast, thyroid, colon, and parotid gland, hepatocellular carcinoma, and primary CNS malignancies. The study group concluded that it appeared that treatment of these patients with doxorubicin increased the risk of SMN, potentiating the oncogenic effect of the administered ionizing radiation.

Hodgkin's Disease

Patients treated for Hodgkin's disease with chemotherapy, ionizing radiation, or both have a risk of developing a variety of SMNs that, cumulatively, is 2 to 4 times greater than unaffected individuals.[23,27,28,48,69–71] The relative risk of developing specific solid tumors as SMNs shows a great variability, ranging from 2 to more than 50 times greater, depending upon the tissue of origin as well as the chemotherapeutic agents used and whether ionizing radiation was administered con-

comitantly. The cumulative incidence of SMN following the treatment of Hodgkin's disease thus shows a great variability as well, from as low as 2% to as high as 27% within 30 years of treatment.

Specific tissues of origin for these secondary SMNs include thyroid, breast, and skin (melanoma and nonmelanoma). Thyroid cancer remains the most common SMN following the treatment of Hodgkin's and is affected by both chemotherapeutic agents as well as the dose of ionizing radiation.[18] And, although the risks associated with ionizing radiation have already been discussed, the risks associated with alkylating agents apply to patients treated for Hodgkin's disease as well. Indeed, up to 25% of SMNs among these patients are either lymphomas or leukemias.[27,28,48,69,70] The risk of hematologic malignancy as an SMN is, in large part, attributable to the chemotherapeutic agents included in the management of the disease, that is, alkylators versus others. Risks of leukemia, demonstrating the dose–response relationship as discussed, continue to rise with additional chemotherapy, and thus patients requiring retreatment for recurrence of Hodgkin's disease are at higher risk yet of SMN. Given the significant concerns regarding long-term risk of SMNs from therapy, pediatric oncologists have begun modifying treatment regimens, with boys receiving fewer alkylating agents and girls receiving less chest wall irradiation.

Breast Cancer

Women with breast cancer are known to be at higher risk for SMN malignancies within the contralateral breast, as well as at least a slightly elevated risk of primary malignancies of many other organs, including the ovaries, endometrium, and lower gastrointestinal tract; this risk elevation, however, appears to be independent of the treatment modalities used in the primary malignancy.[72–74] These associations suggest that these organs share one or more common risk factors for malignancy with the breast, including hormonal status, diet, and adiposity. A subset of patients with breast cancer carries a heritable risk due to mutations in *BRCA1* and *BRCA2*; these patients are also at greatly increased risk for ovarian neoplasms and second primary breast cancer. Among patients with a history of breast cancer, rigorous screening for SMN within the breast is universally advocated, and many experts argue for screening for both ovarian and endometrial neoplasms as well.[31,74]

The modalities employed in the treatment of breast cancer have the ability to impact the frequency of SMNs within and beyond the breast. However, unlike each of the organs discussed so far, treatments of breast cancer can either raise or lower this risk. There appears to be an increased risk among patients receiving radiotherapy administered for breast cancer of ipsilateral lung cancer, particularly among smokers.[33,75] When alkylating agents or anthracyclines are used in the adjuvant setting, an increased risk of treatment-associated leukemia has been seen, an effect that appears to be augmented by concomitant radiotherapy.[30,76]

Antiestrogenic therapy has been well documented in its ability to both decrease the mortality from primary breast cancer as well as diminish the frequency of second breast cancers.[77–79] This chemoprotective effect has been observed in the high-risk subgroup of patients with *BRCA1* and *BRCA2* mutation-associated primary malignancies, with odds ratios of between 0.4 and 0.6, odds that approach those seen with prophylactic oophorectomy.[80] Data from the largest randomized clinical trial, however, have to date been unable to confirm this observation. Although limited by an extremely small number of incident cancers among BRCA mutation carriers in the trial, the investigators were unable to show a protective effect among BRCA1-positive patients (RR, 1.67; 95% CI, 0.32, 10.7) and only found a trend toward efficacy among BRCA2-positive patients (RR, 0.38; 95% CI, 0.06, 1.56).[81] Newly emerging data suggest that the protective benefit of tamoxifen's antiestrogenic effect on breast tissue can be further prolonged by the use of aromatase inhibitors after the discontinuation of tamoxifen. Tamoxifen, however, acts in certain tissues, such as breast tissue, as an estrogen receptor antagonist, whereas in others as an estrogen receptor agonist, tissues that include the ovaries and endometrium.[82] Research has consistently found that women who undergo long-term tamoxifen therapy are at approximately twice the risk of endometrial cancer, or about 80 excess cases per 10,000 tamoxifen-treated individuals.[83–85] Early suggestions that tamoxifen may confer an additional risk of ovarian, colorectal, and stomach cancers as SMNs have not been borne out by additional investigation.[82,85] Although there is some debate concerning the potential value of screening for endometrial cancer via transvaginal ultrasonography or endometrial biopsy among breast cancer patients taking tamoxifen, experts agree on the value of annual visits to an experienced gynecologist for these patients and on the importance of an expeditious evaluation of abnormal vaginal bleeding.[1,86]

Testicular Cancer

Etoposide is a mainstay of chemotherapy in testicular malignancies, often at high doses, and it comes as little surprise that long-term survivors demonstrate an elevated risk of hematologic malignancy. Estimates have placed the cumulative incidence of AML or non-Hodgkin's lymphoma as SMNs following treatment of testicular cancer at between 1.3% and 2%.[46,87–89] Although the development of metachronous contralateral testicular cancer remains a concern for patients cured of a primary unilateral cancer, the incidence of contralateral testicular cancer as an SMN does not appear to be influenced by the treatments chosen for the first primary malignancy.[90]

Survivors of primary testicular cancer have also been described as having an increased incidence of solid tumors involving the stomach, colon, rectum, pancreas, prostate, kidney, bladder, and thyroid, as well as soft tissue sarcomas and cutaneous malignancies. All of these, with the possible exception of cutaneous malignancies, have been found to be solely associated with the dose of ionizing radiation administered.[91] The association of both melanoma and non-melanoma skin cancers with chemotherapy of testicular cancer has been reported but remains incompletely elucidated.[92]

Lung Cancer

Both non-small cell lung cancer (NSCLC) and small cell lung cancer (SCLC) have been clearly associated with an increased risk of developing SMNs. However, the elevated risk of second upper aerodigestive tract tumors, including head and neck tumors, esophageal cancers, and second primary lung cancers, has been clearly and closely linked to smoking status[93,94] and the field cancerization that can ensue following continuous exposure to the carcinogens present in cigarette smoke.[95,96] No association has been identified to link the treatment of a primary NSCLC with an increased risk of SMN. This stands in contrast to the case of SCLC, for which such an association does appear to exist.

Although long-term survival in SCLC patients with extensive disease (ED) rarely exceeds 5 years, more-favorable results have been reported in patients with limited disease (LD); disease-free survival at 2 years in some reports has approached or exceeded 50%.[97–99] Among SCLC survivors, there has been noted a markedly greater risk of subsequent development of an SMN, as has been noted. However, this risk is not limited to those patients undergoing therapeutic irradiation. An early retrospective analysis of long-term SCLC survivors had found a markedly elevated risk of SMN, with an overall risk of 10.3% per person-year and an 8-year actuarial risk of 50.3%.[100] Although all SCLC patients have an increased rate of second lung cancers (typically NSCLC in histology), this risk rises from approximately 7 times that of unaffected patients to approximately 13 times among patients treated with any of a number of combination chemotherapy protocols.[54]

Prostate Cancer

Although some reports concerning the risk of therapy-associated SMN with radiotherapy of prostate cancer have emerged, far less attention has been either merited or received from the risk of SMN from chemotherapy for prostate cancer. While systemic chemotherapy has a limited role in the treatment of prostate cancer, there is some use of nitrogen mustard, which has been associated with increased risk of myelodysplastic syndrome in patients receiving it for the treatment of prostate cancer.[92] The use of antiandrogenic therapy in controlling this malignancy is far more common than traditional chemotherapeutic agents, and the theoretical possibility exists that such agents could predispose to tumors that are suppressed by the androgenic state. Suggestion of such a possible phenomenon can be found in a recent report of an increased risk of male breast cancer among patients treated for prostate cancer.[101]

Gastrointestinal Cancers

It is interesting to note that among the most prevalent gastrointestinal cancers—colorectal cancer, gastric cancer, and pancreatic cancer—there are no convincing data suggesting linkage between chemotherapy and SMN. The reasons underlying this lack of convincing connections undoubtedly vary by malignancy.

Gynecologic Cancers

Analyses of the common gynecologic malignancies—cervical, uterine, and ovarian—have established some patterns of increased risk of SMNs. However, there lacks a robust literature addressing the attributable risk of systemic chemotherapy in patients with cancer of either the uterine cervix or the corpus uteri; that chemotherapy has at this time a limited role in the treatment of these malignancies both makes the identification of such an association difficult and renders any findings clinically unimportant.

Ovarian cancer presents a different scenario altogether, as it is often treated with a multimodal regimen that includes systemic chemotherapy. Historically, associations had been seen between melphalan-based chemotherapeutic regimens that would now be considered outdated and risk of secondary leukemia in patients treated for ovarian cancer.[43,102] A Swedish record-linkage study from 1995 found a relative risk of 7 for leukemia among patients with ovarian cancer, likely reflecting the common use of melphalan during the time period under investigation, 1958–1992.[40] Although an elevated risk of acute nonlymphocytic leukemia has been suggested to exist for patients treated for ovarian cancer with cyclophosphamide, chlorambucil, or regimens containing doxorubicin and cisplatin,[102–105] a retrospective analysis stratified by decade demonstrated that the risk of leukemia following treatment of ovarian cancer has decreased from 40 during the 1970s to 17 from 1980 to 1992.[41] While this suggests that more modern regimens, largely cisplatin based, may be less leukemogenic, clearly more data are needed to more thoroughly clarify this risk relationship more thoroughly.

Transplantation and Oncogenesis

An additional predisposing factor toward treatment-induced SMN that has recently emerged is immunosuppression (see Chapter 15). Over the past two decades we have seen a dramatic improvement in the ability to suppress immunologic transplant rejection thanks to new, potent immunosuppressive agents, including cyclophosphamide, cyclosporine A, tacrolimus, and mycophenolate mofetil, but it has become apparent that the long-term administration of such medications can dramatically increase the risk of developing late neoplasia, both hematologic and solid malignancies.[106,107]

Risk of hematologic malignancy has been noted to be dramatically elevated among transplant recipients, both allogeneic bone marrow transplant (BMT) recipients as well as patients receiving solid organ donation. Indeed, the name posttransplantation lymphoproliferative disorder (PTLD) has emerged in the literature to report and describe such patients. PTLD as a diagnostic category includes a spectrum of pathology ranging from atypical marrow hyperplasia to frank non-Hodgkin's lymphoma; what the constituent diagnoses share is a common association with Epstein–Barr virus infection, either acute seroconversion or reactivation of latent infection.[107] Rates of lymphoma are dramatically increased by bone marrow ablation and hematopoietic stem cell transplant in the treatment of malignancy; these rates are higher yet when the stem cell transplant was given for an indication of an underlying immunocompromised condition, such as Hodgkin's disease or chronic myelogenous leukemia (CML).[108] These PTLDs can occur quite rapidly following BMT, with a median time to onset of 2.5 months, whereas secondary leukemias have an almost equally rapid arrival, with a median time to onset of 6.7 months.[109,110] PTLD complicates solid organ transplant as well; while most studies place the cumulative "de novo" tumor incidence among recipients of solid organs at between 5% and 15%, PTLD accounts for 15% to 25% of these malignancies, a marked elevation of risk as compared to the general population.[111,112]

Although the rise in risk of lymphoproliferative disorders among transplant recipients is striking, there have been noted elevated risks of a number of solid tumors as well in this population. Kaposi's sarcoma, another malignancy with a viral pathogenesis (human herpesvirus 8), is seen among transplant recipients, as are hepatomas among patients with chronic infection by hepatitis B or C virus. And while some solid tumors (renal carcinoma in renal transplant patients, for example) are largely attributable to the underlying conditions necessitating transplantation (e.g., analgesic nephropathy), it is clear that others are strongly associated with the induction of an immunocompromised state. This connection is most clear in the case of squamous cell skin cancer: the cumulative incidence of this malignancy 10 years after transplant is 10% and 20 years after transplant rises to 40%. In Australia, where the baseline incidence is higher than that in the United States because of more-intense solar UV exposure, these numbers rise to 45% and 70%, respectively.[113]

References

1. Neugut AI, Meadows AT, Robinson E (eds). Multiple primary cancers. Philadelphia: Lippincott Williams & Wilkins, 1999.
2. Goolden WG. Radiation cancer of the pharynx. Br Med J 1951;2:1110–1117.
3. Sherrill DJ, Grishkin BA, Galal FS, Zajtchuk R, Graeber GM. Radiation associated malignancies of the esophagus. Cancer (Phila) 1984;54(4):726–728.
4. Shimizu T, Matsui T, Kimura O, Maeta M, Koga S. Radiation-induced esophageal cancer: a case report and a review of the literature. Jpn J Surg 1990;20(1):97–100.
5. Ribeiro U Jr, Posner MC, Safatle-Ribeiro AV, Reynolds JC. Risk factors for squamous cell carcinoma of the oesophagus. Br J Surg 1996;83(9):1174–1185.
6. Neugut AI, Weinberg MD, Ahsan H, Rescigno J. Carcinogenic effects of radiotherapy for breast cancer. Oncology (Huntingt) 1999;13(9):1245–1256; discussion 57, 61–65.
7. Boice JD Jr. Studies of atomic bomb survivors. Understanding radiation effects. JAMA 1990;264(5):622–623.
8. Pierce DA, Preston DL. Radiation-related cancer risks at low doses among atomic bomb survivors. Radiat Res 2000;154(2):178–186.
9. UNSCEAR (United Nations Scientific Committee on the Effects of Atomic Radiation). 2000 Report to the General Assembly, with Scientific Annexes. Volume II: Effects. New York: United Nations, 2000.
10. Tucker MA, Meadows AT, Boice JD Jr, et al. Leukemia after therapy with alkylating agents for childhood cancer. J Natl Cancer Inst 1987;78(3):459–464.
11. Hawkins MM, Wilson LM, Stovall MA, et al. Epipodophyllotoxins, alkylating agents, and radiation and risk of secondary leukaemia after childhood cancer. BMJ 1992;304(6832):951–958.
12. Tucker MA, D'Angio GJ, Boice JD Jr, et al. Bone sarcomas linked to radiotherapy and chemotherapy in children. N Engl J Med 1987;317(10):588–593.
13. de Vathaire F, Francois P, Hill C, et al. Role of radiotherapy and chemotherapy in the risk of second malignant neoplasms after cancer in childhood. Br J Cancer 1989;59(5):792–796.
14. Neglia JP, Meadows AT, Robison LL, et al. Second neoplasms after acute lymphoblastic leukemia in childhood. N Engl J Med 1991;325(19):1330–1336.

15. Tucker MA, Jones PH, Boice JD Jr, et al. Therapeutic radiation at a young age is linked to secondary thyroid cancer. The Late Effects Study Group. Cancer Res 1991;51(11):2885–2888.

16. Ron E, Lubin JH, Shore RE, et al. Thyroid cancer after exposure to external radiation: a pooled analysis of seven studies. Radiat Res 1995;141(3):259–277.

17. Olsen JH, Garwicz S, Hertz H, et al. Second malignant neoplasms after cancer in childhood or adolescence. Nordic Society of Paediatric Haematology and Oncology Association of the Nordic Cancer Registries. BMJ 1993;307(6911):1030–1036.

18. Neglia JP, Friedman DL, Yasui Y, et al. Second malignant neoplasms in five-year survivors of childhood cancer: childhood cancer survivor study. J Natl Cancer Inst 2001;93(8):618–629.

19. Boice JD Jr. Radiation and non-Hodgkin's lymphoma. Cancer Res 1992;52(19 suppl):5489s–5491s.

20. Curtis RE, Rowlings PA, Deeg HJ, et al. Solid cancers after bone marrow transplantation. N Engl J Med 1997;336(13):897–904.

21. Socie G, Curtis RE, Deeg HJ, et al. New malignant diseases after allogeneic marrow transplantation for childhood acute leukemia. J Clin Oncol 2000;18(2):348–357.

22. Clemons M, Loijens L, Goss P. Breast cancer risk following irradiation for Hodgkin's disease. Cancer Treat Rev 2000;26(4):291–302.

23. Bhatia S, Robison LL, Oberlin O, et al. Breast cancer and other second neoplasms after childhood Hodgkin's disease. N Engl J Med 1996;334(12):745–751.

24. Travis LB, Gospodarowicz M, Curtis RE, et al. Lung cancer following chemotherapy and radiotherapy for Hodgkin's disease. J Natl Cancer Inst 2002;94(3):182–192.

25. Birdwell SH, Hancock SL, Varghese A, Cox RS, Hoppe RT. Gastrointestinal cancer after treatment of Hodgkin's disease. Int J Radiat Oncol Biol Phys 1997;37(1):67–73.

26. Ron E, Preston DL, Mabuchi K, Thompson DE, Soda M. Cancer incidence in atomic bomb survivors. Part IV: Comparison of cancer incidence and mortality. Radiat Res 1994;137(2 suppl):S98–S112.

27. Swerdlow AJ, Barber JA, Hudson GV, et al. Risk of second malignancy after Hodgkin's disease in a collaborative British cohort: the relation to age at treatment. J Clin Oncol 2000;18(3):498–509.

28. Metayer C, Lynch CF, Clarke EA, et al. Second cancers among long-term survivors of Hodgkin's disease diagnosed in childhood and adolescence. J Clin Oncol 2000;18(12):2435–2443.

29. Curtis RE, Boice JD Jr, Stovall M, Flannery JT, Moloney WC. Leukemia risk following radiotherapy for breast cancer. J Clin Oncol 1989;7(1):21–29.

30. Curtis RE, Boice JD Jr, Stovall M, et al. Risk of leukemia after chemotherapy and radiation treatment for breast cancer. N Engl J Med 1992;326(26):1745–1751.

31. Boice JD Jr, Harvey EB, Blettner M, Stovall M, Flannery JT. Cancer in the contralateral breast after radiotherapy for breast cancer. N Engl J Med 1992;326(12):781–785.

32. Inskip PD, Stovall M, Flannery JT. Lung cancer risk and radiation dose among women treated for breast cancer. J Natl Cancer Inst 1994;86(13):983–988.

33. Neugut AI, Murray T, Santos J, et al. Increased risk of lung cancer after breast cancer radiation therapy in cigarette smokers. Cancer (Phila) 1994;73(6):1615–1620.

34. Travis LB, Curtis RE, Inskip PD, Hankey BF. Re: Lung cancer risk and radiation dose among women treated for breast cancer. J Natl Cancer Inst 1995;87(1):60–61.

35. Zablotska LB, Neugut AI. Lung carcinoma after radiation therapy in women treated with lumpectomy or mastectomy for primary breast carcinoma. Cancer (Phila) 2003;97(6):1404–1411.

36. Rubino C, de Vathaire F, Diallo I, Shamsaldin A, Le MG. Increased risk of second cancers following breast cancer: role of the initial treatment. Breast Cancer Res Treat 2000;61(3):183–195.

37. Ahsan H, Neugut AI. Radiation therapy for breast cancer and increased risk for esophageal carcinoma. Ann Intern Med 1998;128(2):114–117.

38. Curtis RE, Boice JD Jr, Stovall M, et al. Relationship of leukemia risk to radiation dose following cancer of the uterine corpus. J Natl Cancer Inst 1994;86(17):1315–1324.

39. BEIR V (Committee on the Biological Effects of Ionizing Radiations). Health effects of exposure to low levels of ionizing radiation. Washington, DC: National Academy Press, 1990.

40. Bergfeldt K, Einhorn S, Rosendahl I, Hall P. Increased risk of second primary malignancies in patients with gynecological cancer. A Swedish record-linkage study. Acta Oncol 1995;34(6):771–777.

41. Travis LB, Curtis RE, Boice JD Jr, Platz CE, Hankey BF, Fraumeni JF Jr. Second malignant neoplasms among long-term survivors of ovarian cancer. Cancer Res 1996;56(7):1564–1570.

42. Travis LB, Holowaty EJ, Bergfeldt K, et al. Risk of leukemia after platinum-based chemotherapy for ovarian cancer. N Engl J Med 1999;340(5):351–357.

43. Kaldor JM, Day NE, Pettersson F, et al. Leukemia following chemotherapy for ovarian cancer. N Engl J Med 1990;322(1):1–6.

44. Kaldor JM, Day NE, Kittelmann B, et al. Bladder tumours following chemotherapy and radiotherapy for ovarian cancer: a case-control study. Int J Cancer 1995;63(1):1–6.

45. van Leeuwen FE, Stiggelbout AM, van den Belt-Dusebout AW, et al. Second cancer risk following testicular cancer: a follow-up study of 1,909 patients. J Clin Oncol 1993;11(3):415–424.

46. Travis LB, Andersson M, Gospodarowicz M, et al. Treatment-associated leukemia following testicular cancer. J Natl Cancer Inst 2000;92(14):1165–1171.

47. Boice JD Jr, Blettner M, Kleinerman RA, et al. Radiation dose and leukemia risk in patients treated for cancer of the cervix. J Natl Cancer Inst 1987;79(6):1295–1311.

48. Kaldor JM, Day NE, Clarke EA, et al. Leukemia following Hodgkin's disease. N Engl J Med 1990;322(1):7–13.

49. Preston DL, Kusumi S, Tomonaga M, et al. Cancer incidence in atomic bomb survivors. Part III. Leukemia, lymphoma and multiple myeloma, 1950–1987. Radiat Res 1994;137(2 suppl):S68–S97.

50. Pawlish KS, Schottenfeld D, Severson R, Montie JE. Risk of multiple primary cancers in prostate cancer patients in the Detroit metropolitan area: a retrospective cohort study. Prostate 1997;33(2):75–86.

51. Movsas B, Hanlon AL, Pinover W, Hanks GE. Is there an increased risk of second primaries following prostate irradiation? Int J Radiat Oncol Biol Phys 1998;41(2):251–255.

52. Johnstone PA, Powell CR, Riffenburgh R, Rohde DC, Kane CJ. Second primary malignancies in T1-3N0 prostate cancer patients treated with radiation therapy with 10-year followup. J Urol 1998;159(3):946–949.

53. Neugut AI, Ahsan H, Robinson E, Ennis RD. Bladder carcinoma and other second malignancies after radiotherapy for prostate carcinoma. Cancer (Phila) 1997;79(8):1600–1604.

54. Tucker MA, Murray N, Shaw EG, et al. Second primary cancers related to smoking and treatment of small-cell lung cancer. Lung Cancer Working Cadre. J Natl Cancer Inst 1997;89(23):1782–1878.

55. Salminen E, Pukkala E, Teppo L, Pyrhonen S. Risk of second cancers among lung cancer patients. Acta Oncol 1995;34(2):165–169.

56. Hoar SK, Wilson J, Blot WJ, McLaughlin JK, Winn DM, Kantor AF. Second cancer following cancer of the digestive system in Connecticut, 1935–82. Natl Cancer Inst Monogr 1985;68:49–82.

57. Knudson AG. Karnofsky Memorial Lecture. Hereditary cancer: theme and variations. J Clin Oncol 1997;15(10):3280–3287.

58. Pui CH, Ribeiro RC, Hancock ML, et al. Acute myeloid leukemia in children treated with epipodophyllotoxins for acute lymphoblastic leukemia. N Engl J Med 1991;325(24):1682–1687.

59. Kimball Dalton VM, Gelber RD, Li F, Donnelly MJ, Tarbell NJ, Sallan SE. Second malignancies in patients treated for childhood acute lymphoblastic leukemia. J Clin Oncol 1998;16(8): 2848–2853.

60. Loning L, Zimmermann M, Reiter A, et al. Secondary neoplasms subsequent to Berlin-Frankfurt-Munster therapy of acute lymphoblastic leukemia in childhood: significantly lower risk without cranial radiotherapy. Blood 2000;95(9):2770–2775.

61. Relling MV, Yanishevski Y, Nemec J, et al. Etoposide and antimetabolite pharmacology in patients who develop secondary acute myeloid leukemia. Leukemia 1998;12(3):346–352.

62. Meadows AT, Baum E, Fossati-Bellani F, et al. Second malignant neoplasms in children: an update from the Late Effects Study Group. J Clin Oncol 1985;3(4):532–538.

63. Kuttesch JF Jr, Wexler LH, Marcus RB, et al. Second malignancies after Ewing's sarcoma: radiation dose-dependency of secondary sarcomas. J Clin Oncol 1996;14(10):2818–2825.

64. Dunst J, Ahrens S, Paulussen M, et al. Second malignancies after treatment for Ewing's sarcoma: a report of the CESS-studies. Int J Radiat Oncol Biol Phys 1998;42(2):379–384.

65. Rich DC, Corpron CA, Smith MB, Black CT, Lally KP, Andrassy RJ. Second malignant neoplasms in children after treatment of soft tissue sarcoma. J Pediatr Surg 1997;32(2):369–372.

66. Raney RB, Asmar L, Vassilopoulou-Sellin R, et al. Late complications of therapy in 213 children with localized, nonorbital soft-tissue sarcoma of the head and neck: A descriptive report from the Intergroup Rhabdomyosarcoma Studies (IRS)-II and -III. IRS Group of the Children's Cancer Group and the Pediatric Oncology Group. Med Pediatr Oncol 1999;33(4):362–371.

67. Heyn R, Haeberlen V, Newton WA, et al. Second malignant neoplasms in children treated for rhabdomyosarcoma. Intergroup Rhabdomyosarcoma Study Committee. J Clin Oncol 1993; 11(2):262–270.

68. Breslow NE, Takashima JR, Whitton JA, Moksness J, D'Angio GJ, Green DM. Second malignant neoplasms following treatment for Wilm's tumor: a report from the National Wilms' Tumor Study Group. J Clin Oncol 1995;13(8):1851–1859.

69. Green DM, Hyland A, Barcos MP, et al. Second malignant neoplasms after treatment for Hodgkin's disease in childhood or adolescence. J Clin Oncol 2000;18(7):1492–1499.

70. van Leeuwen FE, Klokman WJ, Veer MB, et al. Long-term risk of second malignancy in survivors of Hodgkin's disease treated during adolescence or young adulthood. J Clin Oncol 2000; 18(3):487–497.

71. Swerdlow AJ, Schoemaker MJ, Allerton R, et al. Lung cancer after Hodgkin's disease: a nested case-control study of the relation to treatment. J Clin Oncol 2001;19(6):1610–1618.

72. Boice JD Jr, Storm H, Curtis RE. Multiple primary cancers in Connecticut and Denmark. Monogr Natl Cancer Inst 1985; 68(1):1–437.

73. Schatzkin A, Baranovsky A, Kessler LG. Diet and cancer. Evidence from associations of multiple primary cancers in the SEER program. Cancer (Phila) 1988;62(7):1451–1457.

74. Bergfeldt K, Nilsson B, Einhorn S, Hall P. Breast cancer risk in women with a primary ovarian cancer: a case-control study. Eur J Cancer 2001;37(17):2229–2234.

75. Inskip PD, Boice JD Jr. Radiotherapy-induced lung cancer among women who smoke. Cancer (Phila) 1994;73(6):1541–1543.

76. Saso R, Kulkarni S, Mitchell P, et al. Secondary myelodysplastic syndrome/acute myeloid leukaemia following mitoxantrone-based therapy for breast carcinoma. Br J Cancer 2000;83(1): 91–94.

77. Cook LS, Weiss NS, Schwartz SM, et al. Population-based study of tamoxifen therapy and subsequent ovarian, endometrial, and breast cancers. J Natl Cancer Inst 1995;87(18):1359–1364.

78. Curtis RE, Boice JD Jr, Shriner DA, Hankey BF, Fraumeni JF Jr. Second cancers after adjuvant tamoxifen therapy for breast cancer. J Natl Cancer Inst 1996;88(12):832–834.

79. Li CI, Malone KE, Weiss NS, Daling JR. Tamoxifen therapy for primary breast cancer and risk of contralateral breast cancer. J Natl Cancer Inst 2001;93(13):1008–1013.

80. Narod SA, Brunet JS, Ghadirian P, et al. Tamoxifen and risk of contralateral breast cancer in BRCA1 and BRCA2 mutation carriers: a case-control study. Hereditary Breast Cancer Clinical Study Group. Lancet 2000;356(9245):1876–1881.

81. King MC, Wieand S, Hale K, et al. Tamoxifen and breast cancer incidence among women with inherited mutations in BRCA1 and BRCA2: National Surgical Adjuvant Breast and Bowel Project (NSABP-P1) Breast Cancer Prevention Trial. JAMA 2001;286(18):2251–2256.

82. Rutqvist LE, Johansson H, Signomklao T, Johansson U, Fornander T, Wilking N. Adjuvant tamoxifen therapy for early stage breast cancer and second primary malignancies. Stockholm Breast Cancer Study Group. J Natl Cancer Inst 1995;87(9):645–651.

83. Fisher B, Costantino JP, Redmond CK, Fisher ER, Wickerham DL, Cronin WM. Endometrial cancer in tamoxifen-treated breast cancer patients: findings from the National Surgical Adjuvant Breast and Bowel Project (NSABP) B-14. J Natl Cancer Inst 1994;86(7):527–537.

84. Fisher B, Costantino JP, Wickerham DL, et al. Tamoxifen for prevention of breast cancer: report of the National Surgical Adjuvant Breast and Bowel Project P-1 Study. J Natl Cancer Inst 1998;90(18):1371–1388.

85. Fisher B, Dignam J, Wolmark N, et al. Tamoxifen in treatment of intraductal breast cancer: National Surgical Adjuvant Breast and Bowel Project B-24 randomised controlled trial. Lancet 1999;353(9169):1993–2000.

86. Shapiro CL, Recht A. Side effects of adjuvant treatment of breast cancer. N Engl J Med 2001;344(26):1997–2008.

87. Kollmannsberger C, Beyer J, Droz JP, et al. Secondary leukemia following high cumulative doses of etoposide in patients treated for advanced germ cell tumors. J Clin Oncol 1998;16(10): 3386–3391.

88. Kollmannsberger C, Hartmann JT, Kanz L, Bokemeyer C. Therapy-related malignancies following treatment of germ cell cancer. Int J Cancer 1999;83(6):860–863.

89. Ruther U, Dieckmann K, Bussar-Maatz R, Eisenberger F. Second malignancies following pure seminoma. Oncology 2000;58(1): 75–82.

90. Hale GA, Marina NM, Jones-Wallace D, et al. Late effects of treatment for germ cell tumors during childhood and adolescence. J Pediatr Hematol Oncol 1999;21(2):115–122.

91. Travis LB, Curtis RE, Storm H, et al. Risk of second malignant neoplasms among long-term survivors of testicular cancer. J Natl Cancer Inst 1997;89(19):1429–1439.

92. Hartmann JT, Nichols CR, Droz JP, et al. The relative risk of second nongerminal malignancies in patients with extragonadal germ cell tumors. Cancer (Phila) 2000;88(11):2629–2635.

93. Warren S, Gates DC. Multiple primary malignant tumors: a survey of the literature and statistical study. Am J Cancer 1932; 16:1358–1414.

94. Lippman SM, Lee JJ, Karp DD. Phase III intergroup trial of 13-cis-retinoic acid to prevent second primary tumors in stage I non-small cell lung cancer (SNCLC): interim report of NCI No. I19-0001. Proc Am Soc Clin Oncol 1998;17:1753.

95. Vokes EE, Weichselbaum RR, Lippman SM, Hong WK. Head and neck cancer. N Engl J Med 1993;328(3):184–194.

96. Tepperman BS, Fitzpatrick PJ. Second respiratory and upper digestive tract cancers after oral cancer. Lancet 1981; 2(8246):547–549.

97. Johnson BE, Bridges JD, Sobczeck M, et al. Patients with limited-stage small-cell lung cancer treated with concurrent twice-daily chest radiotherapy and etoposide/cisplatin followed by cyclophosphamide, doxorubicin, and vincristine. J Clin Oncol 1996; 14(3):806–813.

98. Jeremic B, Shibamoto Y, Acimovic L, Milisavljevic S. Carboplatin, etoposide, and accelerated hyperfractionated radiotherapy for elderly patients with limited small cell lung carcinoma: a phase II study. Cancer (Phila) 1998;82(5):836–841.

99. Turrisi AT III, Kim K, Blum R, et al. Twice-daily compared with once-daily thoracic radiotherapy in limited small-cell lung cancer treated concurrently with cisplatin and etoposide. N Engl J Med 1999;340(4):265–271.

100. Heyne KH, Lippman SM, Lee JJ, Lee JS, Hong WK. The incidence of second primary tumors in long-term survivors of small-cell lung cancer. J Clin Oncol 1992;10(10):1519–1524.

101. Thellenberg C, Malmer B, Tavelin B, Gronberg H. Second primary cancers in men with prostate cancer: an increased risk of male breast cancer. J Urol 2003;169(4):1345–1348.

102. Greene MH, Harris EL, Gershenson DM, et al. Melphalan may be a more potent leukemogen than cyclophosphamide. Ann Intern Med 1986;105(3):360–367.

103. Kaldor JM, Day NE, Pettersson F, et al. Leukemia following chemotherapy for ovarian cancer. N Engl J Med 1990;322(1):1–6.

104. Haas JF, Kittelmann B, Mehnert WH, et al. Risk of leukaemia in ovarian tumour and breast cancer patients following treatment by cyclophosphamide. Br J Cancer 1987;55(2):213–218.

105. Greene MH, Boice JD Jr, Greer BE, Blessing JA, Dembo AJ. Acute nonlymphocytic leukemia after therapy with alkylating agents for ovarian cancer: a study of five randomized clinical trials. N Engl J Med 1982;307(23):1416–1421.

106. Ciancio G, Siquijor AP, Burke GW, et al. Post-transplant lymphoproliferative disease in kidney transplant patients in the new immunosuppressive era. Clin Transplant 1997;11(3):243–249.

107. Andreone P, Gramenzi A, Lorenzini S, et al. Posttransplantation lymphoproliferative disorders. Arch Intern Med 2003;163(17):1997–2004.

108. Gross TG, Steinbuch M, DeFor T, et al. B cell lymphoproliferative disorders following hematopoietic stem cell transplantation: risk factors, treatment and outcome. Bone Marrow Transplant 1999;23(3):251–258.

109. Deeg HJ, Socie G. Malignancies after hematopoietic stem cell transplantation: many questions, some answers. Blood 1998;91(6):1833–1844.

110. Socie G, Kolb HJ. Malignant diseases after bone marrow transplantation: the case for tumor banking and continued reporting to registries. EBMT Late-Effects Working Party. Bone Marrow Transplant 1995;16(4):493–495.

111. Catena F, Nardo B, Liviano d'Arcangelo G, et al. De novo malignancies after organ transplantation. Transplant Proc 2001;33(1–2):1858–1859.

112. Valero JM, Rubio E, Moreno JM, Pons F, Sanchez-Turrion V, Cuervas-Mons V. De novo malignancies in liver transplantation. Transplant Proc 2003;35(2):709–711.

113. Dreno B. Skin cancers after transplantation. Nephrol Dial Transplant 2003;18(6):1052–1058.

114. Hancock SL, Tucker MA, Hoppe RT. Breast cancer after treatment of Hodgkin's disease. J Natl Cancer Inst 1993;85(1):25–31.

115. Tinger A, Wasserman TH, Klein EE, et al. The incidence of breast cancer following mantle field radiation therapy as a function of dose and technique. Int J Radiat Oncol Biol Phys 1997;37(4):865–870.

116. Hudson MM, Poquette CA, Lee J, et al. Increased mortality after successful treatment for Hodgkin's disease. J Clin Oncol 1998;16(11):3592–3600.

117. Wolden SL, Lamborn KR, Cleary SF, Tate DJ, Donaldson SS. Second cancers following pediatric Hodgkin's disease. J Clin Oncol 1998;16(2):536–544.

118. Dores GM, Metayer C, Curtis RE, et al. Second malignant neoplasms among long-term survivors of Hodgkin's disease: a population-based evaluation over 25 years. J Clin Oncol 2002;20(16):3484–3494.

18

Psychosocial Rehabilitation in Cancer Care

Richard P. McQuellon and Suzanne C. Danhauer

Prevalence data on psychosocial morbidity indicate that from 30% to 50% of cancer patients may experience distress significant enough to warrant professional intervention at some time during survivorship.[1,2] These patients may require professional attention to manage the debilitating effects of diagnosis, treatment, and morbidity that can wax and wane over time depending upon a host of other variables. It is in this group that some form of psychosocial rehabilitation may be useful.[3,4]

Psychosocial Rehabilitation in Cancer Care

The formal definition of rehabilitation is "the process by which physical, sensory and mental capacities are restored or developed in (for) people with disabling conditions."[5] This definition implies some type of disabling condition that requires rehabilitation. Not all cancer patients experience a disability and not all cancer patients require rehabilitation of any sort. The founders of cancer rehabilitation were physicians trained in rehabilitative medicine largely focused on physical needs of cancer patients with interdisciplinary teams.[6,7] The Oncology Nursing Society in 1989 defined cancer rehabilitation as "a process by which individuals within their environments are assisted to achieve optimal functioning within limits imposed by cancer."[8] Psychosocial rehabilitation in cancer care has a more specific focus than rehabilitation in general[9] and is often described by the broader term psychosocial intervention.

The diagnosis, treatment and survivorship of cancer often involves much more varied rehabilitation needs than those experienced following most other medical problems.[10] There are more than 100 cancer diagnoses that can elicit a multitude of psychosocial responses. Hence, there may be wide variability in the needs for rehabilitative intervention in the psychosocial area. For example, the patient with radical head and neck surgery left with significant disfiguration is very different than the early-stage breast cancer patient expected to have complete cure with no significant appearance alteration who may require minimal or no psychosocial intervention. The irony of this situation is that although we would expect one patient to experience intensive psychosocial distress and

the other not, depending upon a host of mediating variables (social support, natural resilience, effective communication with healthcare team, etc.), the outcome may be not what one would predict. This variability of psychosocial needs and experiences illustrates but one challenge for the psychosocial care of patients: How can patients who need and want services be identified?

The National Comprehensive Cancer Center Network has developed definitions and guidelines to help treat distressed cancer patients.[11] Distress has been defined as "a multifactorial, unpleasant experience of an emotional, psychological, social, or spiritual nature that interferes with the ability to cope with cancer, its physical symptoms, and its treatment. Distress extends along a continuum ranging from normal feelings of vulnerability, sadness and fear to disabling conditions such as clinical depression, anxiety, panic, isolation and existential or spiritual crisis" (p. 369). In the context of cancer care, the term psychosocial refers to the psychologic and social adaptation and reaction of the patient to the diagnosis of cancer, treatment, and survivorship.[12]

Scope of the Field

Psychosocial rehabilitation could include all psychosocial interventions that are designed to positively influence patient psychosocial adaptation and adjustment to diagnosis, treatment, and survivorship. For example, physical and occupational therapists play a significant role with patients undergoing debilitating treatment. To illustrate, bone marrow transplantation and cytoreductive surgery plus intraperitoneal hyperthermic chemotherapy often leave patients deconditioned physically and distressed psychologically.[13,14] Such patients might benefit significantly from a physical rehabilitation program without explicit emphasis on psychosocial care or intervention. An example of a physical rehabilitation program (walking) following bone marrow transplantation has been reported as effective.[15] Such interventions do not explicitly focus on psychologic outcomes with the use of targeted psychosocial interventions but may measure them as secondary endpoints. This chapter focuses primarily on randomized clinical trials specifically designed to address psychosocial deficits in patients that have been the result of initial diagnosis, treatment, and morbidities of treatment and survivorship.

Models for Understanding Psychosocial Rehabilitation

The biopsychosocial model of medical care is most useful in conceptualizing the rehabilitation of the patient with cancer and holds that health or illness outcomes are a consequence of the relationship between biologic, psychological, and social factors.[16,17] Both macro forces (e.g., culture–subculture, family) and micro forces (e.g., organ systems, cells) interact with the person to determine health outcomes. For example, attention to the psychologic and social aspects of a patient's life can direct attention to macro-level processes such as the existence of social support or the presence of a helpful caregiver. The presence or absence of caregiver support can interact with micro-level events (cellular disorders) such as anemia. Low hemoglobin may result in significant fatigue, mild depression, and/or waning social support associated with a failure to return to normal functioning following hematopoietic cell transplantation.[13] The biopsychosocial model takes account of both health and illness and provides the conceptual framework for understanding patient adaptation following rigorous medical treatments. In this situation, a biopsychosocial approach would direct providers to test for anemia and inquire about social support in the home, perhaps leading to both a medical (e.g., epoetin alpha injection) and a behavioral intervention (e.g., caregiver consultation).

The Kornblith Vulnerability Model of Psychosocial Adaptation of Cancer Survivors suggests that adaptation to cancer (psychologic, vocational, sexual, and social) and its treatment is influenced by a host of mediating variables, medical management of late effects, and psychosocial interventions[17] (Figure 18.1). Patients who adapt well will not need rehabilitation. It is likely that mediating variables such as the patient's communication with the medical team can have a powerful effect on the patient's need for psychosocial rehabilitation.[18] For example, the patient who is upset by the way the diagnosis was conveyed can experience debilitating anxiety and depressive symptoms that require psychologic intervention. Also, fear of recurrence, which is heightened by an obsessive-compulsive personality style, can hinder healthy adaptation.

Historical Perspective

One of the earliest studies to assess cancer rehabilitation needs identified 805 patients who were comparable to a national study sample.[19] This group was screened to identify (1) rehabilitation problems experienced with different cancer diagnoses; (2) need for rehabilitation services; and (3) significant gaps in the delivery of rehabilitation care. Psychologic problems were found to be fairly common and appeared to be more severe in patients with concomitant physical disabilities. The percentage of patients with psychologic problems varied from a low of 30% in patients with bladder cancer to a high of 78% in patients with central nervous system tumors. The authors concluded that psychologic and physical rehabilitation problems were common in patients with most cancer diagnoses and that many of these problems would likely be amenable to therapeutic intervention. However, at the time of the study there were many barriers to optimal rehabilitative care.

Over a decade ago, Ivan Barofsky provided an eloquent description of the status of psychosocial research in the rehabilitation of the cancer patient.[20] A basic assumption in the literature is that the patient sustains some type of loss (physical, psychologic, social). Rehabilitation involves an attempt to restore the person to previous functioning. The definition of rehabilitation implies that restoration is possible; how and if restoration can occur becomes the fundamental issue in rehabilitation research.

Much of the research on the psychosocial dimension of cancer care involves the management of anxiety and depressive symptoms as well as distress, a term favored by many researchers because it is less stigmatizing. Not all patients with cancer need psychosocial rehabilitation in the form of a systematic intervention delivered by a professional. However,

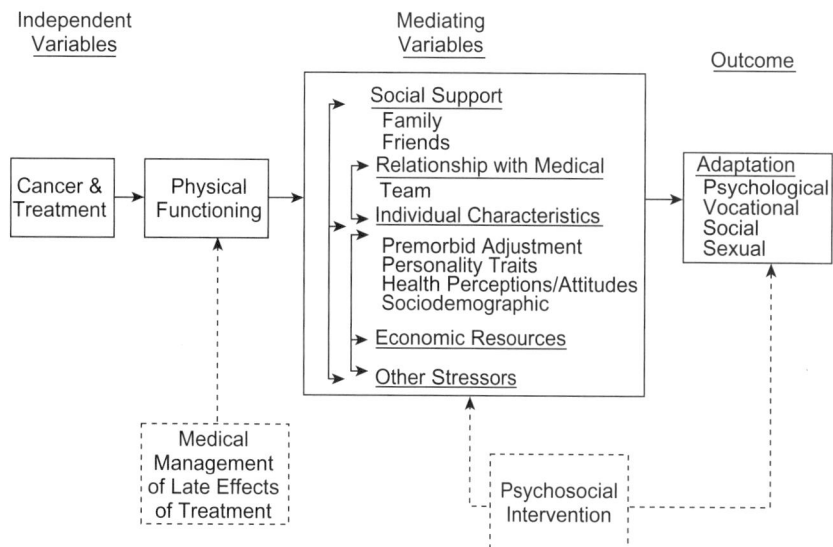

FIGURE 18.1. Kornblith vulnerability model. (From Kornblith,[17] by permission of Oxford University Press.)

it is likely that all patients will require a time period to be restored to normal functioning following the diagnosis and treatment of their illness. Moreover, the psychosocial rehabilitative process is further complicated by the fact that the treatment of cancer is rarely a single event but often consists of a series of different treatments over time.

The most economical approach may be to assume that a certain percentage of patients will develop psychosocial distress over the course of diagnosis, treatment, and survivorship. Some patients may be more or less vulnerable depending upon a host of individual factors.[21] Some researchers have proposed a screening process early in treatment to detect those experiencing abnormal levels of distress[22,23] to be targeted for interventions.

Systematic Reviews and Meta-Analyses of Psychosocial Interventions

There are a number of excellent reviews[24–26] as well as meta-analyses[27–29] of the effects of psychosocial interventions in cancer care. Newell and colleagues[24] conducted a comprehensive, systematic review and analysis of psychologic therapies for cancer patients. They identified 627 relevant papers that reported on 329 intervention trials. More specifically, they identified 34 trials with psychosocial outcomes. These trials were aimed at reducing patient anxiety or depression or at improving functional ability (e.g., overall quality of life) or the interpersonal relationships of patients. The authors applied a rigorous criteria of evidence that has been established by the Cochrane Collaboration.[30] The Cochrane Collaboration recommends that randomized trials should be assessed on 10 methodologic quality indicators that specify whether potential threats to the trial's internal validity have been adequately controlled. Largely due to the failure of nearly all trials to gain a good rating based on this assessment, the authors' recommendations for psychological therapies are somewhat guarded. This review applied the most rigorous standards for evidence and, unfortunately, only one trial evaluated achieved a quality rating of good for its methodology. This study, a pilot project on reducing patient anxiety,[31] was followed by a larger RCT with a similar methodology[32] that was not reported in the review. The dearth of findings suggests that the evidence supporting the effectiveness of psychological therapies with cancer patients needs further development.

The authors used a method they term "decision process" to analyze the results and to produce recommendations for or against each intervention strategy. This method of analysis

resulted in the following five outcome recommendations: (1) strong recommendation for the intervention strategy, (2) a tentative recommendation for it, (3) a tentative recommendation against it, (4) a strong recommendation against it, or (5) no recommendation for or against it. With regard to patient anxiety, the authors concluded that music therapy can be tentatively recommended for reducing a patient's anxiety levels. Additionally, a number of therapist-delivered interventions (e.g., individual therapy, cognitive behavior therapy, communication skills training, guided imagery, and self-practice of a cognitive intervention) warrant further exploration before a recommendation for or against their use can be made. The authors concluded that no intervention strategy reviewed could be recommended for reducing a patient's levels of depression. However, group therapy, education, structured counseling, cognitive behavior therapy, communication skills training, and self esteem building warrant further assessment before recommendation either for or against could be made.

A widely cited meta-analysis by Meyer and Mark yielded a more positive conclusion regarding psychosocial interventions.[27] They identified 45 studies that reported 62 treatment–control comparisons. This sample of studies included only published randomized experiments conducted on adult cancer patients receiving a psychosocial, behavioral, or psychoeducational intervention. Five categories of dependent measures were developed in this analysis: (1) emotional adjustment, (2) functional adjustment, (3) treatment or disease-related symptoms, (4) medical measures category, and (5) global measures, which combine core aspects of more than one of the preceding categories. The results and effect sizes reported by Meyer and Mark are shown in Table 18.1.

While all five of the categories of dependent measures have relevance for psychosocial rehabilitation, it is emotional adjustment that is most relevant to this chapter. The overall average effect size was 0.31 (95% confidence interval defined by –0.13 ~ 0.31 ~ 0.75), for emotional adjustment, was recorded. A score in the 0.20 to 0.40 range is considered typical of effective psychologic interventions. The authors were cautious in their conclusions, particularly because the studies included in their meta-analysis were made up predominantly of white women from the United States. It is difficult to know just to what extent the results of these studies can be generalized to the broader population. A further limitation of Meyer and Mark's study was that they grouped all psychological therapies (in this case five different categories) into one and further reduced all possible outcomes increasing overall sample size and thereby the chance of significant findings.

Another meta-analysis of studies examined the effects of psychosocial interventions on quality of life in adult cancer

TABLE 18.1. Weighted effect sizes for dependent measure categories.

Measure	Studies	Comparisons	Total N	d	d 95% CI
Emotional Adjustment	41	56	2,840	0.24	0.17/0.32
Functional Adjustment	16	21	940	0.19	0.06/0.32
Treatment- and disease-related symptoms	28	39	1,606	0.26	0.16/0.37
Medical	5	7	232	0.17	0.10/0.44
Compound and global	5	7	373	0.28	0.08/0.49

CI, confidence interval; d, weighted average effect sizes.

Source: Data from Meyer and Mark.[27]

patients.[33] The stated hypothesis was that cancer patients treated with adjuvant psychosocial intervention experienced a higher level of subjective quality of life (QOL) compared to those without additional psychosocial intervention. The authors identified 37 studies that included a total of 3,120 cancer patients. The overall effect size on QOL in this study was 0.31 [95% confidence interval (CI), $0.13 \leq 0.31 \leq 0.75$]. The authors concluded that psychosocial interventions have a positive impact on quality of life in adult cancer patients, and the effect was moderated by duration of treatment, suggesting that psychosocial interventions should be planned for at least 12 weeks.

A study of psychological interventions for patients with symptoms of anxiety and depression has particular relevance for this chapter.[28] In this study, two meta-analyses were conducted with anxiety and depression examined as separate outcome measures. Even though the majority of trials included in the analysis were preventive (i.e., not targeted to patients with identified abnormal symptoms of anxiety or depression), these studies can shed some light on the rehabilitation process. Nineteen trials on anxiety had a combined effect size of 0.42 favoring treatment against "no treatment controls" (95% CI, 0.08–0.74; $n = 1,023$). Twenty trials on depression had a combined effect size of 0.36 as well, favoring the treatment (95% CI, 0.06–0.66; $n = 1,101$). Four trials focusing on patients who were identified as "at risk" had particularly significant effects, suggesting that targeted interventions were more likely to demonstrate beneficial effects. However, the mean effect size for depression was weak to negligible (0.19), prompting the authors to state that preventive psychological interventions with cancer patients may have a moderate effect on anxiety but little effect on depression. The authors concluded that resources should be directed toward those patients demonstrating psychological or psychosocial deficits, and that group therapy trials appear to be equally effective relative to individual interventions and are likely more economical. Finally, relatively short, intensive interventions delivered by more-experienced counselors appear to be more effective than interventions delivered by less-experienced counselors over a long period of time.

Measurement Tools in Psychosocial Rehabilitation

A number of assessment tools are widely used by researchers and clinicians for examining the psychosocial impact of cancer and its treatment as well as the impact of psychosocial interventions on patient functioning. These tools include measures of general mood (e.g., Profile of Mood States, Positive and Negative Affect Scale), depression (e.g., Center for Epidemiologic Studies Depression, Beck Depression Inventory, Hamilton Depression Inventory), anxiety (e.g., State-Trait Anxiety Inventory), and general mental health symptoms (e.g., Brief Symptom Inventory).[22] These instruments have been used largely because of their psychometric properties and ease of administration.

The interest in overall patient QOL has spawned the Functional Assessment of Cancer Therapy (FACT) and the European Organization for Research and Treatment of Cancer (EORTC) questionnaires. These instruments include modules that measure symptoms of specific cancers or characteristics

of treatment situations (e.g., bone marrow transplantation). For example, the FACT includes many disease site-related subscales (breast, colon, brain, etc.)[34,35] and treatment- or symptom-related modules (bone marrow transplantation, etc.).[36–38] The SF-36 has also been used in the assessment of cancer patients because it provides normative values for the nonmedical patient population;[39] this allows for comparison of patients undergoing treatment with normative samples in the U.S. adult population. Such comparisons can be helpful when patients ask what they might expect in terms of healthy functioning following specific treatments.[40–42] These instruments have been particularly useful as they allow for comparisons over time because of their sensitivity to change. Thus, one would be able to look at baseline levels of emotional well-being with the FACT or mental health functioning on the EORTC and compare these with posttreatment functioning in longitudinal studies. These instruments, however, were not developed with the intent of measuring outcomes of psychosocial rehabilitation following cancer treatment.

In contrast, the Cancer Rehabilitation Evaluation System (CARES) allows patients to identify problems and to indicate with which problems they want help.[43] For example, one item on the CARES reads something like the following, "I have difficulty doing physical activity such as running." Patients are asked to answer on a 5-point scale from "not at all" to "very much" and then to indicate "yes" or "no" to the question, "Do you want help?" The 139 items on the CARES cover nearly every conceivable problem situation. It has been used in a number of studies attempting to assess rehabilitation needs and success in patients.[44–46] Because of the depth of coverage of items in the CARES, it is not typically used in clinical trials where the emphasis must necessarily be on rapid assessment and fewer items, but one of the most significant strengths of the CARES is that it directs patients to identify problems (including psychosocial problems) that they want to address. This coverage can be very useful to providers trying to focus scarce resources, because as few as one-third of patients actually are interested in a counseling intervention[47] even though a significant number of cancer patients may experience psychosocial distress.[1]

Randomized Controlled Trials

We systematically searched Pub Med and PsychInfo with the following descriptors: psychosocial rehabilitation and cancer, psychosocial intervention and cancer, psychological intervention and cancer, and behavioral intervention and cancer. After compiling this list we also looked for relevant studies in the reference sections of studies identified in the searches. We selected studies based on two criteria: (1) for the most part, the intervention was targeted toward a current or anticipated need or deficit exhibited by the patient (e.g., high distress, anxiety, or depression); and (2) assignment to treatment was made randomly. We have selected representative studies that provide evidence for the effectiveness of psychosocial interventions in modifying and potentially improving outcomes for patients in the psychological and social domains. The studies reviewed, including caregiver studies, are summarized in Table 18.2.

TABLE 18.2. Randomized control trials.

Reference	Year	n/dx	Intervention/source/duration	Measures/timing	Outcomes
Gordon et al.[48]	1980	217/Breast = 71 Lung = 37 Melanoma = 109	Three interventions: (1) patient education re: how to live with disease; (2) general counseling; (3) environmental manipulation, e.g., consultation with other professionals vs. usual care/a single oncology counselor Average of 11 20-minute sessions	Problems (number, intensity severity); MAACL; LPIS; SREs; HLC; ADL (modified version); API. Hospital admit., hosp. d/c, 3 and 6 months post d/c.	Intervention group showed improvement of some problems, more rapid decline of neg. affect, more realistic outlook, return to previous vocational status and more active pattern of time usage.
Cheung et al.[49]	2003	59/Colorectal	Progressive muscle relaxation training (PMRT) vs. standard care/therapist and audiotape/two face-to-face teaching sessions before intervention of listening to tape Two to three times/1-week interval period	STAI; QOL-Colostomy; WHO QOL measure abbreviated version (all instruments Chinese version for Chinese population). Within 1 week of surgery, week 5, and week 10 postsurgery.	Reduced state anxiety; no significant difference between groups over time on disease-specific QOL; both groups improved with time. Improved general QOL for experimental group.
Mishel et al.[51]	2002	239/Prostate	Three intervention groups: uncertainty management direct, uncertainty management supplemented (family support person received phone call also), and control/trained nurse Eight consecutive weekly phone calls	Mishel Uncertainty in Illness scale, Self-Control scale (problem solving and cognitive reframing subscales), the Symptom distress scale, and two study specific measures, i.e., the Cancer Knowledge Scale and a measure of patient–provider communication. Baseline, 4 and 7 months.	Improvement in cognitive reframing and problem solving at 4 mos. for intervention groups; decrease in symptom intensity for all groups, no difference by intervention. Impact of impotence was modified for some in intervention group. Some differences between African-Americans and Caucasians described.
Lepore et al.[52]	2003	250/prostate	Three groups: group education (GE); group education + discussion (GED); usual care control/content experts, i.e., oncologist, urologist, etc. Six weekly 1-hour sessions	Prostate cancer knowledge; ratings of lectures; health behavior index; SF-36; CES-D; UCLA Prostate Cancer Index. Baseline, 2 weeks, 6 months, and 12 months.	Both interventions increased prostate ca. knowledge. GED group had fewer sexual problems than controls. Among noncollege graduates, GED and GE results in better physical functioning than controls and GED resulted in more positive health behaviors. No differences in these variables for college graduates.
Goodwin et al.[53]	2001	235/breast	Two groups: supportive expressive group therapy or usual care control/two professional counselors Weekly group sessions of 90 minutes for 1 year	POMS; LASA pain; EORTC-QLQ-30; Survival. Baseline, 4, 8, and 12 months.	No increased survival; improved mood and reduced pain for intervention group.
Molassiotis et al.[55]	2002	71/breast	Two groups: progressive muscle relaxation training, including individual audiocassettes and 30-minute video training program or control/therapist trained in PMRT Thirty-minute sessions daily beginning 1 hour before chemotherapy and for 6 days following	POMS; STAI; MANE; Karnofsky Performance Index/baseline (POMS, STAI, Karnofsky). At 7 and 14 days postchemotherapy (MANE).	Significant decrease in duration and trend toward lower frequency of N/V in intervention group; significant decrease in total mood disturbance.

TABLE 18.2. Randomized control trials. (*continued*)

Reference	Year	n/dx	Intervention/source/duration	Measures/timing	Outcomes
McArdle et al.[56]	1996	272/breast	Three groups: support from breast care nurse; support from voluntary organization; support from both nurse and organization; routine care control/breast care nurse and Tak Tent (Take Care) volunteer organization Variable	GHQ; HADS. First postoperative visit, 3, 6, and 12 months.	Psychological morbidity fell for all groups over 12 months. Compared to other groups, support from breast care nurse resulted in significant declines in depression, anxiety, and insomnia.
Winzelberg et al.[57]	2003	72/breast	Two groups: internet-based social support group with moderator; wait-list control health care professional Twelve weeks	CES-D, PCL-C, STAI, PSS, Cancer Behavior Inventory, Mini-MAC. Baseline (before randomization), post termination of group session.	Significantly greater decreases in depression, cancer-related trauma, and perceived stress in intervention compared to control group.
Helgeson et al.[58]	2001	312/ breast	Four groups: education; peer discussion; education + peer discussion; control/ facilitators and content experts Eight weekly 45-minute sessions	SF-36/six assessments. Baseline (after diagnosis, before randomization). Time 6 was mean 3.6 years postdiagnosis.	Long-term follow-up (mean, 3.6 years): higher vitality and physical functioning and lower bodily pain in education group. No long-term benefits on health-related QOL in peer discussion or education + peer discussion groups.
Antoni et al.[59]	2001	100/ breast	Two groups: cognitive-behavioral stress management group (intervention) and seminar (control)/postdoctoral fellows and graduate students Ten weekly 2-hour sessions (intervention) and 1 day (control)	POMS-SF; CES-D; IES; LOT-R; novel measures of perceived benefits and emotional processing. Baseline; postintervention; 3 and 9 months postintervention.	No overall effects of intervention on distress for intervention group; however, reduced depressive symptoms for those with higher depressive symptoms at baseline. Intervention group increased in benefit finding and optimism, particularly those with lower scores at baseline.
Edelman et al.[60]	1999	121/ breast	Two groups: cognitive-behavioral group intervention; control group/professional therapists Twelve 2-hour sessions	POMS; Coopersmith Self-Esteem Inventory; Survival. Baseline, immediately postintervention, and 3, 6, and 12 months postintervention.	Reduced depression and total mood and disturbance and increased self-esteem in intervention compared to control group. No group differences at 3- or 6-month follow-up. No survival effects.
Fukui et al.[61]	2000	50/ breast	Two groups: cognitive-behavioral therapy group; wait-list control group/ one psychologist and one psychiatrist Six weekly 90-minute sessions	POMS; MAC; HADS Baseline, 6 weeks (postintervention), and 6 months.	Significant decreases in anxiety and depression for tx group but no group differences for these outcomes. Tx group had lower mood disturbance, greater vigor, and greater fighting spirit at both follow-ups compared to control group.
Edmonds et al.[62]	1999	66/ breast	Two groups: psychological intervention, (supportive therapy + cognitive-behavioral techniques); control group (received information on coping and relaxation audio tapes)/ trained therapists Weekly 2-hour sessions for 35 weeks + one weekend	POMS; POMS-SF; FLIC; MAC; RED; DUFSS; RED; M-C. Baseline, 4, 8, and 14 months.	No group differences for mood, QOL, social support, or repression. In intervention group, greater anxious preoccupation and less helplessness; no survival effects.

TABLE 18.2. Randomized control trials. (*continued*)

Reference	Year	n/dx	Intervention/source/duration	Measures/timing	Outcomes
Classen et al.[63]	2001	125/ breast	Two groups: supportive-expressive group + educational materials; educational materials only (control)/a psychiatrist, psychologists, and social workers Weekly 90-minute sessions for 1 year	POMS; IES. Baseline, every 4 months for 1 year, every 6 months thereafter.	Greater decline in traumatic stress symptoms for intervention group but no group difference for mood at 1 year. When data excluded in year preceding death, mood disturbance and traumatic stress symptoms declined more for treatment group.
Bultz et al.[64]	2000	36 breast cancer partners	Two groups: psychoeducational and control/cofacilitated by two psychologists Six weekly 1.5- to 2-hour sessions	POMS; Index of Marital Satisfaction; DUFSS; MAC. Pre- and postintervention, 3 months postintervention.	Partners in intervention group had less mood disturbance than controls 3 months post-intervention. Women whose partners received the intervention reported less mood disturbance, and greater confidant support and marital satisfaction.
Toseland et al.[65]	1995	40 cancer patients and spouses	Two groups: intervention (support, problem-solving, coping skills) and usual treatment (control)/experienced oncology social worker Six 1-hour sessions with patient's spouse	For caregivers: CES-D; STAI; Dyadic Adjustment Scale; Social Functioning Subscale from Health & Daily Living Form; SF-20; Zarit Burden Inventory; Help-Seeking Coping Index; Index of Coping Responses; Pressing problems (cancer caregiving); drug/EtOh use; Personal Change Scale. For patients: FLIC; ECOG Global Performance Scale. Baseline, postintervention.	No significant between-group differences found for any measures. Intervention appeared to be effective only for distressed subsample of caregivers.

n/dx, number of patients/diagnosis; MAACL, Multiple Affect Adjective Checklist—state form; LPIS, Langer Psychiatric Impairment Scale; SRE, Schedule of recent events; HLC, Health Locus of Control; ADL, activities of daily living; ADPI, Activity Pattern Indicators; STAI, State-Trait Anxiety inventory; QOL, quality of life; WHO, World Health Organization; SF-36, Short Form 36 (Rand Medical Outcomes Study); CES-D, Center for Epidemiologic Studies–Depression scale; POMS, Profile of Mood States; LASA, Linear Analog Scale Assessment; EORTC-QLQ-30, European Organization for Research and Treatment of Cancer—Quality of Life Questionnaire–30; PMRT, progressive muscle relaxation training; MANE, Morrow Assessment of Nausea and Emesis; GHQ, General Health Questionnaire; HADS, Hospital Anxiety and Depression Scale; PCL-C, posttraumatic stress disorder (PTSD) Checklist—Civilian Version; PSS, Perceived Stress Scale; Mini-MAC, mini-mental adjustment to cancer scale; SF-36, Medical Outcomes Study Short-Form 36; SF-20, Medical Outcomes Study—20; IES, Impact of Events Scale; LOT-R, Life Orientation Test–Revised; MAC, Mental Adjustment to Cancer Scale; FLIC, Functional Living Index for Cancer; ECOG, Eastern Cooperative Oncology Group performance status scale; DUFSS, Duke-UNC Functional Social Support Questionnaire; RED, Rationality/Emotional Defensiveness Scale; M-C, Marlowe Crowne Social Desirability Scale; N/V, nausea/vomiting.

In one of the earliest randomized clinical trials measuring the efficacy of a psychosocial intervention, cancer patients with diagnoses of breast or lung cancer or melanoma were studied.[48] The intervention group (n = 157) was given one of three types of psychosocial intervention: (1) patient education about how to live with the disease effectively; (2) a more generic counseling intervention focusing on patients' reactions to and feelings about their disease; and (3) environmental manipulation, including consultations with other healthcare personnel and referral for additional services as necessary. The control group (n = 151) received usual care and evaluations only. The most notable effects of the intervention included amelioration of psychosocial problems reported by the patient, a more-rapid decline of negative affect (anxiety, hostility, and depression), a more realistic outlook on life, a greater proportion of return to previous vocational status, and a more-active pattern of time usage.

Another study examined the effect of progressive muscle relaxation training (PMRT) on anxiety and quality of life following stoma surgery in Chinese colorectal cancer patients.[49] Subjects were randomly assigned to a control group (n = 30) and the experimental group utilizing PMRT (n = 29). This procedure significantly decreased state anxiety and improved overall quality of life in the experimental group. These findings are notable particularly because patient baseline state anxiety scores were higher than reported norms.[50] Thus, this sample would constitute one that needed psychosocial rehabilitation, assuming that premorbid state anxiety was lower than that reported at baseline here.

In a unique study with prostate cancer patients, Mishel et al. examined effects of a nurse-delivered psychoeducational intervention over the telephone in helping patients to manage uncertainty and treatment side effects.[51] A total of 239 men were randomly assigned to one of the three treatment conditions: (1) uncertainty management with the patient, (2) uncertainty management with the patient and a family member (supplemented group), and (3) the control group. The intervention consisted of eight weekly telephone calls by a nurse who was trained in this specific intervention. Patients in each of the two treatment groups (individual or supplemented) received the same intervention. However, in the supplemented group, a spouse or designated significant other from the family also received a weekly telephone call and a similar intervention was applied. The majority of intervention effects were seen at 4 months after baseline, a time when treatment side effects were also most intense. Both uncertainty management approaches were useful in producing cognitive reframing and problem solving. When both individual and supplemented intervention groups were combined for analysis, there was measured improvement in control of incontinence at the 4-month assessment. Furthermore, the negative impact of impotence could be modified for some of the men who had received the intervention. This study represents an economical and convenient intervention in a population with significant morbidity, particularly in terms of sexual functioning and incontinence following treatment for localized prostate cancer. The telephone intervention method is also portable and has great potential for psychosocial interventions with cancer patients.

Lepore et al. attempted to improve the QOL of men recently treated for prostate cancer.[52] Two hundred and fifty patients were randomly assigned to a control group, a group education intervention (GE), or a group education-plus-discussion intervention (GED). Both GE and GED increased prostate cancer knowledge. In the year following the intervention, men in the GED condition were less bothered by sexual problems than men in the control condition, and they were more likely to remain steadily employed than men in the GE or control conditions. Both the Mishel and Lepore studies support the idea that relatively straightforward interventions can be useful for improving psychosocial functioning in prostate cancer patients.

Breast Cancer Studies

Breast cancer patients are the most extensively studied group in randomized clinical trials conducted in the area of psychosocial rehabilitation (see also Chapter 11). The literature is extensive, and we only cite representative studies here. There is an excellent review of health-related QOL (HRQOL) results that does include 20 studies with psychosocial outcomes in breast cancer.[53]

In a study of women with newly diagnosed breast cancer (n = 96) about to begin chemotherapy, patients were randomized to an intervention (standard care plus relaxation training and imagery) or to a control condition (standard care only).[54] The goal of this study was to develop and evaluate a simple and easily administered intervention to help women cope with the diagnosis and treatment of breast cancer. Those in the intervention group practiced relaxation and imagery daily for the 18 weeks of their chemotherapy. No significant between-group differences were noted for anxiety and depression. Using intention-to-treat analyses, between-group effects were found with women in the intervention group reporting fewer psychologic symptoms and higher quality of life during chemotherapy.

Molassiotis and colleagues assessed the effectiveness of progressive muscle relaxation training (PMRT) in the management of chemotherapy-related nausea and vomiting, mood disturbance and anxiety.[55] Women diagnosed with nonmetastatic breast cancer (n = 71) were randomized to the PMRT intervention or to a control condition. The PMRT intervention was administered by a trained therapist six times for 30 minutes before receiving chemotherapy. The total mood disturbance score of the POMS decreased in the intervention group and increased in the control group when assessed at 7 and 14 days postintervention. No between-group differences were observed for POMS subscales or for anxiety.

McArdle et al. examined the effects of support from a nurse specialist and from a volunteer support organization in breast cancer.[56] Women under 70 years of age diagnosed with breast cancer (n = 272) were randomized to one of four groups before undergoing surgery for breast cancer: (1) standard support from ward staff and information booklet; (2) standard support from ward staff plus support from a specialist breast care nurse; (3) standard support from ward staff plus support from a voluntary organization (included any combination of information, counseling, and group meetings); and (4) standard support from ward staff plus support from a specialist breast care nurse and from a voluntary organization. Individuals in the treatment group receiving support mainly from the nurse specialist reported improved depressive symptoms, anxiety symptoms, somatic symptoms, and social dysfunction compared to all other groups, including the group that had support from *both* the nurse specialist and the voluntary organization.

Another RCT employed a newer technologic approach to providing psychosocial support to women with breast cancer.[57] Women with breast cancer (n = 72) were randomly assigned to a 12-week internet-based social support group moderated by a healthcare professional or to a wait-list control group. Participants in the intervention group reported significantly decreased depressive symptoms, cancer-related traumatic stress, and perceived overall stress when compared to the control group. No changes were found for anxiety or coping measures.

Helgeson and colleagues examined the long-term effects of participation in a psychosocial group intervention on health-related quality of life (measured with the SF-36)[58] in which 312 women with early-stage breast cancer were randomly assigned to one of four conditions: education, peer discussion, education plus peer discussion, and control. The length of the intervention was 8 weeks with participants meeting once each week. The education group focused on the provision of information to enhance sense of control while the peer discussion group focused on the expression of feelings and self-disclosure. Intent-to-treat analysis was used in this study. Follow-up with those who had no recurrent disease at 3 years revealed that the women in the education-only group retained higher levels of vitality (energy and lack of fatigue) and physical functioning and lower bodily pain than women in the control group. No benefits of the peer discussion group or the education plus peer discussion group were observed at 3-year follow-up.

Antoni et al. examined distress as well as positive outcomes in women who had recently been treated for early-stage breast cancer.[59] Patients were randomly assigned to take part in a 10-week cognitive-behavioral stress management intervention (met weekly for 2 hours over 10 weeks) or to a more-limited control condition (1-day informational seminar). Findings showed that while there were no overall effects of the intervention on measures of distress, participation in the 10-week intervention reduced the prevalence of moderate depressive symptoms for those whose levels were higher at baseline. Also, benefit-finding and optimism increased for those taking part in the intervention, with the effects most pronounced in women with low baseline scores. Findings from this study underscore the notion that psychosocial rehabilitation is most likely to be useful for those patients who report the most psychosocial distress and/or the least psychosocial resources.

In a study with metastatic breast cancer patients, 124 patients were randomized to take part in a group cognitive behavioral therapy (CBT) intervention or to a no-therapy control group condition.[60] Participants in the CBT group attended eight weekly group sessions, followed by a family night and three additional monthly sessions. Immediately following participation in the CBT group, data indicated significant improvements in depression, total mood disturbance, and self-esteem. However, no significant differences between the CBT and control groups were evident at 3- or 6-month follow-up.

A similar study of a short-term psychosocial intervention was conducted with lymph node-positive breast cancer patients in Japan.[61] Patients (n = 50) were randomized to a 6-week structured psychosocial group intervention (included health education, coping skills training, stress management, and support) or to a wait-list control group. Analyses were conducted on the 46 women who completed the intervention. Anxiety and depression decreased significantly over the course of the study for the treatment group; however, no significant between-group differences emerged for these outcomes. Significant between-group differences were found for POMS total mood disturbance score at both the 6-week (immediately following the intervention) and 6-month assessments. The experimental group had significantly lower scores than the controls for total mood disturbance and significantly higher scores for vigor on the POMS, and significantly higher scores for fighting spirit on the MAC at the end of the 6-week intervention. These improvements were sustained over 6 months of follow-up.

Several of the previously described studies demonstrated that short-term psychosocial interventions resulted in improvement in quality of life and psychosocial distress. There has been little evidence, however, for the efficacy of longer-term psychosocial interventions. In a study of longer duration, patients with metastatic breast cancer were randomized to an 8-month weekly psychologic intervention (n = 36; group discussion, emotional support, coping skills training, and relaxation) or to a control group (n = 30; received information on coping and relaxation audio tapes).[62] Study outcomes included mood, quality of life, and adjustment to cancer measured at baseline, 4 months, 8 months, and 14 months. Participation in the long-term psychologic intervention did not result in significantly improved mood or quality of life in comparison to those in the control group, although there were short-term clinical gains reported by therapists that were not quantified.

A group of 125 metastatic breast cancer patients was randomized to a 1-year weekly supportive-expressive group psychotherapy intervention with additional educational materials or to a control group offered only educational materials.[63] Data from all participants who completed at least one follow-up assessment (n = 102) regardless of level of group attendance were included in study analyses. Women in the group intervention reported a significantly greater decline in traumatic stress symptoms at 1 year, but no difference in overall mood when compared with women randomized to

the control condition. However, when data from final assessments that took place during the year before participants' deaths were excluded, both mood disturbance and traumatic stress symptoms declined significantly more for those in the treatment compared to the control condition.

Caregiver Studies

The patient has long been the primary focus for psychosocial rehabilitation or psychosocial interventions. However, the diagnosis and treatment of cancer can have far-reaching effects, evoking distress and feelings of helplessness in spouses/partners and other close family members. Role transitions in spousal and family relationships are often required. Relatively few interventions and even fewer RCTs to date have focused on psychosocial rehabilitation issues in close family members of cancer patients. The following several studies are representative examples of high-quality research that has sought to empirically validate methods for helping family members increase their understanding of cancer and treatment, normalize their responses to a loved one's cancer, and provide a safe place for relatives to express emotional distress.

One RCT examined the effects of a brief psychoeducational support group intervention for male partners of women with early-stage breast cancer (n = 36 pairs).[64] The intervention was offered to partners of breast cancer patients weekly for six sessions by two experienced psychologists and focused on two primary components: education and support. Results indicated that total mood disturbance score had improved by 3-month follow-up for both patients and partners who in the intervention group; however, these findings did not reach statistical significance.

Another RCT offered a six-session intervention to spouses (n = 40 male, n = 40 female) of patients with various types of cancer.[65] Spouses were randomly assigned to the intervention that included support, problem-solving, and coping skills or to a usual care condition. At baseline and within 2 weeks of completing the intervention, spousal caregivers completed measures of depression, anxiety, marital satisfaction, social support, health status, burden, help-seeking behavior, coping (perceived stressfulness of 17 cancer-related caregiving problems), and drug/alcohol use. At the same time points, patients completed measures of functional and physical status. Taking part in the group did not significantly improve any of the psychosocial outcomes for those in the intervention versus the control group. However, post hoc subgroup analyses revealed that for those caregivers who were more distressed at baseline (lower marital satisfaction, higher burden), greater improvements were found in the intervention group compared to the control group. This type of result, once again, highlights the usefulness of targeting psychosocial rehabilitation interventions to those individuals most in need of them.

Rehabilitation Programs

A number of programs have been developed and tested over the past 15 years directed at psychosocial care of patients.[66-68] Examples of such programs include Gilda's House, The Wellness Community, and the Commonweal Help Program. Even though there are programs for posttreatment cancer survivors that have a psychosocial component (e.g., the posttreatment resource center at Memorial Sloan Kettering Cancer Center), there is a need for dissemination of research outcomes so that programs can integrate evidence-based rehabilitation strategies. Additionally, specific programs have been developed to attend to particular difficulties of patients.

In a review article, Ronson and Body described the psychosocial rehabilitation of cancer patients after curative therapy.[69] They reported that even though the majority of cancer survivors do quite well, there is a substantial minority of patients who have significant psychosocial distress and/or psychiatric disturbance. A number of factors seem to predict psychosocial difficulty or adjustment, including a past history of psychiatric disturbance (especially depression), comorbid physical problems, poor social support, low social or economic status, and individual psychologic factors (including certain coping styles and personality traits). An important observation they make is that "no effective psychosocial rehabilitation can be achieved without simultaneous efforts to promote improvement of the physical condition." Physical and psychosocial functioning may be so closely related that it is impossible to talk about one without reference to the other. It is safe to say that patients returning to predisease physical functioning are less likely to experience severe psychosocial distress, although this cannot be stated with 100% certainty. Under the best of conditions, when patients return to health, fear and anxiety can act to rob the patient of the present when a feared future looms ahead in the form of recurrent disease.

Specific psychologic disorders and symptom entities that were summarized from the literature by Ronson and Body with estimated prevalence rates were posttraumatic stress disorder (as high as 14% to 21%), fear of recurrence (ranging from 10% to 89%), conditioned nausea/vomiting (no estimates given; highly dependent on emetogenic potential of chemotherapy and antiemetic agents used), treatment-related body image disturbances (no estimates given; related to area of surgery, timing of assessment, and premorbid functioning), and general psychosocial functioning (ranging from 18% to 40% depending on tumor type and treatment). They also identified aspects of physical functioning that have a psychosocial impact. Although attention to the literature on physical functioning is beyond the scope of this paper, it is important that the reciprocal relationship between physical and psychosocial functioning in general be understood, as well as the psychosocial issues related to specific tumor types and their treatment.

There are few randomized prospective studies of rehabilitation programs described in the literature. One such study is the "Starting Again Group Rehabilitation Program"[67] that enrolled a total of 199 patients (n = 98 intervention; n = 101 control) in the program. The intervention (called the "Starting Again Program") consisted of eleven 2-hour sessions that emphasized physical training, information, and coping skills. Outcomes that improved following the intervention included appraisal of having received sufficient information, physical strength, and fighting spirit. The psychosocial area of this study consisted of coping skills training and role playing (employed to help study participants understand the issues of returning to work, as well as problem situations that may

arise with return medical appointments). One session devoted to anxiety management included coping strategies such as relaxation, distraction, and cognitive techniques. Depressive symptoms for program participants diminished significantly over time. The authors pointed out that the study included patients at low risk for psychosocial disturbance, thereby making it more difficult to measure appreciable change. Furthermore, spontaneous recovery is common for those experiencing psychosocial morbidity in low-risk patients, and it would be difficult for an intervention to achieve superior results under these circumstances. In other words, many people simply improve with time with regard to sadness and depressive symptoms related to the diagnosis and treatment of cancer.

The Tapestry Program is an example of a novel method for providing psychosocial support for persons living with cancer.[68] It consists of a 5-day residential retreat program focusing on the following areas: creating a safe environment for patients, providing a daily narrative group, the use of arts and medicine therapy, providing yoga and meditation sessions, discussions about complementary therapies and pain control, death and dying, and use of rituals to foster a supportive collegial atmosphere. A primary method within this group involves general support provided by patients undergoing similar difficulties together. The Tapestry group has attempted to measure patient improvement following participation in the program with pre- and posttest measures that generally favor the impact of this program. There have been other promising reports of the effectiveness of these types of programs.[70]

Returning to Normal

Returning to "normal" is a prominent theme in the clinical care of patients. Although there has been some work in this area,[71] there is little research on returning to normal from a psychosocial standpoint only. Indeed, some patients comment that "things will never be normal again," because the issue of recurrence is always present even after a declaration of survival at the 5-year posttreatment time point. However, although some patients may carry a constant sense of foreboding and worry about cancer recurring, others may claim not only a return to normality but a deeper appreciation for life.[72–74] Such patients not only return to normal but actually find some benefits and, perhaps, improved psychosocial functioning in the form of deeper appreciation and meaning in everyday living. This finding has been incidental, although researchers are now focusing more on benefits that patients experience following a cancer diagnosis and treatment.[74] Typically, such benefit finding is in the area attitudinal shifts and/or improved social relations. For example, one attitudinal shift might be reflected in a change of career or a change of work habits in the direction of increasing time with family or friends as a consequence of recognition of mortality. Even though benefit finding is not a particularly common approach in psychosocial rehabilitation, it is an important area to consider because it could be that one psychosocial deficit such as fear of recurrence is balanced by a benefit in the form of deeper meaning noted by the patient or other family members.

Concluding Comments

There is a growing body of literature supporting the effectiveness of psychosocial interventions in the rehabilitation of cancer patients. Interest in this area is driven by the increasing number of cancer survivors living 5 years or longer, less stigma attached to utilizing psychosocial services such as support groups or individual coaching/counseling, research initiatives of the National Cancer Institute (NCI) emphasizing psychosocial care, efforts of the National Coalition for Cancer Survivorship and Office of Cancer Survivorship of the NCI, growing consumer interest, effective intervention techniques, and validated measurement tools for assessing the usefulness of such interventions. Another force operating within the community of cancer medicine is the emphasis on quality of life as an important outcome in addition to survival.

There are specific types of treatments that have been shown to be effective for a variety of patients for reasons of their ease of administration as well as face validity. These interventions include cognitive behavioral therapy, progressive muscle relaxation, structured psychoeducational interventions including problem solving, and supportive-expressive therapy. For the most part, such interventions have been demonstrated with breast cancer patients, possibly because of funding opportunities provided by the Department of Defense and the Komen Foundation. There are few RCTs with psychosocial interventions in most other cancer sites. Patients with head and neck and pancreatic cancer, as well as those with brain tumors, remain little researched for a variety of reasons. Most of the excellent randomized clinical trials that have been conducted are associated with major medical centers. However, the vast majority of cancer care is delivered in communities. Patients treated in community settings are most likely to find psychosocial care with mental health counselors and the clergy, American Cancer Society programs, and in Wellness Communities. These settings are hard pressed to devote the resources necessary to conduct a clinical trial on psychosocial care.

If psychosocial rehabilitation is to move forward, more clinical trials with a broader range of patients need to be developed and conducted. There has been progress made. Cognitive behavior therapy and structured supportive educational approaches have promise, as do telephone interventions. Yet, the central question remains: What interventions for what patients along what point of their trajectory of survivorship and care, delivered by what type of professional, can offer the promise of reduced suffering and return to full-quality living following the diagnosis and treatment for cancer?

References

1. Zabora J, BrintzenhofeSzoc K, Curbow B, Hooker C, Piantadosi S. The prevalence of psychological distress by cancer site. Psycho-Oncology 2001;10(1):19–28.
2. Derogatis LR, Morrow GR, Fetting J, et al. The prevalence of psychiatric disorders among cancer patients. JAMA 1983; 249(6):751–757.
3. American Cancer Society: Facts and Figures. Atlanta, GA: American Cancer Society, 2003.
4. Psychosocial care improves quality of life but half of US cancer patients do not receive essential interventions. In: The Clinical Cancer Letter: A Research Guide for Clinicians. The Cancer Letter, Inc. 1995:1–9.
5. Enabling America: Assessing the Role of Rehabilitation, Science and Engineering. Washington, DC: National Academy Press, 1997.
6. Dietz JH. Rehabilitation Oncology. New York: Wiley, 1981.
7. Gunn AE. Cancer Rehabilitation. New York: Raven, 1984.
8. Mayer D, O'Connor L. Rehabilitation of persons with cancer: an ONS position statement. Oncol Nurs Forum 1989;16(3):433.
9. Ganz PA. Current issues in cancer rehabilitation. Cancer (Phila) 1990;65(3 suppl):742–751.
10. McQuellon RP, Hurt GJ. The psychosocial impact of the diagnosis and treatment of laryngeal cancer. Otolaryngol Clin N Am 1997;30(2):231–241.
11. Distress management: clinical practice guidelines. J Natl Comprehens Cancer Network 2003;1(3):344–374.
12. Holland JC. Update: NCCN Practice Guidelines for the Management of Psychosocial Distress. Oncology 1999;13(5A): 113–147.
13. McQuellon RP, Russell GB, Rambo TD, et al. Quality of life and psychological distress of bone marrow transplant recipients: the "time trajectory" to recovery over the first year. Bone Marrow Transplant 1998;21(5):477–486.
14. McQuellon RP, Loggie BW, Fleming RA, Russell GB, Lehman AB, Rambo TD. Quality of life after intraperitoneal hyperthermic chemotherapy (IPHC) for peritoneal carcinomatosis. Eur J Surg Oncol 2001;27(1):65–73.
15. Dimeo F, Bertz H, Finke J, Fetscher S, Mertelsmann R, Keul J. An aerobic exercise program for patients with haematological malignancies after bone marrow transplantation. Bone Marrow Transplant 1996;18(6):1157–1160.
16. Engel GL. The need for a new medical model: a challenge for biomedicine. Science 1977;196(4286):129–136.
17. Kornblith AB. Psychosocial adaptation of cancer survivors. In: Holland JC, Breitbart W, Jacobsen PB, et al. (eds). Psycho-Oncology. New York: Oxford University Press, 1998:223–254.
18. Fallowfield L, Jenkins V. Effective communication skills are the key to good cancer care. Eur J Cancer 1999;35(11):1592–1597.
19. Lehmann JF, DeLisa JA, Warren CG, deLateur BJ, Bryant PL, Nicholson CG. Cancer rehabilitation: assessment of need, development, and evaluation of a model of care. Arch Phys Med Rehabil 1978;59(9):410–419.
20. Barofsky I. The status of psychosocial research in the rehabilitation of the cancer patient [review]. Semin Oncol Nurs 1992; 8(3):190–201.
21. Andersen BL, Kiecolt-Glaser JK, Glaser R. A biobehavioral model of cancer stress and disease course [review]. Am Psychologist 1994;49(5):389–404.
22. Zabora JR, Smith-Wilson R, Fetting JH, Enterline JP. An efficient method for psychosocial screening of cancer patients. Psychosomatics 1990;31(2):192–196.
23. Zabora JR. "Development of a self-administered psychosocial cancer screening tool" [letter]. Cancer Pract 1995;3(2):117–118.
24. Newell SA, Sanson-Fisher RW, Savolainen NJ. Systematic review of psychological therapies for cancer patients: overview and recommendations for future research. J Natl Cancer Inst 2002;94(8):558–584.
25. Andersen BL. Psychological interventions for cancer patients to enhance the quality of life. J Consult Clin Psychol 1992;60(4): 552–568.
26. Fawzy FI, Fawzy NW, Arndt LA, Pasnau RO. Critical review of psychosocial interventions in cancer care [review]. Arch Gen Psychiatry 1995;52(2):100–113.
27. Meyer TJ, Mark MM. Effects of psychosocial interventions with adult cancer patients: a meta-analysis of randomized experiments [see comments]. Health Psychol 1995;14(2):101–108.

28. Sheard T, Maguire P. The effect of psychological interventions on anxiety and depression in cancer patients: results of two meta-analyses. Br J Cancer 1999;80(11):1770–1780.

29. Rehse B, Pukrop R. Effects of psychosocial interventions on quality of life in adult cancer patients: meta analysis of 37 published controlled outcome studies. Patient Educ Counsel 2003;50(2):179–186.

30. Mulrow CD OA. Cochrane Collaboration Handbook. Oxford (UK): Cochrane Collaboration, 1997.

31. Wells ME, McQuellon RP, Hinkle JS, Cruz JM. Reducing anxiety in newly diagnosed cancer patients: a pilot program. Cancer Pract 1995;3(2):100–104.

32. McQuellon RP, Wells M, Hoffman S, et al. Reducing distress in cancer patients with an orientation program. Psycho-Oncology 1998;7(3):207–217.

33. Rehse B, Pukrop R. Effects of psychosocial interventions on quality of life in adult cancer patients: meta analysis of 37 published controlled outcome studies. Patient Educ Counsel 2003;50(2):179–186.

34. Brady MJ, Cella DF, Mo F, et al. Reliability and validity of the Functional Assessment of Cancer Therapy-Breast quality-of-life instrument. J Clin Oncol 1997;15(3):974–986.

35. Cella DF, Bonomi AE, Lloyd SR, Tulsky DS, Kaplan E, Bonomi P. Reliability and validity of the Functional Assessment of Cancer Therapy–Lung (FACT-L) quality of life instrument. Lung Cancer 1995;12:199–220.

36. Cella DF. Manual for the Functional Assessment of Cancer Therapy (FACT) Measurement System (version 3): 1994. Chicago: Rush Cancer Center, 1994.

37. Yellen SB, Cella DF, Webster K, Blendowski C, Kaplan E. Measuring fatigue and other anemia-related symptoms with the Functional Assessment of Cancer Therapy (FACT) measurement system. J Pain Symptom Manag 1997;13(2):63–74.

38. Cella DF, Tulsky DS, Gray G, et al. The Functional Assessment of Cancer Therapy scale: development and validation of the general measure. J Clin Oncol 1993;11(3):570–579.

39. Ware JE Jr, Snow KK, Kosinski M, Gandek B. SF-36 health survey. Manual and interpretation guide. Boston: Nimrod Press, 1993.

40. Hann DM, Jacobsen PB, Martin SC, Kronish LE, Azzarello LM, Fields KK. Quality of life following bone marrow transplantation for breast cancer: a comparative study. Bone Marrow Transplant 1997;19(3):257–264.

41. Hann DM, Jacobsen PB, Martin SC, Kronish LE, Azzarello LM, Fields KK. Fatigue in women treated with bone marrow transplantation for breast cancer: a comparison with women with no history of cancer. Support Care Cancer 1997;5(1):44–52.

42. McQuellon RP, Loggie BW, Lehman AB, et al. Long-term survivorship and quality of life after cytoreductive surgery plus intraperitoneal hyperthermic chemotherapy for peritoneal carcinomatosis. Ann Surg Oncol 2003;10(2):155–162.

43. Ganz PA, Schag CA, Lee JJ, Sim MS. The CARES: a generic measure of health-related quality of life for patients with cancer. Qual Life Res 1992;1(1):19–29.

44. Schag CA, Ganz PA, Polinsky ML, Fred C, Hirji K, Petersen L. Characteristics of women at risk for psychosocial distress in the year after breast cancer. J Clin Oncol 1993;11(4):783–793.

45. Ganz PA, Greendale GA, Petersen L, Zibecchi L, Kahn B, Belin TR. Managing menopausal symptoms in breast cancer survivors: results of a randomized controlled trial. J Natl Cancer Inst 2000;92(13):1054–1064.

46. Schag CA, Ganz PA, Wing DS, Sim MS, Lee JJ. Quality of life in adult survivors of lung, colon and prostate cancer. Qual Life Res 1994;3(2):127–141.

47. Worden JW, Weisman AD. Do cancer patients really want counseling? Gen Hosp Psychiatry 1980;2(2):100–103.

48. Gordon WA, Freidenbergs I, Diller L, et al. Efficacy of psychosocial intervention with cancer patients. J Consult Clin Psychol 1980;48(6):743–759.

49. Cheung YL, Molassiotis A, Chang AM. The effect of progressive muscle relaxation training on anxiety and quality of life after stoma surgery in colorectal cancer patients. Psycho-Oncology 2003;12(3):254–266.

50. Spielberger CD, Gorsuch RL, Lushene RD. STAI: Manual for the State-Trait Anxiety Inventory. Palo Alto: Consulting Psychologists Press, 1970.

51. Mishel MH, Belyea M, Germino BB, et al. Helping patients with localized prostate carcinoma manage uncertainty and treatment side effects: nurse-delivered psychoeducational intervention over the telephone. Cancer (Phila) 2002;94(6):1854–1866.

52. Lepore SJ, Helgeson VS, Eton DT, Schulz R. Improving quality of life in men with prostate cancer: a randomized controlled trial of group education interventions. Health Psychol 2003;22(5):443–452.

53. Goodwin PJ, Black JT, Bordeleau LJ, Ganz PA. Health-related quality-of-life measurement in randomized clinical trials in breast cancer: taking stock. J Natl Cancer Inst 2003;95(4):263–281.

54. Walker LG, Walker MB, Ogston K, et al. Psychological, clinical and pathological effects of relaxation training and guided imagery during primary chemotherapy. Br J Cancer 1999; 80(1–2):262–268.

55. Molassiotis A, Yung HP, Yam BM, Chan FY, Mok TS. The effectiveness of progressive muscle relaxation training in managing chemotherapy-induced nausea and vomiting in Chinese breast cancer patients: a randomised controlled trial. Support Care Cancer 2002;10(3):237–246.

56. McArdle JM, George WD, McArdle CS, et al. Psychological support for patients undergoing breast cancer surgery: a randomised study. BMJ 1996;312(7034):813–816.

57. Winzelberg AJ, Classen C, Alpers GW, et al. Evaluation of an internet support group for women with primary breast cancer. Cancer (Phila) 2003;97(5):1164–1173.

58. Helgeson VS, Cohen S, Schulz R, Yasko J. Long-term effects of educational and peer discussion group interventions on adjustment to breast cancer. Health Psychol 2001;20(5):387–392.

59. Antoni MH, Lehman JM, Kilbourn KM, et al. Cognitive-behavioral stress management intervention decreases the prevalence of depression and enhances benefit finding among women under treatment for early-stage breast cancer. Health Psychol 2001;20(1):20–32.

60. Edelman S, Bell DR, Kidman AD. A group cognitive behaviour therapy programme with metastatic breast cancer patients. Psycho-Oncology 1999;8(4):295–305.

61. Fukui S, Kugaya A, Okamura H, et al. A psychosocial group intervention for Japanese women with primary breast carcinoma. Cancer (Phila) 2000;89(5):1026–1036.

62. Edmonds CV, Lockwood GA, Cunningham AJ. Psychological response to long-term group therapy: a randomized trial with metastatic breast cancer patients. Psycho-Oncology 1999;8(1):74–91.

63. Classen C, Butler LD, Koopman C, et al. Supportive-expressive group therapy and distress in patients with metastatic breast cancer: a randomized clinical intervention trial. Arch Gen Psychiatry 2001;58(5):494–501.

64. Bultz BD, Speca M, Brasher PM, Geggie PH, Page SA. A randomized controlled trial of a brief psychoeducational support group for partners of early stage breast cancer patients. Psycho-Oncology 2000;9(4):303–313.

65. Toseland RW, Blanchard CG, McCallion P. A problem solving intervention for caregivers of cancer patients. Soc Sci Med 1995; 40(4):517–528.

66. McQuellon RP, Hurt GJ, DeChatelet P. Psychosocial care of the patient with cancer: a model for organizing services. Cancer Pract 1996;4(6):304–311.

67. Berglund G, Bolund C, Gustafsson UL, Sjoden PO. One-year follow-up of the "Starting Again" group rehabilitation programme for cancer patients. Eur J Cancer 1994;30A(12):1744–1751.

68. Angen MJ, MacRae JH, Simpson JS, Hundleby M. Tapestry: a retreat program of support for persons living with cancer. Cancer Pract 2002;10(6):297–304.

69. Ronson A, Body JJ. Psychosocial rehabilitation of cancer patients after curative therapy. Support Care Cancer 2002;10(4):281–291.

70. Walsh-Burke K. Family communication and coping with cancer: impact of the We Can Weekend. J Psychosocial Oncol 1992; 10(1):63–81.

71. Andrykowski MA, Brady MJ, Greiner CB, et al. 'Returning to normal' following bone marrow transplantation: outcomes, expectations and informed consent. Bone Marrow Transplant 1995;15(4):573–581.

72. Andrykowski MA, McQuellon RP. Readaptation to normal life following bone marrow transplantation. In: Barrett J, Treleaven J (eds). The Clinical Practice of Stem Cell Transplantation. Oxford: Isis Medical Media, 1997:828–835.

73. Fromm K, Andrykowski MA, Hunt J. Positive and negative psychosocial sequelae of bone marrow transplantation: implications for quality of life assessment. J Behav Med 1996;19(3): 221–240.

74. Sears SR, Stanton AL, Danoff-Burg S. The yellow brick road and the emerald city: benefit finding, positive reappraisal coping and posttraumatic growth in women with early-stage breast cancer. Health Psychol 2003;22(5):487–497.

Reproductive Complications and Sexual Dysfunction in Cancer Survivors

Leslie R. Schover

Defining the Population at Risk for Reproductive Complications

This chapter will review risk factors and management for three types of reproductive complications of cancer treatment: infertility, menopausal symptoms, and sexual dysfunction. Each problem area affects unique, albeit overlapping, populations of cancer patients and survivors.

Risk Factors for Cancer-Related Infertility

The demographics of cancer survivorship and delayed childbearing ensure that increasing numbers of patients will have their family-building disrupted by cancer treatment. The success of cancer treatment for malignancies that affect young people, such as pediatric cancers, testicular cancer, and Hodgkin's Disease, has yielded a large population of cancer survivors. According to the National Health Information Survey of 2001,[1] 2.2% of adults aged 18 to 44 in the United States have been diagnosed with cancer. Extrapolating based on statistics for this age group from the United States 2000 Census,[2] approximately 2.5 million adults of childbearing age are cancer survivors. It is more difficult to specify how many have faced infertility, but most probably had treatment with gonadotoxic chemotherapy, and smaller numbers would be at risk for infertility because of surgery or radiation therapy affecting the reproductive system.

Another trend that increases the salience of cancer and fertility is delayed childbearing in American families. Birth rates for women in their thirties have been climbing steadily, reaching a high in 2001 of 95.6 per 1,000 women aged 30–34 and 41.4 per 1,000 women aged 35–39.[3] Births to women aged 40–44 have more than doubled since 1981 to 8.1 per 1,000 women. According to the United States Census report for 2000, the percentage of childless women age 30–34 has jumped from 19.8% in 1980 to 28.1% in 2000, and for women aged 35–39 from 12.1% in 1980 to 20.1% in 2000.[4] When these women are ready to conceive, some will receive the unwelcome news of a malignancy. Data on paternal age are not readily available, but in 1995 in the United States, men at marriage were on the average 2.7 years older than their brides so that men, too, would be more at risk currently to have cancer interfere with their fertility.[5]

Infertility Related Directly to a Malignancy

For a few types of malignancy, for example testicular cancer, the risk of infertility and risk of cancer are related. In a cohort of 3,530 Danish men who were born between 1945 and 1980 and developed testicular cancer from 1960 to 1993, the standardized fertility rate was significantly lower (ratio 0.93) than for all 1,488,957 Danish men born in the same era.[6] Fertility was particularly reduced in the two years leading up to cancer diagnosis, and for men with nonseminomatous tumors (ratio 0.87). Furthermore, men who developed testicular cancer were less likely than men in the general population to conceive male children, possibly indicating a genetic or environmental factor.

Skakkebæk and his colleagues believe that a testicular dysgenesis syndrome (TDS) is increasing in frequency in Western countries because of environmental influences in utero, perhaps combined with a genetic susceptibility factor. The syndrome includes testicular cancer, undescended testes, hypospadias, and decreased semen quality.[7] Although the evidence for TDS, and in particular the influence of endocrine disrupting pollutants, remains controversial, it is clear that men with testis cancer have a high percentage of abnormalities in the contralateral testis suggesting abnormal fetal development of these tissues.[8] The standardized incidence ratios of testis cancer in 32,442 men who had a semen analysis at the laboratory in Copenhagen between the years of 1963 and 1995 were compared with rates in the general population of Danish men.[9] Parameters of poor semen quality, including low count, poor motility, and abnormal morphology, were all associated with increased risk of testis cancer (standardized incidence ratios of 2.3–3.0).

In women, a recent evidence-based review of the link between infertility and cancer risk concluded that borderline ovarian tumors are slightly more common in women diagnosed with infertility.[10] It is less clear whether infertile women are at increased risk for invasive ovarian cancer, but rates may be elevated in those who never achieve a pregnancy or among women with endometriosis. In contrast, infertility does not appear to be a risk factor for breast cancer.[10] Although most cohort and case-control studies have not demonstrated a link between using ovarian stimulating drugs to treat female infertility and subsequent cancer risk for any site,[11] a recent comparison of 4,575 women with breast cancer and 4,682 controls found that women who used human menopausal gonadotropin for at least 6 cycles had a greater relative risk of breast cancer (2.7–3.8).[12]

Infertility Caused by Cancer Treatment

Many cancer patients are put at risk for infertility by the therapies used to eradicate or control their malignancy. Surgical treatment for pelvic cancer may remove a critical part of the reproductive organ system, e.g. bilateral orchiectomy for prostate cancer or for asynchronous testicular tumors, or bilateral oophorectomy as part of treatment for gynecological malignancies or as prevention for breast or ovarian cancer in women with BRCA mutations.[13] Treatment of prostate or bladder cancer may entail removal of the prostate and seminal vesicles and the vagina or uterus may be removed to treat vaginal, cervical, or uterine cancer. Nerves controlling antegrade ejaculation of semen may be damaged in retroperitoneal lymphadenectomy for testicular cancer[14] or in surgery for colorectal cancer.[15]

Radiation therapy to the pelvis damages fertility because developing gametes and ovarian follicles, like cancer cells, are more likely to be in the genetically vulnerable, proliferative state.[16] Patients treated for prostate or cervical cancer, or those who have total body irradiation as preparation for bone marrow transplant, are the most common groups to experience radiation-associated infertility.

Chemotherapy drugs also interfere with gametogenesis because maturing sperm and oocytes are vulnerable to the toxins that damage rapidly-growing cancer cells.[17,18] Alkylating drugs (including the platinum-based chemotherapies) are most likely to damage fertility. The likelihood of permanent ovarian failure in women increases with cumulative dose and age, and is manifested as decreased numbers of follicles, atretic follicles, and fibrotic changes in the ovary.[19] Spermatogenesis is even more vulnerable to disruption by chemotherapy, with a similar pattern of risk factors in terms of dosage and type of drugs.[20] The impact of male age on fertility after cancer is unclear, but in general men over age 45 take longer to establish a pregnancy and have decreased conception rates.[21]

Preventing and Managing Cancer-Related Infertility

Preserving fertility is highly important to men and women diagnosed with cancer before completing their families. Although research on the psychosocial aspects of cancer-related infertility is limited, surveys and qualitative interview studies concur that most survivors feel healthy enough to be ~od parents, believe that their experience of cancer has ~ased the value they place on family closeness, are par-

ticularly distressed about infertility if childless, and are not getting enough information on options to spare or treat fertility.[22–26]

Utilization of infertility services in the United States is limited even for the population at large. Less than 50% of women with infertility seek medical consultation and only 1.6% use assisted reproductive technology.[27] Although male factors explain roughly half of infertility, no statistics are available on men's use of infertility services.[28] This gives some context for help-seeking among cancer survivors with infertility.

Preventing Cancer-Related Infertility

Obviously, it is preferable to prevent cancer-related infertility rather than to try treating it after the fact. Hormonal manipulation during chemotherapy may be used to try to minimize damage to the gonads. In addition, when treatment of a particular malignancy has become highly successful, efforts have been made to spare fertility in younger patients by using less toxic chemotherapy drugs or by limiting cancer surgery. Several options are available to cryopreserve gametes or embryos before cancer treatment for later use in conception, although assisted reproductive technology is typically required. Each of these options will be reviewed, and the level of evidence for its efficacy examined.

HORMONAL PREVENTION

In men, efforts during chemotherapy to protect the spermatogonia A cells that produce mature spermatozoa have included prescribing GnRH analogues with or without accompanying testosterone. Despite promising results in animals, human trials have been uniformly disappointing.[29] Howell and Shalet speculate that continuing hormonal treatment for several months after finishing chemotherapy might have more success, allowing surviving stem cells to recover and renew spermatogenesis. If no spermatogonia survive chemotherapy or radiation therapy, however, continuing hormonal treatment will be fruitless. Even in the prepubertal testis, cancer therapies damage fertility because the Leydig, Sertoli, and germ cells are not truly quiescent, but continue to develop,[30] making them vulnerable to toxic cancer therapies.

Efforts at hormonal protection of the ovaries during chemotherapy in women have had more promising results, but double-blind randomized trials are still lacking. The largest case-control cohort has been followed by Blumenfeld in Israel.[31] An injectable GnRH agonist was administered, beginning 1 to 2 weeks before chemotherapy and continuing for up to 6 months, to a group of 60 women aged 15 to 40 being treated for lymphoma. All but 3 of the surviving women resumed menstruation by the end of the first year, compared to only 45% of 60 women treated with chemotherapy alone, without hormonal protection. Inhibin –A and –B levels decreased during GnRH administration, normalizing only in the women who resumed menstruation.[18] Although the GnRH and comparison groups did not differ on age, tumor type, cumulative dose of chemotherapy drugs, or exposure to radiation therapy, the comparison group consisted either of historical controls or women who were not seen in time to start the GnRH-agonist before chemotherapy.[31] Obviously, selection bias is possible.

The use of a GnRH-agonist during adjuvant chemotherapy for breast cancer is attractive because it not only may protect against ovarian failure in young women, but could potentially add to cancer control. In a Phase II pilot study, a group in Rome administered the long-acting GnRH analog goserelin for one year during adjuvant chemotherapy to 64 newly diagnosed women with breast cancer, aged 18 to 50 and without distant metastases.[32] Dosage and drug regimen depended on cancer stage. At a median follow-up time of 55 months, 86% of women had resumed menstruation after chemotherapy, including five who had stem cell transplantation. Although this was a lower rate of ovarian failure than would be expected, no comparison group was provided.

Chemoprotection Strategies

Even if hormonal protection helps preserve a greater number of primordial follicles during chemotherapy, many of those remaining would be damaged.[33] Another type of chemoprotection is suggested by advances in understanding how toxins like chemotherapy influence signaling pathways in the testis and ovary. A small lipid molecule, sphingosine 1-phosphate, may be able to prevent damage to the follicles as well as protecting against genetic damage to the oocyte.[34] Even more tantalizing is the recent discovery of stem cells in the human ovary, suggesting that females are not limited to the number of oocytes that survive fetal development, but have ongoing replenishment of primordial follicles.[35]

Cryopreservation of Reproductive Tissue for Future Conception

The most well-established form of reproductive tissue cryopreservation in cancer patients is sperm banking. Measures of the effectiveness of sperm banking include the success of using sperm cryopreserved by cancer patients in conceiving healthy offspring and the utilization of stored samples by cancer survivors.

Conception rates from banked sperm have increased radically since the advent of intracytoplasmic sperm injection (ICSI) in 1992. In this technique, only one live sperm is injected into each oocyte retrieved from in vitro fertilization (IVF). Rates of fertilization with ICSI do not differ when using sperm that was cryopreserved versus from a fresh ejaculate, nor has the use of cryopreserved sperm resulted in increased birth defects.[36]

Although many men diagnosed with cancer have impaired semen quality, samples from patients with suboptimal semen parameters survive freezing and thawing just as well as sperm from men of normal fertility.[37,38] Several prospective case series of men who cryopreserved sperm are presented in Table 19.1. Only about 6% to 18% of cancer patients are azoospermic and unable to bank at the time of attempted semen collection.[39,41,42,44] The most efficient use of stored samples is to attempt to conceive with IVF-ICSI,[41,43] unless the semen quality is unusually good.

It appears that less than 10% of men who store semen actually use their samples to try to conceive, but this rate may be accelerating with the availability of IVF-ICSI.[42-44] The percentage of couples who use their cryopreserved sperm with assisted reproductive technology (ART) and actually have a live birth varies widely from center to center, but is comparable to results for the general population of infertile couples.[41,43] With all cohorts in Table 19.1 combined, 37 healthy babies were born, with only one pregnancy terminated because a major fetal malformation was detected.[42]

Although specific rates of impaired fertility have been reported for a variety of chemotherapy combinations or radiation therapy doses and fields,[29] it is not possible to accurately predict recovery of fertility in any one man treated for cancer.[36] Therefore, sperm banking should be routinely offered when men are about to begin treatments that put fertility at risk. An adequate number of specimens can be banked without delaying cancer treatment in all but the most

TABLE 19.1. Long-term follow-ups of cohorts of consecutive cancer patients who cryopreserved sperm.

Reference	Year	Number of Patients	Years follow-up	% able to store sperm	% using samples	Cycles of ART	Pregnancies per cycle	Live births	% couples attempting conception who achieved parenthood	Birth defects
Lass et al.[39]	1998	191	8	83%	3%	IUI: 2 IVF: 9 ICSI: 4	100% 22% 50%	7	83%	0
Audrins et al.[40]	1999	258*	20	—	2%	IUI: 53 IVF: 14	4% 36%	7	33%	0
Kelleher et al.[41]	2001	930	22	90%	10%	IUI: 28 IVF: 28 ICSI: 35	43% 31% 21%	39	45%	2
Blackhall et al.[42]	2002	122*	22	94%	27%	—	—	11	27%	1
Agarwal et al.[43]	2002	318**	20	—	9% (26% in past 4 yrs.)	IUI: 37 IVF: 23 ICSI: 20	8% 26% 35%	12	44%	0
Ragni et al.[44]	2003	776	15	88%	5%***	IUI: 40 IVF: 6 ICSI: 42	8% 0% 26%	14	43%	1

*Hodgkin's disease only.

**Only N cryopreserving sperm was reported.

***Rates increase with duration of follow-up to 12% at 12 years.

emergent cases. A study of 95 cancer patients found that acceptable post-thaw semen quality could be obtained when men abstained for only 24 to 48 hours between collecting ejaculates.[45]

Despite low rates of usage of stored sperm, men do not appear to regret the trouble or expense. Hallak and colleagues examined the reasons that 56 (16%) of 342 cancer men who had banked sperm before cancer treatment in their clinic discarded their cryopreserved specimens.[46] Out of the 56 men, 21 had died and the families discarded the samples, 23 had already conceived all the children they wanted without using their stored sperm, 8 had a return of good semen parameters, and 4 had decided not to have children. The cost of banking sperm was not a factor in these decisions.

Unfortunately, recent surveys of oncologists reveal that many fail to give men information about sperm-banking, underestimating its importance to their male patients and overestimating the barriers of cost and availability of sperm banking facilities.[47–49] For those cancer patients interested in having future children, the most common reason cited for failure to bank sperm is lack of timely information. In our recent survey of young male survivors, only half recalled their oncology health care providers discussing the possibility of banking sperm.[23]

The pediatric oncology community has shown an increasing interest in giving teens with cancer the option of banking sperm. Out of 238 boys aged 12 to 19 referred to one center in London, 87% were able to produce an ejaculate for semen storage, with semen quality similar to that in adult cancer survivors.[50] A new experimental technique uses testicular biopsies to obtain spermatogonia from prepubertal boys for cryopreservation before cancer treatment, in the hope that they can be replaced through autografting to restore fertility later. Attempts at replacement in adult men have been disappointing, however, since it is not possible to inject the thawed suspension of cells directly into the fibrous seminiferous tubules.[29] Cryopreserved human spermatogonial stem cells have been transplanted into mouse testes and survived for up to 6 months, suggesting that xenotransplantation could some day be another option for producing mature sperm cells for IVF-ICSI, or at least for providing a research model.[51]

In women, progress is also being made with the use of a rapid freezing technique called *vitrification* to freeze mature, unfertilized oocytes, although pregnancy rates still do not approach those with cryopreserved embryos.[52] Another promising avenue is the use of sugars as cryoprotectants during freezing.[53] To have a true analogue to sperm banking in men, it would be necessary to cryopreserve primordial follicles and then to mature them in the laboratory. Although such techniques remain years away,[54] researchers are having some preliminary success with in vitro maturation of freshly retrieved antral follicles that are approaching full maturity.[55]

A number of centers around the world are removing and cryopreserving ovarian tissue for women about to undergo cancer treatment that could impair fertility.[54] Several cases of auto-transplantation have taken place, with promising results.[56,57] Technical problems include minimizing injury to ovarian tissue during the freezing itself and ischemia causing damage to follicles while the graft grows a new vascular system.[58] For some malignancies, concern about reintroducing cancer cells along with the ovarian tissue may limit this option.[58] An alternative use of the tissue could be in xeno-transplantation to immunodeficient mice with subsequent harvest of mature oocytes. Recently an embryo was produced using an oocyte retrieved from transplanted ovarian tissue in a female cancer survivor, but no pregnancy resulted when the embryo was transferred to the woman's uterus.[59] Furthermore, the first primate has been born using this technique—a rhesus monkey.[60] Still, an ethical dilemma is that women facing cancer treatment and desperate to protect their future fertility are paying several thousand dollars in out-of-pocket costs to harvest, freeze, and store ovarian tissue with very low odds that a pregnancy will ever result.

Ovarian Transposition During Pelvic Radiation Therapy

When radiation therapy fields include the pelvis, the ovaries can be moved surgically to a more protected location. Although both medial positioning behind the uterus and lateral movement to the pelvic sidewall have been used, currently the most common procedure is to use laparoscopy to move the ovaries laterally just prior to starting radiotherapy. Although ovarian transposition can be performed during a staging laparotomy, it is less effective because the ovaries tend to migrate back to their original position.[61] The ideal position is above the pelvic brim, with the fallopian tubes remaining attached to the uterus.[62]

A recent literature review of the outcome of laparoscopic lateral ovarian transposition included only 44 cases of women under age 40 with a variety of malignancies. However, 89% had preserved menstrual function.[62] Oophoropexy can be complicated by vascular injury, infarction of the fallopian tube, or ovarian cyst formation. IVF is often required to conceive. Women with adenocarcinoma of the cervix or with more advanced stage disease may be at some risk for metastasis to a transposed ovary or to the site of trocar insertion for the laparoscopy.[63] Successful transposition may still be followed by early menopause because of reduced ovarian reserve after radiation therapy.[64]

Fertility-Sparing Surgery for Early-Stage Gynecological Malignancies

Young women diagnosed with early stage cervical or ovarian cancer may opt for conservative surgical procedures that allow them to retain fertility. For women with squamous cell carcinoma of the cervix that is invasive but still early stage, a trachelectomy can be substituted for a radical hysterectomy.[65–68] After the majority of the cervix is removed, the vaginal cuff is sewn back to the cervical remnants. As long as lymph nodes and surgical margins are clear, recurrence rates are comparable to those after radical hysterectomy. Although many women are able to become pregnant after trachelectomy, rates of miscarriage and prematurity are higher than normal. The cervical mucous plug that prevents infection of the amniotic membranes may be inadequate and there is an increased risk of cervical incompetence.

Women with adenocarcinoma of the cervix that is either in situ or very early stage can be treated with conization alone to preserve fertility, as long as surgical margins are clear.[69,70] Adenocarcinoma of the cervix is often multifocal or located high in the endocervical canal, however, and about 20% of women with negative margins at the time of conization will have local recurrences.

In conservative surgery for young women with borderline or germ cell ovarian tumors, only the affected ovary is removed, preserving the uterus and contralateral ovary.[66] Results have been good, both in terms of fertility and cancer control, but only small case series have been published.[71,72] Recurrence rates after conservative surgery for borderline tumors are higher than after radical surgery, but survival rates remain similar.[71] Conservative surgery has also been utilized for Stage I epithelial tumors.[73] The largest cohort study included women treated for germ cell tumors with a median follow-up of 122 months.[74] Of those who tried to conceive (N = 38), 76% have become pregnant.

Other Fertility-Sparing Modifications of Cancer Treatment

Other modifications made to cancer treatment to spare fertility have not been evaluated in randomized clinical trials, but instead have been compared to historical controls. Examples include the less gonadotoxic chemotherapy regimens for Hodgkin's disease[75]; surveillance protocols and nerve-sparing retroperitoneal lymphadenectomy for early stage testicular cancer[76]; and orthotopic bladder reconstruction with fertility preservation for men with bladder cancer.[77]

The Safety of Pregnancy After Cancer Treatment

It would be of little utility to promote fertility in women after cancer if pregnancy were a risk factor for cancer recurrence. However, evidence has accumulated that becoming pregnant after successful cancer treatment does not affect women's survival, even those who have had breast cancer.[78] Women diagnosed with breast cancer during pregnancy often have more advanced disease but do not have a survival disadvantage when matched to nonpregnant controls on medical factors such as cancer stage and histology.[79]

An area much in need of study is the psychosocial impact of experiencing cancer during pregnancy, and the development of supportive interventions for women in this predicament.[80] One recent survey found that reproductive concerns remain salient in women successfully treated for gestational trophoblastic disease and that 75% would have attended support groups if they had been available during treatment.[81] Young survivors often lack accurate information about pregnancy after cancer. In our pilot survey, 20% of breast cancer survivors and 18% of women with other cancer sites worried at least "a fair amount" that pregnancy could trigger a recurrence of cancer. Only 53% of women recalled any discussion by their oncology team of pregnancy after cancer.[22]

Survivors also lack knowledge about potential pregnancy complications related to impaired cardiac, pulmonary, or uterine function after cancer treatment. Few would plan evaluation by a high-risk obstetrician before trying to conceive.[22] In the largest study to date, 4,029 pregnancies of participants in the Childhood Cancer Survivor Study were reviewed.[82] A woman's history of chemotherapy was not associated with adverse outcomes, but women who had pelvic irradiation were more likely to have low birthweight infants. A higher than expected rate of voluntary pregnancy termination was observed, again suggesting that women may be worried about the safety of pregnancy or about the likelihood of having healthy offspring. Some women may also have been told in error that they were infertile, and thus did not use contraception to prevent an unwanted pregnancy. Higher rates of miscarriage and prematurity have also been observed in women with uterine exposure to radiotherapy as young adults, although the damage from childhood exposure is more severe.[83]

The Use of Assisted Reproductive Technology (ART) and Cancer

Although cryopreservation of embryos is far more successful than freezing unfertilized oocytes or ovarian tissue, undergoing IVF before cancer treatment presents some difficulties.[84,85] Women with a very aggressive malignancy such as acute leukemia may not have time to delay chemotherapy for several weeks of ovarian stimulation. Women who do not have a committed male partner have to use an anonymous sperm donor to create embryos. Women recently diagnosed with cancer often do not produce many mature oocytes in response to IVF. Women with untreated breast cancer risk exacerbating their disease by taking hormones for IVF. One alternative is natural cycle IVF, in which the one or two oocytes that mature without exogenous hormones are harvested and fertilized. Recently Oktay and colleagues developed an IVF protocol especially for women newly diagnosed with breast cancer, using tamoxifen for ovarian stimulation. The average number of embryos per cycle was 1.6 compared to 0.6 with a natural cycle, yielding a higher chance of an eventual pregnancy.[86] Ovarian stimulation regimens combining tamoxifen and follicle stimulating hormone (FSH) are yielding even better results.[87]

Women who wait until after chemotherapy to try IVF typically have a suboptimal response to the hormone stimulating drugs.[85] Creating embryos with oocytes from a donor is another option for the woman who has diminished fertility or is in ovarian failure after cancer treatment, but can still carry a pregnancy.[88,89] The cancer survivor herself does not undergo the risks of ovarian stimulation. If she is in ovarian failure, she may need some hormonal support to prepare her uterus for embryo transfer, as well as during the first weeks of a pregnancy, until the placenta begins to produce its own hormones. The hormone levels during these intervals are similar to those in a natural pregnancy. Pregnancy rates per cycle with donated oocytes are high, especially when both egg donor and recipient are under age 35. Women who have had pelvic irradiation still suffer the risk of prematurity and miscarriage, however. Along with survivors who have lost their uterus to cancer but have stored embryos or ovarian tissue, they may work with a gestational carrier to have a child. Only isolated case reports are available in the literature, however.[90]

For men with poor semen quality after cancer, IVF with ICSI is the preferred method of treatment. Some men do not have any mature spermatozoa in their semen, or no longer ejaculate seminal fluid after their cancer treatment. If they did not bank sperm before treatment, some options are still open to them. Men who do not ejaculate after node dissection for testis cancer or surgery for colorectal tumors may respond to medications that temporarily restore antegrade ejaculation. Viable sperm may also be retrieved from urine voided just after orgasm. Perhaps the most reliable means of obtaining sperm from these men is via electrical stimulation of ejaculation with a probe in the anal canal.[91] This procedure must be performed under anesthesia, but yields samples that typically can be used for IVF with ICSI.[92] Some urologists have used electroejaculation to obtain ejaculates from young teens who are unable to collect semen through masturbation due to anxiety or religious constraints.[93]

About half of men with no sperm in their semen after chemotherapy do have islands of spermatogenesis in their testes. A few viable sperm can be retrieved in testicular biopsies and used for successful IVF with ICSI.[94,95] Although increased aneuploidy has been observed in the sperm of men recently treated for cancer,[96] and aneuploidy has been associated with poorer fertilization rates with ICSI,[97] the pregnancy rates using ICSI with testicular sperm from cancer survivors have been comparable to those with other causes of male factor infertility, with a quarter to a third of cycles resulting in a healthy baby.[94,95] In a recent case series of 33 male childhood cancer survivors, only 33% of had normal semen quality but the integrity of DNA in their spermatozoa did not differ from that in a group of control men, suggesting that offspring would not be at increased risk of birth defects or other health problems.[98]

Health of Offspring of Cancer Survivors

Despite concerns that children born to men or women who had been treated for cancer would have unusual rates of genetic abnormalities or fetal malformations,[99] the available data suggest reasonable cause for optimism. Karyotypes of 2,630 live-born children with a parent who had survived childhood cancer were available from the Danish Cytogenetic Registry.[100] The rate of abnormal karyotypes was not significantly greater than those in the children born to the siblings of the childhood cancer patients. No study has thus far documented an excess rate of birth defects in children born after one parent's cancer treatment, with the caveats that (1) a limited number of offspring have been studied; and (2) the nature and duration of follow-up of offspring has been limited.

Genetic damage from cancer treatment may impact rates of early miscarriage or the gender of surviving infants. In addition to the results of pregnancies from the females in the Childhood Cancer Survivor Study,[82] 2,323 pregnancies sired by the male cancer survivors were documented. The live birth rate of 69% was significantly less than that for the survivors' brothers, and a deficit of male offspring born to the survivors was also observed.[101] Partners of men exposed to more than $5,000 \, mg/m^2$ of procarbazine had an increased risk of miscarriage. A large Scandinavian registry study did not document any increased lifetime cancer risk in offspring, except in families with known, autosomal dominant inherited cancer syndromes.[102] Most offspring in these studies have been born to childhood cancer survivors long removed from their active treatment when they conceived. On the other hand, some types of chemotherapy can be administered to pregnant women in the second and third trimesters without causing fetal malformations.[103]

A new issue is the impact on young adults' childbearing decisions of knowing they carry a mutation that increases lifetime cancer risk. For example, women with BRCA mutations increase their risk of breast cancer by having a pregnancy before age 40 and decrease their risk by early

oophorectomy without estrogen replacement.[104,105] Technologies such as prenatal diagnosis and preimplantation genetic diagnosis are also available to identify known autosomal dominant mutations responsible for hereditary cancer syndromes,[106] bringing potential ethical dilemmas, especially whether they should be used for those syndromes with a relatively late onset.

Risk Factors for Cancer-Related Menopausal Symptoms

Since the incidence of cancer increases with aging, menopausal symptoms are probably of high concern for more survivors than infertility. Women treated for breast cancer and men receiving hormonal therapy for advanced prostate cancer are particularly at risk for troublesome hot flashes (see Chapters 11 and 12). Vaginal atrophy and dyspareunia are the major sexual consequences of menopause for women[107] and will be discussed in the sections on sexual function. Menopause-related risks for cardiovascular disease and osteoporosis fall outside of the scope of this chapter.

Psychosocial Factors and Hot Flashes

It is unclear whether cancer survivors experience more severe menopause symptoms than women in the community without a cancer history. The prevalence of menopausal symptoms has generally been overestimated. The Massachusetts Women's Health Study followed a large cohort of women through the transition to menopause.[108,109] Most women did not have hot flashes or depression, had neutral or positive attitudes to menopause, and did not seek any medical attention for menopausal symptoms. Women who had hysterectomy were a more distressed group, with indications that women with pre-existing psychological problems are more likely to have this surgery.[110] An analysis of sexual function in 200 of the participants found that estrogen levels were significantly correlated with reports of dyspareunia, but not with any other sexual problem. A woman's perceptions of her overall health and the quality of her dyadic relationship were stronger predictors of her sexual function than was her menopausal status.[111]

Psychosocial factors play an important role in women's menopause complaints. The best predictors of depression, general health, and utilization of medical services after menopause are a woman's physical and psychological health and history of medical consultation before menopause.[109,110,112,113] Hot flashes and the use of hormone replacement therapy (HRT) are both correlated with psychological distress.[114,115] More educated women are consistently less likely to report hot flashes,[114,115] and cultural beliefs and expectations about menopause affect women's symptom reporting.[116]

The Prevalence of Hot Flashes After Breast Cancer

Women with breast cancer are the group most at risk for troublesome hot flashes after cancer treatment because they are advised not to use systemic estrogen replacement. No large case-control study has compared hot flashes in breast cancer survivors and other women. Carpenter and colleagues surveyed breast cancer survivors from a tumor registry, with about a third responding (N = 69), and compared them to a convenience sample of women with no history of breast cancer but similar age. Hot flashes were more frequent, severe, and distressing for the breast cancer sample. This finding may reflect selection bias in women who chose to participate, as well as the fact that women in the breast cancer group were significantly more likely to be menopausal and less likely to be using estrogen replacement.[117] Within the breast cancer group, hot flash severity and indices of emotional distress were related, parallel to findings in the general population of postmenopausal women.[117,118]

Among 860 breast cancer survivors surveyed by Ganz and colleagues at an average of 3 years post-diagnosis, 55% reported problems with hot flashes, a higher rate than expected from similar studies in healthy postmenopausal non-users of HRT.[119] Women who are premenopausal at breast cancer diagnosis and become menopausal because of cancer treatment are at highest risk to have hot flashes.[119–121] Although women taking tamoxifen experience hot flashes, they decrease after therapy ceases if women resume menses.[122,123] When adjuvant chemotherapy causes permanent menopause, however, hot flashes, vaginal dryness, and decreased quality of life persist even at long-term follow-up.[122,124]

Menopause Symptoms After Other Malignancies

Very little information is available on the prevalence and severity of menopausal symptoms in young women treated for other malignancies with chemotherapy or pelvic radiation that causes ovarian failure, although hot flashes and vaginal dryness are classic symptoms in women who become menopausal after treatment for gynecological cancer[125,126] or after intensive chemotherapy for hematological malignancies.[127] Women whose tumors are not hormone-sensitive may be less reluctant than breast cancer survivors to use estrogen replacement,[127] although publicity about the results of the Women's Health Initiative[128] has many women questioning the benefits of estrogen to manage all but the most short-term menopausal symptoms.

Hot Flashes in Male Cancer Survivors

A final group of cancer survivors at risk for menopausal symptoms are men who have androgen ablation to treat prostate cancer or take hormonal therapy for male breast cancer. Whether prostate cancer treatment involves orchiectomy or administration of a gonadotropin-releasing-hormone (GnRH) agonist, half to three-quarters of men report troublesome hot flashes.[129] As in the literature on menopausal women, there is not convincing evidence that androgen ablation increases depression in men, although sexual dysfunction is quite common.[129] Although in the year 2002, 189,000 new cases of prostate cancer were expected compared to only 1,500 men diagnosed with breast cancer,[130] the symptoms of hot flashes and sexual dysfunction are also common when men are treated with tamoxifen for advanced breast malignancies.[131]

Managing Menopausal Symptoms in Cancer Survivors

A variety of treatments are available for menopausal symptoms, ranging from relaxation treatment to antidepressant medication or hormonal replacement therapy. Only a few have been validated in double-blind randomized trials, a crucial design given the large and enduring placebo effect observed when breast cancer survivors are presented with a credible treatment for hot flashes.[132] Most intervention studies have used breast cancer survivors, the principal group at risk because of their concern about using estrogen replacement and their high rates of hot flashes. Men on hormonal therapy for prostate cancer have been another target group.

Estrogen Replacement for Hot Flashes

Estrogen replacement has consistently been shown to reduce hot flashes in 80% to 90% of postmenopausal women.[132] Nevertheless, an estimated 56% of all American women on HRT tried to stop within the first 8 months after publication of the Women's Health Initiative findings.[133] This randomized trial not only failed to confirm health benefits of HRT[128] but showed that HRT increases the risk of breast cancer.

The literature on using estrogen replacement after treatment for breast cancer also showed clear benefits in alleviating menopausal symptoms.[134–136] Case control studies failed to find an impact on survivors' cancer recurrence or decreased survival,[134,135,137–143] including a meta-analysis comparing 717 breast cancer survivors using some form of HRT to 2,545 nonusers. The relative risk of recurrence for women on HRT was 0.72 (95% confidence interval 0.47–1.10).[144] The relative risk of death for women on HRT after breast cancer was 0.18 (95% confidence interval, 0.10–0.31).

The first randomized trial[145] to be conducted confirmed these results, but included only 56 women in the estrogen-treated group. Women who agree to participate in such a trial may be a very select sample, since most survivors of breast cancer are highly anxious about the risks of taking estrogen.[145,146] More recently, the HABITS trial of the safety of hormone replacement therapy after breast cancer was stopped after 345 women had been followed for a median of about 2 years. An excess of new breast cancer events showed up in the hormone-treated group.[147]

One alternative hormonal therapy for hot flashes is to use progestins alone. Depomedroxyprogesterone acetate was effective in reducing hot flashes in a randomized clinical trial of breast and prostate survivors, and 45% continued using the medication for up to three years, despite some side effects.[148]

Nonhormonal Therapies for Hot Flashes

Trials of nonhormonal approaches to treating hot flashes are summarized in Table 19.2, with a focus on trials that include cancer survivors. Newer antidepressants appear to be the most promising nonhormonal therapy for both breast and prostate cancer survivors with hot flashes, producing greater relief and fewer side effects than older treatments such as progestins, clonidine, or bellergal.[132] Some other widely touted remedies such as isoflavones, black cohosh, and magnetic therapy have proved disappointing when tested in placebo-controlled trials.[153–155,158,159]

TABLE 19.2. Trials of nonhormonal therapies for hot flashes.

Reference	Year	Type of trial	Number of patients	Type of treatment	Type of patients	Average length of follow-up	Impact on hot flashes
Pandya et al.[149]	2000	Randomized, double-blind trial	194	Oral clonidine, 0.1 mg./day	Postmenopausal women on tamoxifen for breast cancer	12 weeks	38% reduction on clonidine vs. 24% on placebo
Stearns et al.[150]	2003	Randomized, double-blind trial	165	Paroxetine, 12.5 or 25.0 mg./day	Postmenopausal women without active cancer or cancer treatment	6 weeks	62% reduction on 12.5-mg./day and 65% on 25.0 mg./day
Loprinzi et al.[151]	2000	Randomized, double-blind trial	191	Venlaxafine, 75 mg./day or 150 mg/day	Breast cancer survivors or women scared to use HRT	4 weeks	37% reduction on 75 mg./day, 49% on 150 mg./day and 27% on placebo
Quella et al.[152]	1999	Pilot trial	16	Venlaxafine, 25 mg./day	Prostate cancer patients on androgen ablation with hot flashes	4 weeks	54% reduction in hot flashes
Quella et al.[153]	2000	Randomized, double-blind trial	149	50 mg. soy isoflavone/day	Breast cancer survivors with severe hot flashes	9 weeks	24% of women had 50% reduction on soy, 36% on placebo
Tice et al.[154]	2003	Randomized, double-blind trial	246	57 mg. or 82 mg. of isoflavone/day	Recently postmenopausal with severe hot flashes	12 weeks	No significant group differences
Nikander et al.[155]	2003	Randomized, double-blind trial	62	114 mg.isoflavone/day	Postmenopausal breast cancer survivors with hot flashes	12 weeks	No significant group differences
Muñoz et al.[156]	2003	Random, open-label trial	136	20 mg. *Cimicifuga racemosa*	Premenopausal breast cancer survivors on tamoxifen	52 weeks	Treatment group improved significantly more than usual care group in number and frequency of hot flashes
Wuttke et al.[157]	2003	Randomized, double-blind placebo-controlled	62	40 mg. *Cimicifuga racemosa* vs. 6 mg. conjugated estrogens vs. placebo	Postmenopausal women	13 weeks	Herbal preparation and estrogen gave equal symptom relief and both were better than placebo
Jacobson et al.[158]	2001	Randomized placebo-controlled, stratified on tamoxifen use	69	Black cohosh	Breast cancer survivors who had completed primary treatment	8 weeks	No significant group differences
Carpenter et al.[159]	2002	Randomized, placebo-controlled crossover study	11	Magnetic device	Breast cancer survivors	3 days	Placebo group improved more than magnet group
Porzio et al.[160]	2002	Pilot trial	15	Acupuncture	Breast cancer patients on tamoxifen	26 weeks	Emotional distress and hot flashes decreased significantly

Given the magnitude of the placebo effect, promising results using herbal remedies or acupuncture must be confirmed with randomized, placebo-controlled trials. For example, acupuncture using clinically recommended points could be tested against acupuncture using sites judged inactive according to traditional Chinese medicine. The duration of therapies tested has also been quite short, particularly given the stubborn nature of hot flashes in breast and prostate cancer survivors. Since some studies focused on cancer survivors with severe symptoms while others used unselected samples, the efficacy of various treatments cannot be directly compared. Although not yet tested in cancer survivors, behavioral modalities such as relaxation training[132,161] and engaging in regular aerobic exercise[162] show promise in decreasing hot

flashes in postmenopausal women unselected for cancer history.

One small, randomized trial has examined the efficacy of a brief, nursing intervention in reducing menopausal symptoms in 76 postmenopausal breast cancer survivors chosen because they had at least one severe problem of hot flashes, vaginal dryness, or urinary stress incontinence.[163] Women were randomized to receive usual care or to have a special session with a nurse practitioner to assess symptoms and apply treatment algorithms such as prescribing medication or advising on the use of vaginal lubricants and moisturizers. Telephone follow-up calls were included. All three target symptoms improved in the treated group compared to the usual care group. This type of inexpensive, brief intervention should be replicated, and then tested in further studies to evaluate its effectiveness and dissemination into a variety of healthcare settings.

Risk Factors for Cancer-Related Sexual Dysfunction

To understand the prevalence of sexual dysfunction after cancer, it is important to realize how common these problems are in otherwise healthy adults.

Prevalence of Sexual Dysfunction in the General Population

The National Health and Social Life Survey (NHSLS) conducted in 1992 still provides the best estimates of the prevalence of sexual problems in American adults 18 to 59, because the researchers used probability sampling and achieved a high response rate (79%).[107,164] Thirty-one percent of men and 43% of women had experienced a sexual dysfunction in the past year. Factors associated with sexual problems included poor physical and mental health, aging, past sexual trauma, and relationship satisfaction.

More recently, the Pfizer Global Study of Sexual Attitudes and Behaviors has used similar interview techniques to sample over 26,000 men and women aged 40 to 80 in 28 countries around the world. Although response rates were much lower than in the NHSLS, the sheer volume of data is impressive. Again, one-third to one-half of men and women reported having sexual dysfunctions during the past year.[165] In the data subsets from the United States, Canada, Australia and New Zealand, lack of sexual desire was the most frequent female problem (29%) whereas premature ejaculation was the most common male dysfunction (26%)[166] Overall, women were twice as likely as men to experience difficulty with sexual desire, experiencing pleasure, and reaching orgasm. Most large surveys agree that erectile dysfunction (ED) increases dramatically with age and cardiovascular risk factors in men, so that by age 70, about half of men experience it.[167-168] In contrast, sexual problems in sexually active women (other than vaginal dryness) do not increase consistently with age or ill health.[107,166] Elderly women are more likely than men of the same age to be without a sexual partner, however.[169]

Risk Factors for Sexual Dysfunction After Cancer

Within groups of cancer survivors, sexual dysfunction is usually related to the impact of cancer treatment, rather than being a function of the cancer itself, with a few notable exceptions. Prostate cancer that is locally advanced may damage nerves essential for erection.[170] Women with gynecological cancer, especially cancer of the cervix, vagina, or vulva, may experience pain and bleeding with sexual activity as a presenting symptom of their malignancy.[171] Cancer survivors most at risk for treatment-related sexual dysfunction are those with pelvic tumors and/or those whose treatments damage the hormonal systems mediating sexual desire and pleasure.

Psychosocial factors are also crucial. The risk of sexual dysfunction for any individual cancer survivor is heightened by overall emotional distress, relationship conflict, and having a partner who is sexually dysfunctional. It is also important to remember that medications used to treat depression, anxiety, pain, and nausea during and after cancer treatment frequently have sexual side effects.[167-169]

Treatment-Related Sexual Problems in Men

Men treated for prostate cancer are the group at highest risk for sexual dysfunction. In a prospective study of 31,742 nonphysician health professionals aged 53 to 90, rates of ED for the 2,109 men who had been diagnosed with prostate cancer were 10 to 15 times higher than for men of comparable age.[168] Despite attempts to modify surgery or radiation therapy for prostate cancer to spare sexual function, recent large cohort studies suggest that 75% to 85% of men treated for localized disease have long-term problems with ED.[172-175] Rates of ED are similar after radical cystectomy[176] but somewhat lower with treatment for colorectal cancer.[177] Men on hormonal therapy for advanced prostate cancer have even more severe sexual dysfunction because of the impact of androgen ablation on sexual desire and arousability.[129,175]

Men treated for testicular cancer are often assumed to be at increased risk for sexual problems. Two extensive recent reviews of the literature on this topic concur that few studies of high quality are available.[178,179] Nevertheless, both reviews conclude that the only clear sexual morbidity of treatment for testicular cancer is the interference of retroperitoneal node dissection with antegrade ejaculation. When the lymph nodes are fully dissected along the bifurcation of the aorta, nerves are disrupted that control the smooth muscle contractions of the prostate and seminal vesicles during the emission phase of male orgasm. The result is that men experience the pleasure of orgasm, but with no expulsion of semen. Most retroperitoneal lymphadenectomies now spare crucial nerves by limiting the dissection, preserving normal ejaculation of semen in 75% to 90% of patients.[180,181]

Prospective data on sexual function from a very recent Norwegian randomized trial of chemotherapy for 666 men with metastatic germ cell tumors found that sexual problems rose somewhat 3 months after treatment began, but by 2-year follow-up had subsided to normal levels.[182] The quality of the sexual relationship with a partner had also not suffered. In the longer term, however, testicular cancer survivors who had higher doses of external beam radiation therapy may have an increased risk of ED with aging[178] because of the potential for reduced blood flow in an irradiated pelvic vascular bed.

Higher than expected rates of sexual dysfunction have been reported in longer-term survivors of renal cell carcinoma[183] and bone marrow transplantation.[184] Low-normal to frankly low levels of testosterone are common in young men treated with high-dose chemotherapy for lymphoma or Hodgkin's Disease, which could be a factor in loss of sexual interest and arousal.[29]

Treatment-Related Sexual Problems in Women

Breast cancer is often assumed to be the site most associated with female sexual dysfunction. Although sexual problems are present in about half of long-term survivors of breast cancer, rates are comparable to those in age-matched women who have not had cancer.[119] Frequency of sexual activity is also similar to that of community-dwelling women of similar age.[119,123,185] Premenopausal women whose chemotherapy results in ovarian failure cancer do have unusually high rates of sexual dysfunction, however,[119,123,186] including a long-term loss of desire for sex, increased vaginal dryness, and dyspareunia. In a sample of 153 women interviewed 20 years after having chemotherapy for premenopausal breast cancer, 29% attributed current sexual problems to past cancer treatment.[187] In contrast to chemotherapy, tamoxifen is not associated with decreased desire for sex or impaired lubrication with sexual arousal.[119,186–188] Breast loss is not a crucial factor in these problems, contrary to conventional wisdom. Comparisons of women after various breast surgeries have been highly consistent in showing that breast conservation and reconstruction are not superior to mastectomy in preserving women's sexual function or satisfaction.[119,123,188,189]

Indeed, young women treated for leukemia or Hodgkin's disease are as likely as breast cancer survivors to report sexual dysfunction.[187] About a quarter to a third of women have sexual dysfunction after treatment for hematological malignancies. Although both psychosocial trauma and ovarian failure can contribute to their sexual problems,[190,191] in at least one, small randomized trial, a less gonadotoxic chemotherapy was not superior in sparing sexual function.[192]

A gender difference in sexual function seen both in unselected, healthy women[193] and in cancer survivors[119,194] is that women's sexual satisfaction is not tightly linked to physical functioning like men's, but rather to overall well-being and the quality of intimacy and affection with the sexual partner. For example, in women treated for vulvar cancer, the extent of the tissue excised is less important than relationship happiness in predicting sexual satisfaction.[194] Among breast cancer survivors, those who had found new partners after their cancer treatment had the happiest sex lives.[119]

Nevertheless, it is clear that treatment for gynecological malignancies, including cancer of the cervix, vulva, or uterus, does increase the prevalence of sexual dysfunction beyond that seen in healthy, community-dwelling peers, particularly rates of vaginal dryness and pain with sexual activity.[195] In women treated for localized cervical cancer, pelvic radiation therapy has a more negative impact than radical hysterectomy in reducing vaginal lubrication and expansion with sexual arousal, as seen in two small, but carefully monitored, prospective studies.[196,197] The literature on hysterectomy for benign disease also demonstrates no detriment of surgery to sexual function, even when the cervix is removed, as long as the woman's hormonal status remains unchanged.[198,199] The risk of painful sex and loss of erotic pleasure increases when bilateral oophorectomy is included, or if pelvic surgery affects vaginal caliber or depth, as in abdomino-perineal resection,[177] radical cystectomy,[200] or total pelvic exenteration.[201]

Management of Sexual Symptoms in Cancer Survivors

Despite increased attention in the past 20 years to sexual dysfunction as a consequence of cancer treatment, pitifully little progress has been made in developing cost-effective treatment programs to alleviate these symptoms. The entire field of behavior therapy for sexual dysfunction has seen scant innovation in techniques or new outcome research since the 1970s.[202] Although standard sex therapy programs have been modified for cancer patients,[203] prospective studies of efficacy are lacking.

In 1987, we published a retrospective chart review of detailed clinical notes on consultations in a sexual rehabilitation program within a cancer center over a 4-year period.[203] Out of 384 individuals or couples, 73% were seen only once or twice. Of the index patients seen, 308 were men and 76 were women. Male cancer patients were older, and were more likely to include a partner in their visits (56%) than were the women (28%). Seventy-nine percent of the patients had pelvic malignancies, but this probably reflected referral bias, since the program was located within a urology department and also had strong ties to gynecology. According to their retrospective reports, the prevalence of sexual dysfunctions had increased after cancer treatment in the index patients, but not in their partners. Most men sought help for ED whereas women typically had a combination of loss of desire and vaginal dryness/dyspareunia.

About half of patients were seen prior to or during cancer treatment, and half were first evaluated after treatment had been completed. Follow-up data on outcome were available for only 118 cases. The therapist rating of improvement was "somewhat to much better" for 63% of this group. Factors correlated with better outcome included having more counseling sessions, younger age, absence of depression, and absence of marital conflict.

Prospective clinical trials of sex therapy for specific types of sexual dysfunctions after cancer, using standardized outcome measures, should have followed this report. They are strikingly absent from the literature, however. The majority of people with sexual dysfunction after cancer never seek professional help. In the Pfizer Global Study of Sexuality, less than 20% of men or women unselected for health who had sexual problems consulted a physician about them, although roughly half discussed the problem with a partner, friend, or family member.[204]

Physicians are often urged to initiate discussions of sexuality with all patients, but an analysis of data from the same survey on 5,250 men aged 40 to 80 from 7 countries in Europe revealed that less than 7% had a physician who initiated an assessment of sexual function in the past year, although the majority of men believed such dialogues should be routine.[205] Medical schools in North America only devote an average of 3 to 10 hours to sexuality in the entire 4-year curriculum,[206] so that a physician who wants to counsel patients on sexual rehabilitation must be essentially self-taught. Qualitative interviews of nurses and physicians on an ovarian cancer treatment unit in England confirmed that less than a quarter ever discussed sexuality with patients,[207] despite knowing that sexual problems were prevalent.

We will discuss evidence-based management of sexual problems after cancer using the minimal empirical evidence that exists in the literature on treatment of dysfunctions in men and women unselected for health, and in the literature on sexual rehabilitation after cancer.

Modifying Cancer Treatment to Spare Male Sexual Function

One approach to managing cancer-related sexual dysfunction is to modify cancer treatment to prevent damage to hormonal, vascular, or neurologic systems needed for a healthy sexual response.

In men, hormonal therapy for advanced prostate cancer results in a profound loss of desire for sex, as well as erectile dysfunction and difficulty reaching orgasm (see also Chapter 12).[175,208,209] Tactics to avoid this morbidity have included delaying treatment in asymptomatic men, using intermittent hormonal therapy to keep prostate specific antigen (PSA) values close to zero while allowing improved sexual function during intervals off treatment, or prescribing an androgen-blocker such as bicalutamide either alone or in combination with finasteride. Unfortunately, delayed treatment may compromise ultimate survival time,[210] and both androgen production and sexual function appear to be permanently impaired by a period of months on androgen ablation.[175,211] Bicalutamide is more promising, but considerable sexual morbidity still occurs.[212]

Perhaps the best-validated attempt to preserve sexual function after cancer is the nerve-sparing modification of radical prostatectomy, cystectomy, and colorectal cancer surgery.[213] Although avoiding damage to the nerves near the prostate and posterior urethra helps preserve penile hemodynamics and erection in some men, up to 80% do not recover erections firm enough to allow vaginal penetration on most attempts.[172–175,214] Success depends on the skill of the surgeon, the ability to spare nerves bilaterally, and younger patient age. Although nerve-sparing may not restore normal erections, it does increase the percentage of men who can effectively use oral medications such as sildenafil.[175,214] Similarly, using brachytherapy instead of external beam irradiation to treat localized prostate cancers is only slightly more successful in preserving erectile function.[175,215]

Modifying cancer surgery to conserve or reconstruct pelvic organs does appear superior in terms of impact on sexuality. For example, conserving the bladder by using a combination of transurethral resection, chemotherapy, and radiation leaves men with better sexual function compared to radical cystectomy.[216] Procedures to reconstruct a continent, internal urinary pouch combined with nerve-sparing also appear to result in better sex lives for men compared to the traditional, radical cystectomy with ileal conduit.[217,218]

Modifying Cancer Treatment to Spare Female Sexual Function

In women, the main approaches that spare hormonal function are aimed at fertility, i.e. the conservative surgical approaches to gynecologic cancers.[66,71–74] The sexual consequences of such modifications have not been examined. Likewise, researchers have not studied the sexual impact of efforts to spare ovarian function by using ovarian transposition prior to radiation therapy, or GnRH agonists during chemotherapy.

In contrast to results after radical cystectomy, women who have orthotopic bladder reconstruction with preservation of the anterior vaginal wall do not report sexual dysfunction.[176,219] Surgery for colorectal cancer that avoids creation of an ostomy also results in better quality of life and sexual satisfaction.[220] Despite some controversy about the value of vaginal reconstruction after total pelvic exenteration for cervical cancer, the majority of women stay sexually active with their neovagina[201] and the use of myocutaneous flaps helps fill in the surgical defect and promotes healing.

Unfortunately, these reports focus on small series of highly selected patients treated at academic centers. It would be virtually impossible to conduct randomized trials of more vs. less radical surgical procedures, keeping patient age, education, socioeconomic status, and tumor variables equal between groups. Yet, when several randomized trials did compare mastectomy to breast conservation, researchers were surprised to find that neither sexual variables nor quality of life differed according to the extent of breast surgery.[119,188]

Treatment of Desire Disorders

Loss of desire for sex is one of the most common sexual problems seen in both male and female cancer survivors. The efficacy of androgen in alleviating these problems is controversial. Decreased androgen levels are an important factor in men on androgen ablation, some men treated for testicular cancer, or men who have sustained gonadal damage from high-dose chemotherapy.[221] Ovarian failure in women and chronic use of opioid therapy[222] in both genders also can reduce circulating androgens and sexual desire.

Unfortunately, androgen replacement therapy remains more of an art than a science. In young men who are clearly hypogonadal, testosterone replacement restores sexual motivation and pleasure.[223,224] Only two double-blinded, randomized, placebo-controlled trials of the newer testosterone gel or patch formulations have been published, however, with contrasting outcomes.[225,226] Androgens were administered to hypogonadal men unselected for cancer history. The study showing no benefit focused on men over age 65 with testosterone in low-normal range.[225] Men in the more successful trial were more hypogonadal.[226]

In men, loss of desire for sex is often linked to frustration and low self-esteem when erectile function is impaired.[175] One research group has had success in treating ED by combining testosterone with sildenafil for men with low circulating androgen levels.[227] The same strategy was helpful to eight severely hypogonadal men who had testicular failure after bone marrow transplant.[221] Whereas testosterone replacement is a viable option for young, hypogonadal, cancer survivors, men treated for prostate cancer are obviously not candidates. Although elevated luteinizing hormone levels combined with low-normal testosterone levels are common in young men after high-dose chemotherapy, a recent trial of the testosterone patch in 35 such survivors failed to document positive changes in mood or sexual function.[228]

Loss of desire for sex is common after systemic treatment for breast cancer,[119,124,188] As reviewed in the previous section of this chapter, there is reasonable evidence for the safety of short-term estrogen replacement in breast cancer survivors, but no studies have examined the impact of androgen replacement in this population, despite suggestions that such treatment might improve women's sexual function.[229] Yet, high androgen levels are clearly associated with breast cancer risk in postmenopausal women, and have also been observed post-diagnosis.[230]

In fact, the level of androgens needed to maintain normal sexual function in women, particularly after menopause, is unknown.[231] Several methodologically sound studies have not found any correlation between endogenous androgen levels and sexual function in naturally postmenopausal women.[232-234] The only randomized, placebo-controlled trials that have shown a sexual benefit of testosterone replacement in women have studied surgically menopausal women and have raised testosterone above the normal physiological level.[235-237] No published trials of testosterone replacement have focused on female cancer survivors, although studies of safety and efficacy would be appropriate in women in ovarian failure after treatment for tumors that are not hormone sensitive. However, female survivors of Hodgkin's disease exposed to radiation would be poor candidates because of their already elevated risk of breast cancer, which appears to be potentiated by ovarian hormones.[238]

In the future, selective androgen receptor modifiers may provide a safer modality to treat desire problems in women with abnormally low testosterone. A recent randomized, double-blind cross-over trial of tibolone vs. placebo in 44 post-menopausal women who did not have sexual complaints found in a laboratory paradigm that women taking tibolone had increased sexual desire, fantasies, and arousability, as well as improved vaginal lubrication.[239] Unfortunately, tibolone also appears to increase the risk of breast cancer in postmenopausal women.[240]

Loss of sexual desire after cancer treatment is often multifactorial, rather than a purely hormonal problem, particularly in women. Risk factors can include lingering post-treatment fatigue, pain, or nausea; perceiving oneself as less attractive after cancer; loss of sexual pleasure because of changes in skin sensitivity or genital blood flow; dreading sex because of dyspareunia; medication side effects; mild depression; and relationship conflict exacerbated by cancer treatment. Empirical studies suggest that sexual desire and arousability are linked in women, not only with each other, but with chronic mood disorders, low self-esteem, and guilt about sexuality.[241] Andersen developed a questionnaire to measure negative sexual self-image and found women's scores correlated with failure to resume sex comfortably after gynecological cancer.[242] Treating low desire in women may involve cognitive-behavioral psychotherapeutic interventions rather than a simple, pharmaceutical approach. Such treatment programs should also be evaluated in randomized, controlled trials.[243,244]

Treatment of Erectile Dysfunction (ED) After Cancer

Most efforts at sexual rehabilitation for men after cancer have had the goal of mechanically restoring erectile rigidity. Despite the revolution in treating ED in the past 20 years, yielding not only the various types of penile prosthesis, medications to inject into the penis, vacuum devices, urethral suppositories, and more recently several oral prostaglandin E5-inhibiting drugs (PDE5-inibitors), the majority of men who seek help for ED are not satisfied in the long term. In three studies of outcome in impotence clinics where men were not selected for health or the etiology of their ED, only 30% to 40% of men were sexually active and considered their problem resolved by one to five years after their initial evaluation despite trying a mean of two treatment modalities.[245-247]

Men prefer noninvasive, "natural" therapies, such as oral medication, and often will not try more invasive treatments for ED if PDE-5 inhibitors do not restore reliable, firm erec-

tions. Men's adherence even to taking a pill is limited. In two case series of men prescribed sildenafil for ED of varied etiology, over half were no longer taking it by 2-year follow-up.[248,249] In a cohort of 197 consecutive patients, the most significant correlate of discontinuing sildenafil was a history of radical prostatectomy, primarily because the drug was less effective for these men.[249] Only 56% of the men who stopped using sildenafil tried a second treatment.

The importance of encouraging men who fail a first-line treatment to try a more invasive method is reinforced by data from 89 men with ED prospectively followed over 12 months.[250] Men tried an average of two treatments for ED, and those who found an effective medical treatment for ED reported better quality of life and less emotional distress about ED. Prostate cancer survivors were more likely to report trying more than one ED treatment.

In our own retrospective cohort study of men in the prostate cancer registry at the Cleveland Clinic Foundation, half of consecutive men surveyed filled out questionnaires.[214] At an average of 4.5 years after cancer treatment, 59% of 1,188 respondents with ED had tried at least one treatment for it. Only 38% of men found a medical treatment that was at least somewhat helpful in improving their sex lives, however, and just 30% of respondents were still using an ED treatment at the time of the survey. Seventy-nine percent of men had stopped using intraurethral prostaglandin suppositories, 66% no longer used penile injections, 61% stopped taking sildenafil, 59% discarded a vacuum erection device, and 19% no longer had sex with their implanted penile prosthesis. The most important factor in men continuing to use a treatment for ED was that it worked effectively. As in the case series above, men who tried a greater number of treatments were more likely to have positive scores on the International Index of Erectile Function.

A man's motivation to progress from taking a pill to trying a more invasive therapy may be a particularly important factor in the ultimate success of sexual rehabilitation. Penile injection therapy is one of the most effective treatments for men after prostate cancer.[214,250] Other correlates of a good sexual outcome in our survey included younger age, having a sexual partner who still enjoyed sex, having a cancer treatment that was more likely to spare some erectile function (e.g., bilateral nerve-sparing prostatectomy or brachytherapy), and no historical or current use of anti-androgen therapy.[175,214]

Surgeons who perform radical prostatectomy frequently encourage men to begin attempts within 6 weeks to get an erection through use of penile injections, a vacuum device, or a PDE5-inhibitor.[251] The theory is that regular increases of blood circulating to the penis will oxygenate the tissues of the cavernous bodies, preventing fibrosis and atrophy and enhancing the chance of nerve regeneration. This popular theory is based on one very small randomized trial using early penile injection therapy after prostatectomy, published in 1997.[252] Despite a number of attempts to replicate the results using oral medication or vacuum devices, no other peer-reviewed randomized trial has been published.

Treating Female Sexual Arousal Disorder (FSAD)

Men can observe their erections, but women are often unaware of vaginal expansion and lubrication, and subjective ratings of sexual arousal do not always correlate well with physiological measures.[253] When women complain of poor sexual arousability after cancer, they typically report a loss of desire for sex, along with a lack of subjective excitement and symptoms of vaginal dryness and tightness. Ovarian failure is a frequent medical factor.

In recent years, researchers testing pharmacological treatments for women's sexual problems have created the "diagnosis" of female sexual arousal disorder (FSAD), an isolated sexual complaint characterized by lack of genital vasocongestion. Nine randomized, placebo-controlled trials of therapies for FSAD in postmenopausal women have been published, including those reviewed above on androgen replacement.[254–257] None focus on cancer populations. Two randomized, placebo-controlled clinical trials of sildenafil for FSAD have not produced convincing results on its efficacy,[255,258] and Pfizer no longer intends to seek approval of the drug for women.[259] Another trial examined the efficacy of alprostadil cream applied to the vulva before intercourse. This is the same medication most commonly used in penile injection therapy, but no significant impact on female sexual function was observed.[256] The remaining trial compared a proprietary vulvar herbal lotion to placebo oil.[257] Only 20 women participated. The outcome measure was a sexual diary created for the study, which was conducted by the company marketing the lotion.

Thinking that FSAD might be caused by inadequate blood flow to the clitoris, researchers created a special vacuum device, the Eros, to increase clitoral engorgement.[260] In a sample of 19 women, use of the Eros over 6 weeks significantly increased reports of erotic sensation, lubrication, ability to reach orgasm, and overall sexual satisfaction, regardless of whether a woman had sexual dysfunction at baseline. The device has received FDA approval and has been shown to increase genital engorgement on repeated use.[261]

Women's subjective pleasure as well as objective changes in genital blood flow should be measured in a randomized trial comparing the Eros device to a handheld vibrator, or even to a woman's own manual self-stimulation. Although a placebo-controlled trial may not be possible, these two other conditions would presumably also induce sexual arousal and increased genital blood flow, as well as giving the woman tacit permission to enjoy genital stimulation. It is possible that these are the active components of the Eros intervention, rather than the vacuum-induced clitoral vasocongestion.

Managing Sexual Pain After Cancer Treatment

For women, pain with sexual activity is one of the most frequent problems after cancer treatment. Postmenopausal vaginal atrophy is frequently the cause. As noted in the previous section on managing menopausal symptoms, systemic or local estrogen replacement is highly effective in reversing vaginal atrophy as well as decreasing hot flashes. Although many female cancer survivors have concerns about using systemic estrogen, new forms of topical estrogen may be safer options.

The Estring® is a vaginal ring delivering a low dose of estradiol time-released over three months. It is effective in reversing vaginal atrophy with little impact on plasma estrogen levels.[262–264] In the dosage that would be used in breast cancer survivors, the Estring® may not reduce hot flashes but has been shown in randomized, placebo-controlled trials to reduce urinary incontinence in about 50% of women.[264] A higher dose could be used in women who had not had a history of hormone-sensitive tumors. Women prefer the Estring® to vaginal suppositories[265] or creams. Many can insert the Estring® themselves but others may need a medical visit to replace the ring. Women with significant vaginal prolapse may not be able to tolerate the ring. Another form of vaginal estrogen replacement that is superior to estrogen cream in patient acceptance and does not elevate plasma estradiol is the Vagifem® suppository[266] which contains 17beta-estradiol.

Trials of these localized estrogen therapies should be conducted specifically in cancer survivors. One goal would be to ascertain the safety of long-term use in women prematurely menopausal after breast cancer. Another would be to test efficacy in women whose vaginal atrophy is not just the result of estrogen deficiency, but is complicated by tissue damage from pelvic radiotherapy[267] or post-transplant graft vs. host disease.[268] These women are particularly vulnerable to dyspareunia. Recently a case report has described successful treatment of vaginal agglutination after allogeneic bone marrow transplant, using a combination of surgical dissection of adhesions, estrogen cream, and vaginal dilation.[269]

Although regular vaginal stretching by intercourse or use of a dilator has been assumed to prevent loss of depth and caliber after pelvic radiation therapy, remarkably little evidence exists to demonstrate this effect. A recent Cochrane Library review of interventions for female sexual dysfunction after pelvic radiotherapy[270] found only two references on dilators. Both were retrospective case series, although they presented evidence that dilators could help maintain or restore vaginal patency. The most recent reference was published in 1999. Furthermore, most women are probably not adherent with the classic recommendation to have sexual intercourse or use a dilator three times weekly. In one small study, 32 cervical cancer survivors were randomized to one session of counseling plus a booklet on sex and cancer, or to a 3-hour psychoeducational group designed to increase adherence to vaginal dilation.[271] Group participation increased the percentage of women under age 41 who met the criterion of dilator/intercourse use from 6% to 44%. About half of the older women met the criterion, whether they were in the intervention or control group. For all women, rates of dilation decreased over the year of the study. Since the fibrosis after radiation therapy continues to progress for several years,[267] long-term adherence to vaginal stretching would be necessary to ensure continued ability to enjoy sexual intercourse and to allow adequate pelvic examinations—assuming that vaginal stretching is indeed physiologically effective.

Perhaps the simplest and most conservative intervention for dyspareunia after cancer is instruction on the use of water-based lubricants during sexual activity. Yet, the only study that evaluates the outcome of giving advice on lubricants is Ganz' nursing intervention, which did reduce vaginal pain and dryness.[163] This trial and several others also included the use of Replens®, a polycarbophil-based vaginal moisturizer that adheres to the vaginal mucosa and is designed to be used three times weekly, independent of any sexual activity. One double-blind, crossover, randomized clinical trial compared 4 weeks of Replens® to a "placebo" water-based lubricant[272] in 45 postmenopausal breast cancer survivors. Although both preparations relieved vaginal dryness, Replens® was signifi-

TABLE 19.3. Treatment algorithms for common reproductive problems after cancer.

Level of intervention	Hot flashes	Loss of sexual desire	Erectile dysfunction	Vaginal dryness/dyspareunia
Written pamphlet, video, internet, or nurse	Education about diet, dress, sleep, hygiene	Assessment of depression, fatigue, and medications with sexual side effects	Education about impact of cancer treatment and availability of medical treatments	Education on use of water-based lubricants and vaginal moisturizers[280]
Peer counseling or counseling by a mental health professional	Stress management with focus on relaxation training	Promote positive body image, permission to have sexual fantasies, activities that increase desire, and erotic material such as stories or films[280]	Intervention to enhance couple's sexual communication, improve partner's sexual satisfaction[280]	Education on positioning, Kegel exercises to gain voluntary control over circumvaginal muscles[280]
Intervention by a physician	Prescription of antidepressant medication, and consideration of risk/benefit ratio of using estrogen replacement	Change medications that may be interfering with desire; Consideration of androgen replacement, but only if survivor's levels are in the clinically hypogonadal range and the survivor is not at high risk for breast or prostate cancer as a recurrence or second primary tumor	Try medical treatments that are acceptable to both partners, starting with least invasive[281]	Prescription of graduated vaginal dilators with instructions on use to maximize control over vaginal muscles[280]; Prescription of local vaginal estrogen replacement if appropriate; Consideration of vaginal reconstructive surgery in rare cases

cantly more effective in reducing dyspareunia scores. In two open-label studies of women unselected for cancer history, Replens® was just as effective as estrogen cream in treating vaginal atrophy and dyspareunia.[273,274]

In women with chronic pelvic pain and dyspareunia unrelated to a history of cancer treatment, successful comprehensive treatment programs have combined sexual counseling with specific biofeedback and physical therapy modalities designed to increase awareness of and control over muscle tension in the pelvic floor.[275] Trials applying these techniques are needed with women who have dyspareunia related to surgical adhesions or anatomic changes, radiation damage to the vagina, or vaginal complications of graft vs. host disease.

Similar treatments have been helpful in a pilot study of men with chronic pelvic pain.[276] Pelvic pain has been reported to be more common than usual after treatment for testicular cancer[277] or after radical prostatectomy.[175,278] This type of pain is very recalcitrant to treatment and may include aching in the testes or groin, and/or urethral pain exacerbated by urination or ejaculation. Non-steroidal anti-inflammatory or alpha-blocking drugs, low-dose antidepressants, and nerve blocks are occasionally helpful, but more extreme surgical procedures do not produce results that justify routine use.[279] Randomized trials of treatments for male pelvic pain have not been published.

Table 19.3 presents treatment algorithms for the most common reproductive symptoms seen in cancer survivors: hot flashes, loss of sexual desire, erectile dysfunction, and vaginal dryness/dyspareunia. The first level of intervention involves giving patient education materials in written, video, or interactive computerized format. If more help is needed, brief counseling can be provided either by a trained peer counselor or by a member of the oncology team, such as a nurse clinician or social worker. At the third level, a health care provider specialist is consulted. Many brief counseling interventions can be found in a self-help format[280] and algorithms for treating ED are also available.[281]

Conclusions

Reproductive health problems, including sexual dysfunction, menopausal symptoms, and infertility are common, long-term consequences of cancer treatment for both men and women. Until targeted cancer therapies are more common, systemic chemotherapy is likely to entail considerable gonadal toxicity. Efforts to modify pelvic surgery and radiation therapy to spare the reproductive system are ongoing, but remain limited in applicability and efficacy. Because sexuality and childbearing are such sensitive issues, psychosocial counseling and education may increase the efficacy of purely physiological interventions As this review highlights, very little evidence-based knowledge is available to guide oncology clinicians in remediating reproductive health issues. For many problems, pilot studies of efficacy of innovative treatments are needed before randomized trials can be justified. Hopefully our increasing knowledge about the prevalence, causes, and impact on quality of life of reproductive health problems will soon generate more research.

References

1. Lucas JW, Schiller JS, Benson V. Summary health statistics for United States adults: National Health Interview Survey, 2001. National Center for Health Statistics, Vital Health Stat 2004; 10(218).
2. United States Census Bureau. US Summary 2000: Census 2000 Profile. Washington, DC: Government publication C2KPROF00US; 2002.
3. MacDorman MF, Minino AM, Strobino DM, et al. Annual summary of vital statistics—2001. Pediatrics 2002;110: 1037–1052.
4. Bachu A, O'Connell M. Fertility of American women: June 2000. Current Population Reports, P20-543RV. U.S. Census Bureau, Washington, DC, 2001.
5. United Nations Population Division of the Department of Economic and Social Affairs. Wall chart: World Marriage

Patterns 2000. http://www.un.org/esa/population/publications/worldmarriage/worldmarriage.htm, accessed 12/7/04.

6. Jacobsen R, Bostofte E, Engholm G, et al. Fertility and offspring sex ratio of men who develop testicular cancer: a record linkage study. Hum Reprod 2000;15:1958–1961.

7. Skakkebæk NE, Rajpert-De Meyts E, Main KM. Testicular dysgenesis syndrome: an increasingly common developmental disorder with environmental aspects. Hum Reprod 2001;16:972–978.

8. Hoei-Hansen, CE, Holm M, Rajpert-De Meyts E, Skakkebæk NE. Histological evidence of testicular dysgenesis in contralateral biopsies from 218 patients with testicular germ cell cancer. J Pathol 2003;200:370–374.

9. Jacobsen R, Bostofte E., Engholm G, et al. Risk of testicular cancer in men with abnormal semen characteristics: cohort study. Brit Med J 2000;321:789–792.

10. Venn A, Healy D, McLachlan R. Cancer risks associated with the diagnosis of infertility. Best Practice & Res Clin Obstet Gynecol 2003;17:343–367.

11. Doyle P, Maconochie N, Beral V, et al. Cancer incidence following treatment for infertility at a clinic in the UK. Hum Reprod 2002;17:2209–2213.

12. Burkman RT, Tang MTC, Malone KE, et al. Infertility drugs and the risk of breast cancer: findings from the National Institute of Child Health and Human Development Women's Contraceptive and Reproductive Experiences Study. Fertil Steril 2003;79:844–851.

13. Kauff ND, Satagopan JM, Robson ME, et al. Risk-reducing salpingo-oophorectomy in women with a BRCA1 or BRCA2 mutation. N Eng J Med 2002;346:1609–1615.

14. Heidenreich A, Albers P, Hartmann M, et al. Complications of primary nerve sparing retroperitoneal lymph node dissection for clinical stage I nonseminomatous germ cell tumors of the testis: experience of the German Testicular Cancer Study Group. J Urol 2003;169:1710–1714.

15. Havenga K, Maas CP, DeRuiter MC, Welvaart K, Trimbos JB. Avoiding long-term disturbance to bladder and sexual function in pelvic surgery, particularly with rectal cancer. Sem Surg Oncol 2000;18:235–243.

16. Meirow D, Nugent D. The effects of radiotherapy and chemotherapy on female reproduction. Hum Reprod 2001;7:535–543.

17. Tilly JL, Kolesnick RN. Sphingolipids, apoptosis, cancer treatments and the ovary: investigating a crime against female fertility. Biochim Biophys Acta 2002;1585:135–138.

18. Blumenfeld Z. Preservation of fertility and ovarian function and minimalization of chemotherapy associated gonadotoxicity and premature ovarian failure: the role of inhibin-A and –B as markers. Molecular Cellular Endocrinol 2002;187:93–105.

19. Minton SE, Munster PN. Chemotherapy-induced amenorrhea and fertility in women undergoing adjuvant treatment for breast cancer. Cancer Control 2002;9:466–472.

20. Thomson AB, Critchley HOD, Wallace WHB. Paediatric update: fertility and progeny. Eur J Cancer 2002;38:1634–1644.

21. Hassan MA, Killick SR. Effect of male age on fertility: evidence for the decline in male fertility with increasing age. Fertil Steril 2003;79 (Suppl 3):1520–1527.

22. Schover LR, Rybicki LA, Martin BA, et al. Having children after cancer: a pilot survey of survivors' attitudes and experiences. Cancer 1999;86:697–709.

23. Schover, LR Brey K, Lichtin A, et al. Knowledge and experience regarding cancer, infertility, and sperm banking in younger male survivors. J Clin Oncol 2002;20:1880–1889.

24. Green D, Galvin H, Horne B. The psycho-social impact of infertility on young male cancer survivors: a qualitative investigation. Psycho-Oncology 2003;12:141–152.

25. Thewes B, Meiser B, Rickard J, et al. The fertility- and menopause-related information needs of younger women with a diagnosis of breast cancer: a qualitative study. Psycho-Oncology 2003;12:500–511.

26. Dow KH. Having children after breast cancer. Cancer Practice 1994;2:407–413.

27. Stephen EH, Chandra A. Use of infertility services in the United States: 1995. Family Planning Perspect 2000;32:132–137.

28. Schover LR, Thomas AJ. Overcoming Male Infertility. New York: John Wiley & Sons, 2000.

29. Howell SJ, Shalet SM. Fertility preservation and management of gonadal failure associated with lymphoma therapy. Curr Oncol Rep 2002;4:443–452.

30. Kelnar CJ, McKinnell C, Walker M, et al. Testicular changes during infantile 'quiescence' in the marmoset and their gonadotrophin dependence: a model for investigating susceptibility of the prepubertal human testis to cancer therapy. Hum Reprod 2002;17:1367–1378.

31. Blumenfeld Z, Dann E, Avivi R, et al. Fertility after treatment for Hodgkin's disease. Ann Oncol 2002;13 (Suppl 1):138–147.

32. Recchia F, Sica G, De Filippis S, et al. Goserelin as ovarian protection in the adjuvant treatment of premenopausal breast cancer: a phase II pilot study. Anti-Cancer Drugs 2002;13:417–424.

33. Familiari G, Caggiati, A, Nottola SA, et al. Ultrastructure of human ovarian primordial follicles after combination chemotherapy for Hodgkin's disease. Hum Reprod 1993;8:2080–2087.

34. Tilly JL. Molecular and genetic basis of normal and toxicant-induced apoptosis in female germ cells. Toxicol Lett 1998;102–103:497–501.

35. Johnson J, Canning J, Kaneko T, Pru JK, Tilly J. Germline stem cells and follicular renewal in the postnatal mammalian ovary. Nature 2004;428:145–150.

36. Anger JT, Gilbert BR, Goldstein M. Cryopreservation of sperm: Indications, methods and results. J Urol 2003;170:1079–1084.

37. Agarwal A, Tolentine MV, Sidhu RS, et al. Effect of cryopreservation on semen quality of patients with testicular cancer. Urol 1995;46:382–389.

38. Padron OF, Sharma RK, Thomas AJ, et al. Effects of cancer on spermatozoa quality after cryopreservation: a 12–year experience. Fertil Steril 1997;67:326–331.

39. Lass A, Akagbosu F, Abusheikha N, et al. A programme of semen cryopreservation for patients with malignant disease in a tertiary infertility centre: lessons from 8 years' experience. Hum Reprod 1998;13:3256–3261.

40. Audrins P, Holden CA, McLachlan RI, Kovacs GT. Semen storage for special purposes at Monash IVF from 1977 to 1997. Fertil Steril 1999;72:179–181.

41. Kelleher S, Wishart SM, Liu PY, et al. Long-term outcomes of elective human sperm cryostorage. Hum Reprod 2001;16:2632–2639.

42. Blackhall FH, Atkinson AD, Maaya MB et al. Semen cryopreservation, utilization and reproductive outcome in men treated for Hodgkin's disease. Brit J Cancer 2002;87:381–384.

43. Agarwal A, Ranganathan P, Kattal N, et al. Fertility after cancer: a prospective review of assisted reproductive outcome with banked semen specimens. Fertil Steril 2004;81:342–348.

44. Ragni G, Somigliana E, Restelli L, et al. Sperm banking and rate of assisted reproduction treatment: insights from a 15–year cryopreservation program for male cancer patients. Cancer 2003;97:1624–1629.

45. Agarwal A, Sidhu RK, Shekarriz M, et al. Optimum abstinence time for cryopreservation of semen in cancer patients. J Urol 1995;54:86–88.

46. Hallak J, Sharma RK, Thomas AJ, et al. Why cancer patients request disposal of cryopreserved semen specimens post-therapy: a retrospective study. Fertil Steril 1998;69:889–893.

47. Schover LR, Brey K, Lichtin A, et al. Oncologists' attitudes and practices regarding banking sperm before cancer treatment. J Clin Oncol 2002;20:1890–1897.

48. Wilford H, Hunt J. An overview of sperm cryopreservation services for adolescent cancer patients in the United Kingdom. Eur J Oncol Nurs 2003;7:24–32.

49. Allen C, Keane D, Harrison, RF. A survey of Irish consultants regarding awareness of sperm freezing and assisted reproduction. Ir Med J 2003;96:23–25.

50. Hallak J, Hendin B, Bahadur G, et al. Semen quality and cryopreservation in adolescent cancer patients. Hum Reprod 2002; 17:3157–3161.

51. Nagano M, Patrizio P, Brinster RL. Long-term survival of human spermatogonial stem cells in mouse testes. Fertil Steril 2002; 78:1225–1233.

52. Yoon TK, Kim TJ, Park SE, et al. Live births after vitrification of oocytes in a stimulated in vitro fertilization-embryo transfer program. Fertil Steril 2003;79:1323–1326.

53. Eroglu A, Toner M, Toth TL. Beneficial effect of microinjected trehalose on the cryosurvival of human oocytes. Fertil Steril 2002;77:152–158.

54. Gosden R, Nagano M. Preservation of fertility in nature and ART. Reprod 2002;123:3–11.

55. Liu J, Ju G, Qian Y, et al. Pregnancies and births achieved from in vitro matured oocytes retrieved from poor responders undergoing stimulation in in vitro fertilization cycles. Fertil Steril 2003;80:447–449.

56. Oktay K, Economos K, Khan M, et al. Endocrine function and oocyte retrieval after autologous transplantation of ovarian cortical strips to the forearm. JAMA 2001;286:1490–1493.

57. Radford JA, Leiberman BA, Brison RB, et al. Orthotopic reimplantation of cryopreserved ovarian cortical strips after high-dose chemotherapy for Hodgkin's lymphoma. Lancet 2001;57:1172–1175.

58. Kim SS. Ovarian tissue banking for cancer patients: to do or not to do? Hum Reprod 2003;18:1759–1761.

59. Oktay K, Buyuk E, Veeck L, et al. Embryo development after heterotopic transplantation of cryopreserved ovarian tissue. Lancet 2004;363:837–840.

60. Lee DM, Yeoman RR, Battaglia DE, et al. Brief Communication: live birth after ovarian tissue transplant. Nature 2004;428: 137–138.

61. Williams RS, Littell RD, Mendenhall NP. Laparoscopic oophoropexy and ovarian function in the treatment of Hodgkin disease. Cancer 1999;86:2138–2142.

62. Bisharah M, Tulandi T. Laparoscopic preservation of ovarian function: an underused procedure. Am J Obstet Gynecol 2003; 188:367–370.

63. Picone O, Aucouturier JS, Louboutin A, et al. Abdominal wall metastasis of a cervical adenocarcinoma at the laparoscopic trocar insertion site after ovarian transposition: case report and review of the literature. Gynecol Oncol 2003;90:446–449.

64. Buekers TE, Anderson B, Sorosky JI, et al. Ovarian function after surgical treatment for ovarian cancer. Gynecol Oncol 2001;80:85–88.

65. Burnett AF, Roman LD, O'Meara AT, Morrow CP. Radical vaginal trachelectomy and pelvic lymphadenectomy for preservation of fertility in early cervical carcinoma. Gyn Oncol 2003; 88:419–423.

66. Plante, M. Fertility preservation in the management of gynecologic cancers. Curr Opin Oncol 2000;12:497–507.

67. Schlaerth JB, Spritos NM, Schlaerth AC. Radical trachelectomy and pelvic lymphadenectomy with uterine preservation in the treatment of cervical cancer. Am J Obstet Gynecol 2003; 188:29–34.

68. Shepherd JH, Mould T, Oram DH. Radical trachelectomy in early stage carcinoma of the cervix: outcome as judged by recurrence and fertility rates. BJOG 2001;108:882–885.

69. McHale MT, Le TD, Burger RA, et al. Fertility sparing treatment for in situ and early invasive adenocarcinoma of the cervix. Obstet Gynecol 2001;98:726–731.

70. Soutter WP, Haidopoulos D, Gornall, RJ, et al. Is conservative treatment for adenocarcinoma in situ of the cervix safe? BJOG 2001;108:1184–1189.

71. Morris RT, Gershenson DM, Silva EG, et al. Outcome and reproductive function after conservative surgery for borderline ovarian tumors. Obstet Gynecol 2000;95:541–547.

72. Brewer M, Gershenson DM, Herzog CE, et al. Outcome and reproductive function after chemotherapy for ovarian dysgerminoma. J Clin Oncol 1999;17:2670–2675.

73. Schilder JM, Thompson AM DePriest PD, et al. Outcome of reproductive age women with stage IA or IC invasive epithelial ovarian cancer treated with fertility-sparing therapy. Gynecol Oncol 2002;87:1–7.

74. Tangir J, Zelterman D, Ma W, Schwartz PE. Reproductive function after conservative surgery and chemotherapy for malignant germ cell tumors of the ovary. Obstet Gynecol 2003;101:251–257.

75. Meistrich ML, Wilson G, Mathur K, et al. Rapid recovery of spermatogenesis after mitoxantrone, vincristine, vinblastine, and prednisone chemotherapy for Hodgkin's disease. J Clin Oncol 1997;15:3488–3495.

76. Ohl DA, Sonksen J. What are the chances of infertility and should sperm be banked? Sem Urol Oncol 1996;14:36–44.

77. Colombo R, Bertini R, Salonia A, et al. Nerve and seminal sparing radical cystectomy with orthotopic urinary diversion for select patients with superficial bladder cancer: an innovative surgical approach. J Urol 2001;165:51–55.

78. Weisz B, Schiff E, Lishner M. Cancer in pregnancy: maternal and fetal implications. Hum Reprod Update 2001;7:384–393.

79. Gwyn KM, Theriault RL. Breast cancer during pregnancy. Curr Treat Options Oncol 2000;1:239–243.

80. Schover LR. Psychosocial issues associated with cancer in pregnancy. Sem Oncol 2000;27:699–703.

81. Wenzel L, Berkowitz RS, Newlands E, et al. Quality of life after gestational trophoblastic disease. J Reprod Med 2002;47:387–394.

82. Green DM, Whitton JA, Stovall M, et al. Pregnancy outcome of female survivors of childhood cancer: a report from the Childhood Cancer Survivor Study. Am J Obstet Gynecol 2002;187: 1070–1080.

83. Critchley HO, Bath LE, Wallace WH. Radiation damage to the uterus: Review of the effects of treatment of childhood cancer. Hum Fertil 2002;5:61–66.

84. Surbone A, Petrek JA. Childbearing issues in breast carcinoma survivors. Cancer 1997;79:1271–1278.

85. Ginsburg ES, Yanushpolsky EH, Jackson KV. In vitro fertilization for cancer patients and survivors. Fertil Steril 2001;75: 705–710.

86. Oktay KH, Buyuk E, Yermakova I, Veeck L, Rosenwaks Z. Fertility preservation in breast cancer patients: IVF and embryo cryopreservation after ovarian stimulation with tamoxifen. Hum Reprod 2003;18:90–95.

87. Oktay K. Further evidence on the safety and success of ovarian stimulation with letrozole and tamoxifen in breast cancer patients undergoing in vitro fertilization to cryopreserve their embryos for fertility preservation. J Clin Oncol 2005;23:3858–3859.

88. Anselmo AP, Cavalieri E, Aragona C, et al. Successful pregnancies following an egg donation program in women with previously treated Hodgkin's disease. Haematologia 2001;86:624–628.

89. Larsen EC, Loft A, Holm K, et al. Oocyte donation in women cured of cancer with bone marrow transplantation including total body irradiation in adolescence. Hum Reprod 2000; 15:1505–1508.

90. Giacalone PL, Laffargue F, Benos P, et al. Successful in vitro fertilization-surrogate pregnancy in a patient with ovarian

transposition who had undergone chemotherapy and pelvic irradiation. Fertil Steril 2001;76:388–389.

91. Ohl DA, Denil J, Bennett CJ, et al. Electroejaculation following retroperitoneal lymphadenectomy. J Urol 1991;145:980–983.

92. Ohl DA, Wolf LJ, Menge AC, et al. Electroejaculation and assisted reproductive technologies in the treatment of anejaculatory infertility. Fertil Steril 2001;76:1249–1255.

93. Hovav Y, Dan-Goor M, Yaffe H, et al. Electroejaculation before chemotherapy in adolescents and young men with cancer. Fertil Steril 2001;75:811–813.

94. Damani MN, Master V, Meng MV, et al. Postchemotherapy ejaculatory azoospermia: fatherhood with sperm from testis tissue with intracytoplasmic sperm injection. J Clin Oncol 2002;20:930–936.

95. Chan PT, Palermo GD, Veeck LL, Rosenwaks Z, et al. Testicular sperm extraction combined with intracytoplasmic sperm injection in the treatment of men with persistent azoospermia postchemotherapy. Cancer 2001;92:1632–1637.

96. Robbins WA, Meistrich ML, Moore D, et al. Chemotherapy induces transient sex chromosomal and autosomal aneuploidy in human sperm. Nat Genet 1997;16:74–78.

97. Burrello N, Vicari E, Shin P, et al. Lower sperm aneuploidy frequency is associated with high pregnancy rates in ICSI programmes. Hum Reprod 2003;18:1371–1376.

98. Thomson AB, Campbell AJ, Irvine DC, et al. Semen quality and spermatozoal DNA integrity in survivors of childhood cancer: a case-control Study. Lancet 2002;360(9330):361–367.

99. Arnon J, Meirow D, Lewis-Roness H, et al. Genetic and teratogenic effects of cancer treatments on gametes and embryos. Hum Reprod 2001;7:394–403.

100. Winther JF, Boice JD, Mulvihill JJ, et al. Chromosomal abnormalities among offspring of childhood-cancer survivors in Denmark: a population-based study. Am J Hum Genet 2004;74:1282–1285.

101. Green DM, Whitton JA, Stovall M, et al. Pregnancy outcome of partners of male survivors of childhood cancer: a report from the Childhood Cancer Survivor Study. J Clin Oncol 2003;21:716–721.

102. Sankila R, Olson JH, Anderson H, et al. Risk of cancer among offspring of childhood-cancer survivors. Association of the Nordic Cancer Registries and the Nordic Society of Paediatric Haematology and Oncology. N Engl J Med 1998;38:1339–1344.

103. Berry DL, Theriault RL, Holmes FA, et al. Management of breast cancer during pregnancy using a standardized protocol. J Clin Oncol 1999;7:855–861.

104. Narod SA. Hormonal prevention of hereditary breast cancer. Ann NY Acad Sci 2001;952:36–43.

105. Rebbeck TR, Lynch HT, Neuhausen SL, et al. The Prevention and Observation of Surgical End Points Study Group. Prophylactic oophorectomy in carriers of BRCA1 or BRCA2 mutations. N Eng J Med 2002;346:1616–1622.

106. Rechitsky S, Verlinsky O, Chistokhina A, et al. Preimplantation genetic diagnosis for cancer predisposition. Reprod Biomed 2002;5:148–155.

107. Laumann EO, Paik A, Rosen RC. Sexual dysfunction in the United States: Prevalence and predictors. JAMA 1999;281:537–544.

108. Avis NE, McKinlay SM. The Massachusetts Women's Health Study: an epidemiologic investigation of the menopause. J Amer Med Women's Association 1995;50:45–49.

109. Avis NE, McKinlay SM. A longitudinal analysis of women's attitudes toward the menopause: results from the Massachusetts Women's Health Study. Maturitas 1991;13:65–79.

110. McKinlay JB, McKinlay SM, Brambilla DJ. Health status and utilization behavior associated with menopause. Amer J Epidemiol 1987;125:111–121.

111. Avis NE, Stellato R, Crawford S, Johannes C, et al. Is there an association between menopause status and sexual functioning? Menopause 2000;7:286–288.

112. McKinlay JB, McKinlay SM, Brambilla D. The relative contributions of endocrine changes and social circumstances to depression in mid-aged women. J Health Soc Behav 1987;28:345–363.

113. Avis NE, Crawford S, McKinlay SM. Psychosocial, behavioral, and health factors related to menopause symptomatology. Womens Health 1997;3:103–120.

114. Sternfeld B, Quesenberry CP Jr., Husson G. Habitual physical activity and menopausal symptoms: a case-control study. J Women's Health 1999;8:115–123.

115. Keating NL, Cleary PD, Rossi AS, et al. Use of hormone replacement therapy by postmenopausal women in the United States. Annals Internal Med 1999;130:545–553.

116. Staropoli CA, Flaws JA, Bush TL, et al. Predictors of menopausal hot flashes. J Women's Health 1998;7:1149–1155.

117. Carpenter JS, Johnson D, Wagner L, et al. Hot flashes and related outcomes in breast cancer survivors and matched comparison women. Oncol Nurs Forum 2002;29:E16–25.

118. Carpenter JS, Andrykowski MA, Cordova M, et al. Hot flashes in postmenopausal women treated for breast carcinoma: prevalence severity, correlates, management, and relation to quality of life. Cancer 1998;82:1682–1691.

119. Ganz PA, Rowland JH, Desmond K, et al. Life after breast cancer: understanding women's health-related quality of life and sexual functioning. J Clin Oncol 1998;16:501–514.

120. Biglia N, Cozzarella M, Cacciari F, et al. Menopause after breast cancer: a survey on breast cancer survivors. Maturitas 2003;45:29–38.

121. Stein KD, Jacobsen PB, Hann DM, et al. Impact of hot flashes on quality of life among postmenopausal women being treated for breast cancer. Pain Symptom Manage 2000;19:436–445.

122. Nystedt M, Berglund G, Bolund C, et al. Side effects of adjuvant endocrine treatment in premenopausal breast cancer patients: a prospective randomized study. J Clin Oncol 2003;21:1836–1844.

123. Mourits MJ, Bockermann I, de Vries EG, et al. Tamoxifen effects on subjective and psychosexual well-being, in a randomized breast cancer study comparing high-dose and standard-dose chemotherapy. Br J Cancer 2002;86:1546–1550.

124. Ganz PA, Desmond KA, Leedham B, et al. Quality of life in long-term disease-free survivors of breast cancer: a follow-up study. J Natl Cancer Inst 2002;94:39–49.

125. Jensen PT, Klee MC, Groenvold M. Validation of a questionnaire for self-rating of urological and gynaecological morbidity after treatment of gynaecological cancer. Radiother Oncol 2002;65:29–38.

126. Denton AS, Maher EJ. Interventions for the physical aspects of sexual dysfunction in women following pelvic radiotherapy (Cochrane Review). In: The Cochrane Library 2003;3:1–26. Oxford: Update Software.

127. Schimmer AD, Quatermain M, Imrie D, et al. Ovarian function after autologous bone marrow transplantation. J Clin Oncol 1998;16:2359–2363.

128. Rossouw JE, Anderson GL, Prentice RL, et al. Risks and benefits of estrogen plus progestin in healthy postmenopausal women: principal results from the Women's Health Initiative randomized controlled trial. JAMA 2002;288:321–333.

129. Thompson CA, Shanafelt TD, Loprinzi CL. Andropause: symptom management for prostate cancer patients treated with hormonal ablation. The Oncologist 2003;8:474–487.

130. American Cancer Society. Cancer facts and figures: 2002. American Cancer Society, Atlanta, GA.

131. Smolin Y, Massie MJ. Male breast cancer: a review of the literature and a case report. Psychomatics 2002;43:326–330.

132. Hoda D, Perez DG, Loprinzi CL. Hot flashes in breast cancer survivors. Breast J 2003;9:431–438.

133. Ettinger B, Grady D, Tosteson ANA, et al. Effect of the Women's Health Initiative on women's decisions to discontinue postmenopausal hormone therapy. Obstet Gynecol 2003;102:1225–1232.

134. Beckmann MW, Jap D, Djahansouzi S, et al. Hormone replacement therapy after treatment of breast cancer: effects on postmenopausal symptoms, bone mineral density and recurrence rates. Oncol 2001;60:199–206.

135. Durna EM, Wren BG, Heller GZ, et al. Hormone replacement therapy after a diagnosis of breast cancer: cancer recurrence and mortality. Med J Australia 2002;177:347–351.

136. Decker DA, Pettinga JE, VanderVelde N, et al. Estrogen replacement therapy in breast cancer survivors: a matched-controlled series. Menopause 2003;10:277–285.

137. Wile AG, Opfell RW, Margileth DA. Hormone replacement therapy in previously treated breast cancer patients. Am J Surg 1993;165:372–375.

138. DiSaia PJ, Grosen EA, Kurosaki T, et al. Hormone replacement therapy in breast cancer survivors: a cohort study. Am J Obstet Gynecol 1996;174:1494–1498.

139. Dew J, Eden J, Beller E, et al. A cohort study of hormone replacement therapy given to women previously treated for breast cancer. Climacteric 1998;1:137–142.

140. Ursic-Vrscaj M, Bebar S. A case-control study of hormone replacement therapy after primary surgical breast cancer treatment. Eur J Surg Oncol 1999;25:146–151.

141. O'Meara ES, Rossing MA, Daling JR, et al. Hormone replacement therapy after a diagnosis of breast cancer in relation to recurrence and mortality. JNCI 2001;93:754–762.

142. Peters GN, Fodera T, Sabol J, et al. Estrogen replacement therapy after breast cancer: a 12-year follow-up. Ann Surg Oncol 2001; 8:828–832.

143. Natrajan PK, Gambrell RD Jr. Estrogen replacement therapy in patients with early breast cancer. Am J Obstet Gynecol 2002; 187:289–294.

144. Meurer LN, Lena S. Cancer recurrence and mortality in women using hormone replacement therapy after breast cancer: meta-analysis. J Fam Pract 2002;51:1056–1062.

145. Vassilopoulou-Sellin R, Cohen DS, Hortobagyi GN, et al. Estrogen replacement therapy for menopausal women with a history of breast carcinoma: results of a 5-year, prospective study. Cancer 2002;95:1817–1826.

146. Ganz PA, Greendale GA, Kahn B, et al. Are older breast carcinoma survivors willing to take hormone replacement therapy? Cancer 1999;86:814–820.

147. Holmberg L, Anderson H. The HABITS steering and data monitoring committee. Lancet 2004;363:453–455.

148. Quella SK, Loprinzi CL, Sloan JA, et al. Long term use of megestrol acetate by cancer survivors for the treatment of hot flashes. Cancer 1998;82:1784–1788.

149. Pandya KJ, Raubertas RF, Flynn PJ et al. Oral clonidine in postmenopausal patients with breast cancer experiencing tamoxifen-induced hot flashes: a University of Rochester Cancer Center Community Clinical Oncology Program study. Ann Inten Med 2000; 32:788–793.

150. Stearns V, Beebe KL, Iyengar M, et al. Paroxetine controlled release in the treatment of menopausal hot flashes: a randomized controlled trial. JAMA 2003;289:2827–2834.

151. Loprinzi CL, Kugler JW, Sloan JA, et al. Venlafaxine in management of hot flashes in survivors of breast cancer: a randomised controlled trial. Lancet 2000;356:2059–2063.

152. Quella SK, Loprinzi CL, Sloan J, et al. Pilot evaluation of venlafaxine for the treatment of hot flashes in men undergoing androgen ablation therapy for prostate cancer. J Urol 1999;162:98–102.

153. Quella SK, Loprinzi CL, Barton DL, et al. Evaluation of soy phytoestrogens for the treatment of hot flashes in breast cancer survivors: a North Center Cancer Treatment Group Trial. J Clin Oncol 2000;18:1068–1074.

154. Tice JA, Ettinger B, Ensrud K, et al. Phytoestrogen supplements for the treatment of hot flashes: the Isoflavone Clover Extract (ICE) Study: a randomized controlled trial. JAMA 2003;290: 207–214.

155. Nikander E, Kilkkinen A, Metsa-Heikkila M, et al. A randomized placebo-controlled crossover trial with phytoestrogens in treatment of menopause in breast cancer patients. Obstet Gynecol 2003;101:1213–1220.

156. Muñoz GH, Pluchino S. Cimicifuga racemosa for the treatment of hot flushes in women surviving breast cancer. Maturitas 2003;44(Suppl 1):S59–65.

157. Wuttke W, Seidlove-Wuttke D, Gorkow C. The Cimicifuga preparation BNO 1055 vs. conjugated estrogens in a double-blind placebo-controlled study: effects on menopause symptoms and bone markers. Maturitas 2003;44(Suppl 1):S67–77.

158. Jacobson J, Traxel AB, Evans J, et al. Randomized trial of black cohosh for the treatment of hot flashes among women with a history of breast cancer. J Clin Oncol 2001;19:2739–2745.

159. Carpenter JS, Wells N, Lambert B, et al. A pilot study of magnetic therapy for hot flashes after breast cancer. Cancer Nurs 2002;25:104–109.

160. Porzio G, Trapasso T, Martelli S, et al. Acupuncture in the treatment of menopause-related symptoms in women taking tamoxifen. Tumori 2002;88:128–130.

161. Irvin JH, Domar AD, Clark C, et al. The effects of relaxation response training on menopausal symptoms. J Psychosom Obstet Gynaecol 1996;17:202–207.

162. Ivarsson T, Spetz AC, Hammar M. Physical exercise and vasomotor symptoms in postmenopausal women. Maturitas 1998; 29:139–146.

163. Ganz PA, Greendale GA, Petersen L, et al. Managing menopausal symptoms in breast cancer survivors: Results of a randomized controlled trial. J Nat Cancer Inst 2000; 92:1054–1064.

164. Rosen RC, Laumann EO. The prevalence of sexual problems in women: How valid are comparisons across studies? Arch Sex Behav 2003;32:209–211.

165. Laumann EO, Nicolosi A, Glasser DB, et al. GSSAB Investigators' Group. Sexual problems among women and men aged 40–80 years: prevalence and correlates identified in the global study of sexual attitudes and behaviors. Int J Impot Res 2005;17:39–57.

166. Nicolosi A, Laumann EO, Glasser DB, et al. Global Study of Sexual Attitudes and Behaviors Investigators' Group. Sexual behavior and sexual dysfunctions after age 40: the global study of sexual attitudes and behaviors. Urology 2004;64:991–997.

167. Feldman HA, Goldstein I, Hatzichristou DG, et al. Impotence and its medical and psychosocial correlates: results of the Massachusetts Male Aging Study. J Urol 1994;151:54–61.

168. Bacon CG, Mittleman MA, Kawachi I, et al. Sexual function in men older than 50 years of age: results from the Health Professionals Follow-Up Study. Ann Intern Med 2003;139: 161–168.

169. Laumann EO, Gagnon JH, Michael RT, et al. The social organization of sexuality. Chicago: The University of Chicago Press, 1994:184–185.

170. Hollenbeck BK, Dunn RL, Wei JT, et al. Determinants of long-term sexual health outcome after radical prostatectomy measured by a validated instrument. J Urol 2003;169:1453–1457.

171. Andersen BL, Lachenbruch PA, Anderson B, et al. Sexual dysfunction and signs of gynecologic cancer. Cancer 1986;7: 1880–1886.

172. Cooperberg MR, Koppie TM, Lubeck DP et al. How potent is potent? Evaluation of sexual function and bother in men who report potency after treatment for prostate cancer. Data from CaPSURE. Urol 2003;61:190–196.

173. Potosky AL, Davis WW, Hoffman RM, et al. Five-year outcomes after prostatectomy or radiotherapy for prostate cancer: the prostate cancer outcomes study. J Natl Cancer Inst 2004;96:1358–1367.

174. Steineck G, Helgesen F, Adolfsson J, et al. Quality of life after radical prostatectomy or watchful waiting. N Eng J Med 2002; 347:790–796.

175. Schover LR, Fouladi RT, Warneke CL, et al. Defining sexual outcomes after treatment for localized prostate cancer. Cancer 2002;95:1773–1778.

176. Henningsohn L, Steven K, Kallestrup EB, et al. Distressful symptoms and well-being after radical cystectomy and orthotopic bladder substitution compared with a matched control population. J Urol 2002;168:168–175.

177. Havenga K, Maas CP, DeRuiter MC, Welvaart K, Trimbos JB. Avoiding long-term disturbance to bladder and sexual function in pelvic surgery, particularly with rectal cancer. Sem Surg Oncol 2000;18:235–243.

178. Jonker-Pool G, Van de Wile HBM, Hoekstra HJ, et al. Sexual functioning after treatment for testicular cancer: review and meta-analysis of 36 empirical studies between 1975–2000. Arch Sex Behav 2001;30:55–74.

179. Nazareth I, Lewin J, King M. Sexual dysfunction after treatment for testicular cancer: a systemic review. J Psychosom Res 2001; 51:735–743.

180. Coogan CL, Hejase MJ, Wahle FR, et al. Nerve sparing post-chemotherapy retroperitoneal lymph node dissection for advanced testicular cancer. J Urol 1996;156:1656–1658.

181. Jacobsen KD, Ous S, Waehre H, et al. Ejaculation in testicular cancer patients after post-chemotherapy retroperitoneal lymph node dissection. Br J Cancer 1999;80:249–255.

182. Fossa SD, de Wit R, Roberts T, et al. Quality of life in good prognosis patients with metastatic germ cell cancer: a prospective study of the European Organization for Research and Treatment of Cancer Genitourinary Group/Medical Research Council Testicular Cancer study Group (30941/TE20). J Clin Oncol 2003;21:1107–1118.

183. Anatasiadis AG, Davis AR, Sawczuk IS, et al. Quality of life aspects in kidney cancer patients: data from a national registry. Supportive Care in Cancer 2003;11:700–706.

184. Syrjala KL, Roth-Roemer SL, Abrams JR, et al. Prevalence and predictors of sexual dysfunction in long-term survivors of marrow transplantation. J Clin Oncol 1998;16:3148–3157.

185. Dorval M, Maunsell E, Deschenes L, et al. Long-term quality of life after breast cancer: comparison of 8-year survivors with population controls. J Clin Oncol 1998;16:487–494.

186. Berglund G, Nystedt M, Bolund C, et al. Effect of endocrine treatment on sexuality in premenopausal breast cancer patients: a prospective randomized study. J Clin Oncol 2001;19: 2788–2796.

187. Kornblith AB, Herndon JE II, Weiss RB, et al. Long-term adjustment of survivors of early-stage breast carcinoma, 20 years after adjuvant chemotherapy. Cancer 2003;98:679–689.

188. Schover LR, Yetman RJ, Tuason LJ, et al. Partial mastectomy and breast reconstruction: a comparison of their effects on psychosocial adjustment, body image, and sexuality. Cancer 1995;75:54–64.

189. Rowland JH, Desmond KA, Meyerowitz BE, et al. Role of breast reconstructive surgery in physical and emotional outcomes among breast cancer survivors. J Ntl Cancer Inst 2000;92: 1422–1429.

190. Abrahamsen AF, Loge JH, Hannisdal E, et al. Socio-medical situation for long-term survivors of Hodgkin's disease: a survey of 459 patients treated at one institution. Eur J Cancer 1998;34: 1865–1870.

191. van Tulder MW, Aaronson NK, Bruning PF. The quality of life of long-term survivors of Hodgkin's disease. Ann Oncol. 1994; 5(2):153–158.

192. Kornblith AB, Anderson J, Cella DF, et al. Comparison of psychosocial adaptation and sexual function of survivors of advanced Hodgkin disease treated by MOPP, ABVD, or MOPP alternating with ABVD. Cancer 1992;15:2508–2516.

193. Bancroft J, Loftus J, Long JS. Distress about sex: a national survey of women in heterosexual relationships. Arch Sex Beh 2003; 32:193–208.

194. Weijmar Schultz WCM, Van De Wiel HBM, Hahn DEE, et al. Psychosexual functioning after treatment for gynecological cancer: an integrative model, review of determinant factors and clinical guidelines. Int J Gynecol Cancer 1992;2:281–290.

195. Andersen BL, Anderson B, deProsse C. Controlled prospective longitudinal study of women with cancer: I. Sexual functioning outcomes. J Consult Clin Psychol. 1989;57:683–691.

196. Grumann M, Robertson R, Hacker NF, et al. Sexual functioning in patients following radical hysterectomy for stage IB cancer of the cervix. Int J Gynecol Cancer 2001;11:372–380.

197. Schover LR, Fife M, Gershenson DM. Sexual dysfunction and treatment for early stage cervical cancer. Cancer 1989; 63:204–212.

198. Rhodes JC, Kjerulff KH, Langenberg PW, et al. Hysterectomy and sexual functioning. JAMA 1999;282:1934–1941.

199. Thakar R, Ayers S, Clarkson P, et al. Outcomes after total versus subtotal abdominal hysterectomy. N Engl J Med 2002;347: 1318–1325.

200. Schover, LR, von Eschenbach, AC. Sexual function and female radical cystectomy: a case series. J Urol 1985;134:465–468.

201. Ratliff CR, Gershenson DM, Morris M, et al. Sexual adjustment in patients undergoing gracilis myocutaneous flap vaginal reconstruction in conjunction with pelvic exenteration. Cancer 1996; 78:2229–2235.

202. Heiman JR. Sexual dysfunction: overview of prevalence, etiological factors, and treatments. J Sex Res 2002;39:73–78.

203. Schover LR, Evans RB, von Eschenbach AC. Sexual rehabilitation in a cancer center: diagnosis and outcome in 384 consultations. Arch Sex Beh 1987;16:445–461.

204. Moreira ED Jr, Brock G, Glasser DB, et al. GSSAB Investigators' Group. Help-seeking behaviour for sexual problems: the global study of sexual attitudes and behaviors. Int J Clin Pract 2005;59:6–16.

205. Gingell C, Nicolosi A, Buvat J, et al. Preliminary results from the Global Study of Sexual Attitudes and Behaviors: patient-physician communication. Presented at the 18th Congress of the European Association of Urology, February 2002, Birmingham, UK.

206. Solursh DS, Ernst JL, Lewis RW, et al. The human sexuality education of physicians in North American medical schools. Int J Impot Res 2003;15(Suppl 5): S41–45.

207. Stead ML, Brown JM, Fallowfield L, et al. Lack of communication between healthcare professionals and women with ovarian cancer about sexual issues. Br J Cancer 2003;88:666–667.

208. Fossa SD, Woehre H, Kurth KH, et al. Influence of urological morbidity on quality of life in patients with prostate cancer. Eur Urol 1997;31(Suppl 3):S3–8.

209. Helgason AR, Adolfsson J, Dickman P, et al. Factors associated with waning sexual function among elderly men and prostate cancer patients. J Urol 1997;158:155–159.

210. Messing E. The timing of hormone therapy for men with asymptomatic advanced prostate cancer. Urol Oncol 2003;21: 245–254.

211. Shahidi M, Norman AR, Gadd J, et al. Recovery of serum testosterone, LH and FSH levels following neoadjuvant hormone cytoreduction and radical radiotherapy in localized prostate cancer. Clin Oncol 2001;13:291–295.

212. Iversen P. Bicalutamide monotherapy for early stage prostate cancer: an update. J Urol 2003;170:S48–52.

213. Schover LR. Lesson 24: sexuality after pelvic cancer. AUA Updates, 2005.

214. Schover LR, Fouladi RT, Warneke CL, et al. Utilization of medical treatments for erectile dysfunction in prostate cancer survivors. Cancer 2002;95:2397–2407.

215. Merrick GS, Butler WM, Galbreath RW, et al. Erectile function after permanent prostate brachytherapy. Int J Radiation Oncology Biol Phys 2002;52:893–902.

216. Zietman AL, Sacco D, Skowronski U, et al. Organ conservation in invasive bladder cancer by transurethral resection, chemotherapy and radiation: results of a urodynamic and quality of life study on long-term survivors. J Urol 2003;170:1772–1776.

217. Bjerre BD, Johansen, C, Steven K. Sexological problems after cystectomy: bladder substitution compared with ileal conduit diversion. A questionnaire study of male patients. Scand J Urol Nephrol 1998;32:187–193.

218. Spitz A, Stein JP, Lieskovsky G, et al. Orthotopic urinary diversion with preservation of erectile and ejaculatory function in men requiring radical cystectomy for nonurothelial malignancy: a new technique. J Urol 1999;161:1761–1764.

219. Horenblas S, Meinhardt W, Ijzerman W, et al. Sexuality preserving cystectomy and neobladder: initial results. J Urol 2001;166:837–840.

220. Engel J, Kerr J, Schlesinger-Raab A, et al. Quality of life in rectal cancer patients: A four-year prospective study. Ann Surg 2003;238:203–213.

221. Chatterjee R, Kottaridis PD, McGarrigle HH, et al. Management of erectile dysfunction by combination therapy with testosterone and sildenafil in recipients of high-dose therapy for haematological malignancies. Bone Marrow Trans 2002;29:607–610.

222. Rajagopal A, Vassilopoulou-Sellin R, Palmer JL, et al. Hypogonadism and sexual dysfunction in male cancer survivors receiving chronic opioid therapy. J Pain Symptom Manage 2003;26:1055–1061.

223. Wang C, Swerdloff SR, Iranmanesh A, et al. Transdermal testosterone gel improves sexual function, mood, muscle strength, and body composition parameters in hypogonadal men. J Clin Endocrinol Metab 2000;85:2839–2853.

224. McNicholas TA, Mulder DH, Carnegie C, et al. A novel testosterone gel formulation normalizes androgen levels in hypogonadal men, with improvements in body composition and sexual function. BJU Int 2003;91:69–74.

225. Snyder PJ, Peachey H, Hannoush P, et al. Effect of testosterone treatment on body composition and muscle strength in men over 65 years of age. J Clin Endocrinol Metab 1999;84:2647–2653.

226. Steidle C, Schwartz S, Jacoby K, et al. for the North American AA2500 T Gel Study Group. AA2500 testosterone gel normalizes androgen levels in aging males with improvements in body composition and sexual function. J Clin Endocrinol Metab 2003;88:2673–2681.

227. Aversa A, Isidori AM, Spera G, et al. Androgens improve cavernous vasodilation and response to sildenafil in patients with erectile dysfunction. Clin Endocrinol (Oxf) 2003;58:632–638.

228. Howell SJ, Radford JA, Adams JE, et al. Randomized placebo-controlled trial of testosterone replacement in men with mild Leydig cell insufficiency following cytotoxic chemotherapy. Clin Endocrinol (Oxf) 2001;55:315–324.

229. Kaplan HS. A neglected issue: the sexual side effects of current treatments for breast cancer. J Sex Marital Ther 1992;18:3–19.

230. Lillie EO, Bernstein L, Ursin G. The role of androgens and polymorphisms in the androgen receptor in the epidemiology of breast cancer. Breast Cancer Res 2003;5:164–173.

231. Padero MC, Bhasin S, Friedman TC. Androgen supplementation in older women: too much hype, not enough data. J Am Geriatr Soc 2002;50:1131–1140.

232. Cawood EHH, Bancroft J. Steroid hormones, the menopause, sexuality and well-being of women. Psychol Med 1996;26:925–936.

233. Bachmann GA, Leiblum SR, Kemmann E, et al. Sexual expression and its determinants in the post-menopausal woman. Maturitas 1984;6:19–29.

234. Dennerstein L, Dudley EC, Hoppel JL. Sexuality, hormones and the menopausal transition. Maturitas 1977;26:83–93.

235. Sherwin BB. Use of combined estrogen-androgen preparations in the postmenopause: evidence from clinical studies. Int J Fertil 1998;43:98–103.

236. Shifren JL, Braunstein GD, Simon JA, et al. Transdermal testosterone treatment in women with impaired sexual function after oophorectomy. N Eng J Med 2000;343:682–688.

237. Floter A, Nathorst-Boos J, Carlsrom K, et al. Addition of testosterone to estrogen replacement therapy in oophorectomized women: effects on sexuality and well-being. Climacteric 2002;5:357–365.

238. van Leeuwen FE, Klokman WJ, Stovall M, et al. Roles of radiation dose, chemotherapy, and hormonal factors in breast cancer following Hodgkin's disease. J Natl Cancer Inst 2003;95:971–980.

239. Laan E, van Lunsen RHW, Everaerd W. The effects of tibolone on vaginal blood flow, sexual desire and arousability in postmenopausal women. Climacteric 2001;4:28–41.

240. Stahlberg C, Tønnes Pedersen A, Lynge E, et al. Increased risk of breast cancer following different regimens of hormone replacement therapy frequently used in Europe. Int J Cancer 2004;109:721–727.

241. Hartmann U, Heiser K, Ruffer-Hesse C, et al. Female sexual desire disorders: subtypes, classification, personality factors and new directions for treatment. World J Urol 2002;20:79–88.

242. Andersen BL. Surviving cancer: the importance of sexual self-concept. Med Pediatr Oncol 1999;33:15–23.

243. Schover LR, LoPiccolo J. Treatment effectiveness for dysfunctions of sexual desire. J Sex Marital Therapy 1982;8:179–197.

244. Hawton K, Catalan J, Fagg J. Low sexual desire: sex therapy results and prognostic factors. Behav Res Ther 1992;29:217–224.

245. Dewire DM, Todd E, Meyers P. Patient satisfaction with current impotence therapy. Wis Med J 1995;94:542–544.

246. Jarow JP, Nana-Sinkam P, Sabbagh M, et al. Outcome analysis of goal directed therapy for impotence. J Urol 1996;155:1609–1612.

247. Hanash KA. Comparative results of goal oriented therapy for erectile dysfunction. J Urol 1997;157:2135–2138.

248. El-Galley R, Rutland H, Talic R, et al. Long-term efficacy of sildenafil and tachyphylaxis effect. J Urol 2001;166:927–931.

249. Gonzalgo ML, Brotzman M, Trock et al. Clinical efficacy of sildenafil citrate and predictors of long-term response. J Urol 2003;170:503–506.

250. McCullough AR, Kau EL, Kaci L, et al. A 12-month longitudinal study of treatment seeking behavior in 200 men after radical retropubic prostatectomy. American Urological Association Abstracts (#1418), 2003.

251. Gontero P, Fontana F, Bagnasacco A, et al. Is there an optimal time for intracavernous Prostaglandin E1 rehabilitation following nonnerve sparing radical prostatectomy? Results from a hemodynamic prospective study. J Urol 2003;169:2166–2169.

252. Montorsi F, Guazzoni G, Strambi LF, et al. Recovery of spontaneous erectile function after nerve-sparing radical retropubic prostatectomy with and without early intracavernous injections of alprostadil: results of a prospective, randomized trial. J Urol 1997;158:1408–1410.

253. Brody S, Laan E, van Lunsen RH. Concordance between women's physiological and subjective sexual arousal is associated with consistency of orgasm during intercourse but not other sexual behavior. J Sex Marital Ther 2003;29:15–23.

254. Modelska K, Cummings S. Female sexual dysfunction in postmenopausal women: Systematic review of placebo-controlled trials. Am J Obstet Gynecol 2003;188:286–293.

255. Berman JR, Berman LA, Toler SM, et al. Safety and efficacy of sildenafil citrate for the treatment of female sexual arousal disorder: a double-blind placebo-controlled study. J Urol 2003;170:2333–2338.

256. Padma-Nathan H, Brown C, Fendl J, et al. Efficacy and safety of topical alprostadil cream for the treatment of female sexual

arousal disorder (FSAD): a double-blind, multicenter, randomized, and placebo-controlled clinical trial. J Sex Marital Ther 2003;29:329–344.

257. Ferguson DM, Steidle CP, Singh GS et al. Randomized, placebo-controlled, double blind, crossover design trial of the efficacy and safety of Zestra for Women in women with and without female sexual arousal disorder. J Sex Marital Ther 2003; 29(Supple 1):33–44.

258. Basson R, McInnes R, Smith MD, et al. Efficacy and safety of sildenafil citrate in women with sexual dysfunction associated with female sexual arousal disorder. J Womens Health Gend Base Med 2002;11:367–377.

259. Mayor S. News roundup: Pfizer will not apply for a licence for sildenafil for women. BMJ 2004;328:542.

260. Wilson SK, Delk JR, Billups KL. Treating symptoms of female sexual arousal disorder with the Eros-Clitoral Therapy Device. J Gend Specif Med 2001;4:54–58.

261. Munarriz R, Maitland S, Garcia Sp, et al. A prospective duplex Doppler ultrasonographic study in women with sexual arousal disorder to objectively assess genital engorgement induced by EROS therapy. J Sex Marital Ther 2003;29(Suppl 1):85–94.

262. Bachmann G. Estradiol-releasing vaginal ring delivery system for urogenital atrophy. Experience over the past decade. J Reprod Med 1998;43:991–998.

263. Gabrielsson J, Wallen beck I, Birgerson L. Pharmacokinetic data on estradiol in light of the estring concept. Estradiol and estring pharmacokinetics. Acta Obstet Gynecol Scand Suppl 1996; 163:26–34.

264. Buckler H, Al-Azzawi F for the UK VR Multicentre Trial Group. The effect of a novel vaginal ring delivering oestradiol acetate on climacteric symptoms in postmenopausal women. BJOG 2003;110:753–759.

265. Casper F, Petri E. Local treatment of urogenital atrophy with an estradiol-releasing vaginal ring: a comparative and a placebo-controlled multicenter study. Vaginal Ring Study Group. Int Urogynecol J & Pelvic Floor Dysfunct 1999;10:171–176.

266. Rioux JE, Devlin C, Gelfand MM, et al. 17beta-Estradiol vaginal tablet versus conjugated equine estrogen vaginal cream to relieve menopausal atrophic vaginitis. Menopause 2000;7: 156–161.

267. Bruner DW, Lanciano R, Keegan M, et al. Vaginal stenosis and sexual function following intracavitary radiation for the treatment of cervical and endometrial carcinoma. Int J Radiat Oncol Biol Phys 1993;27:825–830.

268. Balleari E, Garre S,Van Lint MT, et al. Hormone replacement therapy and chronic graft-versus-host disease activity in women treated with bone marrow transplantation for hematologic malignancies. Ann N Y Acad Sci 2002;966:187–192.

269. Hayes EC, Rock JA. Treatment of vaginal agglutination associated with chronic graft-versus-host disease. Fertil Steril 2002; 78:1125–1126.

270. Denton AS, Maher EJ. Interventions for the physical aspects of sexual dysfunction in women following pelvic radiotherapy. Cochrane Library 2003;3:1–26.

271. Robinson JW, Faris PD, Scott CB. Psychoeducational group increases vaginal dilation for younger women and reduced sexual fears for women of all ages with gynecological carcinoma treated with radiotherapy. Int J Radiation Oncology Biol Phys 1999;44:497–506.

272. Loprinzi CL, Abu-Ghazaleh S, Sloan JA, et al. Phase III randomized double-blind study to evaluate the efficacy of a polycarbophil-based vaginal moisturizer in women with breast cancer. J Clin Oncol 1997;15:969–973.

273. Nachtigall LE. Comparative study: replens versus local estrogen in menopausal women. Fertil Steril 1994;61:178–180.

274. Bygdemen M, Swahn ML. Replens versus dienoestrol cream in the symptomatic treatment of vaginal atrophy in postmenopausal women. Maturitas 1996;23:259–263.

275. Beji NK, Yalcin O, Erkan HA. The effect of pelvic floor training on sexual function of treated patients. Int Urogynecol J Pelvic Floor Dysfunct 2003;14:234–238.

276. Clemens JQ, Nadler RB, Schaeffer AJ, et al. Biofeedback, pelvic floor re-education, and bladder training for male chronic pelvic pain syndrome. Urol 2000;56:951–955.

277. Schover LR, von Eschenbach AC. Sexual and marital relationships after treatment for nonseminomatous testicular cancer. Urol 1985;25:251–255.

278. Sall M, Madsen FA, Rhodes PR, et al. Pelvic pain following radical retropubic prostatectomy: A prospective study. Urol 1997;49:575–579.

279. Masarani M, Cox R. The aetiology, pathophysiology and management of chronic orchialgia. BJU International 2003;91: 435–437.

280. Schover LR. Sexuality and fertility after cancer. New York, John Wiley & Sons, 1997:122–130.

281. Padma-Nathan H. Diagnostic and treatment strategies for erectile dysfunction: the 'Process of Care' model. Int J Impot Res 2000;12 (Suppl 4):S119–121.

The Employment and Insurance Concerns of Cancer Survivors

Barbara Hoffman

The employment and insurance concerns of cancer survivors have changed dramatically during the past generation. In the 1970s, fewer than one-half of those diagnosed with cancer survived more than 5 years. Treatment options were few, often disabling, and commonly ineffective. Myths about cancer prevailed. Consequently, many survivors experienced substantial problems obtaining and retaining employment and adequate health insurance.

Significant medical, social, and legal progress has extended and enhanced the lives of millions of cancer survivors. Advances in cancer treatment have fostered changes in attitudes about cancer. This in turn has led to a considerable expansion of the legal rights of cancer survivors in the workplace. Far less progress has been realized, however, in the rights of cancer survivors to have health insurance that pays for medically necessary cancer screening, preventive care, treatment, and follow-up care.

Cancer Survivorship: Myths and Facts

In the 1970s, a cancer diagnosis was often construed as a death sentence.[1,2] Most individuals, the media, governments, and survivors themselves commonly referred to cancer victims.[1,3] To employers and insurers, a cancer diagnosis meant potential lost profits and productivity.[3] A cancer survivor was the spouse who was left behind to cope alone with unpaid bills and unfulfilled dreams. A cancer diagnosis was seldom discussed publicly.[1,3] Many feared cancer was contagious.[1,4] Physicians expected survivors to be satisfied with achieving medical remission; few considered or responded constructively to psychosocial sequelae, such as the impact of cancer on work.[5] The 5-year survival rate for the top 15 cancers as identified in SEER data from 1975 to 1979 was only 42.7% for men and 56.6% for women.[6]

A generation of medical progress has brought a sea of change in opinions about cancer. The 5-year survival rate for the top 15 cancers from 1995 to 2000 improved to 64% for men and to 64.3% for women.[6] Cancer is no longer considered a death sentence. More than 87% of 957 respondents to a national survey taken in 2002 recognized as false the statement: Cancer is something that cannot be effectively treated.[7]

Only one percent of 1,002 individuals believed that cancer is contagious.[8] All aspects of American society, including the media, research literature, state and federal governments, treatment centers, and millions of Americans who have been diagnosed with cancer, have replaced the passive word victim with the active term survivor.[9] As cancer survivors have become greater advocates for themselves, their healthcare providers have responded to their demands for greater flexibility in scheduling medical care to accommodate survivors' work schedules.[10] These medical and societal changes have contributed to dramatic improvements in cancer survivors' quality of life at work and have encouraged survivors to demand fundamental health insurance reforms.

Cancer Survivors at Work

Although the attitudes of cancer survivors and their coworkers have changed, one factor has remained constant over the past generation: cancer survivors want to, and are able to perform their jobs and return to work after diagnosis in large numbers. Cancer treatment does, however, limit the ability of a minority of survivors to work as they did prior to diagnosis. Using data from the 2000 National Health Interview Survey (NHIS), Yabroff et al. found that cancer survivors have poorer outcomes across all employment-related burden measures relative to matched control subjects without a cancer diagnosis.[9] One estimate is that 16.8% of working-age survivors (compared with 5% of matched controls) are unable to work because of a physical, mental, or emotional problem. Of those who could work, 7.4% (compared with 3.2% of matched controls) were limited in the kind or amount of work they could do.[11]

Whether a survivor continues to work during treatment or returns to work after treatment, and if so, whether that survivor's diagnosis or treatment will result in working limitations, depends on many factors. They include the survivor's age, stage at diagnosis, financial status, education, access to health insurance and transportation, as well as the physical demands of the job and the presence of any other chronic health conditions.[12,13,14] For example, survivors in physically demanding jobs have higher disability rates than those in more sedentary jobs; survivors with advanced education have higher return to work rates than those with less education.[13,14] Medical treatment decisions that consider quality of life and the shift towards providing cancer treatment in outpatient settings have contributed to the increasing number of survivors who can work during their treatment.[15]

For more than 30 years, the vast majority of working-age adults who were diagnosed with cancer have returned to work. A 1972 Bell Telephone survey of 800,000 Bell employees found that of the 1351 employees with a cancer history, 77% returned to work after their diagnosis and treatment.[16] Other efforts to obtain information on unemployment in the 1980s reported that approximately 80% of survivors return to work after diagnosis.[17] Mor found that a higher percentage of white collar workers (78%) than blue collar workers (63%) remained in their jobs twelve months after diagnosis.[18]

Studies of cancer survivors since 1995 have reported similar findings. A survey of ten studies that assessed return-to-work rates of a total of 1,904 cancer survivors from 1986 to 1999 found that a mean of 62% returned to work.[19] A study of 1,763 survivors who were first diagnosed between January 1997 and December 1999 found that of the 1,433 who were working at diagnosis, 73% returned to work within 1 year of diagnosis and 84% returned to work within 4 years:[13] Bradley interviewed 253 long-term survivors in 1999 and found that 67% were employed 5 to 7 years later.[12] Bloom found that young breast cancer survivors had the same employment rates five years after diagnosis as they had at the time of diagnosis.[20]

Most cancer survivors are able to continue working or return to work without limitations resulting from their diagnosis or treatment. In one of the earliest studies of cancer survivors in the workplace, Wheatley surveyed Metropolitan Life Insurance employees between 1959 and 1972.[21] He concluded that the work performance of employees who were treated for cancer differed little from that of others hired at the same age for similar assignments.[21] When compared with similar employees, the turnover, absence, and work performance rates of cancer survivors were so satisfactory that Wheatley concluded that hiring individuals with a cancer history was sound industrial practice.[21]

In 1992, Cerenex Pharmaceuticals commissioned Yankelovich Clancy Shulman to conduct a study of cancer survivors, employees and supervisors. Of 503 cancer survivors, 60% reported that cancer did not affect their performance and an additional 21% reported that cancer had "very little" effect on their performance.[22] In Short's study conducted during 2001, only 16% of men and 21% of women working at diagnosis reported limitations in their ability to work related to cancer.[13]

Cancer has a greater impact on survivors' physical rather than mental capabilities. Of the 253 long-term survivors in Bradley's study, 18% reported problems completing some physical tasks.[12] The effects of cancer treatment, especially fatigue, can also impact some survivors' ability to perform mental tasks, such as concentrating for longer periods of time (12%), learning new things (14%), and analyzing data (11%).[12,23] For example, survivors of thyroid cancer reported that work productivity, concentration, and quality of life changed dramatically within a few weeks of going off thyroid hormone medication.[24]

During the past 30 years, cancer survivors have reported decreasing incidences of work problems attributable to their cancer. In the 1970s, the California Division of the American Cancer Society sponsored a 5-year study of the work experiences of 344 white-collar workers, blue-collar workers, and youths with cancer histories.[25] Feldman found that 54% of white-collar and 84% of blue-collar respondents reported discrimination at work.[25]

In the 1980s, Fobair found that 43% of 403 Hodgkin's disease survivors experienced difficulties at work that they attributed to their cancer history.[26] Eight of the forty (20%) survivors of childhood/adolescent Hodgkin's disease surveyed by Wasserman reported job discrimination.[4] Koocher and O'Malley studied 60 survivors of childhood cancer and found that 25% reported employment discrimination (10 persons were refused a job at least once, 3 were denied benefits, 3 experienced illness related conflict with supervisor, 4 reported job task problems, and 11 were rejected by the military).[27]

Of the 503 cancer survivors surveyed in the 1992 Yankelovich survey, 1 in 5 of the survivors who told their employer of their cancer reported discrimination, including changed job responsibilities, forced early retirement, denial of expected promotion, and termination.[22] A study of long-term breast cancer survivors reported only minor difficulties with work.[28] Thirteen percent reported difficulty getting time off from work for medical appointments, eight percent reported difficulty with their employer in regard to their breast cancer experience, and six percent reported difficulties with their coworkers in regard to their breast cancer experience.[28] Almost all of the 253 long-term survivors interviewed in 1999 by Bradley reported that employers were completely cooperative in accommodating reduced schedules and absenteeism during treatment.[12]

The Impact of Cancer on Survivors' Current Employment Opportunities

Never before has cancer affected so many employed adults. In 2001, 38% of all cancer survivors—approximately 3.7 million Americans—were of working age (age 20 to 64).[29] For most survivors, work is a financial and emotional necessity. Most survivors work not only for the obvious financial benefit, but also for the accompanying health insurance, self-esteem, and social support. In quality of life assessments, survivors have reported that being able to work full-time and having an enjoyable job contribute to a better quality of life.[30] Work provides a sense of normalcy and control during a period when cancer strips survivors of control over life's routines.[31]

A cancer diagnosis may affect any type of job action, including dismissal, failure to hire, demotion, denial of promotion, undesirable transfer, denial of benefits and hostility in the workplace.[32] Though cancer survivors today experience fewer blatant barriers to job opportunities, many Americans still fear that cancer will have a negative impact on their ability to obtain and keep a job. A 1997 telephone survey of 662 employed adult Americans who did not have cancer found that 40% feared losing their job if they were diagnosed with cancer.[33] A survey of Hodgkin's disease and leukemia survivors indicated that more than one-third attributed at least one negative vocational (employment, income, or education) problem to their cancer.[34]

One reason survivors fear problems at work is because many supervisors and coworkers have misconceptions about survivors' abilities to work during and after treatment. A 1992 survey of 200 supervisors found that 66% were concerned that employees with cancer could no longer perform their jobs adequately.[22] Of 200 supervisors surveyed in 1996, 33% believed that a survivor could not handle the job and cancer, and 31% thought that the survivor needed to be replaced.[35] Yet after working with a survivor, 34% of the supervisors and 43% of coworkers said that they would be less concerned about working with a survivor in the future.[35] Nearly one-half admitted that a current cancer diagnosis would affect their decision to hire a qualified applicant.[22] Of 662 employees surveyed by Ferrell, 14% believed that coworkers with cancer probably would not be able to do their jobs.[31] Twenty-seven percent of coworkers thought they would have to work harder to pick up the slack.[31]

When Cancer-Based Discrimination Is Illegal

Under federal law and many state laws, an employer cannot treat a survivor differently from other workers in job-related activities because of his or her cancer history, as long as the survivor is qualified for the job. Individuals are protected by these laws only if

(1) they can do the major duties of the job in question

  and

(2) their employer treated them differently from other workers in job-related activities because of their cancer history.

FEDERAL LAW

Four federal laws provide some job protection to cancer survivors: the Americans with Disabilities Act, the Federal Rehabilitation Act, the Family and Medical Leave Act, and the Employee Retirement and Income Security Act.

THE AMERICANS WITH DISABILITIES ACT ("ADA")

The Americans with Disabilities Act prohibits some types of job discrimination by employers, employment agencies, and labor unions against people who have or have had cancer. The ADA covers private employers with 15 or more employees, state and local governments, the legislative branch of the federal government, employment agencies, and labor unions. Most cancer survivors, regardless of whether their cancer is cured, is in remission, or is not responding to treatment, are considered persons with a disability under the ADA. From July 26, 1992, through September 30, 2004, 2.5% of all charges brought under the ADA were cancer-based discrimination claims.[36]

The ADA prohibits employment discrimination against individuals who have a disability, have a record of a disability, or are regarded as having a disability. A disability is a major health problem that substantially limits the ability to do everyday activities, such as drive a car or walk. Because most cancer survivors, even those who do not consider themselves to be limited by their cancer, fit under at least one of these three groups, most cancer survivors are protected by the ADA from the time of diagnosis. For example, the ADA covers survivors

- whose cancer currently substantially limits their ability to do everyday activities, such as climbing stairs; a tem-

porary, nonchronic impairment, such as a broken bone, usually is not considered a disability;

- whose cancer, at one time, substantially limited the ability to do everyday activities, but no longer does; the ADA protects most cancer survivors who have completed treatment from discrimination based on their medical histories; and

- whose employer believes that the employee's cancer substantially limits and his or her ability to do everyday activities, even if the employee believes it does not.

Whether an individual is covered by the ADA is determined on a case-by-case basis. Most federal courts find that cancer survivors who are qualified for their jobs are covered by the ADA.

Some federal courts, however, have misapplied the ADA by placing cancer survivors in a catch-22. They have concluded that a cancer survivor who is sufficiently healthy to work is not a person with a disability as defined by the ADA. A cancer survivor who has never been substantially limited in a major life activity may not be a person with a disability as defined by the ADA. Additionally, cancer survivors who, through medicine or other measures, can alleviate the limitations caused by cancer treatment, may not have a disability as defined by the ADA.

The ADA prohibits discrimination in almost all job-related activities, including, but not limited to

- not hiring an applicant for a job or training program;
- firing a worker;
- providing unequal pay, working conditions, and benefits such as pension, vacation time, and health insurance;
- punishing an employee for filing a discrimination complaint; or
- screening out disabled employees.

In most cases, an employer may not ask prospective employees if they have ever had cancer. An employer has the right to know only if the applicant is able to do the job. An employer may not ask a prospective employee about his or her health history, unless the employee has a visible disability and the employer could reasonably believe that it affects the ability to perform that job. A job offer may be contingent upon passing a relevant medical exam, provided that all prospective employees are subject to the same exam. An employer may ask detailed health questions only after offering a job.

Employers must keep employee medical histories in a file separate from other personnel records. The only people entitled to see employee medical files are supervisors who need to know whether the employee needs an accommodation, emergency medical personnel, and government officials who enforce the ADA.

If a survivor needs extra time or help to do his or her job, the ADA requires an employer to provide a "reasonable accommodation." An "accommodation" is a change in working conditions, such as in work hours or duties. Common accommodations for cancer survivors during and after treatment are

- providing extended leave or flexible work hours to accommodate treatment schedules,

- relocating an employer from a physical area that may compromise his or her health,

- providing a fatigued cancer survivor sufficient time to rest, and
- allowing a survivor to work from home when practical.

An employer does not have to make changes that would be an "undue hardship" on the employer or other workers. "Undue hardship" refers to any accommodation that would be unduly costly, extensive, substantial or disruptive, or that would fundamentally alter the nature or operation of the business. For example, an employer may be permitted to replace a cancer survivor who has to miss a substantial amount of work time and whose work cannot be performed by a temporary employee. Studies of employers with disabilities report that most employees can be accommodated with relatively simple and inexpensive solutions.[37]

The ADA does not prohibit an employer from firing or refusing to hire a cancer survivor under any circumstance. Because the law requires employers to treat all employees similarly, regardless of disability, an employer may fire a cancer survivor who would have been dismissed even if he or she were not a survivor.

The ADA allows employers to establish attendance and leave policies that are uniformly applied to all employees, regardless of disability. Employers must grant leave to cancer survivors if other employees are granted similar leave. They may be required to change leave policies as a reasonable accommodation. Employers are not obligated to provide additional paid leave, but accommodations may include leave flexibility and unpaid leave.

The ADA does not require employers to provide health insurance, but when they choose to provide health insurance, they must do so fairly. For example, an employer who provides health insurance to all employees with similar jobs may violate the ADA by refusing to provide health insurance to a cancer survivor. The employer must prove that the failure to provide health insurance is based on legitimate actuarial data or that the insurance plan would become insolvent or suffer a drastic increase in premiums, copayments, or deductibles.

Most employment discrimination laws protect only the employee. The ADA offers protection more responsive to survivors' needs because it prohibits discrimination against family members, too. Employers may not discriminate against workers because of their relationship or association with a "disabled" person. Employers may not assume that an employee's job performance would be affected by the need to care for a family member who has cancer. For example, employers may not treat an employee differently because they assume that the employee would use excessive leave to care for a spouse who has cancer. Additionally, employers who provide health insurance benefits to dependents of employees may not decrease benefits to an employee solely because that employee has a dependent who has cancer. State laws, however, do not protect an employee who is treated differently because a family member has cancer.

THE FEDERAL REHABILITATION ACT

Before the passage of the Americans with Disabilities Act in 1990, the Federal Rehabilitation Act was the only federal law that prohibited cancer-based employment discrimination. The Rehabilitation Act bans public and private employers who receive public funds from discriminating on the basis of disability. Some employees continue to be covered by the Rehabilitation Act, but *not* the ADA:

- employees of the executive branch of the federal government (covered by Section 501 of the Rehabilitation Act),
- employees of employers who receive federal contracts and have fewer than 15 workers (covered by Section 503 of the Rehabilitation Act), and
- employees of employers who receive federal financial assistance and have fewer than 15 workers (covered by Section 504 of the Rehabilitation Act).

For example, small companies that receive federal grants for research and development, physicians in small groups who receive Medicare Part B funds, and small health agencies that receive Medicaid payments, may be subject to the Rehabilitation Act, but not to the ADA. The military is not covered either by the ADA or the Federal Rehabilitation Act, although retired military personnel and civilian employees of the Department of Defense are protected.

Like the ADA, the Rehabilitation Act protects cancer survivors, regardless of extent of disability. The Rehabilitation Act protects only qualified workers and requires employers to provide reasonable accommodations.

THE FAMILY AND MEDICAL LEAVE ACT ("FMLA")

In 1993, Congress enacted the Family and Medical Leave Act to provide job security to workers who must attend to the serious medical needs of themselves or their dependents. The Family and Medical Leave Act requires employers with 50 or more employees—approximately 60% of American workers—to provide up to 12 weeks of unpaid, job-protected leave for family members who need time off to address their own serious illness or to care for a seriously ill child, parent, spouse, or a healthy newborn or newly adopted child.[38] An employee must have worked at least 25 hours per week for one year to be covered. The law allows employers to exempt their highest paid workers. Many employees who are eligible for leave under the Family and Medical Leave Act, however, are unable to take advantage of it. One survey found that 78% of workers who needed leave did not take it because they could not afford unpaid leave.[38]

The Family and Medical Leave Act affects cancer survivors in the following ways:

- it provides 12 weeks of unpaid leave during any 12 month period;
- it requires employers to continue to provide benefits—including health insurance—during the leave period;
- it requires employers to restore employees to the same or equivalent position at the end of the leave period;
- it allows leave to care for a spouse, child, or parent who has a "serious health condition";
- it allows leave because a serious health condition renders the employee "unable to perform the functions of the position";
- it allows intermittent or reduced work schedule when "medically necessary" (under some circumstances, an employer may transfer the employee to a position with equivalent pay and benefits to accommodate the new work schedule);
- it requires employees to make reasonable efforts to schedule foreseeable medical care so as to not to unduly disrupt the workplace;
- it requires employees to give employers 30 days notice of foreseeable medical leave or as much notice as is practicable;

- it allows employers to require employees to provide certification of medical needs and allows employers to seek a second opinion (at employer's expense) to corroborate medical need;
- it permits employers to provide leave provisions more generous than those required by the Family and Medical Leave Act; and
- it allows employees to "stack" leave under the Family and Medical Leave Act with leave allowable under state medical leave law.

THE EMPLOYEE RETIREMENT AND INCOME SECURITY ACT ("ERISA")

The Employee Retirement and Income Security Act may provide the answer for an employee who has been denied full participation in an employee benefit plan because of a cancer history. ERISA prohibits an employer from discriminating against an employee for the purpose of preventing him or her from collecting benefits under an employee benefit plan. All employers who offer benefit packages to their employees are subject to ERISA.

Some employers fear that participation of a cancer survivor in a group medical plan will drain benefit funds or increase the employer's insurance premiums. A violation of ERISA may occur when an employer, upon learning of a worker's cancer history, dismisses that worker for the purpose of excluding him or her from a group health plan.

An employer may violate ERISA by firing an employee for the purpose of cutting off that employee's benefits, regardless of whether the employee is considered disabled under the statute. An employer may also violate ERISA by encouraging a person with a cancer history to retire as a "disabled" employee. Most benefits plans define disability narrowly to include only the most debilitating conditions. Individuals with a cancer history often do not fit under such a definition and should not be compelled to label themselves so.

Under certain circumstances, ERISA may provide grounds for a lawsuit by workers with a cancer history. ERISA covers both participants (employees) and beneficiaries (spouses and children). Thus, if the employee is fired because his or her child has cancer, the employee may be entitled to file a claim. ERISA, however, is inapplicable to many victims of employment discrimination, including

- individuals who are denied a new job because of their medical status,
- employees who are subjected to different treatment that does not affect their benefits, and
- employees whose compensation does not include benefits.

STATE LAWS

STATE EMPLOYMENT DISCRIMINATION LAWS

Most employers must comply with federal and state employment discrimination laws. Cancer survivors who face discrimination by employers who are not covered by federal law may turn to state laws for relief. Every state has a law that regulates, to some extent, employment discrimination against people with disabilities. The application of these laws to cancer-based discrimination varies widely.

Many state laws have been amended to parallel the requirements of the ADA. Most state laws cover cancer survivors because they prohibit job discrimination against persons who

- have a disability, or
- have a record of a disability, or
- are regarded by others as having a disability.

Different state and federal laws define "disability" in a variety of ways. For example, a cancer survivor may have a "disability" under the ADA, yet not have a "disability" as defined by a state employment discrimination law or by the Social Security Act.

All states except Alabama and Mississippi have laws that prohibit discrimination against people with disabilities in public and private employment. Alabama and Mississippi laws cover only state employees. Several states, such as New Jersey, cover all employers regardless of the number of employees. The laws in most states, however, cover only employers with a minimum number of employees.

In states that do not protect individuals with a record of a disability or those who are regarded by others as having a disability, to be protected by the law a person actually must be disabled from his or her cancer. A few states, such as California and Vermont, expressly prohibit discrimination against cancer survivors.

Although state discrimination laws differ substantially, they all share one requirement in common with the federal law: only "qualified" workers are entitled to relief. Most state laws prohibit discrimination in "terms and conditions of employment," such as salary, benefits, duties, and promotional opportunities. Some state laws require employers to provide reasonable accommodations of an employee's disability and prohibit employers from asking about an applicant's medical history before offering employment.

STATE MEDICAL LEAVE LAWS

Some employers give their employees paid or unpaid medical leave. Employees who do not receive medical leave as a job benefit may have a right to medical leave under state law. Many states have leave laws similar to the federal Family and Medical Leave Act. These laws guarantee employees in the private sector unpaid leave for pregnancy, childbirth, and the adoption of a child. Some state laws provide employees with medical leave to address a serious illness, such as cancer. Several states provide coverage more extensive than the federal law.

GENETIC-BASED DISCRIMINATION

A growing concern among cancer survivors is whether employers will use genetic information as a basis for discrimination. Some people who have tested positively for a genetic change which increases their chances of getting cancer face discrimination because employers fear they will become ill, miss work, and raise insurance costs. Several federal laws provide limited protection to cancer survivors. They are: the Genetic Privacy Act, the Genetic Privacy and Nondiscrimination Act, the ADA, and the Health Insurance Portability and Accountability Act.[39]

Although the ADA does not specifically mention whether it prohibits discrimination based on genetic information, the Equal Employment Opportunities Commission, which enforces the ADA, recognizes that a healthy individual who has a genetic predisposition to a disease is regarded as disabled, and therefore is covered by the law. Thus, an employer may violate the ADA by discriminating against a person because he or she has a genetic marker for cancer. Additionally, the ADA permits employers to test current employees for genetic information that is job-related and consistent with business necessity.

Federal employees have the greatest right to privacy of their genetic information. Executive Order 13,145 prohibits federal departments and agencies from making employment decisions about civilian federal employees based on protected genetic information. The Order also prohibits federal employees from requiring genetic tests as a condition of being hired or receiving benefits.

More than 30 states have genetic nondiscrimination laws. All prohibit discrimination based on the results of genetic tests and many restrict employer access to genetic information.[40] The protection offered by these laws varies widely.

How to Avoid Employment Discrimination

Lawsuits are neither the only, nor usually the best, way to fight employment discrimination. State and federal anti-discrimination laws help cancer survivors by discouraging discrimination and offering remedies when discrimination does occur. These laws, however, are not panaceas because enforcing them can be costly and time-consuming, and does not necessarily result in a fair solution. Indeed, employers prevail in the vast majority of ADA cases.[41]

A survivor's first step is to try to avoid discrimination. If that fails, the next step is to attempt a reasonable settlement with the employer. If informal efforts fail, however, a lawsuit may be the most effective last step. The most constructive efforts against cancer-based discrimination eliminate opportunities for discrimination. Cancer survivors can take several measures to lessen the chance of encountering employment discrimination:

- Do not volunteer information about a cancer history unless it directly affects qualifications for the job.
- Do not lie on a job or insurance application.
- Be aware of legal rights.
- Suggest specific reasonable accommodations where appropriate.
- Keep the focus on current ability to do the job in question.
- Survivors should apply only for jobs for which they are qualified.
- Provide an employer with a physician's letter that explains the survivor's current health status, prognosis, and ability to perform the essential duties of the job in question.
- Seek help from a job counselor with resume preparation and job interviewing skills.
- If interviewing for a job, do not ask about health insurance until after receiving a job offer.
- If possible, look for jobs with state or local governments or with large employers (50+ employees) because they are less likely than small employers to discriminate.
- Seek information and assistance from organizations that advocate for cancer survivors. See Figure 20.1.

(1) The National Coalition for Cancer Survivorship
1010 Wayne Avenue, 7th Floor
Silver Spring, MD 20910
(888) 650-9127
www.canceradvocacy.org

Provides publications, answers to questions about cancer survivorship, including employment and in surance rights, and assistance locating legal resources. Publications include Working It Out: Your Employment Rights as a Cancer Survivor (booklet), What Cancer Survivors Need to Know About Health Insurance (booklet),and A Cancer Survivor=s Almanac: Charting Your Journey (Wiley:2004) (paperback book).

(2) Cancer Care, Inc.
275 Seventh Avenue
New York, NY 10001
(800) 813-HOPE or (212) 302-2400
www.cancercare.org

Provides assistance by oncology social workers, including answers to questions about employment, insurance and finances. Provides help in locating local resources.

FIGURE 20.1. Cancer advocacy organizations and resources.

Health Insurance: Paying for Cancer Care

Second only to heart disease, cancer is the most expensive disease for an American to endure.[42] Only one-third of the financial costs of cancer are covered by either Medicare or private health insurance.[42] Survivors and their families pay for the other two-thirds of cancer care, including direct medical costs, such as surgery or chemotherapy, and indirect costs, such as lost wages.[42]

These costs can be staggering. In 2003, the direct medical expenses of cancer in the United States were $64.2 billion.[43] Approximately one-half of all bankruptcies filed in 2001 were attributed to medical costs, 10% of which were for cancer care.[44] Of those who filed for bankruptcy, out-of-pocket medical spending for cancer cost more than $35,000 per family.[44] The lack of adequate health insurance contributes to this crisis. Almost 40% of those who filed for bankruptcy because of medical costs experienced a lapse in health insurance coverage during the two years before filing.[44] One study found that one-third of families lost most or all of their savings after a family member was diagnosed with cancer and one-fifth of families saw a family member quit work or experience a similar lifestyle change to provide care.[42]

Where Cancer Survivors Obtain Health Insurance

Like millions of Americans, many cancer survivors have insufficient access to adequate health insurance. Approximately 45,000,000 Americans are uninsured at any point in time; many more experience substantial gaps in health insurance coverage.[44] The majority of uninsured Americans are so because they cannot afford effective coverage.[44] Many of those who are fortunate enough to have health insurance face substantial gaps in coverage.[44] Each year, approximately 200,000 of the 4,000,000 survivors receiving cancer treatment lack health insurance.[45]

Where a survivor obtains insurance is primarily determined by age and employment. Because the incidence of cancer increases with age, approximately 60% of all new cancer diagnoses are among those age 65 and older.[45] Thus, 56% of cancer survivors are covered by Medicare.[45] Of those survivors not covered by Medicare, 33% have private health insurance, 4% are covered by Medicaid, and 2% have other public health insurance.[45] Five percent of all cancer survivors have no insurance at all.[45] Hispanic (12%) and black (8%) survivors are uninsured at higher rates.[45]

Cancer survivors under the age of 65 obtain health insurance primarily through group plans provided by an employer.[46] Seventy percent of survivors under the age of 65 have private health insurance, 4% receive Medicare, 6% receive Medicaid, 9% have other public insurance, and 11% have no insurance at all.[45]

Only about 7% of persons under age 65 in the United States purchase individual health insurance.[47] Individual insurance is a poor option for cancer survivors because it is more costly than group insurance and provides fewer benefits per premium dollar than group plans.[47]

Cancer Survivors' Obstacles to Obtaining Health Insurance

Cancer survivors experience two types of obstacles to obtaining health insurance. First, many survivors are unable to purchase affordable, effective coverage. Because most adults obtain health insurance through their or their spouses' employment,[46] cancer survivors can lose health coverage when they or their spouse or parent becomes unemployed. Those who are not covered by group policies or a patchwork of legal protection are the most vulnerable to insurance problems.

Studies report a variety of barriers to insurance, including refusal of new applications, policy cancellations or reductions, higher premiums, waived or excluded preexisting conditions, and extended waiting periods.[46] Hays found that the more years that have passed since treatment, the better the chances that survivors can obtain health insurance on the same terms as nonsurvivors.[48] Nearly one-half of Hodgkin's disease and leukemia survivors in Kornblith's study reported insurance problems due to cancer.[34] These problems included the denial of health insurance, increased insurance rates, problems changing from a group to an individual plan, and lost health insurance.[34]

Survivors of childhood cancer also experience problems obtaining health insurance. Like adults, the more years that have passed since treatment, the better the chances that childhood cancer survivors can obtain health insurance on the same terms as those who did not have cancer. Vann found that young adult survivors of childhood cancer in North Carolina were more likely to be denied health insurance than their siblings.[49] Hays found that 81% to 91.9% of long-term childhood survivors were covered as adults by health insurance policies without cancer-related restrictions (compared with 82.3% to 94.6% of the controls).[48] Among survivors, 6.9% to 14.3% described difficulties experienced by their parents in obtaining affordable health insurance for the entire family group during or after the survivor's illness (compared with 5.1% to 9.7% of the controls).[48]

The lack of adequate health insurance can have a detrimental impact on survivors' physical, emotional, financial, social, and occupational health.[50] Uninsured individuals are less likely to receive cancer screening and other preventative care than those with insurance.[51] Many uninsured survivors delay diagnosis of symptomatic cancer because of the costs of doctors' appointments and screening tests.[51] Thus, uninsured survivors are diagnosed at later stages than those with insurance.[51] For example, one study found that breast cancer patients who have inadequate health insurance receive fewer medical services, lower quality hospital care, fewer major procedures, and less state-of-the-art cancer treatment.[52] Survivors who have private health insurance and higher income experience better cancer screening, treatment, and access to medical care.[50] This discrepancy is so great that survivors who have no or inadequate health insurance experience poorer health and higher mortality risks.[50]

The type of health insurance also affects cancer survival rates and quality of life. Most health insurance is provided through traditional fee-for-service plans, managed care plans, or public insurance. Under each of these, survivors find that their screening, treatment, and posttreatment care can be compromised by the providers' failure to pay for care recommended by their physicians. With the growth of managed care, survivors are increasingly forced to make decisions regarding their choice of type of treatment, treatment site, and provider, based on whether their insurance plan will cover treatment rather than whether their choices satisfy their medical and personal needs.[50]

Approximately 4% of all cancer survivors are covered by Medicaid.[45] To qualify for Medicaid, an adult who is not pregnant or caring for young children must have a disabling condition that is expected to last at least one year and must meet asset and income requirements.[53] Thus, most Medicaid enrollees who have cancer as their disabling condition are diagnosed with later stages of cancer relative to survivors who are not insured by Medicaid.[51,53] The likelihood of dying from cancer is 2 to 3 times greater for survivors who are insured by Medicaid than for other survivors.[53] Survivors who enroll in Medicaid before diagnosis survive twice as long as those who enroll in Medicaid after diagnosis.[53]

Cancer Survivors' Health Insurance Rights

Cancer survivors who have health insurance are entitled to all of the rights described in their policies. Insurers who fail to pay for treatment in accordance with the terms of the policies may be sued for violating the contract between the survivor and the insurer. In addition to contractual rights, a growing but insufficient patchwork of state and federal laws offer cancer survivors very limited remedies to barriers to securing adequate health insurance.

FEDERAL HEALTH INSURANCE LAWS

Four federal laws provide survivors some opportunities to keep health insurance that they obtain through work.

AMERICANS WITH DISABILITIES ACT

The ADA prohibits employers from denying health insurance to cancer survivors, if other employees with similar jobs receive insurance. The ADA does not require employers to provide health insurance, but when they choose to provide health insurance, they must do so fairly. An employer who does not provide a person with cancer or a history of cancer that the same health insurance provided to employees with similar jobs must prove that the failure to provide insurance is based on legitimate actuarial data or that the insurance plan would become insolvent or suffer a drastic increase in premiums, copayments, or deductibles. An employer, such as a small business, that can prove it is unable to obtain an insurance policy to cover the survivor, may not have to provide him or her with the same health benefits provided to other employees. Because the ADA protects employees from discrimination based on their association with a person with a disability, an employer may not refuse to provide a family health policy solely because one of the employee's dependents has cancer.

HEALTH INSURANCE PORTABILITY AND ACCOUNTABILITY ACT

The Health Insurance Portability and Accountability Act (HIPAA) alleviates job-lock by allowing individuals who have been insured for at least 12 months to change jobs without losing coverage, even if they previously have been diagnosed with cancer. Additionally, in the case of previously uninsured individuals, group plans cannot impose preexisting condition exclusions of more than 12 months for conditions for which medical advice, diagnosis, or treatment was received or recommended within the previous 6 months. HIPAA prevents group health plans from denying coverage based on health status factors such as current and past health, claims experience, medical history, and genetic information. Insurers, may, however, uniformly exclude coverage for specific conditions and place lifetime caps on benefits.

HIPAA specifically helps cancer survivors retain their health insurance by

- alleviating job-lock by allowing individuals who have been insured for at least 12 months to change to a new job without losing coverage, even if they previously have been diagnosed with cancer,
- increasing insurance portability for employees who change from a group policy to an individual one,
- requiring insurers of small groups to cover all interested small employers and to accept every eligible individual under the employer's plan who applies for coverage when first eligible,
- requiring health plans to renew coverage for groups and individuals in most cases, and
- increasing the tax deduction for health insurance expenses available to self-employed individuals.

COMPREHENSIVE OMNIBUS BUDGET RECONCILIATION ACT

The Comprehensive Omnibus Budget Reconciliation Act (COBRA) requires employers to offer group medical coverage to employees and their dependents who otherwise would have lost their group coverage due to individual circumstances. Public and private employers with more than 20 employees are required to make continued insurance coverage available to employees who quit, are terminated, or work reduced hours. Coverage must extend to surviving, divorced, or separated spouses, and to dependent children.

By allowing survivors to keep group insurance coverage for a limited time, COBRA provides valuable time to shop for long-term coverage. Although the survivor, and not the former employer, must pay for the continued coverage, the rate may not exceed by more than 2% the rate set for the survivor's former coworkers. Not all survivors, however, can shoulder the cost of these premiums.

Eligibility for the employee, spouse, and dependent child varies under COBRA. The employee becomes eligible if he or she loses group health coverage because of a reduction in hours or because of termination due to reasons other than gross employee misconduct.

The spouse of an employee becomes eligible for any of four reasons:

(1) the death of a spouse,
(2) the termination of a spouse's employment (for reasons other than gross misconduct) or reduction in a spouse's hours of employment,
(3) a divorce or legal separation from a spouse, or
(4) a spouse becomes eligible for Medicare.

The dependant child of an employee becomes eligible for any of five reasons:

(1) the death of a parent,
(2) the termination of a parent's employment or reduction in a parent's hours,
(3) a parent's divorce or legal separation,
(4) a parent becomes eligible for Medicare, or
(5) a dependent ceases to be a dependent child under a specific group plan.

The continued coverage under COBRA must be identical to that offered to the families of the employee's former coworkers. If employment is terminated for any reason other than gross misconduct, the employee and his or her dependents can continue coverage for up to 18 months. A qualified beneficiary who is categorized as disabled for Social Security purposes at the time of the termination of employment or reduction in employment hours can continue COBRA coverage for a total of 29 months. Dependents can continue coverage for up to 36 months if their previous coverage will end because of any of the above reasons.

Continued coverage may be cut short if

- the employer no longer provides group health insurance to any of its employees,
- the continuation coverage premium is not paid,
- the survivor becomes covered under another group health plan, or
- the survivor becomes eligible for Medicare.

EMPLOYEE RETIREMENT AND INCOME SECURITY ACT

The Employee Retirement and Income Security Act (ERISA) regulates employee-benefit or self-insured plans. ERISA prohibits an employer from discriminating against an employee for the purpose of preventing him or her from collecting benefits under an employee benefit plan. Employee benefit plans are defined broadly, and include any plan with the purpose of providing medical, surgical, or hospital care benefits, or benefits in the event of sickness, accident, disability, death, or unemployment.

Unlike commercial insurance plans that employers purchase to provide health insurance as a benefit for their employees, self-insured plans are funds set aside by employers to reimburse employees for their allowable medical expenses. By 2000, approximately one-third of all privately insured Americans were covered by self-insured plans.[54] The claims employees file to obtain reimbursement through these plans are likely to be administered by commercial insurance companies. Generally, large employer groups or unions find it to their benefit to self-insure, while smaller employer groups choose to finance employee health benefits through commercial insurers. Employee-benefit plans are regulated by federal law only and are not subject to state insurance laws and regulations.

STATE INSURANCE LAWS

Additionally, every state regulates policies sold by insurance companies in the state. These laws vary significantly. Some states require insurance policies to cover off-label chemotherapy, minimum hospital stays for cancer surgery, and benefits for certain types of cancer treatment and screening. Most states provide the right to convert a group health insurance policy to an individual policy. The specific rules of open enrollment periods vary from state to state. Many states guarantee the right to purchase health insurance to individuals who are barred from the marketplace due to their medical history.

Approximately 30 states offer high-risk pools as an alternative source of health insurance for those who cannot purchase an individual plan.[47] High-risk pools have had only a minor impact on the ability of survivors to obtain health insurance. In 2002, less than one percent of the individual health insurance market was enrolled in high-risk pools; 60% were enrolled in just five states—California, Minnesota, Illinois, Wisconsin, and Texas.[47]

CHALLENGING DENIAL OF AN INSURANCE CLAIM

Cancer treatment often involves numerous bills from different parties: hospitals, physicians (such as surgeons, anesthesiologists, oncologists, and radiologists), support services (such as nurses, social workers, nutritionists, and therapists), radiology groups, pharmacies (drugs and medical supplies), and consumer businesses (such as wigs, breast inserts, and special clothing). Insurance companies will pay some of these parties directly, in part or in whole. The survivor must pay other bills and submit copies to the company for reimbursement.

Keeping track of dozens of expenses, often amounting to tens of thousands of dollars, can be confusing and exhausting. The key to collecting the maximum benefits covered by the insurance policy is to keep accurate records of all medical expenses by

- making photocopies of everything sent to the insurance provider, including letters, claim forms, and bills;
- keeping all correspondence received from the insurance provider;
- submitting a bill for every potential claim; and
- keeping accurate records of expenses, claim submissions, and payment vouchers.

A policyholder has a right to appeal a claim denial by a public or private insurer. Because claims are frequently delayed or rejected in part or in full because of errors in filling out the claims forms, care should be taken in accurately providing all the information requested by the insurance company. The following steps could help survivors who are having trouble collecting on their claims:

- Contact the insurance company in writing and insist on a written response.
- Keep original documents in organized files. Send copies of documents to the provider.
- Keep a record of all contacts with the insurance company, including copies of letters and notes from telephone calls. Written records of telephone calls should include the names of the provider's representatives, date of each call, and other relevant facts.
- Contact the state or federal agency that regulates the insurance provider if the provider fails to provide a satisfactory and timely response. Most state insurance departments or commissions help consumers with complaints.
- Contact cancer advocacy organizations. See Figure 20.1.
- Consider legal action as a last resort.

How Healthcare Professionals Can Help Survivors Advocate for Their Employment and Health Insurance Needs

The primary burden of cancer advocacy rests with cancer survivors themselves. Cancer survivors must seek information about their rights and communicate with those who can best understand and meet their needs.[55] Though family members, friends, and other survivors are often the most immediate and direct assistance to survivors, healthcare providers are a critical part of a survivor's advocacy network. Most survivors want to discuss with their providers the impact of their cancer on all aspects of their lives, not just the medical impact.[56] Yet a minority of survivors report actually having this communication with their providers.[56]

Physicians, nurses, social workers, therapists, pharmacists, home health professionals, and rehabilitation specialists can help survivors advocate for their employment and health insurance needs.[57] Healthcare providers are usually a survivor's first and most influential source of information. Providers' primary responsibility is to provide quality cancer care; medical providers cannot be expected to be experts in all nonmedical aspects of cancer care. They must, however, be aware of survivors' needs and rights so that they can inform survivors of the employment and insurance consequences of cancer and guide them to the resources that provide more information and assistance.

Employment Advocacy

Healthcare providers can increase survivors' opportunities to obtain and protect employment. Providers can write letters to prospective and current employers that explain a survivor's abilities and limitations at work. Such letters can also explain an individual's prognosis in a way that may dispel myths about the survivor's current and projected future abilities. Survivors who seek accommodations at work are more likely to obtain those accommodations if they are endorsed by the survivor's healthcare provider. Physicians, nurses, social workers, therapists, and rehabilitation specialists can suggest specific accommodations to help survivors adjust to their workplace.

Many survivors want to use medical leave from work judiciously to mitigate the impact of their cancer on their actual, as well as perceived, ability to work. The fact that most cancer treatment is now provided in outpatient settings permits greater flexibility in scheduling treatment to avoid workplace disruption. For example, many survivors prefer to have chemotherapy on Friday afternoons to minimize the impact of chemotherapy's side effects on their ability to work.

Survivors who have physical or mental limitations resulting from their cancer can benefit from therapy designed to enhance their ability to work. Physical, occupational, and rehabilitation therapists can teach survivors how to adjust to limitations that affect work performance. Oncology social workers and therapists can help survivors who are unable to work during treatment reenter the job market with resume preparation, interviewing skills, and psychosocial support.

Insurance Advocacy

All oncology providers are keenly aware of the significant costs of cancer care. In recommending a treatment plan, providers must consider the survivor's insurance coverage and ability to pay for the recommended care. For those survivors who do not have adequate health insurance, providers should help survivors find alternate ways to pay for treatment. For example, providers should have available contact information for resources that provide assistance such as financial grants, discounted pharmaceutical programs, wigs, prosthetic devices, and transportation.

For those survivors who have health insurance, providers must give survivors the accurate and detailed documentation necessary for them to successfully apply for benefits. Like the survivors themselves, healthcare providers must be willing to follow-up claims to health insurance providers to ensure that all legitimate claims are reimbursed.

Conclusion

A generation ago, most cancer resources were directed towards medical treatment. Few healthcare providers considered playing any role in helping survivors meet their employment and insurance needs.

In the past thirty years, significant changes in cancer treatment, employment rights, and the cost and payment systems of cancer care have transformed survivors' options and expectations. Healthcare providers should be able to evaluate survivors' employment and insurance needs and offer timely information and referrals.[58] Beginning with their initial diagnosis, survivors should have team-based, long-term support in managing their employment and insurance concerns.

Acknowledgments. A substantial portion of the section on employment is based on Hoffman B. Cancer Survivors at Work: A Generation of Progress. *CA: A Cancer Journal for Clinicians*, 2005 (in press).

References

1. McKenna RJ. Employment Discrimination Against Cancer Victims and the Handicapped: Hearings on H.R. 370 and H.R. 1294, Before the Subcommittee on Employment Opportunities of the House Committee on Education and Labor, 99th Cong. 15 1985.

2. Mellette S. The Semantics of Cancer and Disability. In: Proceedings of the Workshop on Employment, Insurance and the Patient with Cancer. New Orleans: American Cancer Society 1986;24–26.

3. Hoffman B. Employment Discrimination Based on Cancer History: The Need for Federal Legislation. 59 Temple Law Quarterly 1 1986.

4. Wasserman AL, Thompson ET, Wilmas JA, et al. The psychosocial status of survivors of childhood/adolescent Hodgkin's disease. Arch Pediatr Adolesc Med 1987;141:626–631.

5. Leigh S. Cancer Rehabilitation: a consumer perspective. Seminars in Oncology Nursing 1992;8(3):164–166.

6. Jemal, Ahmedin. Annual report to the nation on the status of cancer, 1975–2001, with a special feature regarding survival. Cancer 2004;101(1):3–27.

7. Gansler T, Henley SJ, Stein K, Nehl EJ, Smigal C, Slaughter E. Sociodemographic determinants of cancer treatment health literacy. Cancer (in press).

8. Gansler, Ted. Personal communication, May 5, 2005.

9. Yabroff KR, Lawrence WF, Clauser S, et al. Burden of illness in cancer survivors: findings from a population-based national sample. Journal National Cancer Institute 2004;96(17):1322–1330.

10. Clark E, Stovall E. Advocacy: the cornerstone of cancer survivorship. Cancer Practice 1996;4(5):239–244.

11. Hewitt M, Rowland J, Yancik R. Cancer survivors in the United States: age health, and disability. The Journals of Gerontology, Series A: Biological Sciences 2003;58(1):82–91.

12. Bradley C, Bednarek H. Employment patterns of long-term cancer survivors. Psycho-Oncology 2002;11:188–198.

13. Short P, Vasey J, Tunceli K. Employment pathways in a large cohort of adult cancer survivors. Cancer 2005;103(6):1292–1301.

14. Steiner J, Cavender T, Main D, et al. Assessing the impact of cancer on work outcomes: what are the research needs? Cancer 2004;101(8):1703–1711.

15. Messner C, Patterson D. The challenge of cancer in the workplace. Cancer Practice 2001;9(1):50–51.

16. Stone RW. Employing the recovered cancer patient. Cancer 1975;36(1):285–286.

17. Crothers H. Employment problems of cancer survivors: local problems and local solutions. In: American Cancer Society: Proceedings of the Workshop on Employment, Insurance and the Patient with Cancer. New Orleans: American cancer Society, 1986;51–57.

18. Mor V. Work loss, insurance coverage, and financial burden among cancer patients. In: American Cancer Society: Proceedings of the Workshop on Employment, Insurance and the Patient with Cancer. New Orleans: American Cancer Society, 1986: 5–10.

19. Spelten E, Sprangers M, Verbeek J. Factors reported to influence the return to work of cancer survivors: a literature review. Psycho-Oncology 2002;11:124–131.

20. Bloom J, Stewart S, Chang S, et al. Then and now: quality of life of young breast cancer survivors. Psycho-Oncology 2004;13: 147–160.

21. Wheatley GM, Cunnick WR, Wright BP, et al. The employment of persons with a history of treatment for cancer. Cancer 1974;33(2):441–445.

22. Yankelovich Clancy Shulman, Cerenex Survey on Cancer Patients in the Workplace: Breaking Down Discrimination Barriers (1992).

23. Ferrell B, Grant M, Dean G, et al. Bone tired: the experience of fatigue and its impact on quality of life. Oncol Nurs Forum 1996;23(10):1539–1547.

24. Dow K, Ferrell B, Anello C. Balancing demands of cancer surveillance among survivors of thyroid cancer. Cancer Practice 1997;5:289–295.

25. Feldman FL. Work and Cancer Health Histories. American Cancer Society, California Division 1982 (five-year study of the work experiences of 344 white collar workers, blue collar workers, and youths with cancer histories between 1975 and 1980).

26. Fobair P, Hoppe RT, Bloom J, et al. Psychosocial problems among survivors of Hodgkin's disease, J Clin Oncol 1986;4(5):805–814.

27. Koocher GP, O'Malley JE. The Damocles Syndrome: Psychosocial Consequences of Surviving Childhood Cancer. New York: McGraw-Hill, 1982.

28. Polinsky M. Functional status of long-term breast cancer survivors: demonstrating chronicity. Health Soc Work 1994;19(3): 165–174.

29. National Cancer Institute, 2004. http://www.dccps.nci.gov/ocs/prevalence/index.html accessed May 10, 2005.

30. Ferrell B, Schmidt G, Rhiner M, et al. The meaning of life for bone marrow transplant survivors, party 2: improving quality of life for bone marrow survivors. Cancer Nursing 1992;15:247–253.

31. Ferrell B, Dow K. Quality of life in breast cancer survivors as identified by focus groups. Psycho-Oncology 1997;6(13):20–21.

32. Hoffman B. Between a disability and a hard place: the cancer survivors' catch-22 of proving disability status under the Americans with Disabilities Act, 59. Maryland Law Review 2000;352.

33. National Coalition for Cancer Survivorship, Amgen, National Survey on Cancer and the Workplace, (random telephone survey of 662 employed adult Americans interviewed from June 13 to June 15, 1997).

34. Kornblith A, Herndon JE, Zuckerman E, et al. Comparison of psychosocial adaptation of advanced stage Hodgkin's disease and acute leukemia survivors. Ann Oncol 1998;9:297–306.

35. Working Women, Amgen, Cancer in the Workplace Survey (conducted by CBD Research & Consulting: random telephone survey of 500 survivors employed at time of their treatment, 100 supervisors, and 100 co-workers in May 1996).

36. Equal Employment Opportunities Commission, ADA Charge Date by Impairments/Bases—Receipts, http://www.eeoc.gov/stats.ada=receipts.html. Accessed May 10, 2005.

37. Blanck P. The Economics of the Employment Provisions of the Americans with Disabilities Act: Part I. Workplace Accommodations, 46 DePaul Law Review 877, 1997.

38. Grant J, Hatcher T, Patel N. Expecting Better: A State-by-State Analysis of Parental Leave Programs, National Partnership for Women and Families, accessed at www.nationalpartnership.org, May 10, 2005.

39. Nicoll R. Long-Term Care Insurance and Genetic Discrimination Get It While You're Young and Ignorant: An Examination of Current Discriminatory Problems in Long-Term Care Insurance Through the Use of Genetic Information. 13 Albany Law Journal of Science & Technology 751 2003.

40. National Conference of State Legislatures, State Genetics Employment Laws, http://www.ncsl.org/programs/health/genetics/ndiscrim.htm. Accessed May 10, 2005.

41. Colker R. The Americans with Disabilities Act: A Windfall for Defendants. 34 Harvard Civil Rights Civil Liberties Law Review 99 1999.

42. Arozullah A, Calhoun E, Wolf M, et al. The financial burden of cancer: estimates from a study of insured women with breast cancer, Journal of Supportive Oncology 2004;2:271–278.

43. Centers for Disease Control and Prevention, Comprehensive Cancer Control: Collaborating to Conquer Cancer, Fact Sheet 2004/2005.

44. Himmelstein D, Warren E, Thorne D, et al. Illness and injury as contributor to bankruptcy, February 2, 2005, Health Affairs, Web Exclusive, W5-63 to W5-73.

45. Thorpe K, Howard D. Health Insurance and Spending Among Cancer Patients, April 9, 2003, Health Affairs, Web Exclusive, W3-189 to W3-198.

46. Crothers HM. Health insurance: problems and solutions for people with cancer histories. In American Cancer Society: Proceedings of the Fifth National Conference on Human Values and Cancer. San Francisco, California Division of the American Cancer Society, 1987;100–109.

47. Fuchs B. Expanding the Individual Health Insurance Market: Lessons from the State Reforms of the 1990s. The Robert Wood Johnson Foundation, Research Synthesis Report No. 4, 2004.

48. Hays DM, Landsverk J, Sallan SE, et al. Educational, occupational, and insurance status of childhood cancer survivors in their fourth and fifth decades of life. J Clin Oncol 1992; 10(9):1397–1406.

49. Vann JC, Biddle AK, Daeschner CW, et al. Health insurance access to young adult survivors of childhood cancer in North Carolina. Medical Pediatric Oncology 1995;25(5):389–395.

50. Glajchen M. Psychosocial consequences of inadequate health insurance for patients with cancer. Cancer Practice 1994; 2(2):115–120.

51. Roetzheim R, Pal N, Tennant C, et al. J Nat Cancer Inst 1999;91(16):1409–1415.

52. Ayanian JZ, Kohler BA, Abe T, et al. The relation between health insurance coverage and clinical outcomes among women with breast cancer. N Engl J Med 1993;329:326–331.

53. Bradley C, Gardiner J, Given C, et al. Cancer, Medicaid enrollment, and survival disparities. Cancer 2005;103(8):1712–1718.

54. Politz K, Tapay N, Hadley E, et al. Early experience with "New Federalism" in health insurance regulation. Health Affairs 2000;19(4):7–22.

55. Stovall E, Clark E. Survivors as Advocates. In: Hoffman B, ed. Charting Your Journey: A Cancer Survivor's Almanac. Wiley: Hoboken, NJ 2004;302–308.

56. Back A, Baile W. Communication skills: myths, realities, and new developments. Journal of Supportive Oncology, 2003;1: 169–171.

57. Clark E. You and Your Health Care Team. In: Hoffman B, ed. Charting Your Journey: A Cancer Survivor's Almanac, Wiley: Hoboken, NJ 2004;56–68.

58. Kattlove H, Winn R. Ongoing care of patients after primary treatment for their cancer. CA Cancer J Clin 2003;54:172–196.

Cancer Advocacy

Ellen L. Stovall

Thousands of individual citations using the expression *cancer advocacy* can be found in contemporary medical and scientific literature as well as in the popular press and on Internet websites. For purposes of this chapter, the term *cancer advocacy* is used to describe a skill set that has been documented in previously published work by Clark and Stovall.[1] This chapter also includes specific examples of how self-described advocacy organizations are involved with research organizations and how they influence cancer research and related health policy.

In 1996, Clark and Stovall described a cancer-related advocacy skill set that could be acquired through a learning process and would ideally be incorporated into care plans for cancer patients. Their article proposed a definition of cancer advocacy that most easily correlated with the terms "cancer survivor" and "cancer survivorship" first used by the founders of the National Coalition for Cancer Survivorship (NCCS) in 1986.[2] NCCS defines a cancer survivor as anyone with a diagnosis of cancer—from the time of its discovery and for the balance of life. NCCS further defines cancer survivorship as a process that begins when an individual is diagnosed with cancer and continues until their death. NCCS believes that, at the time of diagnosis, an individual with cancer [and/or a significant person in his or her life—known as the "other survivor"(s)] can play a very active role in assuring that they receive quality care. This is the first step in the cancer advocacy continuum and is further defined by Clark and Stovall as "personal advocacy or self-advocacy." The next step in the continuum is "advocacy for others." This is where some of the most effective advocacy occurs for individuals with cancer, and it is where many people with cancer find a role for themselves as advocates in their own community. The third part of the advocacy paradigm described by Clark and Stovall is national advocacy, or public interest advocacy.

Over the past decade, relative survival data for all cancer types have ranged from 6 to 10 million survivors in any given year, and estimates are that of that number, more than half are living 5 years or more postdiagnosis.[3] With this epidemiology alone, it is likely that this cohort (and their primary caregivers and healthcare providers) could be the most likely beneficiaries of a greater understanding of the role that advocacy can play as part of a successful adjustment to a cancer diagnosis. To accept the notion that advocacy can play a role in enhancing the quality of one's survivorship, a shared understanding of cancer advocacy and its relationship to cancer survivorship among healthcare professionals and sig-

nificant others involved with a cancer patient's adjustment postdiagnosis is desirable.

The term *cancer survivorship* was a term of art rather than science when the founders of NCCS used it to describe the condition of living with the consequences of a diagnosis of cancer. Now commonly referred to as the cancer survivorship movement, several of its early founders and adopters crafted the language and gave definition to terminology frequently used today for what has become a burgeoning field of study called *cancer survivorship research*. Mullan wrote about cancer survivorship as the "act of living on."[4] Carter and Leigh have written about survivorship in terms of "going through" and "the experience of living with, through or beyond cancer."[5,6] These dynamic concepts of survivorship suggested that more research was needed to focus on cancers whose prognosis could be defined as protracted and/or episodic, rather than as an acute diagnosis followed by death. It was also noted that the degree to which a history of cancer affects the life of an individual is largely dependent on many qualitative variables with respect to how they experience their illness. These variables include, but are not limited to, their familial and cultural relationships, their religious beliefs, how their cancer is treated, and how their disease progresses or is resolved.

Previous chapters in this book elaborate on the survivorship issues and deal specifically with the myriad of medical and psychosocial sequelae of many cancers. The challenges posed by these changes in one's biologic and psychologic condition suggest that although each person's cancer is an individual experience, there are overarching issues with which many survivors contend.[7] We also know from the literature and from the cancer survivorship movement that the skills necessary for positive adaptation to cancer have been identified and that survivors must become self-advocates and viewed by health professionals as partners in making the very important decisions that will impact on their medical, social, psychologic, and vocational well-being. What follows is a suggestion by Clark and Stovall that successful adaptation to cancer involves acquiring advocacy skills that will enhance each survivor's sense of self-determination throughout his or her survivorship. The skill set is neither gender- nor age-specific and does not suggest an impact on longevity, but rather on quality of life across several domains.

Using advocacy as an approach to adjusting to cancer calls for establishing a competency model that has skill-building and coping strategies at its core. This approach is suggested as a way of preventing or overcoming psychosocial limitations and promoting expectations for effective living.[8,9] The notion of learning an advocacy skill set is especially useful if one agrees that the psychosocial dimensions of a cancer diagnosis may cause a time-limited state of diminished functioning. Maher[10] defines a diagnosis of cancer as an anomic situation for many, suggesting it is "a temporary state of mind occasioned by a sudden alteration in one's life situation, and characterized by confusion and anxiety, uncertainty, loss of purpose, and a sense of separateness from one's usual social support system." Clark[11] suggests that the concept of crisis is useful for adaptation to cancer in terms of both situational requirements and the various phases over time of the mobilization of resources. The tasks facing the individual, as well as the strategies selected for attempted management of these tasks, become important parts of the process for resolving crises. These tasks and the strategies for managing them, such as seeking information or support, can be integrated into a method of skills training.

Skills training is used across many diverse professional settings, including education, psychology, sociology, and social work, and is distinguished from competence by McFall,[12,13] who associates skills with the specific underlying component processes that enable a person to perform in a manner which has been identified as competent. Skills are task specific and are acquired through a learning process.

Skills training is especially useful because of the complexities of the cancer experience. Drawing from a body of evidence found largely in the psychosocial research literature and derived from educational programs developed by cancer advocacy organizations, four interrelated skills have been identified as integral to the advocacy skills model: (1) information-seeking skills,[14–16] (2) communication skills,[17–21] (3) problem-solving skills,[22–28] and (4) negotiation skills.[29–31]

The founders of many patient advocacy organizations widely agree that providing reliable and timely information as well as providing decision support to people with cancer are among the most pressing needs of the public who are in touch with them when dealing with a diagnosis of cancer. Information needs are variable among cancer patients and change over the course of their illness. Also variable are the methods used by people when they seek health- and medical-related information. Books and articles about cancer can be found in public, university, hospital, and medical school libraries, and public access to the Internet is widely available. If anything, the amount of cancer information is daunting, and there are few compendia that annotate the information available, often making it difficult to identify what are the most suitable and reliable cancer-related resources. The Internet Health Care Coalition[32] offers an excellent guide for evaluating the reliability of online health information and advice, including cancer information. Being a wise medical consumer involves asking questions, seeking answers, gathering and organizing data, and the ability to access resources. Training for the development of information-seeking skills involves well-developed communication and negotiation skills.

Communication skills-building is an aspect of medical consumerism that is frequently complicated by the patient's need to learn a new lexicon of terms to increase his or her comprehension and understanding of cancer. At the critical time of learning about and understanding the diagnosis, the goals of treatment, and decision making about which treatment is most suitable, shared responsibility for communicating clearly between the healthcare provider and patient is important. The quality of communication should be characterized by equity, reciprocity, and a mutual understanding of hope and goals, wherein both patient and professional have input into care decisions.[33]

The literature on effective communication skills is widely available and adaptable to a clinical setting. The American Society of Clinical Oncology (ASCO) and the Oncology Nursing Society (ONS) are excellent resources of information on patient/provider communications skills building, and both associations provide workshops to their members on effective communication strategies.

Problem-solving skills are especially helpful when utilized to more carefully consider a situation with no clear and evident resolution. A diagnosis of cancer is one of those situations that can benefit from employing a number of problem-solving methods including modeling and role-playing.[34] Modeling is a form of observational learning in which the behavior of an individual or group acts as a stimulus for similar thoughts, attitudes, and behavior on the part of another individual. Role-playing relies on the re-creation of real or hypothetical situations. Cancer survivors use role-playing effectively in group settings where peer support and critique for their interactions with role-playing professionals can be supported.

It is common to hear cancer survivors use words such as "powerless" or "out of control" when describing how they felt when diagnosed with cancer. Because these feelings of temporary impotence frequently accompany a diagnosis of cancer, how one advocates for one's own needs during this time may be compromised. Especially relevant to a diagnosis of cancer is negotiation skills training if one must contend with employment, insurance, and financial institutions. Advocating in the occupational setting or with insurers often includes negotiations that go beyond anyone's ordinary mastery of skills and requires the involvement of legal counsel.[35,36] Because conflict is inherent in many well-intended interactions, conflict resolution through negotiation bears attention as part of a good self-advocacy model. Effective communication, resourcefulness, open-mindedness, and understanding alternative positions are central to all negotiation efforts.[37]

The advocacy continuum as described by Clark and Stovall may begin at a personal level wherein the previously outlined skill sets are most relevant. As the survivorship continuum changes, so do the advocacy needs of the individual and his/her support system. Self-advocacy may evolve into wanting to participate or interact with small groups or organizations at the community level, and, for some, public policy activities at the national level. Succinctly stated, Clark and Stovall describe an advocacy paradigm as follows: (1) Personal Advocacy; (2) Advocacy for Others; and (3) Public Interest Advocacy.

Personal advocacy or self-advocacy is a way of taking charge in an otherwise portentous environment of tests, surgery, radiation, chemotherapy, and office visits. From arming oneself with good information about one's diagnosis, to seeking second opinions, to locating resources for identifying and obtaining support, to knowing how to ask the right questions and negotiate the terms of one's employment while undergoing treatment, a cancer patient can become self-efficacious. This type of self-determination can mean the difference between maintaining a positive future outlook and enhancing one's quality of life or feeling helpless and less certain of the desirability of survival.[38,39]

For many cancer survivors, the 5 years following diagnosis and treatment mark a time of reentry and reevaluation of one's life. Many significant relationships in the lives of survivors change during this time as family and friends cannot understand why survivors are not simply jubilant with their survival. Support systems that were intact during the initial workup and treatment period may diminish or disappear. It is at this time in survivorship that many seek out others with whom they can identify. This transitional period, whether at age 20 or 70, calls for another kind of self-advocacy. With the notion that they may want to "give something back" in gratitude for their survival, many survivors seek to share their experiences with others.[40] The idea that shared information can be both powerful and validating—the veteran helping the rookie—is what the survivorship movement is largely about. When occurring in the context of a support group, this transmission of wisdom from a more-seasoned survivor to the newcomer provides a strong foundation for people who have had cancer to play a more-proactive role in making the myriad decisions that will follow them the rest of their lives.

The second part of the advocacy paradigm is characterized by cancer survivors going on to relay their experiences beyond one-on-one counseling interventions or small group interactions. Involvement in one's community can range from speaking to civic or religious groups and to the local media, participating in runs/walks for cancer awareness and cancer research, enrolling in advocacy training courses such as the National Breast Cancer Coalition's Project LEAD, to inquiring about participation on local Institutional Review Boards, etc. By speaking about one's experience to groups of medical students, for example, cancer survivors have an opportunity to educate them about the complex interpersonal and psychosocial issues that dominate their lives after treatment. This public speaking becomes a testimony that affirms one's survival, defies the myths and stigmas about cancer, and perhaps reaches others who are silently struggling with similar issues.

The last part of the cancer advocacy paradigm is Public Interest Advocacy. Largely a consequence of improved diagnostic tools and treatments for cancer that resulted in months and years of survival beyond initial diagnosis, issues related to adult cancer survivorship emerged as an agenda for advocacy and activism in the mid-1980s. These issues principally fall into three areas: economic/vocational, psychosocial/spiritual, and physiologic.

Compared with the number of cancer survivors, relatively very few engage in this type of advocacy, although breast cancer survivors have been visible and notable in the way they have brought about policy change through political advocacy and activism. A distinction is being made between the visibility or awareness of breast and other cancers through mass cause-related marketing campaigns and the work of cancer advocates and activists who participate in focused activities to change or initiate public policies.

Although *cancer advocacy* is not a contemporary phenomenon and includes much public education and outreach to diverse constituencies, *cancer activism* is in its relative infancy. Cancer survivors as advocates became very visible during the mid-1980s and 1990s when national breast cancer activists petitioned the federal government to target research in breast cancer and petitioned Congress to earmark funds

through an unprecedented appropriation from the Department of Defense. Their petitioning not only increased federal funding for research, but led to a change in the peer-review process for granting monies to research under this program. The distinguishing characteristic of this example was the involvement of cancer survivors at every step of designing the Department of Defense Breast Cancer Program. Their activism laid the groundwork and set an example for participation of advocates at all levels of government-funded cancer research programs.

The 1990s and the new millennium ushered in an era that witnessed the creation of many organizations that self-identify themselves as cancer advocacy groups. Often founded by survivors and/or their supporters, these groups represent the voices of people with commonly diagnosed cancers, for example, breast, colon, lung, lymphatic, and prostate, as well as less-common cancers, such as ovarian, head and neck, brain, pancreatic, and kidney, and provide a valuable resource for people with cancer and their families. Increasingly, their representation can be found sitting on review groups, on the boards of cancer centers, on federal advisory commissions, and walking the halls of Congress to educate their elected officials about the needs of those they represent.

References

1. Clark EJ, Stovall E. Advocacy: the cornerstone of cancer survivorship. Cancer Pract 1996;5:239–244.
2. National Coalition for Cancer Survivorship. Charter. Silver Spring, MD: National Coalition for Cancer Survivorship, 1986.
3. American Cancer Society. Cancer Facts and Figures: 1994–2003. Atlanta, GA: The American Cancer Society, 2003.
4. Mullan F, Hoffman B (eds). Charting the Journey: An Almanac of Practical Resources for Cancer Survivors. Mount Vernon, NY: Consumers Union, 1990.
5. Carter B. Going through: a critical theme in surviving breast cancer. Innov Oncol Nurs 1989;5:2–4.
6. Leigh S. Myths, monsters, and magic: personal perspectives and professional challenges of survival. Oncol Nurs Forum 1992;19:1475–1480.
7. Loescher L, Clark L, Atwood J, Leigh S, Lawl G. The impact of the cancer experience on long-term survivors. Oncol Nurs Forum 1990;17:223–229.
8. Rowland JH. Intrapersonal resources: coping. In: Holland JC, Rowland JH (eds). Handbook of Psychooncology. New York: Oxford University Press, 1990:44–57
9. Seeman J. Toward a model of positive health. Am Psychologist 1989;44:1099–1109.
10. Maher EL. Anomic aspects of recovery from cancer. Soc Sci Med 1982;16:907–912.
11. Clark EJ. Social assessment of cancer patients. Proceedings of the National Conference on Practice, Education, and Research in Oncology Social Work—1984. Philadelphia: American Cancer Society, 1984.
12. McFall R, Dodge K. Self-management and interpersonal skills learning. In: Karoly P, Kanfer F (eds). Self-Management and Behavior Change. New York: Pergamon Press, 1982:353–392.
13. McFall R. A review and reformulation of the concept of social skills. Behav Assess 1082;4:1–33.
14. Tabak ER. Encouraging patient question-asking: a clinical trial. Patient Educ Counsel 1988;12:37–49.
15. Blanchard CG, Labrecque MS, Ruckdeschel JC, Blanchard EB. Information and decision-making preferences of hospitalized adult cancer patients. Soc Sci Med 1988;27:1139–1145.

16. Messerli M, Garamendi C, Romano J. Breast cancer information as a technique of crisis intervention. Am J Orthopsychiatry 1980;50:728–731

17. Mullan F, Hoffman B (eds). Charting the Journey: An Almanac of Practical Resources for Cancer Survivors. Mount Vernon, NY: Consumers Union, 1990.

18. Sharf B. Teaching patients to speak up: past and future trends. Patient Educ Counsel 1988;11:95–108.

19. Knapp ML, Miller GR. Handbook of Interpersonal Communication. Newbury Park, CA: Sage Publications, 1994.

20. Moore LG. Teamwork: The Cancer Patient's Guide To Talking With Your Doctor (booklet). Silver Spring, MD: National Coalition for Cancer Survivorship, 1991.

21. Telch C, Telch M. Group coping skills instruction and supportive group therapy for cancer patients: a comparison of strategies. J Consult Clin Psychol 1986;54:802–808.

22. Mullan F, Hoffman B (eds). Charting the Journey: An Almanac of Practical Resources for Cancer Survivors. Mount Vernon, NY: Consumers Union, 1990.

23. Gray RE, Doan B, Church K. Empowerment issues in cancer. Health Values 1991;15:22–28.

24. Tabak ER. Encouraging patient question-asking: a clinical trial. Patient Educ Counsel 1988;12:37–49.

25. Hoffman B. Employment discrimination: another hurdle for cancer survivors. Cancer Invest 1991;9:589–595.

26. Fawzy F, Cousins N, Fawzy N, Kemeny M, Elashoff R, Morton D. A structured psychiatric intervention for cancer patients: changes over time in methods of coping and affective disturbance. Arch Gen Psychiatry 1990;47:720–725.

27. Roter D. An exploration of health education responsibility for a partnership model of client-provider relations. Patient Educ Counsel 1987;9:25–31.

28. Welch-McCaffrey D, Hoffman B, Leigh S, Loescher L, Meyskans F. Surviving adult cancers. Part 2: psychosocial implications. Ann Intern Med 1989;111:517–524.

29. Kauffman DB. Surviving Cancer. Washington, DC: Acropolis, 1989.

30. Rowland JH. Intrapersonal resources: coping. In: Holland JC, Rowland JH (eds). Handbook of Psychooncology. New York: Oxford University Press, 1990:44–57.

31. Callan DB. Hope as a clinical issue in oncology social work. J Psychosoc Oncol 1989;7:31–46.

32. http://www.ihealthcoalition.org/.

33. Thoits P. Stressors and problem-solving: the individual as social activist. J Health Soc Behav 1994;35:293–304.

34. Anderson L, DeVellis B, DeVellis F. Effects of modeling on patient communication, satisfaction, and knowledge. Med Care 1987;25:1044–1056.

35. Hoffman B. Working It Out: Your Employment Rights As A Cancer Survivor (booklet). Silver Spring, MD: National Coalition for Cancer Survivorship, 2002.

36. Calder K, Pollitz K. What Cancer Survivors Need To Know About Health Insurance (booklet). Silver Spring, MD: National Coalition for Cancer Survivorship, 2002.

37. Volpe M, Maida P. Sociologists and the processing of conflicts. Sociol Pract 1992;10:13–25.

38. Clark EJ. You Have The Right To Be Hopeful (booklet). Silver Spring, MD: National Coalition for Cancer Survivorship, 1995.

39. Farran CJ, Herth KA, Popovich JM. Hope and Hopelessness: Critical Clinical Constructs. Thousand Oaks, CA: Sage, 1995.

40. Ferrell BR, Dow KH. Portraits of cancer survivorship: a glimpse through the lens of survivors' eyes. Cancer Pract 1996;4:76–80.

The Survivorship Care Plan: What, Why, How, and for Whom

2 2

Craig C. Earle, Deborah Schrag, Steven H. Woolf, and Patricia A. Ganz

Overview

This chapter highlights the recent call by the Institute of Medicine for the use of a cancer survivorship plan to be provided to patients and their primary care providers at the end of cancer treatment. The need for evidence-based guidance on surveillance regimens after cancer treatment, how best to communicate what cancer treatments were received, and what care should be provided after treatment, as well as mechanisms to share care between oncology specialists and primary care providers is discussed. With the expanding number of cancer survivors each year, oncologists must find creative ways to ensure that the gains obtained through successful cancer treatment are not lost when patients transition to this phase of their care.

Introduction

In the past two decades, the 5-year survival rate for the top 15 cancers has increased from 42.7% for men and 56.6% for women, to 64% for men and to 64.3% for women.[1] Figures 22.1 through 22.4 provide the most recent statistics available on cancer survivors from the National Cancer Institute Office of Cancer Survivorship, with an estimate that there were more than 10.1 million cancer survivors in the United States in 2001.[2] With this medical and demographic imperative, the Institute of Medicine (IOM), under the auspices of the National Cancer Policy Board, undertook a detailed study of adult cancer survivors, with a focus on "the period following first diagnosis and treatment before the development of a recurrence of cancer or death."[3] This distinct phase in the trajectory of cancer care has not been well described or addressed by the healthcare system previously.[3]

Recommendation number two of this IOM report states, "Patients completing primary treatment should be provided with a comprehensive care plan summary and follow-up care plan that is clearly and effectively explained. The 'Survivorship Care Plan' should be written by the principal provider(s) who coordinated oncology treatment. This service should be reimbursed by third-party payors of health care."[3] To this end,

this article provides a framework and rationale for the survivorship care plan, including important information about surveillance care after primary cancer treatment ends, how oncologists can prepare a treatment summary and survivorship care plan, and a description of the shared care model between specialists and primary care providers as a way to enhance the quality of care for cancer survivors. We realize that, practically speaking, a formal survivorship care plan will take some time to implement and make a routine part of oncology care. Nevertheless, the findings and recommendations of the IOM report suggest that many cancer survivors are "lost in transition" and that the quality of care suffers when patients and providers do not know what is expected at the end of treatment. This article and educational session are one among many educational efforts that the American Society of Clinical Oncology (ASCO) has embarked on to inform ASCO members about the needs of cancer survivors and how oncology professionals can make a difference in their care.

Surveillance After Cancer

Most oncologists focus on surveillance for recurrent cancer after primary treatment, but it is important to recognize that surveillance may also need to be considered for new primary cancers in the same organ or for secondary cancers or treatment-induced late effects. In addition, cancer survivors are also an important audience for healthpromotion and disease-prevention activities.[4,5] As an example, this article focuses on recent changes in ASCO guidelines for colorectal cancer surveillance, to initiate a discussion of the general issues involved regarding surveillance and the evidence behind specific recommendations.

Among the recently updated ASCO recommendations for surveillance after primary treatment of stage II and III colorectal cancer,[6] the recommendation for "annual computerized tomography of the chest and abdomen for 3 years after primary therapy for patients who are at higher risk of recurrence and who could be candidates for curativeintent surgery" is most notable. This statement brings up several issues. It

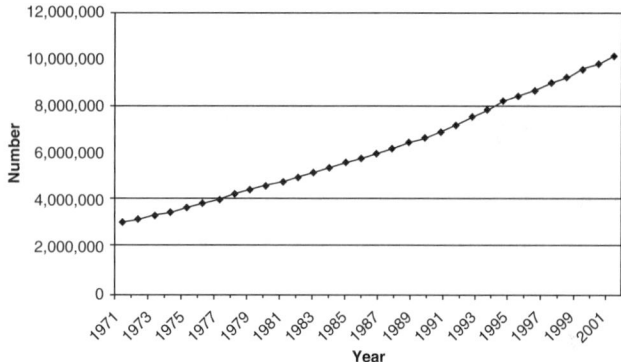

FIGURE 22.1. Estimated number of cancer survivors in the United States from 1971 to 2002. Prevalence counts were estimated by applying U.S. populations to SEER 9 and historical Connecticut Limited Duration Prevalence proportions and adjusted to represent complete prevalence. Populations from January 2002 were based on the average of the July 2001 and July 2002 population estimates from the U.S. Census Bureau. Abbreviations: SEER, Surveillance, Epidemiology and End Results.

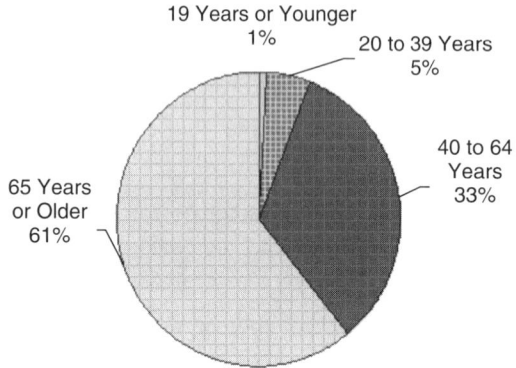

FIGURE 22.2. Estimated number of people alive in the United States diagnosed with cancer by current age (Invasive/First primary case only, 10.1 million survivors).

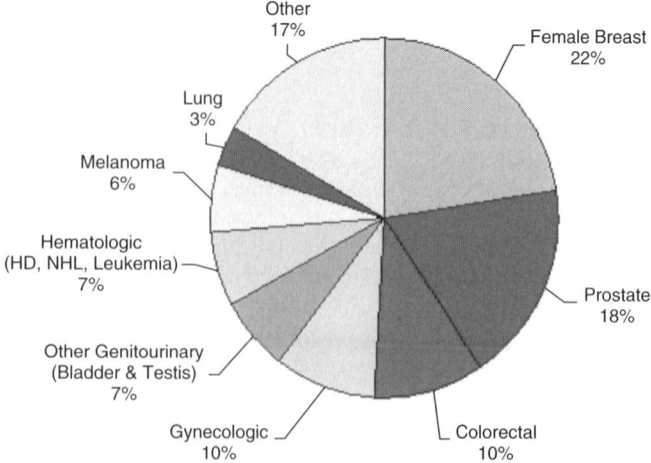

FIGURE 22.3. Estimated number of people alive in the United States diagnosed with cancer by site (10.1 million). Abbreviation: HD, Hodgkin's disease; NHL, non-Hodgkin's lymphoma.

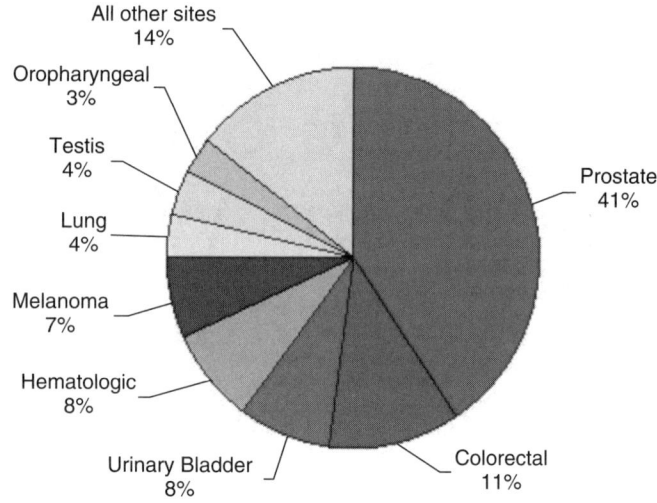

A. Men

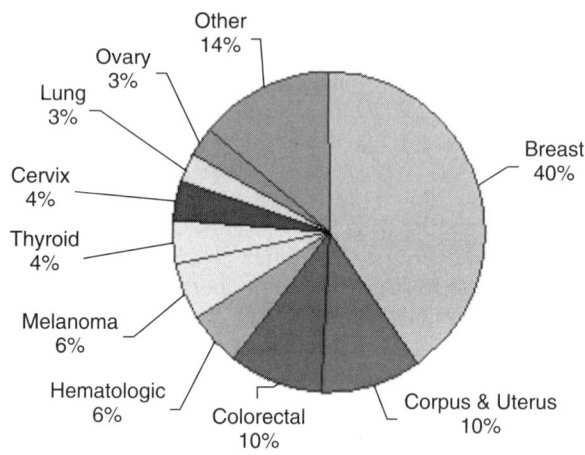

B. Women

FIGURE 22.4. Estimated number persons alive in the United States diagnosed with cancer on January 1, 2002 by time from diagnosis and sex (Invasive/First primary cases only, 10.1 million survivors).

selection of patients for follow-up based on their presumed fitness levels for further therapy.

Patients are willing to accept the notion of surveillance.[7] Having gone through regimented cancer treatments and constant contact with their oncology providers, many are reassured by the sense of control that a follow-up regimen can provide—somebody knows what should be done. Physicians also desire this, but does this provide false reassurance?[8] In most cases physicians do not have high-quality evidence on which to decide what constitutes optimal surveillance, and there is little agreement on recommendations among experts.[9] In many situations, there is not even a plausible rationale for intense monitoring of patients who are asymptomatic to find incurable recurrence.

The reason usually offered for following patients with cancer is to increase their survival by detecting local or distant disease at a time when it is still curable or when palliative treatment can be more effective. Surveillance strategies generally consist of some combination of office visits

prompts reflection on the more general rationale for, evidence behind, and sometimes unintended effects of intensive follow-up strategies for patients with cancer. It also alludes to the incorporation of risk prediction in surveillance and with history and physical examination, blood work including tumor markers, imaging studies, and visualization of the primary organ, for example, with endoscopy or second-look surgery. Surveillance of the primary tumor site can occasionally detect treatable local recurrences, for example, in rectal as well as breast and head and neck malignancies. However, in other examples, second-look surgeries for ovarian and pancreatic cancers have not been associated with improved outcomes because such recurrences are generally not curable.[10] In colon cancer, local recurrences are uncommon. Colonoscopy, therefore, is primarily used to find synchronous or metachronous second primaries.

The media have persuaded the public that if cancer is found early, it can be cured. However, patients often do not understand that the same does not pertain to early detection of incurable distant metastases. Unfortunately, there is a paucity of evidence that early institution of palliative chemotherapy in asymptomatic patients provides benefit.[7,11] An exception might be surveillance for metastases in colorectal cancer, where a small proportion of patients who recur with oligometastatic disease can receive local therapy for cure.[12] There have been seven randomized trials comparing different surveillance strategies in colorectal cancer.[13–19] Although most were underpowered to show benefit individually, meta-analyses have indicated that trials in which patients received more intensive surveillance showed a greater survival advantage than trials with less intensive surveillance.[20,21]

The use of imaging studies is often the most controversial aspect of surveillance because these studies are relatively expensive and are usually only able to find distant, often incurable, recurrence. Even in examples with a strong rationale where salvage therapies are clearly more effective when the tumor burden is low, the majority of relapses present with signs, symptoms, or abnormalities on blood work (e.g., lactate dehydrogenase in lymphoma).[22] The new colorectal surveillance recommendation to image the liver and lungs annually in patients at higher risk is based on recent meta-analyses demonstrating 25% lower mortality for patients undergoing surveillance schedules that include imaging.[21,23,24]

Tailoring surveillance to risk seems logical. Concentrate on following high-risk patients at a time when they are most likely to experience recurrence. However, there is little evidence that following high-risk patients more intensively is either more effective or more cost effective than following all patients similarly in most cases. Because high-risk patients are more likely to experience recurrence, surveillance will certainly find more recurrences in these patients.[25] However, it is possible that those recurrences will tend to become clinically evident relatively quickly anyway, and curative therapy may be less likely to succeed than in the case of more indolent cancers that relapse. Indeed, it has been observed that patients with node-negative primaries who relapse late are more likely to be cured with metastatectomy.[12] Consequently, it may be best to follow lower-risk patients more closely and to do so in later years in order to pick up those indolent relapses that may be most amenable to curative therapy. However, there is no direct evidence supporting this approach.

The common caveat that surveillance need only be applied to patients willing and able to undergo aggressive surgery also can be challenged. Patient preferences can change dramatically with the passage of time from initial therapy and once recurrence is a reality. Further, new technologies

for management of oligometastases, such as percutaneous radiofrequency ablation and stereotactic radiosurgery,[26] are increasing the options for medically-frail patients. As a result, it is not clear that such patients should necessarily be excluded from surveillance recommendations.

In cases in which we cannot reasonably expect survival to be improved, we tend to think that surveillance at least provides important reassurance to patients. However, even this benefit is debatable.[27,28] Although being told that there is no sign of cancer recurrence can understandably decrease anxiety,[29] the stress leading up to it, the inconvenience and often the discomfort of testing, and the not infrequently detected incidental abnormalities are instances in which surveillance causes harm.[25,30] False-positive results cause mental anguish and usually lead to further tests, possibly invasive ones such as biopsy, that add expense and can lead to other complications. Indeed, randomized trials have not been able to consistently find positive psychologic effects associated with surveillance.[7,28]

There are many other reasons to follow patients with cancer, including monitoring for long-term or late effects of treatment (e.g., hypothyroidism, lymphedema, new cancers), detecting and preventing potentially catastrophic complications of recurrence, or providing general primary care. Instituting a surveillance program can be less time consuming and emotionally charged than explaining the evidence and rationale behind a less-aggressive strategy. Moreover, even fully informed patients who relapse may direct their anger at physicians who they may feel missed something if follow-up monitoring was not done.[20] Most compelling, however, can be patient preference—some patients may want to know that their cancer has recurred, even if they are asymptomatic and their survival cannot be prolonged, to best make life decisions going forward.

Current surveillance practices are based more on consensus, tradition, patient demands, medical and legal concerns, and the constraints of third-party payors than on a large body of evidence. Follow-up after cancer seems like a good idea, and in some cases can be important. However, it also comes with costs, both economic and otherwise. Physicians must be aware of its limitations and be honest with patients about its worth. Decisions about posttreatment surveillance strategies are sometimes complex and involve weighing knowledge of patients' preferences and their ability to withstand intensive medical interventions should recurrence be detected. Specifically, communicating with patients at the completion of treatment to specify the surveillance plan may be quite valuable.

Rationale for a Treatment Summary and Survivorship Care Plan

When physicians want to know what surgical treatment a patient with cancer has had they now to ask for two critical documents: the operative report and the pathology report. Thus, even when faced with a thick stack of medical records, these physicians are able to navigate quickly to key information. Although these documents do not provide a summary of postoperative complications, they use a standardized format to describe the reason for performing the operation, the procedure planned and actually performed, and any immediate complications. Similarly, in radiation oncology, the concept of a radiation treatment summary is widely accepted; this succinct document describes the reason for radiation, the area irradiated, the treatment planned, and the treatment actually delivered. Radiation oncologists may use different templates for this summary, some providing more or less accompanying narrative detail. However, the culture of radiation oncology is for all providers to prepare some version of this key document. Other providers recognize this and know to ask for it.

In contrast to radiation and surgical treatments, which are more discrete episodes of cancer care, a chemotherapy regimen has less distinct boundaries. A regimen may be given once or more during a period of years, and thus the amount of information that needs to be summarized may vary tremendously. In some instances, patients may initiate a three-drug regimen, develop an allergy to one drug, and have a component of the initial regimen discontinued or substituted for an alternative. Patients sometimes take holidays from treatment to attend to personal obligations. In this fashion, the boundaries surrounding what constitutes an episode of administration of a chemotherapy regimen or course of treatment is less distinct. Nevertheless, it is possible to identify what is meant by a "chemotherapy treatment regimen" and to develop consensus standards.

Currently, there are three main reasons for medical oncologists to consider a cancer treatment plan, treatment summary, and survivorship care plan. The first reason is the need to communicate with other oncology and nononcology providers about the patient's past care. For example, a cardiologist must know how much doxorubicin a patient received, or a primary care physician must know that the patient received radiation therapy to the neck and is at risk for hypothyroidism in the future. A cancer treatment plan outlining the planned regimen (including chemotherapy radiation, surgery, or other therapies) and a treatment summary describing how treatment was tolerated and the outcomes of care, could streamline communication among cancer providers as well as with primary care providers who subsequently follow cancer survivors.

The second reason for these plans is to facilitate communication with the patient/survivor. Review of the information in the treatment plan may help the patient understand the purpose of treatment and structure conversations about the response to therapy and subsequent decision making. Later, this same document can be amended into a treatment summary—what treatments were completed as planned, what toxicities were experienced, and what potential late effects should be anticipated. Furthermore, in a forward-looking component—the survivorship care plan—the oncology provider can communicate the surveillance needs (as known at the moment) and any areas that need ongoing psychosocial care or follow-up.

Finally, having an explicit document that initially describes the treatment plan and follows with the treatment summary and survivorship care plan facilitates ongoing monitoring of quality of care. To evaluate the quality of cancer care, it is not necessary to know the exact number of milligrams of every treatment dose, nor is it necessary to know the specifics of every single dose delay and reduction. Simply knowing what drugs were delivered, with what purpose and what outcomes, would move the field far ahead of where it is today. Withdrawal of drugs from the market and the emergence of safety concerns for new chemotherapy drugs after regulatory approval highlight the need for monitoring beyond registration trials. When a chemotherapy drug is noted

to have a new or unexpected effect, it would prove invaluable to quickly characterize the experience of large numbers of patients who have been exposed to a particular agent or combination of agents. The ability to obtain this information expeditiously from the medical record would be greatly enhanced if summary documents were standardized and electronically searchable. This would stand in stark contrast to the current system of myriad chronologically organized clinical notes with minimal consistency across practice sites.

A chemotherapy treatment plan is conceived of as a succinct summary document that should typically require a single side of a page. It should indicate the cancer site, histology and stage, and the reason for chemotherapy administration. If treatment is delivered for advanced disease, the plan should indicate whether the patient is symptomatic or is receiving treatment for biochemical or radiographic evidence of disease. The summary should include the name of the regimen, the name of the component drugs in the regimen, and the starting dosages. The number of planned cycles and the strategy for assessing response should be included.

A chemotherapy treatment summary is conceived of as a succinct summary document that also should require no more than a single side of a page. It should be prepared at the end of a course of treatment. This may include at completion of adjuvant therapy, at disease progression through a chemotherapy agent, or at discontinuation of a regimen secondary to toxicity. The treatment summary should indicate how many cycles were delivered and whether any drugs were dropped from the regimen. This summary should review major toxicity, such as the need for hospitalization or complications such as febrile neutropenia. The treatment summary should describe the response to treatment (based on radiographic, biochemical, or clinical criteria or combinations thereof). The document should also provide the reason for treatment discontinuation and the planned next steps (e.g., hospice care, an alternative regimen).

The survivorship care plan should synthesize all the treatments received as part of the initial cancer treatment (surgery, radiation, chemotherapy, other) and should include the following: date of diagnosis, stage of cancer, diagnostic tests performed and results, acute toxicities on treatment, expected late effects from treatment, psychosocial and supportive care needs in follow-up, and identification of providers who will coordinate specific aspects of continuing care. In addition, the plan should include recommended surveillance for recurrence and new cancers, specific recommendations for health behaviors, and, when appropriate, genetic testing and screening for first-degree relatives.[3]

Changing the culture of medical records documentation will not be easy and, ultimately, will only be successful if it is linked to reimbursement and requirements from healthcare payors. Preparation of these documents should be valued as a visit of high care complexity, as it necessarily involves coordination and specific consultation time with the patient. With a modicum of change and restructuring, it should be possible to facilitate coordination and communication about cancer care and the ability to more readily track cancer treatment histories in medical records. This initiative would be easiest to implement if standardized forms, ideally in electronic digitized format, are made freely available. As a first step, extensive pilot work will be necessary to develop forms that work across practice sites.

The Role of Primary Care in Cancer Survivorship

Primary care physicians play an important role in the delivery of survivorship care. The largest proportion of physician office visits for cancer care—32%—is made to primary care physicians, compared with 18% for oncologists.[31] Cancer care specialists lack the time and workforce size to provide follow-up care to the nation's growing population of cancer survivors. Primary care clinicians are better positioned and qualified to ensure that the full spectrum of cancer survivors' health needs are addressed, including not only issues surrounding their cancer(s) but also health maintenance (prevention), the management of concurrent comorbid disease (e.g., heart disease, diabetes), mental health, and acute care.

Primary care physicians face formidable challenges, however, in providing survivorship care. The fact that the patient was previously diagnosed with cancer may itself be unknown to the primary care clinician, and even when this history is obtained, records of the specific diagnosis and treatment regimen may be unavailable. Even if the diagnosis and treatment are clear, evidence-based practice guidelines on recommended follow-up are lacking, leaving clinicians in doubt about what they should do. Primary care clinicians lack expertise in specialized aspects of survivorship care, and their responsibilities of dealing comprehensively with a range of healthcare issues leaves limited time to focus on survivorship issues.[32,33]

When faced with similar challenges in managing other complex diseases, primary care clinicians work closely with specialist colleagues to obtain guidance on appropriate follow-up and to refer patients to specialists when the patients' needs exceed their capabilities and expertise. This model does not always work well in collaborations between primary care and cancer specialists, in part because of the complexity of cancer care and the inadequate communication of treatment plans and summaries noted earlier. Primary care clinicians frequently report a fear of "losing" their patients to cancer specialists and limited correspondence or communication regarding the care their patients receive from specialists, and they often discover—once patients do return to the primary care setting—that other health needs unrelated to cancer have "fallen through the cracks" during the patient's absence.

Recommendations issued by the IOM Committee on Adult Cancer Survivorship[3] provide an important starting point for addressing many of these challenges:

- The visibility given to the committee report and other cancer survivorship initiatives should make primary care clinicians more aware of survivorship as an important, but neglected, clinical entity.
- The difficulty that primary care clinicians face in obtaining details about the prior diagnosis and treatment would be mitigated by the proposed survivorship care plan. The IOM report provides recommendations on strategies to make the plan accessible to clinicians who are separated by geography or time from the setting in which the cancer was first treated, thereby providing details to new clinicians, even decades later.
- The lack of clear guidelines on the optimal content of survivorship care would be addressed by the effort of medical specialty societies, especially primary care organizations, to develop consensus recommendations for primary care practice. Support for randomized trials of regimens in survivorship care is essential to produce the data on which evidence-based guidelines can be developed.
- The need for primary care clinicians to collaborate with cancer specialists to ensure the delivery of highquality survivorship care is addressed by the "shared care" model discussed in the IOM report. Under the shared care model, both the primary care clinician and the cancer specialist merge their resources and talents to offer the patient a combination of comprehensive and expert care. The respective roles of the primary care clinician and cancer specialist are outlined in Table 22.1.

TABLE 22.1. Roles under shared care model.

Primary care clinician	Cancer care specialist
Attend to the breadth of patients' physical and mental health issues. Ensure that the cancer survivor receives care for all health conditions and for preventive care, thereby imporving cancer survivorship and preventing and reducing complications from cancer and other important diseases.	**Provide guidance and specialized treatment, as indicated.** See the cancer survivor for periodic evaluations at recommended intervals, provide guidance to the primary care clinician as questions or concerns arise, and see patients for circumstances or complications that exceed the capabilities of the primary care clinician.
Deliver chronic care needs that are feasible in the primary care setting. Take responsibility for conducting examinations and ordering tests that are recommended for the cancer survivor and that can be performed or arranged in the primary care settling. These tasks generally do not require the dired involvement of cancer specialists, whose time can be better applied toward dealing with new patients and those with complications.	**Keep the primary care clinician informed of the treatment plan.** Provide written guidance to the primary care clinician to include in the chart as a reference for next steps, both at the time of initial discharge, when the cancer survivorship care plan is first developed, and as treatment needs evolve with time.
Refer patient to cancer specialist(s) for periodic evaluations and issues requiring focused expertise. Identify circumstances or complications that require cancer survivors to be seen by specialists and refer patients for periodic evaluations at on agreed frequency.	**Return the patient to primary care for ongoing needs.** Both during and after the period when the patient is being seen by the cancer specialist, ongoing primary care is important to maintain treatment of other comorbid conditions and to follow up on implemenliation of the care plan initiated by the cancer specialist.
Consult with specialists in areas of uncertainty. Whether referrals become necessary, contact specialty colleagues to discuss questions or concerns and to determine which follow-up steps should be taken, either by the primary care practice or by the specialist.	

- To fulfill the ideals of the shared care model, several challenges must be overcome. Chief among these is that primary care clinicians and cancer specialists must reach a common understanding about expected components of care and their respective roles. To some extent, this understanding requires specialists to acquire greater confidence in the ability of primary care clinicians to manage components of care. Primary care clinicians, in turn, must be conscious of their limitations and engage specialty colleagues when they need help. The collaboration requires a common playbook—for both parties to agree on what must be done and who will do it—and clear communication. Primary care clinicians should copy cancer specialists on relevant progress notes, test results, and correspondence. Cancer specialists should copy the primary care clinician with similar information and should provide a standard consultation report when patients are referred from primary care. Shared care works best when it is supported by the infrastructure of the healthcare delivery system in which the clinicians operate and by the managers responsible for the system. Features of such a system include easy transfer of medical records, streamlined referrals, seamless "handoffs," and other features that spare patients the disruption caused by fragmented care.

- These features are evident in certain communities that exhibit excellent coordination between primary and specialty care of cancer survivors, but elsewhere in the United States there is more work to be done to cultivate these conditions, in particular to shift attitudes and expectations about the acceptability of shared care. This stands in contrast to the standard practice of shared care of other diseases, which is hardly a novel concept in primary care. According to the 2002 National Ambulatory Care Outcomes Survey, 18% of office visits to primary care clinicians involve shared care.[31]

- Primary care clinicians and specialists are accustomed to working together in familiar roles in the management of other complex conditions. For example, on a daily basis, primary care clinicians manage coronary artery disease and heart failure, know when to consult cardiology colleagues when a coronary event occurs, and work together in shared roles as patients are hospitalized or suffer complications. Primary care clinicians manage other chronic conditions that, like cancer, involve complex medical concepts, rapidly evolving guidelines, and the need for expert input when problems arise. Examples include human immunodeficiency virus infection, diabetes, chronic renal insufficiency, bipolar disorder, Parkinson's disease, inflammatory bowel disease, and seizure disorders. Building similar working relationships to care for cancer survivors provides a promising model for integrating the best assets of primary and specialty care to ensure optimal delivery of quality service to patients.

Conclusion

The IOM report on adult cancer survivors[3] provides a challenge as well as potential strategies for helping patients with cancer successfully transition into the phase of survivorship care beyond initial treatment. ASCO is well positioned to respond to this challenge through the development of cancer survivorship guidelines, the promotion of tools and strategies to facilitate the implementation of the survivorship care plan in clinical practice, and educational collaboration with the professional organizations of primary care providers and other clinicians who share in the ongoing care of cancer survivors. At the local level, individual ASCO members in clinical practice can work to implement the shared care model within their own practice communities. With the expanding number of cancer survivors each year, we must find creative ways to ensure that the gains obtained through successful cancer treatment are not lost when patients transition to this phase of their care. What is outlined in this article is a suggested beginning.

References

1. Jemal A, Clegg LX, Ward E, et al. Annual report to the nation on the status of cancer, 1975–2001, with a special feature regarding survival. Cancer. 2004;101:3–27.
2. Cancer survivorship—United States, 1971–2001. MMWR Morb Mortal Wkly Rep. 2005;53:526–529.
3. Hewitt M, Greenfield S, Stovall E. From Cancer Patient to Cancer Survivor: Lost in Transition. Washington, DC, The National Academies Press, 2005.
4. Demark-Wahnefried W, Aziz N, Rowland JH, et al. Riding the crest of the teachable moment: Promoting long-term health after the diagnosis of cancer. J Clin Oncol. 2005;23:5418–5430.
5. Ganz PA. A Teachable Moment for Oncologists: Cancer Survivors, 10 Million Strong and Growing! J Clin Oncol. 2005;23:5458–5460.
6. Desch CE, Benson AB, Somerfield MR, et al. Colorectal cancer surveillance: 2005 update of an American Society of Clinical Oncology practice guideline. J Clin Oncol. 2005;23:8512–8519.
7. Impact of follow-up testing on survival and health-related quality of life in breast cancer patients. A multicentre randomized controlled trial. The GIVIO Investigators. JAMA. 1994;271:1587–1592.
8. Muss HB, Tell GS, Case LD, et al. Perceptions of follow-up care in women with breast cancer. Am J Clin Oncol. 1991;14:55–59.
9. Johnson FE. Overview. In: Johnson FE, Virgo KS (eds). Cancer Patient Follow-Up. St. Louis: Mosby, 1997;4.
10. NIH consensus conference. Ovarian cancer. Screening, treatment, and follow-up. NIH Consensus Development Panel on Ovarian Cancer. JAMA. 1995;273:491–497.
11. Nordic Gastrointestinal Tumor Adjuvant Therapy Group. Expectancy or primary chemotherapy in patients with advanced asymptomatic colorectal cancer: A randomized trial. J Clin Oncol. 1992;10:904–911.
12. Fong Y, Cohen AM, Fortner JG, et al. Liver resection for colorectal metastases. J Clin Oncol. 1997;15:938–946.
13. Northover JM, Houghton J, Lennon T. CEA to detect recurrences of colon cancer (letter). JAMA. 1994;272:31.
14. Ohlsson B, Breland U, Ekberg H, et al. Follow-up after curative surgery for colorectal carcinoma. Randomized comparison with no followup. Diseases of the Colon & Rectum. 1995;38:619–626.
15. Makela JT, Laitinen SO, Kairaluoma MI. Five-year follow-up after radical surgery for colorectal cancer. Results of a prospective randomized trial. Archives of Surgery. 1995;130:1062–1067.
16. Kjeldsen BJ, Kronborg O, Fenger C, et al. A prospective randomized study of follow-up after radical surgery for colorectal cancer. Br J Surg. 1997;84:666–669.
17. Schoemaker D, Black R, Giles L, et al. Yearly colonoscopy, liver CT, and chest radiography do not influence 5-year survival of colorectal cancer patients. Gastroenterology. 1998;114:7–14.

18. Pietra N, Sarli L, Costi R, et al. Role of follow-up in management of local recurrences of colorectal cancer: A prospective, randomized study. Diseases of the Colon & Rectum. 1998;41: 1127–1133.

19. Secco GB, Fardelli R, Gianquinto D, et al. Efficacy and cost of risk-adapted follow-up in patients after colorectal cancer surgery: A prospective, randomized and controlled trial. Eur J Surg Oncol. 2002;28:418–423.

20. Rosen M, Chan L, Beart RWJ, et al. Follow-up of colorectal cancer: A meta-analysis. Diseases of the Colon & Rectum. 1998;41:1116–1126.

21. Renehan AG, Egger M, Saunders MP, et al. Impact on survival of intensive follow-up after curative resection for colorectal cancer: Systematic review and meta-analysis of randomised trials. BMJ. 2002;324:1–8.

22. Weeks JC, Yeap BY, Canellos GP, et al. Value of follow-up procedures in patients with large-cell lymphoma who achieve a complete remission. J Clin Oncol. 1991;9:1196–1203.

23. Jeffrey GM, Hickey BE, Hider P. Follow-up strategies for patients treated for non-metastatic colorectal cancer (Cochrane Review). The Cochrane Library 3: Oxford-Update Software, 2002.

24. Figueredo A, Rumble RB, Maroun J, et al. Follow-up of patients with "curatively resected" colorectal cancer: A practice guideline. BMC Cancer. 2003;3:26.

25. Loprinzi CL, Hayes D, Smith T. Doc, shouldn't we be getting some tests? J Clin Oncol. 2000;18:2345–2348.

26. Ben-Josef E, Lawrence TS. Radiotherapy for unresectable hepatic malignancies. Semin Radiat Oncol. 2005;15:273–278.

27. Stiggelbout AM, de Haes JC, Vree R, et al. Follow-up of colorectal cancer patients: Quality of life and attitudes towards follow-up. Br J Cancer. 1997;75:914–920.

28. Grunfeld E, Mant D, Yudkin P, et al. Routine follow-up of breast cancer in primary care: Randomised trial. BMJ. 1996;313:665–669.

29. Kjeldsen BJ, Thorsen H, Whalley D, et al. Influence of follow-up on health-related quality of life after radical surgery for colorectal cancer. Scand J Gastroenterol. 1999;34:509–515.

30. Lampic C, Wennberg A, Schill JE, et al. Anxiety and cancer-related worry of cancer patients at routine follow-up visits. Acta Oncol. 1994;33:119–125.

31. Woodwell DA, Cherry DK. National Ambulatory Medical Care Survey: 2002 Summary. Advance Data from Vital and Health Statistics, No. 346. Hyattsville, MD, National Center for Health Statistics, 2004.

32. Beasley JW, Hankey TH, Erickson R, et al. How many problems do family physicians manage at each encounter? A WReN study. Ann Fam Med. 2004;2:405–410.

33. Jaen CR, Stange KC, Nutting PA. Competing demands of primary care: A model for the delivery of clinical preventive services. J Fam Pract. 1994;38:166–171.

Index

*Page numbers followed by f indicate figures; t, tables; b, boxes.

Printed in the United States of America.